315

CONTROL OF NEOPLASIA
BY
MODULATION OF THE IMMUNE SYSTEM

Progress in
Cancer Research and Therapy
Volume 2

Control of Neoplasia
by
Modulation of the Immune
System

Edited by

Michael A. Chirigos, Ph.D.

Assistant Lab Chief
Laboratory of RNA Tumor Viruses
National Cancer Institute
National Institutes of Health
Bethesda, Maryland

Raven Press ▪ New York

Raven Press, 1140 Avenue of the Americas, New York, New York 10036

Raven Press, New York, 1977.

Made in the United States of America

International Standard Book Number 0-89004-125-3
Library of Congress Catalog Card Number 76-5665

Preface

We have a much clearer understanding of the response manifested by a tumor-bearing host toward malignant cells than existed only a few years ago. During the past decade, an impressive literature has developed concerning mechanisms by which the immune response can be stimulated to effect a "last cell kill," thus preventing relapses resulting from outgrowth of residual, as well as drug-resistant, cancerous cells that have escaped surgery or primary cytoreductive therapy. The immunological surveillance of the cancer patient is suppressed both by the disease itself and the intensive cytoreductive therapy required to manage it. Secondary infectious disease resulting from this immune suppression may also present a life-threatening situation. The return of host immune function is thus of major importance for the successful control and, hopefully, the cure of cancer. A sizeable body of evidence exists to demonstrate a variety of immune responses to tumor-cell antigens. "Killer," thymus-derived (T) lymphocytes primed to destroy tumor cells have been identified in patients who do not show a markedly reduced reactivity to antigens; similarly, macrophages have been shown to possess a nonspecific tumoricidal activity. Antibodies may exert either a beneficial or a detrimental effect.

The ability to modulate host immunity is now a reality, and the rapidly developing field of immunotherapy is becoming an important aspect of cancer therapy.

The Second Conference of Host Immune Resistance in the Prevention or Treatment of Induced Neoplasias was devoted to a consideration of the modes of action through which specific chemical and biological adjuvants act on both cell-mediated and humoral immune responses to increase tumor immunity and control tumor growth. Experimental and clinical evidence is presented, showing that these adjuvants act through their effects on macrophages and/or thymus-derived or bone marrow-derived lymphocytes. The kinetics of cellular stimulation by the chemical adjuvant levamisole is discussed in detail, as is its protective effects in experimental animal model systems. The use of levamisole is discussed both for use in cancer patients and in treating conditions other than cancer. Similar experimental and clinical results are presented for thymosin, a biological material that exerts immunomodulatory activity. The role of other biologicals and chemicals on the modulation of viruses and tumors is also considered.

This volume will be of interest to immunologists and immunochemists as well as to clinicians concerned with cancer immunotherapy.

The editor and contributors of this volume wish to express their gratitude to Dr. J. B. Moloney, Associate Director for Viral Oncology, Division of Cancer

Cause and Prevention, National Cancer Institute, National Institutes of Health, and to Dr. Milo D. Leavitt, Jr., Director of Fogarty International Center, National Institutes of Health, and his staff for their encouragement and invaluable support that made the conference, on which this volume is based, possible.

Michael A. Chirigos
Editor

Contents

vii

MODULATION OF HOST RESISTANCE BY OTHER AGENTS

THYMOSIN

Experimental

Clinical

Glucan

Polynucleotides

Neuraminidase

Contributors

Amery, Willem K., 197
Ammann, Arthur, 315

Badger, Alison M., 25
Baird, Lynn G., 461
Balk, Melvin W., 107
Barker, Anna D., 289
Basch, Christa M., 217
Bekesi, J. George, 369, 573
Bergoc, Rosa M., 57
Biniaminov, M., 239
Browder, William, 475
Burrone, Oscar, 57

Caro, Ricardo A., 57
Casagrande, John, 391
Cavallo, G., 501
Chang, Esther H., 347
Chang, Sandra P., 107
Chirigos, Michael A., 421, 437
Chretien, Paul B., 305
Cohen, Geraldine H., 241
Cook, James A., 475
Cooperband, Sidney R., 25, 43
Crumrine, Martin H., 107

Dau, Peter C., 81
Dauphinee, Michael J., 279
Debois, J. M., 175
Di Luzio, Nicholas R., 475
Doller, Elizabeth W., 97
Dougherty, Mary, 391
Drake, Walter P., 563

Elias, E. George, 265
Engleman, Ephraim P., 217
Estes, John D., 391

Feierstein, Julio N., 57, 159
Fischer, Gerald W., 107
Fleminger, Raphael, 573
Forni, G., 501
Friedman, Herman, 255
Friedman, Robert M., 347
Fye, Kenneth M., 279

Gallin, John I., 227
Gardner, Murray B., 391
Gibson, J. P., 409
Gilden, Raymond B., 381
Glait, Horacio M., 57, 159
Glogau, Richard G., 217
Goldstein, Allan G., 241, 329
Gordon, Benjamin L., II, 205
Gordon, David S., 121
Gutterman, Jordan U., 183, 329

Hall, Linda S., 121
Henderson, Brian E., 391
Henderson, Edward S., 573
Hersh, Evan M., 183, 329
Hieter, Philip A., 517
Hill, Paul R., 381
Hirshaut, Yashar, 147
Hoffmann, Ernesto O., 475
Hokama, Yoshitsugi, 107
Holland, James F., 369, 573
Huebner, Robert J., 381, 391

Ibrahim, Ali Bin, 81
Ihlo, Jorge E., 57

Jay, Francis T., 347

Kaiser, C. William, 25

Wanebo, Harold, 147
Wara, Diane W., 315
Wheelock, E. Frederick, 531
Whitcomb, Michael E., 43
Wiernik, Peter H., 135

Wong, Paul K. Y., 347
Woods, Wilna A., 437
Wright, Daniel G., 227

Yates, Jerome, 573

Control of Neoplasia by Modulation of the Immune System, edited by M. A. Chirigos. Raven Press, New York 1977.

LEVAMISOLE, AN ANTIANERGIC CHEMOTHERAPEUTIC AGENT: AN OVERVIEW

J. Symoens

Janssen Pharmaceutica, Research Laboratoria, B-2340 Beerse, Belgium

INTRODUCTION

Five years ago Renoux for the first time described that the anthelmintic levamisole increased the protective effect of a bacterial vaccine in mice (90, 93).

This was the start of a large, coordinated research effort to investigate the immunological properties of this compound. Many scientists from many countries joined forces because they found the issues that were raised very challenging.

Today I shall try to summarize the data that came to our attention and that have been described in 257 reports and publications from all over the world.

RESISTANCE TO EXPERIMENTAL INVASION BY BACTERIA, VIRUSES, PROTOZOA, AND TUMORAL CELLS

The first observation of Renoux on the potentiation of Brucella vaccination in mice has been confirmed by others and extended to other species, other bacteria (32,36,61) or protozoa (29), and tumoral cells (32,106).

Fischer demonstrated that with levamisole (immunologically immature) newborn rats became significantly more resistant to primary infections with pyogenic bacteria or herpes virus (6,40,41). Many other studies, however, showed that (immunologically mature) adult animals do not become more resistant to a primary invasion by virulent bacteria, viruses, or protozoa after treatment with levamisole (110). The drug is not toxic to bacteria, protozoa, and viruses, nor to normal and tumoral cells in concentrations up to 100µg/ml (17,33,41,44,68,82,111).

Numerous experiments have been performed to determine whether levamisole influences the primary growth and dissemination of experimental tumors

1

TABLE 1. The effect of levamisole on primary growth and dissemination of tumors

Model	Effect	Reference
P 388 leukemia transplanted in mice	0	62
L 5178 X leukemia transplanted in mice	0	104
Moloney LSTRA leukemia transplanted in mice	0	13
Moloney MCAS-10 leukemia transplanted in mice	0	15
Moloney virus induced lymphoma transplanted in mice	0	86
Melanoma B 16 (s.c. or i.p.) transplanted in mice	0	39, 62, 75
Madison 109 lung tumor transplanted in mice	0	62
Spontaneous mammary carcinoma transplanted in mice	0	43
Meth-A tumor transplanted in mice	0	49
Sarcoma MO_4 transplanted in mice	0	17
Sarcoma 180 transplanted in mice	0	4, 43
Sarcoma MC-1 transplanted in rats	0	113, 114
Sarcoma MC-7 transplanted in rats	0	58
Sarcoma MC-57 transplanted in rats	0	58
Rhabdomyosarcoma BA 1112 transplanted in rats	0	43
Walker 256 tumor transplanted in rats	0	42
RD-3 tumor transplanted in rats	0	86
CELO-virus induced tumor transplanted in hamsters	0	86
Spontaneous mammary carcinoma in mice	0	43
DMBA-induced mammary tumor in rats	0	45, 46
Spontaneous leukemia in elderly mice	↓	94
Melanoma B 16 transplanted IV in mice	↑↓	39
HSV-1 transformed tumor 14-012-8-1 transplanted in hamsters	↓	98
HSV-2 transformed tumor 333-8-9 transplanted in newborn hamsters	↓	112
L 1210 leukemia transplanted in mice	(↓)	30, 62, 75, 81, 107
Lewis lung carcinoma transplanted in mice	(↓)	4, 62, 81, 91, 106, 107, 108
Ehrlich tumor transplanted in mice	(↓)	4, 43
Rhabdomyosarcoma induced by Moloney sarcoma virus in mice	(↑↓)	62, 104
L 1210 leukemia transplanted in allogeneic mice	↑	74
Adenovirus-12 induced tumor of mice transplanted in hamsters	↑	86
Adenocarcinoma 15091 transplanted in mice	↑	39

0 = no change; ↓ = decrease; ↑ = increase; ( ) = not reproducible.

in animals. They are listed in Table 1. A detailed analysis of these data shows us that levamisole has no systematic, significant effect on primary growth and dissemination of experimental tumors in normal animals.

But when the tumor mass is first reduced by specific cytoreductive therapy, levamisole may significantly and systematically prevent relapse. This concept, illustrated in Fig. 1, was first demonstrated by Chirigos and his collaborators (14,15), who have shown that this effect is closely related to a faster recovery of the immune capacity after cytostatic therapy (84,107,141).

The effect of levamisole on stabilization of tumor remission has been reproduced in several models including leukemias, carcinomas, and sarcomas (Table 2). It became evident, however, in animals that after cytoreductive therapy there is a critical and limited period during which levamisole should be given.

IMMUNOLOGICAL PROFILE

Soon after Renoux published his experience on <u>Brucella</u> vaccination, studies were designed to find out whether levamisole affected humoral or cellular immunity or both.

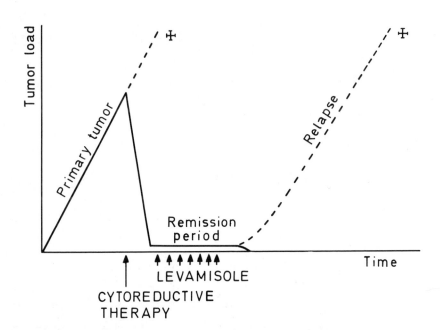

FIG. 1. Concept of the effect of levamisole on stabilization of tumor remission.

TABLE 2. Stabilization of tumor remission with levamisole

Model	Species	Cytoreductive therapy	Effect	Reference
L 1210 leukemia	Mice	Me CCNU	+	81
Moloney LSTRA lymphoid leukemia	Mice	BCNU, cyclo [a]	+	13, 14, 75
Moloney MCAS-10 lymphoid leukemia	Mice	BCNU	+	15
Graffi L leukemia	Mice	BCNU, cyclo [a]	+	14
Lewis lung carcinoma	Mice	Me CCNU	+	106, 107
3-MC induced fibrosarcoma	Mice	BCNU, cyclo [a]	+	14
Meth-A tumor	Mice	Cyclo [a]	+	49
Spontaneous mammary tumor KSP-1	Mice	Me CCNU	+	81
MC-1 sarcoma	Rat	Cyclo [a]	+	114
L 1210 leukemia	Mice	Various [b]	–	31, 75, 105
Lewis lung carcinoma	Mice	Surgery	–	107
MO₄ sarcoma	Mice	Cyclo [a]	–	17
L 311 lymphoid leukemia	Rat	Adriamycine	–	73
ISIS 208 and ISIS 130 leucosarcoma	Rat	Cyclo [a]	–	73
Epithelioma Spl	Rat	Surgery	–	58

+ Effect; – no effect.

[a] Cyclophosphamide.

[b] Cyclophosphamide, BCNU, 5-fluorouracil, methotrexate, adriamycine.

TABLE 3. The boosting and restorative effects of levamisole on skin delayed hypersensitivity in man (summarizing table)

Condition	Antigen	Control			Levamisole			Reference
		No. tested	Percent B	Percent R	No. tested	Percent B	Percent R	
Cancer	DNCB	273	7	6	298	23	22	8, 54, 55, 57, 78, 97, 118, 119, 121, 130, 132
	PPD	14	0	0	24	25	21	12, 35, 78, 95, 118
	Various	—	—	—	57	23	26	66, 78
Various diseases	PPD	43	0	9	68	0	35	8
Leprosy	DNCB	—	—	—	45	4	13	80, 120
	Lepromin	10	0	0	75	1	3	10, 65, 77, 120
	Various	—	—	—	20	55	15	80
Healthy elderly	DNCB	—	—	—	26	42	0	128
	PPD	20	5	10	24	0	42	92, 129
	Various	—	—	—	68	12	15	128

B = boosted; R = restored.

It is now clear that levamisole has little or no effect on antibody production in healthy subjects or animals (25, 26, 64, 71, 87, 99, 110). However, skin delayed hypersensitivity to various antigens is boosted, and even restored in cases of anergy. Approximately 50% of all patients tested responded. These included cancer patients, healthy elderly subjects, and patients with various nonmalignant diseases who were anergic or who had a reduced skin reactivity to antigenic stimulation (Table 3).

The finding that levamisole stimulated or restored a cell-mediated immune reaction fostered research on phagocyte and lymphocyte functions. The results can be summarized as follows. Levamisole normalizes the function of phagocytes and T-lymphocytes when their function is depressed (Table 4). Stimulation above normal does not occur. Cells from normal healthy animals or man can be stimulated slightly, but often there is no response at all and sometimes there is slight depression. Alterations in normal cells are small and insignificant when compared with those in depressed cells.

The restorative effect of levamisole on various cell functions is illustrated in Figs. 2, 3, and 4. It occurs when levamisole is given to animals or man in vivo, or when it is added to their cells in vitro.

In the population of rats used for a carbon clearance test, some animals eliminated carbon efficiently and others did not; 24 hr after treatment with levamisole, all animals efficiently removed the particles. They were not stimulated above normal (Fig. 2).

The chemotaxis of polymorphonuclear cells from patients with recurrent herpes was restored to normal when levamisole was added to these cells in vitro (Fig. 3).

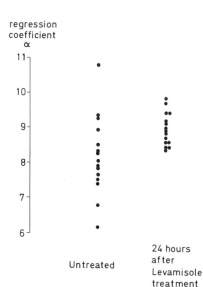

FIG. 2. Carbon clearance in rats (Hoebeke, unpublished data).

TABLE 4. Effects of levamisole on phagocytes and lymphocytes

Restoration to normal	Reference
Phagocytosis	18, 19, 21, 38, 41, 60, 69, 96, 101, 127, 135, 136
Blood clearance of colloidal particles	56, 123, 124, 130
Chemotaxis	2, 17, 53, 88
Migration inhibition	83, 88, 116, 129
T-lymphocyte DNA or protein synthesis	5, 7, 9, 10, 11, 16, 21, 52, 66, 68, 72, 76, 82, 95, 116, 129, 138, 139, 140, 141
E-rosette number	24, 37, 66, 89, 95, 115, 125, 134

This was also the case for migration inhibition of mononuclear cells from patients with Hodgkin's disease, advanced tuberculosis, and sarcoidosis (Fig. 4). This experiment suggests that anergic lymphocytes are stimulated by levamisole in vitro to produce lymphokines.

Table 5 shows that levamisole does not augment noticeably the response to PHA of lymphocytes from healthy donors. These lymphocytes, of course, respond normally to PHA. When, however, lymphocytes from patients with cancer or tuberculosis are taken, their response to PHA is increased by levamisole. This increase is greater in lymphocytes that are hyporesponsive to PHA than in those that respond normally.

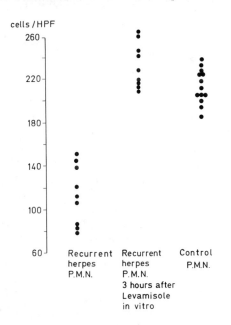

FIG. 3. Chemotaxis of human polymorphonuclear cells (ref. 88).

TABLE 5. Protein synthesis by human lymphocytes. Levamisole in vitro[a]

	Lymphocyte response to PHA	No. augmented by levamisole (percent)
Normal controls	Normal	0
Cancer	Normal	67
	Hyporesponsive	100
Tuberculosis	Normal	18
	Hyporesponsive	69

[a](See ref. 11.)

Figure 5 beautifully illustrates the effects of levamisole. Levamisole treatment restored to normal the more or less reduced number of E-rosette-forming cells of patients with various diseases. Patients who already had normal rosettes remained normal and did not increase above normal.

CLINICAL APPLICATIONS

The clinical situations in which levamisole has been used successfully can be classified into four groups.

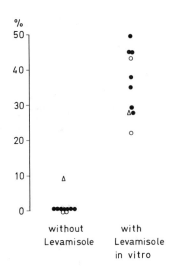

FIG. 4. Migration inhibition of human mononuclear cells (ref. 88). Filled circles, Hodgkin's disease; open circles, advanced tuberculosis; triangles, sarcoidosis.

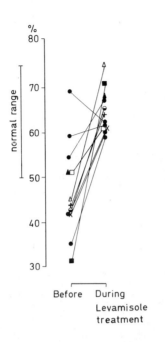

Δ acne conglobata
x atopic dermatitis
□ ataxia telectangiectasia
■ Crohn's disease
⊕ persistent chronic hepatitis
▲ furonculosis adenitis
+ multiple sclerosis
• rheumatoid arthritis

FIG. 5. Number of human E-rosette-forming cells (ref. 24).

1. <u>Recurrent and chronic infections</u>, including skin, mucous membrane, eye, respiratory, and systemic infections caused by viruses, bacteria, or fungi. Here may also be mentioned chronic conditions of unknown etiology such as Crohn's disease.

2. <u>Postviral anergy</u>, by which is meant the period immediately following a virus infection such as influenza or measles, which is often characterized by a slow recovery and prolonged physical and psychic asthenia.

3. <u>Rheumatic diseases</u>, including rheumatoid arthritis, systemic lupus erythematosus, and Reiter's syndrome.

4. <u>Cancer</u>: stabilization of remission.

I will limit my summary to the clinical experience gained in nononcological indications (Table 6).

So far placebo-controlled evidence of clinical efficacy has been gained in four indications.

Huskisson in London compared levamisole to placebo and to penicillamine in patients with rheumatoid arthritis. The patients received only one of the test drugs and minor analgesics. Levamisole was at least as effective as penicillamine, and both were significantly more effective than placebo. Objective as well as subjective parameters improved (Table 7).

Other indications where double-blind proof of activity exists are recurrent upper respiratory tract infections in children, recurrent aphthous ulceration, and intertrigo inguinalis. Levamisole was ineffective in warts.

TABLE 6. Therapeutic profile of levamisole in nononcological indications

	Immune defect restored					Reference
	DH	P	C	T	L	
Double-blind proof						
Rheumatoid arthritis	x			x	x	3,34,37,59*,100,117,137, 122*
Recurrent upper respiratory tract infections in children						23*,28,79,109,131
Recurrent aphthous ulceration						20*
Intertrigo inguinalis						
(Warts: ineffective in 4 studies)						
Effect probable						
Recurrent herpes labialis, genitalis, corneae	x		x	x		27,48,63,70,102,103,109
Pyogenic skin infections, acne conglobata		x		x		24,60,115
Recurrent systemic infections in children	x	x		x	x	21,22,115,133,135
Primary immune deficiency syndromes	x			x	x	51
Chronic brucellosis	x					115
Postviral anergy and asthenia	x			x		126*
Reiter syndrome		x				60,117
Systemic lupus erythematosus					x	50
Crohn's disease	x			x	x	5,24

References with an asterisk concern controlled studies; references underlined concern studies in which immunological assessments have been made. The other references concern open pilot studies; DH = delayed skin hypersensitivity; P = phagocytosis; C = chemotaxis; T = E-rosettes; L = lymphocyte stimulation.

TABLE 7. Levamisole versus penicillamine versus placebo in patients with rheumatoid arthritis [a]

	Levamisole n = 12	Penicillamine n = 12	Placebo n = 10
Pain	↓ +++	↓ +	-
Morning stiffness (min)	↓ | |	↓ ++	-
Joint size (mm)	↓ +++	-	-
Technetium index	↓ ++	↓ +	-
Sedimentation rate (mm/hr)	↓ +++	↓ +++	-
Latex titre	↓ +++	↓ +++	-
IgG	↓ ++	↓ +++	-
IgM	-	↓ ++	-

Statistical significance of the observed changes in clinical and laboratory measurements after 6-months treatment: +++ $p < 0.01$; ++ $0.01 < p < 0.05$; + $0.05 < p < 0.10$; - $p > 0.10$.

[a] (See ref. 59.)

Most of these studies were clinical. But in rheumatoid arthritis patients, delayed skin hypersensitivity, E-rosettes, and lymphoblast transformation were also restored or greatly increased after treatment with levamisole.

In many other conditions, clinical improvement after treatment with levamisole paralleled restoration of one or more immunological tests. Such indications are listed in Table 6.

There is little doubt that levamisole is effective in recurrent herpes infections. It reduces the duration and the severity of the outbreaks, and prolongs the disease-free intervals. Restoration of delayed hypersensitivity, chemotaxis, and the percentage of E-rosettes after treatment occurred especially in protracted herpes corneae.

Patients with acne conglobata, recurrent furonculosis, and other pyogenic skin infections had their lesions cleared after levamisole treatment. This was also the case in children with Job-like syndrome, with lazy leukocyte syndrome, or with cyclic neutropenia who all suffered from recurrent respiratory tract and skin infections for several years. In most of these patients, restoration of one or more phagocyte or lymphocyte functions has been demonstrated. Similar results have been obtained in patients with various primary immune deficiency syndromes, including Wiskott Aldrich, ataxia telectangiectasia, and chronic granulomatous disease. Patients with chronic brucellosis, who were anergic to DNCB, had their skin response restored after treatment with levamisole and recovered clinically.

Levamisole seems to affect postviral anergy. In a double-blind trial, skin delayed hypersensitivity to tuberculin was measured in patients vaccinated against influenza. The patients who were treated with levamisole had a normal skin response. In the patients who received placebo, it was depressed.

In a pilot study in African children with measles, 20 levamisole-treated children had a classical evolution of the disease without complications (which is rare in Africa); of six controls, three had complications which were lethal in one (Barbaix, unpublished data).

Finally, some very encouraging results have been obtained in patients with Reiter's syndrome, with systemic lupus erythematosus, and with Crohn's disease. Phagocytic and lymphocytic defects were restored.

SAFETY

So far, experience with approximately 1,500 patients has been reported (Table 8). Treatment has been daily or intermittent, that is, 2 to 4 days every week or every other week. The longest observation, in a child, is 3 years of treatment for 2 consecutive days every week.

Side effects were not frequent (Table 9). Gastrointestinal complaints were mainly nausea, gastric intolerance, and inappetence.

CNS stimulation consisted of nervousness, irritability, insomnia, and sensory stimulation with alteration in taste and smell.

Some patients had combined symptoms that remind one of a flu-like syndrome, with fatigue, muscle and joint pain, fever, shiverings and chills, and malaise.

Skin rashes were seen in 26 patients and transient granulocytopenia in 7; these were mainly seen in rheumatoid arthritis patients on prolonged daily treatment. The skin rashes were relatively mild in most cases. Seven patients stopped treatment, the others continued without relapse after temporary cessation of medication. Rashes generally occurred after some weeks or months of continuous or intermittent therapy, sometimes after the first days of treatment.

TABLE 8. Number of patients treated with levamisole and reported until December 1975

Treatment scheme	No. of patients
Daily treatment	
3 days	622
1 week	50
1 to 3 months	100
> 3 months	159
Intermittent treatment	
< 3 months	100
3 to 6 months	188
> 6 months up to 3 years	320
Total	1,439

TABLE 9. Side effects reported during levamisole treatment

	No. of patients	No. stopped
Gastrointestinal complaints	<5%	5
CNS stimulation	<5%	0
Flu-like syndrome	<5%	7
Skin rash, urticaria	26 (18 in R.A.[a])	7
Transient granulocytopenia	7 (5 in R.A.)	7

[a]R.A. = rheumatoid arthritis.

Transient granulocytopenia appears to be a completely, rapidly, and spontaneously reversible condition, suggesting that it is due to an allergic reaction. Only granulocytes are affected, while bone marrow shows no evidence of damage.

DOSAGE AND TREATMENT SCHEME

Some remarks must be made with regard to dosage and treatment schedules.

Two hours after the intake of a single oral dose of 150 mg, plasma levels peak to 0.5 μg/ml. After 24 hr, they are a hundred times lower (Fig. 6).

Dose response studies showed levamisole to be consistently effective at 10^{-5} to 10^{-9} M concentrations in vitro (2, 19, 52, 68, 76, 85, 125, 139, 140). This is at the same range of concentrations that are found in vivo. One may question the relevance of effects obtained at higher concentrations in vitro.

In man, a daily standard dose of 150 mg for adults has been used in most studies. Recent data, however, suggest that in heavy patients this dose might be too low (1, 122).

The validity of frequently repeated dosing is not established. The immune reactivity increases promptly after the administration of levamisole (2, 52, 85, 89), and is sometimes abolished after repeated dosing (67, 141). Little is known about the duration of the restorative effect of a single dose.

The time of administration may be very important too. In certain cancer studies, for instance, the time between tumor reductive therapy and levamisole treatment was critical to obtaining optimal restoration (13, 15, 66, 141). In bacterial and protozoal immunization studies (29, 90, 93), and in lymphocyte cytotoxicity studies (85), levamisole had to be administered just before or together with the antigen and not thereafter.

The optimal treatment scheme to be used in man is still a matter of debate. For some indications a more intensive treatment schedule seems to be required than for others. However, certain side effects occur mainly after a period of prolonged continuous daily treatment; and in some studies

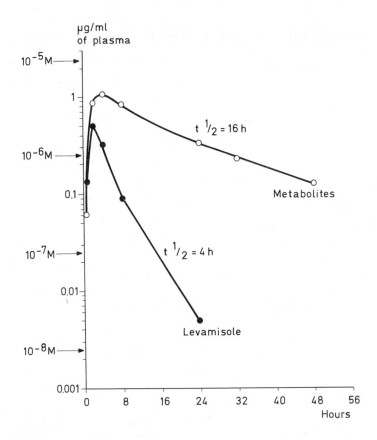

FIG. 6. Levamisole blood levels in man after 150 mg per os (Heykants, unpublished data).

the impression was gained that the immune reactivity waned after excessively intense and prolonged therapy. For these reasons, intermittent therapy is preferred to continuous daily treatment whenever possible.

CONCLUSION

What have we learned from the impressive amount of work done over the last five years?

We have learned that levamisole is an immunologically active compound that normalizes the function of phagocytes and T-lymphocytes without stimulating them above normal. Thus, levamisole is not an immunostimulant. It restores to normal.

The variety of cell functions that are affected makes it likely that levamisole restores a basic mechanism common to all cells involved. There are enough experimental data and theoretical arguments to believe that levamisole acts on these cells by increasing their cyclic GMP and decreasing their cyclic AMP (52).

Levamisole seems to be the first member of a potentially new class of compounds that resemble thymosin. They could, for instance, be called antianergic agents.

SUMMARY

Levamisole is an antianergic chemotherapeutic agent. It restores to normal the function of phagocytes and lymphocytes when this is depressed. Cell functions are not stimulated above normal.

The effect seems to be confined to cells involved in cell-mediated immune reactions. Antibody production is virtually not augmented.

Restoration of immune functions with levamisole results in an increased protective effect of bacterial, viral, protozoal, or tumoral vaccines in animals, and in an increased stabilization of tumor remission.

Levamisole has been used successfully in the treatment of a variety of diseases in man, including recurrent and chronic infections, rheumatic diseases, and postviral anergy. Side effects are not frequent.

REFERENCES

1. Amery, W. (1975): Double blind levamisole trial in resectable lung cancer. Presented at the International Conference on Immunotherapy of Cancer, New York Academy of Sciences, November 5-7, 1975.

2. Anderson, R., Glover, A., Koornhof, H. J., and Rabson, A. R. (1975): In vitro stimulation of neutrophil motility by levamisole. Maintenance of cGMP levels in chemotactically stimulated levamisole treated neutrophils. J. Immunol. (in press).

3. Basch, C. M., Spitler, L. E., and Engleman, E. P. (1975): The effects of levamisole in rheumatoid arthritis. Arthritis Rheum., 18:385.

4. Benazet, F., Guy-Loe, H., Maral, R., Werner, G., Berteaux, S., and Godard, C. (1973): Bilan actuel des résultats obtenus au cours de l'étude de l'action immunostimulante du tétramisole (16535 R.P.) et du lévamisole (20605 R.P.). Unpublished report, March 1973.

5. Bertrand, J., Renoux, G., Renoux, M., and Palat, A. (1974): Maladie de Crohn et levamisole. Nouv. Presse Med., 3:2265.

6. Böhm, K. H. (1975): Prüfung von Levamisol auf resistenzsteigernde Effekte gegenüber bakteriellen Infektionen. Unpublished report, April 1975.

7. Brugmans, J., Schuermans, V., De Cock, W., Thienpont, D., Janssen, P., Verhaegen, H., Van Nimmen, L., Louwagie, A. C., and Stevens, E. (1972): Immunostimulating potential of tetramisole. St. Bartolomeus-Tijdingen, No. 2:83-89.

8. Brugmans, J., Schuermans, V., De Cock, W., Thienpont, D., Janssen, P., Verhaegen, H., Van Nimmen, L., Louwagie, A. C., and Stevens, E. (1973): Restoration of host defense mechanisms in man by levamisole. Life Sci., 13:1499-1504.

9. Cappel, R., Henry, C., and Thiry, L. (1975): Experimental immuno-suppression induced by herpes simplex virus. Arch. Virol., 49:67-72.

10. Cardama, J. E., Gatti, J. C., Balina, L. M., Cabrera, H. N., and Fliess, E. L. (1973): Study of the immunostimulating action of levamisole in leprosy. Int. J. Lepr., 16:567-568.

11. Chan, S. H., and Simons, M. J. (1975): Levamisole and lymphocyte responsiveness. Lancet, i:1246-1247.

12. Chan, S. H., and Simons, M. J. (1975): Levamisole augmentation of lymphocyte hyporesponsiveness to PHA. Unpublished report, July 1975.

13. Chirigos, M. A., Pearson, J. W., and Pryor, J. (1973): Augmentation of chemotherapeutically induced remission of a murine leukemia by a chemical immuno-adjuvant. Cancer Res., 33:2615-2618.

14. Chirigos, M. A., Pearson, J. W., and Fuhrman, F. S. (1974): Effect of tumor load reduction on successful immunostimulation. Proc. Am. Assoc. Cancer Res., 15:116.

15. Chirigos, M. A., Fuhrman, F., and Pryor, J. (1975): Prolongation of chemotherapeutically induced remission of a syngeneic murine leukemia by L-2,3,5,6-tetrahydro-6-phenylimidazo[2,1-b]thiazole hydrochloride. Cancer Res., 35:927-931.

16. Copeland, D., Stewart, T., and Harris, J. (1974): Effect of levamisole (NSC-177023) on in vitro human lymphocyte transformation. Cancer Chemother. Rep., Part I, 58:167-170.

17. De Brabander, M., Aerts, F., and Borgers, M. (1973): Effect of levamisole (R 12564) in the MO₄ tumor system. Janssen Pharmaceutica, Biological Research Report on levamisole, October 1973.

18. De Cock, W., De Cree, J., and Verhaegen, H. (1974): The effect of levamisole on phagocytosis of latex particles by human neutrophils in vitro. Janssen Pharmaceutica, Clinical Research Report on levamisole No. 19, May 1974.

19. De Cock, W., Verhaegen, H., and De Cree, J. (1975): The effect of levamisole in vitro on the nitro-blue tetrazolium reduction to formazan by polymorphonuclear neutrophils. Janssen Pharmaceutica, Clinical Research Report on levamisole No. 25, April 1975.

20. De Cree, J. (1974): A placebo-controlled double blind study of levamisole in the treatment of intertrigo inguinalis. Janssen Pharmaceutica, Clinical Research Report on levamisole No. 14, April 1974.

21. De Cree, J., Verhaegen, H., De Cock, W., Vanheule, R., Brugmans, J., and Schuermans, V. (1974): Impaired neutrophil phagocytosis. Lancet, ii:294-295.

22. De Cree, J., Verhaegen, H., and De Cock, W. (1975): Treatment of 6 cases of recurrent infections by levamisole. Janssen Pharmaceutica, Clinical Research Report on levamisole No. 23, March 1975.

23. De Cree, J., Verhaegen, H., Sterckx, M. L., and Verbruggen, F. (1975): Levamisole, an immunologic treatment of recurrent aphthous stomatitis. Preprint manuscript, December 1975.

24. De Cree, J. (1976): Immunological studies in various conditions in man. In preparation.

25. De Diego, A. I., Carillo, C. G., and Trumper, S. J. (1974): Influencia de los antiparasitarios sistemicos sobre las aglutininas antibrucelicas. I Parte: Aglutininas producidas por vacuna. Gac. Vet., 36:164-170.

26. De Diego, A. I., Carrillo, C. G., Suadrome, A., and Castro, H. W. R. (1974): Influencia de los antiparasitarios sistemicos sobre las aglutininas antibrucelicas. II Parte: Aglutininas de vacas enfermas. Gac. Vet., 36:584-588.

27. De Queiroz Carvalho, C. A., Kinue Otuki, T., Poli, M. E., Nogueira, J. L., and Guerrero, J. (1975): Recurrent herpes infections and levamisole. Unpublished report, November 1975.

28. De Queiroz Carvalho, C. A., Kinue Otuki, T., Poli, M. E., Nogueira, J. L., and Guerrero, J. (1975): Recurrent aphthous stomatitis and levamisole. Unpublished report, November 1975.

29. Desowitz, R. S. (1975): Plasmodium berghei: Immunogenic enhancement of antigen by adjuvant addition. Exp. Parasitol., 38:6-13.

30. Desplenter, L. (1972): Activity of R 12564 and R 18134 in L 1210 leukaemia in mice: A preliminary report. Unpublished report, November 1972.

31. Desplenter, L., and Atassi, G. (1973): Influence of tetramisole and its isomers on a chemotherapeutically induced remission of L 1210 leukaemia Janssen Pharmaceutica, Biological Research Report on tetramisole, dexamisole and levamisole, November 1973.

32. Desplenter, L. (1976): Enhancement of host resistance after immunisation against L 1210 leukaemia and Brucella abortus in mice. In: First International Conference on Modulation of Host Immune Resistance in the Prevention or Treatment of Induced Neoplasias, edited by M. A. Chirigos. Fogarty International Center Proceedings, U. S. Government Printing Office, Washington, D. C. (in press).

33. Diamantstain, T. (1973): Einfluss von Levamisol auf Immunologische Funktionen. Unpublished report, September 1973.

34. Dinai, Y., and Pras, M. (1975): Levamisole in rheumatoid arthritis. Lancet, ii:556.

35. Drochmans, A. (1973): Levamisole in anergic patients with Hodgkin's disease. Janssen Pharmaceutica, Clinical Research Report on levamisole No. 13, December 1973.

36. El Chemali, M., and Vas, S. I. (1974): The effect of levamisole on RES clearance and on resistance to S. typhimurium in mice. Presented at the 24th Annual Meeting of the Canadian Society for Microbiology, Montreal, June 1974.

37. Verhaegen, H., De Cree, J., De Cock, W., Schuermans, Y., Engels, M., and Sonk, W. (1976): Immunologic evaluation of rheumatoid arthritis and therapy with levamisole. Unpublished report, April 1976.

38. Eyckmans, L. (1972): Invloed van levamisole (LMZ) op het verloop van de bacteriële infectie bij de muis. Unpublished report, September 1972.

39. Fidler, I. J., and Spitler, L. E. (1975): The effects of levamisole on in vivo and in vitro murine host response to syngeneic transplantable tumor. J. Natl. Cancer Inst., 55:1107-1112.

40. Fischer, G. W., Oi, V. T., Kelley, J. L., Podgore, J. K., Bass, J. W., Wagner, F. S., and Gordon, B. L. (1974): Enhancement of host defense mechanisms against gram-positive pyogenic coccal infections with levo-tetramisole (levamisole) in neonatal rats. Ann. Allergy, 33:193-198.

41. Fischer, G. W., Podgore, J. K., Bass, J. W., Kelley, J. L., and Kobayashi, G. Y. (1976): Enhanced host defense mechanism with levamisole in suckling rats. J. Infect. Dis., 132: 578-581.

42. Flannery, G. R., Rolland, J. M., and Nairn, R. C. (1975): Levamisole. Lancet, i: 750-751.

43. Franchi, G. (1973): The antitumoral activity of tetramisole and its isomers. Unpublished report, March 1973.

44. Franchi, G. (1973): The in vitro cytotoxic and growth inhibition activity of tetramisole and its isomers levamisole and dextramisole. Unpublished report, March 1973.

45. Gallez, G., and Heuson, J. C. (1972): Effet du lévamisole sur la carcinogénèse mammaire chez le rat. Unpublished report, June 1972.

46. Gallez, G., and Heuson, J. C. (1972): Effet du lévamisole sur la carcinogénèse mammaire chez le rat. Unpublished report, December 1972.

47. Gallin, J. I., and Wolff, S. M. (1975): Leucocyte chemotaxis: Physiological considerations and abnormalities. Clin. Haematol., 4:567-607.

48. Glogau, R. G., Spitler, L. E., Hanna, L., and Ostler, H. B. (1975): Levamisole and lymphocyte response in herpes simplex virus infections. Presented at the Antivirals with Clinical Potential Symposium, Stanford, California, August 26-29, 1975.

49. Gordon, D. S., Hall, L. S., and McDougal, J. S. (1975): Levamisole and cytoxan in a murine tumor model: In vivo and in vitro studies. Presented at the Second Conference on Modulation of Host Immune Resistance in the Prevention or Treatment of Induced Neoplasias, Bethesda, Maryland, December 1-3, 1975.

50. Gordon, B. L., and Keenan, J. P. (1975): The treatment of systemic lupus erythematosus (SLE) with the T-cell immunostimulant drug levamisole: A case report. Ann. Allergy, 35:343-355.

51. Griscelli, C. (1975): Traitement des déficits immunitaires congénitaux par le lévamisole. Unpublished report, February 1975.

52. Hadden, J. W., Coffey, R. G., Hadden, E. M., Lopez-Corrales, E., and Sunshine, G. H. (1975): Effects of levamisole and imidazole on lymphocyte proliferation and cyclic nucleotide levels. Cell. Immunol., 20:98-103.

53. Hill, H. R., and Quie, P. G. (1975): Defective neutrophil chemotaxis associated with hyperimmunoglobulinemia E. In: The Phagocytic Cell in Host Resistance, edited by J. A. Bellanti and D. H. Dayton, p. 249. Raven Press, New York.

54. Hirshaut, Y., Pinsky, C., Marquardt, H., and Oettgen, H. F. (1973): Effects of levamisole on delayed hypersensitivity reactions in cancer patients. Proc. Am. Assoc. Cancer Res., 14:109.

55. Hirshaut, Y., Pinsky, C., Fried, J., and Oettgen, H. (1974): Trial of levamisole as immunopotentiator in cancer patients. Proc. Am. Assoc. Cancer Res. Am. Soc. Clin. Oncol., 15:126.
56. Hoebeke, J., and Franchi, G. (1973): Influence of tetramisole and its optical isomers on the mononuclear phagocytic system. Effect on carbon clearance in mice. J. Reticuloendothel. Soc., 14:317-323.
57. Holmes, E. C., and Golub, S. H. (1976): Immunologic defects in lung cancer patients. J. Thorac. Cardiovasc. Surg., 71: 161-168.
58. Hopper, D. G., Pimm, M. V., and Baldwin, R. W. (1975): Levamisole treatment of local and metastatic growth of transplanted rat tumours. Br. J. Cancer, 32:345-352.
59. Huskisson, E. C., Dieppe, P. A., Scott, J., Trapnell, J., Balme, H. W., and Willoughby, D. A. (1976): Immuno-stimulant therapy for rheumatoid arthritis. Lancet, i: 393-395.
60. Ippen, H., and Qadripur, S. A. (1975): Levamisol zur Behandlung von Hautkrankheiten. Dtsch. Med. Wochenschr., 100:1710-1711.
61. Irwin, M. R., and Knight, H. D. (1975): Enhanced resistance to Corynebacterium pseudotuberculosis infections associated with reduced serum immunoglobulin levels in levamisole-treated mice. Infect. Immun., 12:1098-1103.
62. Johnson, R. K., Houchens, D. P., Gaston, M. R., and Goldin, A. (1975): Effects of levamisole (NSC-177023) and tetramisole (NSC-102063) in experimental tumor systems. Cancer Chemother. Rep., Part I, 59:697-705.
63. Kint, A., Coucke, C., and Verlinden, L. (1974): The treatment of recurrent herpes infections with levamisole. Arch. Belg. Dermatol., 30:167-171.
64. Kulkarni, V. B., Mulbagal, A. N., Paranjape, V. L., Khot, J. B., and Manda, A. V. (1973): Immunostimulating effect of tetramisole on antibody formation against Newcastle disease virus in chicks. Indian Vet. J., 50:225-227.
65. Lechat, M. F. (1973): Virage du test de la lépromine après administration du tétramisole. Unpublished report, June 1973.
66. Levo, Y., Rotter, V., and Ramot, B. (1975): Restoration of cellular immune response by levamisole in patients with Hodgkin's disease. Biomedicine, 23:198-200.
67. Liauw, H. L., Heymann, H., and Barclay, R. C. (1975): Levamisole stimulation of a helminth-induced delayed-type hypersensitivity reaction. Unpublished report, March 1975.
68. Lichtenfeld, J. L., Desner, M. R., Wiernik, P. H., and Mardiney, M. R. (1975): The modulating effects of levamisole on human lymphocyte responsiveness in vitro. Cancer Chemother. Rep. (in press).
69. Lima, O. A., Javierre, M. Q., Dias Da Silva, W., and Sette Camara, D. (1974): Immunological phagocytosis: Effect of drugs on phosphodiesterase activity. Experientia, 30:945-946.
70. Lods, F. (1975): Zona ophtalmique chez l'enfant. Essai de traitement par stimulation macrophagique. Bull Soc. Ophthalmol. Fr., 75:37-40.

71. Lods, J. C., Dujardin, P., and Halpern, G. (1975): Action of levamis-
    ole on antibody protection after vaccination with anti-typhoid and para-
    typhoid A and B. Ann. Allergy, 34:210-212.
72. Louwagie, A. C. (1972): Tuberculin test, lymphocyte cultures and ser-
    um analysts during 4-week treatment with levamisole. Janssen Pharma-
    ceutica, Clinical Research Report on levamisole No. 5, April 1972.
73. Mace, F., Deckers-Passau, L., De Halleux, F., and Deckers, C.
    (1974): Action du lévamisole sur les tumeurs expérimentales du rat
    (immunocytome, leucémie). Unpublished report, September 1974.
74. Mantovani, A., and Spreafico, F. (1975): Allogeneic tumor enhance-
    ment by levamisole, a new immunostimulatory compound: Studies on
    cell-mediated immunity and humoral antibody response. Eur. J. Cancer,
    11:537-544.
75. Matsumoto, T. (1973): Effects of phenylimido thiazole (2,3,5,6-thiazole)
    (tetramisole) and its l-isomer (levamisole) upon immune responses.
    Unpublished report, September 1973.
76. Merluzzi, V. J., Badger, A. M., Kaiser, C. W., and Cooperband,
    S. R. (1975): In vitro stimulation of murine lymphoid cell cultures by
    levamisole. J. Clin. Exp. Immunol., 22:486-492.
77. Meyers, W. M., Kvernes, S., and Staple, E. M. (1975): Failure of
    levamisole to alter the lepromin reaction. Am. J. Trop. Med. Hyg.,
    24:857-859.
78. Naspitz, C. K., and Mendes, N. F. (1975): Preliminary results of
    immunological evaluation in patients with acute lymphatic leukemia,
    receiving chemotherapy, before and after the administration of
    levamisole. Unpublished report, April 1975.
79. Olson, J. A., Nelms, D. C., Silverman, S., and Spitler, L. E. (1976):
    Levamisole: A new treatment for recurrent aphthous stomatitis. Oral
    Surg., 41:588-600.
80. Nelson, K. E. (1975): The effect of levamisole on cell-mediated im-
    munity in lepromatous leprosy patients. Unpublished report, July 1975.
81. Okubo, S. (1975): Experiments on levamisole. Unpublished report,
    March 1975.
82. Pabst, H. F., and Crawford, J. A. (1975): L-Tetramisole, enhance-
    ment of human lymphocyte response to antigen. Clin. Exp. Immunol.,
    21:468-473.
83. Pasquier, P., Vidal, M., Couture, J., Niel, G., Floch, F., and
    Werner, G. H. (1975): Action du lévamisole sur la restauration de
    l'immunité cellulaire chez l'homme. Nouv. Presse Med., 4:2736.
84. Perk, K., Chirigos, M. A., Fuhrman, F., and Perrigrew, H. (1975):
    Some aspects of host response to levamisole after chemotherapy in a
    murine leukemia. J. Natl. Cancer Inst., 54:253-256.
85. Persico, F. J., and Potter, W. A. (1975): The effect of levamisole on
    an in vitro model of cellular immunity. Preprint manuscript, February
    1975.
86. Potter, C. W., Carr, I., Jennings, R., Rees, R. C., McGinty, F., and
    Richardson, V. M. (1974): Levamisole inactive in treatment of four
    animal tumours. Nature, 249:567-569.

87. Provost, A., Tacher, G., and Borredon, C. (1974): Recherche de l'activité immunostimulante de trois dérivés à action anthelminthique de l'imidazole sur les immunogénèses bovipestique, péripneumonique et charbonneuse. Rev. Elev. Med. Vet. Pays Trop., 27:39-52.

88. Rabson, R. (1975): The effect of levamisole on chemotaxis, migration inhibition and blast transformation. Unpublished report, October 1975.

89. Ramot, B., Biniaminov, M., Shoham, C., and Rosenthal, F. (1976): The effect of levamisole on E-rosette forming cells in vivo and in vitro in Hodgkin's disease patients. N. Engl. J. Med., 294: 809-811.

90. Renoux, G., and Renoux, M. (1971): Effet immunostimulant d'un imidothiazole dans l'immunisation des souris contre l'infection par Brucella abortus. C. R. Acad. Sci., 272:349-350.

91. Renoux, G., and Renoux, M. (1972): Levamisole inhibits and cures a solid malignant tumour and its pulmonary metastases in mice. Nature (New Biol.), 240:217-218.

92. Renoux, G., Renoux, M., Morand, P., and Dartigues, P. (1973): Action immunostimulante du lévamisole sur les personnes agées. Rev. Med. Tours, 7:797-801.

93. Renoux, G., and Renoux, M. (1973): Stimulation of anti-brucella vaccination in mice by tetramisole, a phenyl-imidothiazole salt. Infect. Immun., 8:544-548.

94. Renoux, G., Kassel, R. L., Renoux, M., Fiore, N. C., Guillaumin, J. M., and Palat, A. (1976): Immunomodulation by levamisole in normal and leukemic mice. Evidences for a serum transfer. In: First International Conference on Modulation of Host Immune Resistance in the Prevention of Induced Neoplasias, edited by M. A. Chirigos. Fogarty International Center Proceedings, U. S. Government Printing Office, Washington, D. C. (in press).

95. Renoux, G., Renoux, M., and Palat, A. (1976): Influences of levamisole on T-cell reactivity and on survival of untractable cancer patients. In: First International Conference on Modulation of Host Immune Resistance in the Prevention of Induced Neoplasias, edited by M. A. Chirigos. Fogarty International Center Proceedings, U. S. Government Printing Office, Washington, D. C. (in press).

96. Renoux, G., Renoux, M., and Aycardi, D. (1976): Levamisole promotes the killing of Listeria monocytogenes by macrophages. Fed. Proc., 35: 366.

97. Rojas, A. F., Feierstein, J. N., Glait, H. M., Varela, O. A., Pradier, R., and Olivari, A. J. (1976): Clinical action of levamisole and effects of radiotherapy on immune response. In: Second International Conference on Modulation of Host Immune Resistance in the Prevention of Induced Neoplasias, edited by M. A. Chirigos. Fogarty International Center Proceedings, U.S. Government Printing Office, Washington, D.C. (in press).

98. Sadowski, J. M., and Rapp, F. (1975): Inhibition by levamisole on metastases by cells transformed by herpes simplex virus type 1 (38776). Proc. Soc. Exp. Biol. Med., 149:219-222.

99. Schmied, L. M., and Rosenbusch, C. (1973): Effectos del levamisole sobre el indice de sueroproteccion en primovacunacion antiaftosa. Rev. Med. Vet., 54:467-471.

100. Schuermans, Y. (1975): Treatment of rheumatoid arthritis patients with levamisole. Preprint manuscript, December 1975.

101. Schulze, H. J., and Raettig, H. J. (1973): Steigerung der Aktivität von Peritonealmakrophagen der Maus durch Levamisole. Verh. Dtsch. Ges. Inn. Med., 79:622-623.

102. Spitler, L. E., Glogau, R. G., Nelms, D. C., Basch, C. M., Olson, J. A., Silverman, S., and Engleman, E. P. (1976): Clinical and immunologic effects of levamisole. Unpublished report, January 1976.

103. Spitler, L. E., Glogau, R., Nelms, D., Silverman, S., Olson, J., O'Connor, R., Ostler, H., Smolin, G., Basch, K., Wong, P., Engleman, E. P., and Grugmans, J. (1975): Clinical and immunologic effects of levamisole. Unpublished report, February 1975.

104. Spreafico, F. (1973): Immunostimulatory activity of levamisole. Unpublished report, July 1973.

105. Spreafico, F. (1973): Further experiments on the characterization of the immunostimulatory activity of levamisole. Unpublished report, July 1973.

106. Spreafico, F., Vecchi, A., Mantovani, A., Poggi, A., Franchi, G., Anaclerio, A., and Garattini, S. (1975): Characterization of the immunostimulants levamisole and tetramisole. Eur. J. Cancer, 11: 537-544.

107. Spreafico, F., Mantovani, A., Vecchi, A., Poggi, A., Tagliabue, A., and Garattini, S. (1975): On the use of levamisole in experimental tumor immunotherapy. Preprint manuscript, September 1975.

108. Stock, C. (1973): Effect of levamisole on Lewis lung tumor. Unpublished report, April 1973.

109. Symoens, J., and Brugmans, J. (1974): Treatment of recurrent aphthous stomatitis and herpes with levamisole. Br. Med. J., 4:592.

110. Symoens, J., and Brugmans, J. (1976): The effects of levamisole on host defense mechanisms. A review. In: First International Conference on Modulation of Host Immune Resistance in the Prevention or Treatment of Induced Neoplasias, edited by M. A. Chirigos. Fogarty International Center Proceedings, U. S. Government Printing Office, Washington, D.C. (in press).

111. Thienpont, D., Vanparijs, O. F. J., Raeymaekers, A. H. M., Vandenberk, J., Demoen, P. J. A., Allewijn, F. T. N., Marsboom, R. P. H., Niemegeers, C. J. E., Schellekens, K. H. L., and Janssen, P. A. J. (1966): Tetramisole (R 8299), a new, potent broad spectrum anthelmintic. Nature, 209:1084-1086.

112. Thiry, L., Sprecher-Goldberger, S., Tack, L., Jacques, M., and Stienon, J. (1975): Comparison of the immunogenicity of hamster cells transformed by adenovirus and herpes simplex virus. Cancer Res., 35:1022-1029.

113. Thomson, D. M. P. (1973): The effect of BCG, levamisole and BCG and tumor cells on the development of MC-1 cancer in rats. Unpublished report, October 1973.

114. Thomson, D. M. P. (1973): The effect of levamisole (R 12564) s.c. on metastasization in rats treated with cyclophosphamide. Unpublished report, October 1973.

115. Thornes, R. D. (1975): Levamisole treatment of chronic brucellosis and recurrent infections. Unpublished report, June 1975.

116. Thulin, H., Thestrup-Pedersen, K., and Ellegaard, J. (1975): In vitro parameters of cell-mediated immune reactions in healthy individuals following immune-stimulation attempts with levamisole. Acta Allergol., 30:9-18.

117. Trabert, U., Rosenthal, M., and Müller, W. (1975): Levamisol bei der Behandlung entzündlich-rheumatischer Erkrankungen und der Sarkoidose. Dtsch. Med. Wochenschr., 100:2297-2298.

118. Tripodi, D., Parks, L. C., and Brugmans, J. (1973): Drug-induced restoration of cutaneous delayed hypersensitivity in anergic patients with cancer. N. Engl. J. Med., 289:354-357.

119. Tripodi, D., and Parks, L. (1976): Restoration of cutaneous delayed hypersensitivity by levamisole. In: First International Conference on Modulation of Host Immune Resistance in the Prevention or Treatment of Induced Neoplasias, edited by M. A. Chirigos. Fogarty International Center Proceedings, U. S. Government Printing Office, Washington, D. C. (in press).

120. Turine, J. B. (1974): Expérience avec le lévamisole chez les lépreux. Unpublished report, March 1974.

121. Vandercammen, R., and Bollen, J. (1975): DNCB-reactivity, as related to survival, in patients with advanced solid cancers. A double blind placebo-controlled pilot study with levamisole. Janssen Pharmaceutica, Clinical Research Report on levamisole No. 24, April 1975.

122. Van Eygen, M., Znamensky, P. Y., Heck, E., and Raymaekers, I. (1976): Levamisole in the prevention of recurrent upper respiratory tract infections in children. Lancet, i:382-385.

123. Van Ghinckel, R., and Hoebeke, J. (1974): Reversal of corticoid-depressed carbon clearance by levamisole in mice. Janssen Pharmaceutica, Biological Research Report on levamisole No. 4, April 1974.

124. Van Ghinckel, R., and Hoebeke, J. (1975): Carbon clearance enhancing factor in serum for levamisole treated mice. J. Reticuloendothel. Soc., 17:65-72.

125. Van Ghinckel, R. F., and Hoebeke, J. (1976): Effects of levamisole on spontaneous rosette-forming cells in murine spleen. Eur. J. Immunol., 6:305-307.

126. Van Hooren, J. (1976): Influenza vaccine and PPD skin-test reactivity. Lancet, i:44.

127. Van Oss, C. J. (1973): Effect of levamisole on contact angle and on phagocytosis by macrophages. Unpublished report, September 1973.

128. Veldhuizen, R. W., Cardozo, E. L., and Van Veelen, H. (1975):
Immune status in the aged and the effect of levamisole on diverse immunological parameters. Preprint manuscript, October 1975.

129. Verhaegen, H., De Cree, J., Verbruggen, F., Hoebeke, J.,
De Brabender, M., and Brugmans, J. (1973): Immune responses in
elderly cuti-negative subjects and the effect of levamisole. Verh.
Dtsch. Ges. Inn. Med., 79:623-628.

130. Verhaegen, H., De Cree, J., De Cock, W., and Verbruggen, F.
(1973): Levamisole and the immune response. N. Engl. J. Med.,
289:1148-1149.

131. Verhaegen, H., De Cree, J., and Brugmans, J. (1973): Treatment of
aphthous stomatitis. Lancet, ii:842.

132. Verhaegen, H., Verbruggen, F., Verhaegen-Declercq, M. L., and
De Cree, J. (1974): Effets du lévamisole sur les réactions cutanées
d'hypersensibilité retardée. Nouv. Presse Med., 3:2483-2485.

133. Verhaegen, H., De Cree, J., De Cock, W., and Brugmans, J. (1976):
Levamisole treatment of a child with severe aphthous stomatitis and
neutropenia. Postgrad. Med. J. (in press).

134. Verhaegen, H., De Cock, W., De Cree, J., Verbruggen, F.,
Verhaegen-Declercq, M., and Brugmans, J. (1975): In vitro restoration by levamisole of thymus-derived lymphocyte function in Hodgkin's
disease. Lancet, i:978.

135. Verhaegen, H., De Cock, W., and De Cree, J., (1976): In vitro
phagocytosis of C. albicans by peripheral polymorphonuclear
neutrophils of patients with recurrent infections. Case reports of
serum-dependent abnormalities. Biomedicine, 24: 164-170.

136. Versijp, G., Van Zwet, T. L., and Van Furth, R. (1975): Levamisole
and functions of peritoneal macrophages. Lancet, i:798.

137. Veys, E. M., Mielants, H., De Bussere, A., Decrans, L., and
Gabriel, P. (1976): Levamisole in rheumatoid arthritis. Lancet,
i:808-809.

138. Wachi, K. K., Kimura, L. H., Perreira, S., Hokama, Y., Perri, S.,
and Palumbo, N. (1974): Effect of levamisole and C-reactive protein
on mitogen-stimulated lymphocytes in vitro. Res. Commun. Chem.
Pathol. Pharmacol., 8:681-694.

139. Woods, W. A., Siegel, M. J., and Chirigos, M. A. (1974): In vitro
stimulation of spleen cell cultures by poly I:poly C and levamisole.
Cell. Immunol., 14:327-331.

140. Woods, W. A., Fliegelman, M. J., and Chirigos, M. A. (1975):
Effect of levamisole on the in vitro immune response of spleen lymphocytes (38686). Proc. Soc. Exp. Biol. Med., 148:1048-1050.

141. Woods, W. A., Fliegelman, M. J., and Chirigos, M. A. (1975):
Effect of levamisole (NSC-177023) on DNA synthesis by lymphocytes
from immunosuppressed C57BL mice. Cancer Chemother. Rep.,
Part 1, 59:531-536.

Control of Neoplasia by Modulation of the Immune System. edited by M. A. Chirigos. Raven Press, New York 1977.

EFFECT OF LEVAMISOLE ON MURINE LYMPHOID POPULATIONS

Vincent J. Mcrluzzi, Alison M. Badger, C. William Kaiser, and
Sidney R. Cooperband

Departments of Medicine, Microbiology, and Surgery, and the
Cancer Research Center, Boston University School of
Medicine, Boston, Massachusetts 02118

INTRODUCTION

It has been shown that levamisole, 2,3,5,6-tetrahydro-6-phenylimidazo-(2,1-b)-thiazole, an antihelminthic drug (1), may possess immunostimulatory properties in vivo. In mice this drug has been reported to enhance the formation of antibody producing cells (2); to restore the impaired immunological system in aged mice (3); to enhance antibacterial immunization (4); and to increase the intensity of the graft versus host reaction in F_1 hybrid recipients following inoculation of parental donor cells (5). In addition, it has been reported that levamisole reduced the incidence of primary tumors and metastases in mice (6), although not always (7), and augmented a chemotherapeutically induced remission of a murine leukemia (8).

In man, levamisole has been reported to reduce the frequency of lesions in patients with recurrent aphthous stomatitis (9), and also to restore delayed skin test responses in anergic cancer patients (10). Because of these multiple effects on immune events, we felt that it was important to understand the mechanism by which levamisole was influencing the various cellular elements of the immune response. We have therefore examined its effect on the proliferative responses of lymphoid cell populations.

MATERIALS AND METHODS

Mice

CBA/J and C57B1/6J male and DBA/J female mice were purchased from the Jackson Laboratory, Bar Harbor, Maine. Nude (nu/nu) (athymic) mice

25

of a Balb/c strain were obtained from breeding laboratories at the Boston University School of Medicine. Mice were 2 weeks to 6 months old at the time of use and were maintained on acidified drinking water and routine mouse chow. Within any given experiment, only mice of the same age, strain, and sex were used.

Culture Media

Culture media for measuring the DNA synthetic response of murine lymphoid cells consisted of Eagle's Minimal Essential Media (MEM) with Earle's salts obtained from Flow Laboratories, Rockville, Maryland. This medium was supplemented with L-glutamine, sodium pyruvate, Eagle's nonessential amino acids, 100 units of penicillin, and 100 µg of streptomycin per milliliter and 5% (v/v) of heat inactivated (56°C for 30 min) fetal calf serum (Grand Island Biological Co., Grand Island, New York).

Mitogens and Antigens

Concanavalin A (Con A) was obtained from Miles Laboratories, Kankakee, Illinois. Phytohemagglutinin (PHA) and E. coli lipopolysaccharide (LPS) (055:B5) were obtained from Difco Laboratories, Detroit, Michigan. Keyhole Limpet Hemocyanin (KLH) was obtained from Pacific Biomarine Supply Co., Venice, California.

Levamisole

A crystalline preparation of levamisole (lot SM15807) was obtained from the Ortho Research Foundation, Raritan, New Jersey. On the day of use the levamisole preparation was dissolved in the appropriate culture media and immediately sterilized by filtration through millipore filters (HA 0.45 µm).

Culture Conditions

Mouse spleen cells, thymus cells, and lymph node cells were prepared by a procedure similar to that described by Mishell and Dutton (11). Following cervical dislocation, the tissues were removed asceptically and the cells were gently extruded with a small curved forceps into Hanks Balanced Salt Solution (HBSS) in a small Petri dish. In the case of bone marrow, femurs were used and the cells were gently removed into HBSS by pressuring one end of the dissected bone with a syringe capped with a 27-gauge needle. Once the lymphoid cell tissue was obtained, it was then dispersed by repeated aspiration with a Pasteur pipette and transferred to a 15-ml conical tube on ice. The larger tissue particles were allowed to settle out for 5 min. The cells remaining in the supernatant were then removed and washed in HBSS by centrifugation (10 min, 100 X g), and resuspended to a final concentration of 20 X 10^6/ml in culture media.

For the measurement of DNA synthesis, cultures were established in microtest plates (IS-FB-96-TC; Linbro Chemical Co., New Haven, Connecticut). Lymphoid cells (20×10^6/ml), culture media, levamisole, and other reagents were added separately to each culture well with 25- or 50-μl droppers (Linbro). The final concentration of nucleated cells per culture well was 1×10^6 in a final volume of 0.2 ml of culture media. The cultures were incubated in a humidified 5% CO_2 atmosphere at 37°C. They were then pulsed with tritiated thymidine (^{3}H-T) (Schwarz/Mann, Orangeburg, New York, sp. act. 1.9 C/M) after 48 hr in culture, and were terminated at 64 to 66 hr.

For antigen studies, mice were immunized with 400 μg of KLH in Complete Freunds Adjuvant (CFA) subcutaneously. Four weeks later, spleen cells were cultured as above with various doses of KLH per culture. One-way mixed lymphocyte reactions were established by incubating C57Bl/6J spleen cells at a concentration of 10×10^6/ml with mitomycin C (25 μg/ml) (Schwarz/Mann) for 30 min at 37°C. These cells were then washed three times in HBSS and brought to the desired concentration in culture media. The C57Bl/6J spleen cells were used as stimulator cells and the CBA/J spleen cells were used as the responding cells.

Harvesting was accomplished on a multiple automated sample harvestor (MASH II) obtained from Microbiological Associates, Bethesda, Maryland. For DNA synthetic responses the procedure consisted of several saline washes followed by precipitation of the DNA onto glass fiber filters (Reeve Angel, 934AH) with 5% trichloroacetic acid. The filters were then counted in a dioxane naphthalene, 2,5-diphenyl oxazole (PPO) mixture in a Beckman Liquid Scintillation Counter. Toxicity in cultures was determined by the technique of trypan blue dye exclusion.

Enriched T-Cell Populations

Enrichment of spleen cells to contain primarily T-cells was accomplished by a method similar to that described by Trizio and Cudkowicz (12). Briefly, 1.5×10^8 CBA/J spleen cells in a volume of 2 ml were added to a nylon wool column that had been previously preincubated with culture medium at 37°C. The columns were incubated for 45 min and the nonadherent spleen cells were eluted with 25 ml of warm culture medium. This effluent fraction contained the T-cell rich population of spleen cells. Success of enrichment was determined by DNA synthetic responses to the T-cell mitogen Con A, and the B-cell mitogen LPS.

RESULTS

The mitogenic effect of levamisole on mouse spleen cells is shown in Fig. 1. CBA/J spleen cells at 1×10^6/culture well were incubated for 3 days with various doses of levamisole. The cultures were pulsed with 0.5 microcuries (μCi) of tritiated thymidine (^{3}H-T) for the last 16 hr of incubation. Within a dose range of 1 to 30 μg of levamisole, there was a stimulation of ^{3}H-T

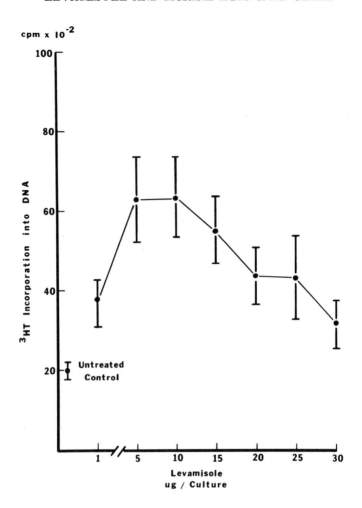

FIG. 1. Effect of various concentrations of levamisole on ^{3}H-T incorporation into DNA of CBA/J mouse spleen cells. Cultures contain a final volume of 0.2 ml. Each point represents the mean cpm $\pm$ SD of the mean.

incorporation into DNA with maximal stimulation occurring between 5 and 15 µg of levamisole/culture well. Similar dose-response curves have been found using the spleen cells from DBA/J female mice. We have at times found that significant stimulation with levamisole can occur with a dose as low as 0.1 µg, whereas at doses approaching 100 µg the drug appears to be toxic; stimulatory doses of levamisole did not increase the number of trypan blue positive cells above that found in untreated controls.

Figure 2 illustrates the data from an experiment designed to determine the optimum time for this stimulatory effect of levamisole on DNA synthesis. In this experiment, untreated spleen cells and spleen cells containing a single dose of levamisole (10 µg) per culture well were established at time 0 and

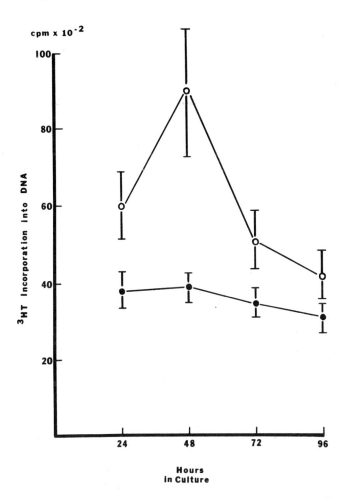

FIG. 2. Effect of an optimal concentration of levamisole (10 μg/culture) on CBA/J spleen cells pulsed with 3H–T at various times after initiation of the culture. The cells were pulsed for 16 hr after 24, 48, 72, or 96 hr in culture. Cultures contain a final volume of 0.2 ml. Each point represents mean cpm ± SD of the mean. O——O levamisole-treated cultures; ●——● untreated cultures.

were pulsed with 0.5 μCi of 3H–T for 16 hr at either 24, 48, 72, or 96 hr after culture initiation. As can be seen, an optimal stimulatory effect occurs when the cultures were pulsed at 48 hr and terminated at 64 hr after culture initiation.

In order to probe which cells levamisole might be stimulating, we looked at the effect of this drug on CBA/J spleen cells stimulated by both T- and B-cell mitogens. Figure 3 illustrates the effect of addition of levamisole to cultures containing a full dose range of the B-cell mitogen E. coli lipopolysaccharide (LPS). Using a single optimally stimulatory dose of levamisole

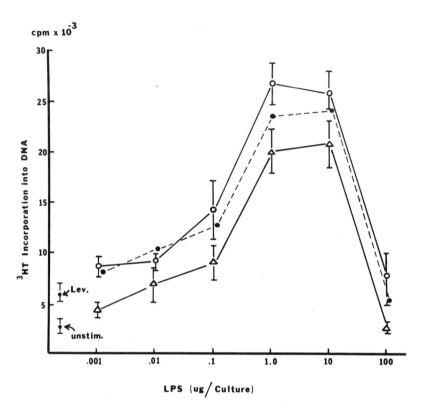

FIG. 3. Effect of an optimal dose (10 µg/culture) of levamisole on the response of CBA/J mouse spleen cells to varying concentrations of E. coli lipopolysaccharide. Cultures contain a final volume of 0.2 ml. Each point represents mean cpm ± SD of the mean. Δ——Δ LPS alone; O——O actual response of LPS + 10 µg of levamisole; ●——● hypothetical response of LPS + 10 µg of levamisole.

(10 µg/culture), it can be seen that there is a simple additive effect of the two agents at all doses of the mitogen LPS. All doses of LPS showed a similar increase in DNA synthesis induced by the addition of levamisole to the cultures. A predicted mathematical summation is presented as a dashed line, and is almost identical to the observed data.

We next performed the same experiment, substituting the T-cell mitogen Con A in place of the B-cell mitogen LPS. Figure 4 depicts DNA synthesis in a series of cultures to which a full dose range of Con A and a maximum stimulatory dose (10 µg) of levamisole were added. It can be seen that levamisole greatly potentiated suboptimal doses of Con A, whereas at the optimum concentration there was no apparent stimulatory effect. That levamisole potentiated at suboptimal doses of Con A rather than acting in a strictly additive manner can be seen from the theoretical line drawn into this figure (dashed line). This line represents the mathematically derived curve one would expect had levamisole been working in an additive manner.

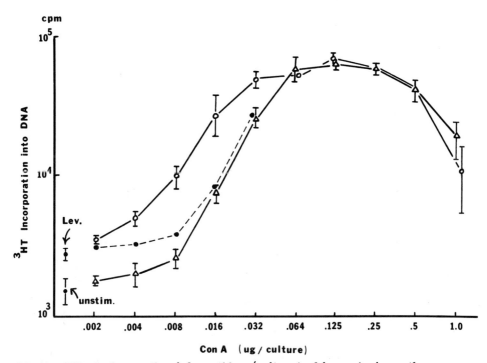

FIG. 4. Effect of an optimal dose (10 μg/culture) of levamisole on the response of CBA/J mouse spleen cells to varying concentrations of Con A. Cultures contain a final volume of 0.2 ml. Each point represents mean cpm ± SD of the mean. Δ———Δ Con A alone; O———O actual response of Con A + 10 μg of levamisole; ●———● hypothetical response of Con A + 10 μg of levamisole.

Figure 5 represents the data from a similar experiment in which a full dose range of the T-cell mitogen phytohemagglutinin (PHA) was employed. Here again, levamisole acted to potentiate the PHA response at suboptimal concentrations of PHA. All optimal and supraoptimal doses of PHA in this experiment were not affected by levamisole.

In place of mitogens, we next attempted to study the in vitro response of spleen cells to antigen stimulation with and without levamisole present in the culture system. CBA/J mice were immunized with 400 μg of Keyhole Limpet Hemocyanin (KLH) in Complete Freund's Adjuvant. Four weeks later the mice were sacrificed, and their spleen cells were incubated with various doses of KLH and a stimulatory dose of levamisole (10 μg/culture). As can be seen from Fig. 6, there was a potentiation of the response to KLH in those cultures that were incubated with levamisole. The dose-response curve of KLH was enhanced throughout the entire experiment except at very high concentrations of the antigen.

In addition to antigen, we have also studied the effect of levamisole on the antigen stimulation induced by allogeneic cells. Figure 7 shows the response of CBA/J spleen cells (0.5 X 10^6/culture) to a dose-response curve of C57B1/6J spleen cells that had been previously treated with mitomycin C. As can be

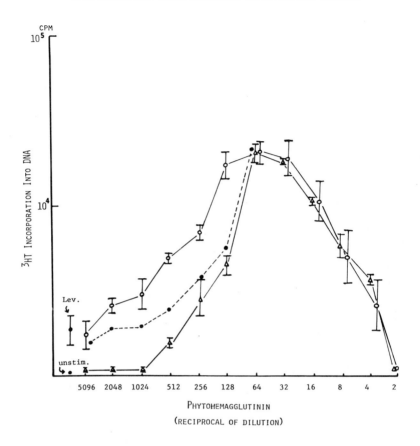

FIG. 5. Effect of an optimal dose (10 μg/culture) of levamisole on the response of CBA/J mouse spleen cells to varying concentrations of phytohemagglutinin (PHA). Cultures contain a final volume of 0.2 ml. Each point represents mean cpm ± SD of the mean. △——△ PHA alone; O——O actual response of PHA + 10 μg of levamisole; ●——● hypothetical response of PHA + 10 μg of levamisole.

seen, there is potentiation by levamisole of the effector cell response to the various doses of stimulator cells (C57B1/6J). At high concentrations of stimulator cells there is no significant enhancement by levamisole.

Since it seemed from the above data that this drug was acting selectively on the T-cell component of the spleen cell cultures, we next attempted to verify if levamisole would stimulate enriched T-cell populations. The nylon wool method was employed as a tool for obtaining the T-cell-rich nonadherent cells. This method has been reported to give a relatively pure population of T-cells with about 5% contamination with other cell types. One million normal spleen cells and 1 X 10^6 nylon wool purified T-cells were incubated separately in the microculture plate as described above, with levamisole (optimum dose of 10 μg/culture) and without. As a check of purity, the

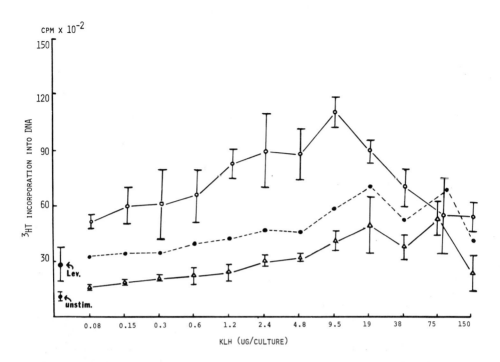

FIG. 6.   Effect of an optimal dose (10 μg/culture) of levamisole on the response of CBA/J mouse spleen cells to varying concentrations of Keyhole Limpet Hemocyanin (KLH).   Cultures contain a final volume of 0.2 ml. Each point represents mean cpm ± SD of the mean.   Δ——Δ KLH alone; O——O actual response of KLH + 10 μg of levamisole; ●——● hypothetical response of KLH + 10 μg of levamisole.

T-cell mitogen Con A and the B-cell mitogen LPS were added to the cultures at doses previously determined to produce optimal stimulation of DNA synthesis.   Table 1 shows that normal spleen cells are stimulated by all three mitogens, Con A, LPS, and levamisole.   The T-cell-rich populations stimulated well with Con A, but very poorly with the B-cell mitogen LPS, indicating that a relatively pure population of T-cells was obtained.   This population of cells was responsive to optimal concentrations of levamisole, giving a greater rate of DNA synthesis than an equal number of whole spleen cells.

Our next experiments were designed to test the responsiveness of spleen cells from nude (athymic) mice to the direct mitogenic effect of levamisole. Since these mice contain relatively few T-cells, it was our assumption that this drug would have little or no effect on the stimulation of spleen cells from these mice.   In the two experiments shown in Table 2, it can be seen that athymic mice (nu/nu) do not respond to stimulatory doses of levamisole, whereas normal, congenitally thymic mice do respond to this drug.

In addition to examining the effect of levamisole on mouse spleen cells, we have also cultured thymic lymphoid cells with varying doses of this drug, both alone and in combination with Con A.   As demonstrated in Fig. 8A, when

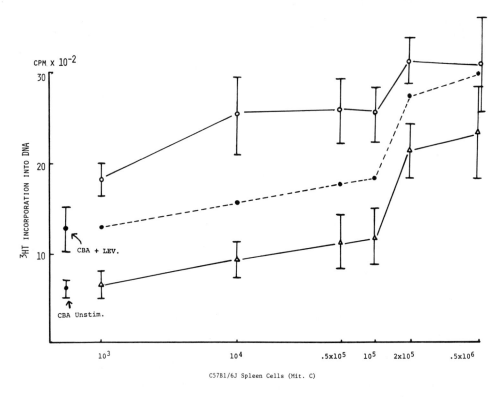

FIG. 7. Effect of an optimal dose (10 μg/culture) of levamisole on the response of CBA/J mouse spleen cells to C57B1/6J mouse spleen cells previously treated with mitomycin C. Cultures contain a final volume of 0.2 ml. Each point represents mean cpm ± SD of the mean. Δ——Δ CBA/J X C57B1/6J; O——O actual response of CBA/J X C57B1/6J + 10 μg of levamisole; ●——● hypothetical response of CBA/J X C57B1/6J + 10 μg of levamisole.

TABLE 1. Stimulation of normal and T-cell-rich spleen cultures as determined by the incorporation of ^{3}H-T into DNA

	Normal spleen cells	T-cell-rich
Unstimulated control	2,401 ± 652[a]	2,602 ± 535
Con A (0.5 μg/culture)	20,521 ± 2,365	29,202 ± 9,681
LPS (10 μg/culture)	28,820 ± 4,021	4,699 ± 1,073
Levamisole (10 μg/culture)	4,594 ± 667	6,750 ± 1,379

[a] Counts/min ^{3}H-T incorporated into DNA ± SD.

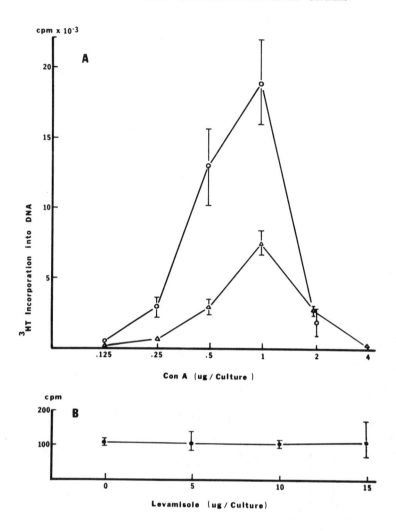

FIG. 8. <u>A</u>: Effect of an optimal dose (10 μg/culture) of levamisole on the response of CBA/J mouse thymocytes to varying concentrations of Con A.
Δ——Δ Con A alone; O——O Con A + 10 μg of levamisole. <u>B</u>: Effect of various
doses of levamisole on CBA/J mouse thymocytes. Cultures contain a final
volume of 0.2 ml. Each point represents mean cpm ± SD of the mean.

levamisole (at the optimal dose for mitogenic stimulation of spleen cells,
10 μg/culture) was added to various doses of Con A-stimulated thymic lymphoid cells, there was an impressive potentiation of the response at both suboptimal and optimal doses of this mitogen. As can be seen from Fig. 8B,
however, there was no direct mitogenic effect of this drug on thymocytes
alone.

TABLE 2. Stimulation of nude spleen cultures by levamisole as determined by the incorporation of ^{3}H-T into DNA

Levamisole (µg/culture)	^{3}H-T incorporation into DNA			
	Exp. 1		Exp. 2	
	Balb/c-nu/nu[a]	Balb/c[b]	Balb/c-nu/nu	Balb/c
—	664 ± 144.1[c]	738 ± 41.8	348 ± 65.3	2,492 ± 470.3
10	686 ± 122.6	1,377 ± 274.6	261 ± 45.9	11,852 ± 2,606.5
20	729 ± 150.8	1,251 ± 245.2	270 ± 54.8	N.D.[d]
30	654 ± 66.3	1,225 ± 229.9	285 ± 102.9	N.D.
Con A[e]	1,082 ± 876.8	7,810 ± 2,879.3	396 ± 133.7	76,570 ± 14,422.8

[a] Balb/c nude (athymic mice).

[b] Balb/c normal littermate control.

[c] cpm ± SD.

[d] N.D. = not done.

[e] Con A = conconavalin A (0.5 µg/culture).

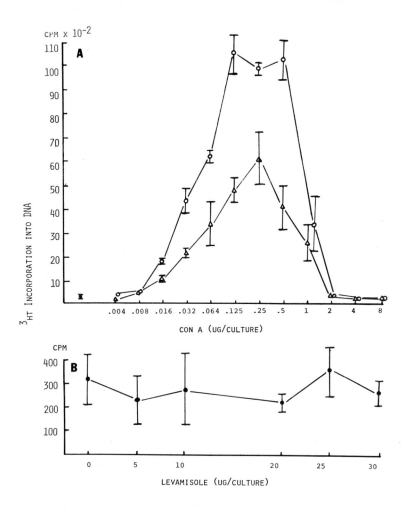

FIG. 9. <u>A</u>: Effect of an optimal dose (10 μg/culture) of levamisole on the response of CBA/J mouse lymph node cells to varying concentrations of Con A. △——△ Con A alone; O——O Con A + 10 μg of levamisole. <u>B</u>: Effect of various doses of levamisole on CBA/J mouse lymph node cells. Cultures contain a final volume of 0.2 ml. Each point represents mean cpm ± SD of the mean.

Figure 9A shows a similar effect of levamisole on murine lymph node cells. Here, as with thymocytes, levamisole potentiated the response of Con A at almost all doses of this mitogen; very high doses of Con A were not enhanced, however. In addition, here there was no direct mitogenic effect of levamisole on murine lymph node cells (Fig. 9B).

Figure 10A illustrates the Con A response of bone marrow cells with levamisole. Bone marrow cells seemed to be totally unresponsive to levamisole; there was no potentiating effect. Figure 10B shows, in addition, that there was no direct mitogenic effect of this drug on cultured bone marrow cells.

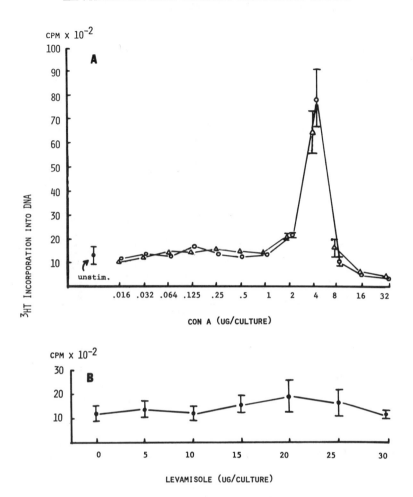

FIG. 10. A: Effect of an optimal dose (10 μg/culture) of levamisole on the response of CBA/J mouse bone marrow cells to varying concentrations of Con A. △——△ Con A alone; O——O Con A + 10 μg of levamisole. B: Effect of various doses of levamisole on CBA/J mouse bone marrow cells. Cultures contain a final volume of 0.2 ml. Each point represents mean cpm ± SD of the mean.

DISCUSSION

Substances which enhance immune responses may act at any of the complex interactions that constitute immune reactivity, but ultimately, a stimulator must act by one of the two following reactions:

1. Altering the responsiveness of the cells capable of reacting to an antigen; or

2.   Altering the interrelationship between immune components or reactive cells essential to the production of an immune response.

We have attempted to determine if levamisole acts by either of these two methods by utilizing in vitro assays.

We have found that levamisole is a selective mitogen for murine splenic T-cells. It is a weak mitogen capable of producing only a mild increase of DNA synthesis above that of untreated spleen cell cultures. This has also been reported by Woods, Siegel, and Chirigos (13). That this substance appears to be a mitogen for splenic T-cells is concluded from two observations:

1.   It is stimulatory in isolated spleen T-cell populations, and has no effect on splenocytes from nude mice; and

2.   There is no additive effect when optimal concentrations of the T-cell mitogens Con A or PHA are used, whereas there is a summation of stimulus when the B-cell mitogen LPS is used.

Thus, a subpopulation of splenic T-cells appears to be capable of reacting to levamisole with a proliferative response. This could imply that levamisole acts to alter a cell population which is involved in the complex cellular interaction involved in the immune response. The observation that immature T-cells (thymus cells) and spleen cells from nude (athymic) mice are not stimulated by levamisole suggests that the target for its direct stimulation is a T-cell population which has undergone further differentiation (or maturation) in the spleen.

We have also found that levamisole acts to potentiate the stimulatory effect of the T-cell mitogens Con A and PHA in splenic cells when these substances are used at concentrations less than optimal. Under these circumstances, levamisole appears to lower the threshold necessary for stimulation of T-cells so that they are activated into DNA synthesis at concentrations of Con A which would not normally be able to do so. Thus, although levamisole appears able to stimulate a subpopulation of T-cells by itself, it also appears to augment the ability of the T-cells to respond to a suboptimal dose of stimulus. This experiment implies that levamisole acts to alter the responsiveness of a reactive cell population. This conclusion was further substantiated with antigen-stimulated lymphoid cells where an increased quantity of DNA synthesis could be induced in the presence of levamisole. The ability of levamisole to augment the response of thymocytes and lymph node cells to optimal doses of Con A suggests that in these populations, the drug allows immature cells, which would not normally respond to a mitogen, to become reactive. This in turn suggests that the augmentation effect on splenic T-cells may also be on a more immature subpopulation of T cells.

It is interesting to note that the augmentation effect of levamisole on Con A responses of murine lymphoid tissues occurs only in the thymus, spleen, and lymph node, and not in the bone marrow cell population. It would thus seem that levamisole will potentiate T-cell responses only if these cells have matured at least to the thymocyte stage of differentiation, and that few if any of these cells are found in the bone marrow. That the potentiation by levamisole is not peculiar to mitogens is demonstrated by the fact that this drug will also enhance stimuli produced by antigen and allogeneic cells.

On the basis of the above experiments we would hypothesize that levamisole acts to stimulate selectively a subpopulation of splenic T-cells, and also acts as an immunological adjuvant on other peripheral T-cells located in the thymus, spleen, and lymph node. On the basis of our experiments, we therefore conclude that levamisole serves in both methods of augmenting the immune response in the murine species.

SUMMARY

Levamisole has been reported to act as an immunological adjuvant. In order to probe the mechanism of action of this drug as an immune stimulator, we have employed several in vitro assays using murine lymphoid tissues.

We have found levamisole to possess a weak mitogenic potential for a subpopulation of murine spleen cells. This mitogenic stimulation induced DNA synthesis is maximal at 48 hr in culture. Levamisole had no direct mitogenic effect on thymocytes, lymph node cells, bone marrow cells, and spleen cells from nude (athymic) mice. This drug also potentiated the response of spleen cells to suboptimal doses of concanavalin A and phytohemagglutinin, but had no enhancing effect when optimal or supraoptimal doses of these mitogens were used. Spleen cells stimulated with antigen or allogeneic cells also exhibited augmentation of DNA synthesis at suboptimal levels of stimuli when levamisole was added to the culture system. In addition, thymus and lymph node cell responses to concanavalin A were greatly potentiated by levamisole, whereas the bone marrow cell response to concanavalin A (Con A) remained unaffected by the addition of the drug to the culture system. Lastly, levamisole had no unusual effect on the lipopolysaccharide stimulation of B-cell DNA synthesis in vitro.

ACKNOWLEDGMENTS

This work was supported in part by research grants CA-12209, CA-15129, and CA-15848 from the U.S. Public Health Service.

REFERENCES

1. Thienpont, D., Vanparijs, O. F. J., Raeymaekers, A. H. M., Vandenberk, J., Demoen, P. J. A., Allewijn, F. T. N., Marsboom, R. P. H., Niemegeers, C. J. E., Schellekens, K. H. L., and Janssen, P. A. J. (1966): Tetramisole, a new, potent broad spectrum antihelminthic. Nature, 209:1084-1086.
2. Renoux, G., and Renoux, M. (1972): Action immunostimulante de dérivés du phénylimidothiazole sur les cellules spléniques formatrices d'anticorps. C. R. Acad. Sci. (D), 274:756-757.

3. Renoux, G., and Renoux, M. (1972): Restaurante par le phenylimidothi-azole de la réponse immunologique des souris Âgées. C. R. Acad. Sci. (D), 274:3034-3035.

4. Renoux, G., and Renoux, M. (1971): Effet immunostimulant d'un imidothiazole dans l'immunisation des souris contre l'infection par Brucella abortus. C. R. Acad. Sci. (D), 272:349-350.

5. Renoux, G., and Renoux, M. (1972): Action du phenylimidothiazole (tétramisole) sur la réaction du Greffon contre l'hôte. Role des macrophages. C.R. Acad. Sci. (D), 274:3320-3323.

6. Renoux, G., and Renoux, M. (1972): Levamisole inhibits and cures a solid malignant tumour and its metastases in mice. Nature, 240:217-218.

7. Potter, C. W., Carr, I., Jennings, R., Rees, R. C., McGinty, F., and Richardson, V. M. (1974): Levamisole inactive in treatment of four animal tumours. Nature, 249:567-569.

8. Chirigos, M. A., Pearson, J. W., and Pryor, J. (1973): Augmentation of a chemotherapeutically induced remission of a murine leukemia by a chemical immunoadjuvant. Cancer Res., 33:2615-2618.

9. Verhaegen, H., DeCree, J., and Brugmans, J. (1973): Treatment of aphthous stomatitis. Lancet, ii:842.

10. Tripodi, D., Parks, L. C., and Brugmans, J. (1973): Drug-induced restoration of cutaneous delayed hypersensitivity in anergic patients with cancer. N. Engl. J. Med., 289:354-357.

11. Mishell, R. I., and Dutton, R. W. (1967): Immunization of dissociated spleen cell cultures from normal mice. J. Exp. Med., 126:423-442.

12. Trizio, D., and Cudkowicz, G. (1974): Separation of T and B lympho-cytes by nylon wool columns: Evaluation of efficacy by functional assays in vivo. J. Immunol., 113:1093-1097.

13. Woods, W. A., Siegal, M. J., and Chirigos, M. A. (1974): In vitro stimulation of spleen cell cultures by po.y I:poly C and levamisole. Cell. Immunol., 14:327-331.

Control of Neoplasia by Modulation of the Immune System, edited by M. A. Chirigos. Raven Press, New York 1977.

EFFECT OF LEVAMISOLE ON HUMAN LYMPHOCYTE MEDIATOR PRODUCTION IN VITRO

Michael E. Whitcomb, Vincent J. Merluzzi, and Sidney R. Cooperband

Thorndike Memorial Laboratory, Department of Medicine,
Boston City Hospital, and Department of Medicine,
Boston University School of Medicine,
Boston, Massachusetts 02118

INTRODUCTION

The administration of levamisole has been reported to increase delayed hypersensitivity reactions in anergic cancer patients and anergic elderly individuals (1-3). Elucidation of the mechanism by which nonspecific immune stimulants such as levamisole augment the immune response in vivo is not only important for further understanding the nature of the immune response, but may also have practical application in the management of the immunosuppression associated with a variety of clinical states. Churchill and David (4) have hypothesized that levamisole might stimulate the immune response by increasing the proliferative response of sensitized lymphocytes or by augmenting defective mediator production by lymphocytes.

Several investigators have studied the effect of levamisole on the proliferative response of human lymphocytes in vitro (3,5,6,7). In all but one of these studies, levamisole had no effect on in vitro lymphocyte proliferation. In order to investigate further the mechanism by which levamisole may stimulate the human immune response in vivo, we have studied the effect of levamisole on both lymphocyte proliferation and lymphocyte mediator production. Our results indicate that in vitro levamisole augments the production of soluble mediators by mitogen-stimulated human lymphocytes, while having no effect on lymphocyte proliferation.

43

METHODS

Levamisole

A stock solution of levamisole (2,3,5,6-tetrahydro-6-phenylimidazo-(2, 1-b)-thiazole) at a concentration of 50 μg/0.1 ml was prepared by dissolving levamisole in minimum essential media containing penicillin (100 units/ml) and streptomycin (100 μg/ml) (MEM). The stock solution was kept frozen until use.

Measurement of Lymphocyte Proliferation

Human mononuclear cell suspensions were prepared as described below. The cells were cultured in microtiter plates at a concentration of 2.5×10^5 cells in 0.2 ml of MEM containing 10% fetal calf serum (MEM-FCS). In different experiments, phytohemagglutinin (PHA) and concanavalin A (Con A) were employed as the stimulating mitogen. A dose-response curve was constructed with each mitogen. Levamisole was added to all cultures at a concentration of 50 μg/ml. In addition, cultures were established in which a peak stimulating dose of Con A (10 μg/ml) was added to each well, and a complete dose-response curve of levamisole (60 to 0.5 μg/ml) constructed. All cultures were incubated for 48 hr in a 5% CO_2-air environment at 37° C. They were then pulsed with 0.5 μCi of tritiated thymidine (Schwartz/Mann, S.A. 1.9) for 24 hr and sacrificed. The cells were collected on a glass fiber filter using a multiple automated sample harvester (MASH II, Microbiologic Ass.) and the incorporation of ^{3}H-thymidine into TCA-precipitable material was measured as an index of DNA synthesis. All cultures were performed in triplicate.

Preparation of Lymphokines

Heparinized blood was obtained from normal human donors by routine venipuncture. After sedimentation in inverted syringes, the cell-rich plasma was removed and centrifuged at 150 X g for 10 min. The cell pellet was resuspended in MEM and the mononuclear cells separated by Ficoll-Hypaque density centrifugation. The mononuclear cell layer was washed three times in MEM and resuspended at a concentration of 1.0×10^6 lymphocytes/ml. The cell suspension was then divided into four equal portions and Con A (10 μg/ml) was added to each. This concentration of Con A was selected because previous studies in our laboratory had demonstrated that this was a suboptimal concentration for stimulating mediator production. Levamisole was added to three of the cultures in concentrations of 25, 50, and 100 μg/ml, respectively. These concentrations of levamisole were selected because they were in the range that had been demonstrated in our laboratory to cause optimal augmentation of the proliferative response of Con A stimulated murine spleen cells. The fourth culture served as a control. In experiments in which the direct effect of levamisole on lymphocyte mediator production was being investigated, no Con A was added to the cultures. All cultures were incubated for 48 hr at 37°C in a 5% CO_2-air environment.

After 48 hr incubation, the cultures were centrifuged at 150 X g for 10 min and the supernatants removed. Residual Con A was removed by passing the supernatants through an inverted syringe containing 15 ml of G-50 Sephadex which had been swollen in MEM. The total volume of the supernatant was collected after passage through Sephadex, dialyzed against 20 volumes of fresh MEM for 48 hr to remove levamisole, and sterilized by passage through a millipore filter (0.45 μm). Fetal calf serum (FCS) was added to a volume of 10%, and the supernatant was frozen until use.

In order to study the effects of levamisole on lymphokine production by antigen-stimulated lymphocytes, blood was obtained from individuals with positive intermediate tuberculin skin tests. Mononuclear cells were separated in an identical fashion, suspended at a concentration of 7.5 X 10^6 lymphocytes/ml, and incubated with PPD (10 μg/ml). The cell suspension was divided into two equal parts, and levamisole was added to one culture at a concentration of 100 μg/ml. The additional culture served as a control. After 48 hr incubation, the supernatants were removed, dialyzed, passed through a millipore filter, and reconstituted with FCS.

Harvesting Macrophages

Five-hundred-gram male Hartley strain guinea pigs were used in all experiments. Pulmonary alveolar macrophages (PAM) were harvested after the animal had been exsanguinated by cardiac puncture under pentobarbital anesthesia. Benadryl was administered intraperitoneally 30 min before the lung lavage to prevent bronchospasm. Following death, the trachea was cannulated and the ventral half of the chest resected. A total lavage of 60 ml was performed by inflating the lung with 5 to 6 cm^3 aliquots of physiologic saline prewarmed to 37°C. The lavage effluent was collected in prechilled glass tubes and placed in an ice bath. The effluent was then centrifuged at 200 X g for 10 min. The cell pellet was washed three times and resuspended at a concentration of 2.0 to 2.5 X 10^6 cells/ml in MEM-FCS.

Peritoneal exudate macrophages (PEC) were harvested 72 hr after intraperitoneal injection of 30 ml of light paraffin oil. The animal was sacrificed by intracardiac air injection and the peritoneal cavity was lavaged with 100 ml of physiologic saline. The lavage effluent was centrifuged at 200 X g for 10 min. The cell pellet was washed three times and the red blood cells lysed by exposure to hypotonic saline for 5 min at 37°C. A 10% suspension (v/v) was then prepared using MEM-FCS.

Lymphokine Assays

Migration Inhibitory Factor (MIF)

Macrophage migration inhibition was measured by the technique of Rocklin, Meyers, and David (8). PEC in capillary tubes were placed in incubation chambers and cultured for 24 hr. The area of migration was traced using projection microscopy and measured planimetrically. The percent of inhibition was calculated in the following way:

$$\% \text{ migration inhibition} = 1 - \frac{\text{area of migration in levamisole supernatant}}{\text{area of migration in control supernatant}} \times 100$$

Macrophage Activating Factor (MAF)

Lymphokine-induced macrophage adherence was measured using a modification of the technique of Nathan, Karnovsky, and David (9). One milliliter of a PAM suspension (2.0 to 2.5 X 10^6 cells/ml) was plated in 10 X 35 mm plastic Petri dishes and incubated for 1 hr. The dishes were then vigorously rinsed in physiologic saline. Control supernatant or levamisole supernatant (1.5 ml) was then added to duplicate dishes. The macrophage monolayer cultures were incubated for 48 hr at 37°C in a 5% CO_2-air environment. The cultures were supplemented with 0.3 ml of MEM-FCS at 24 hr. At 48 hr, the culture dishes were rinsed vigorously in physiologic saline and dried. One milliliter of 1 N NaOH was then added to each dish overnight. A 0.2-ml aliquot of this solution was then assayed for protein content using the method of Lowry et al. (10). Baseline data were obtained by sacrificing monolayers at 1 hr and measuring the protein content as above. The percent adherence was calculated in the following way:

$$\% \text{ adherence} = \frac{\mu\text{g protein} - \text{levamisole supernatant dishes}}{\mu\text{g protein} - \text{baseline supernatant dishes}} \times 100$$

RESULTS

Lymphocyte Proliferation

In six experiments, levamisole had no direct mitogenic effect on human lymphocytes. In addition, levamisole, at a concentration (50 μg/ml) which had been demonstrated to augment Con A-induced lymphokine production, had no augmenting effect on lymphocyte proliferation over the entire dose-response range of Con A or PHA. Finally, in a concentration range from 0.5 to 60 μg/ml, levamisole had no effect on the proliferative response of lymphocytes stimulated with a peak stimulating concentration of Con A (10 μg/ml).

Lymphokine Production

In two experiments, no MIF or MAF activity could be detected in supernatants from lymphocyte cultures containing only levamisole. However, in each of five experiments in which levamisole was added to lymphocyte cultures containing a suboptimal stimulating concentration of Con A, MIF and MAF activity were increased in the supernatants from the cultures stimulated in the presence of levamisole. There was a progressive increase in MIF and

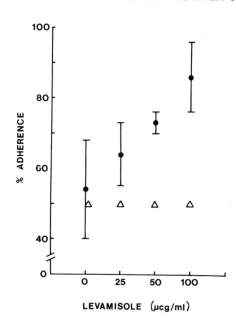

FIG. 1. The effect of increasing concentrations of levamisole on the production of macrophage activating factor in in vitro human lymphocyte cultures is plotted. The closed circle symbols represent the mean ± SD of 5 experiments in which Con A (10 µg/ml) was present in the cultures. The results of a single representative experiment in which no Con A was present in the cultures are depicted by the open triangles for comparative purposes.

MAF activity with increasing concentration of levamisole. Mean MAF activity as measured by macrophage adherence at 48 hr was increased in the levamisole supernatants by 17, 32, and 56% when compared to the control supernatant containing only Con A (Fig. 1). Mean MIF activity was 46, 64, and 80% greater in the three levamisole supernatants than that present in the supernatant from the cultures stimulated with Con A alone (Table 2).

TABLE 1. Effect of levamisole on MIF production

| | Percent migration inhibition of levamisole (µg/ml) | | |
	25	50	100
Supernatants with Con A			
1	2	36	53
2	75	90	100
3	42	67	86
4	69	90	100
5	15	15	59
Supernatants without Con A			
1	0	0	15
2	0	0	0

TABLE 2.   Effect of levamisole on MIF production by antigen-stimulated cells

Exp. no.	Percent migration inhibition
1	100
2	26
3	13
4	23

MIF activity was also increased in the supernatants from antigen-stimulated lymphocyte cultures containing levamisole (Table 2).

Preliminary studies were performed to rule out the possibility that these
results could be due to the effect of residual levamisole in the dialyzed supernatants. The stock solution of levamisole directly inhibited macrophage
migration and augmented lymphokine-induced macrophage adherence. Both
of these effects were lost after dialysis of the stock solution, suggesting that
the small-molecular-weight drug was entirely removed by dialysis or remained in such small concentrations that it could not be responsible for the
results of these experiments.

DISCUSSION

Elucidation of the mechanism by which levamisole stimulates the immune
response is not only of importance for understanding the nature of the immune
response, but also may have practical application in the management of a
variety of immunodeficient stages. Levamisole could stimulate the immune
response either by increasing the proliferative response of stimulated lymphocytes or by augmenting the production of lymphocyte mediators. Several
investigators have studied the effect of levamisole on the proliferative response
of stimulated human lymphocytes. Verhaegen et al. (3) and Glogau et al. (5)
were unable to demonstrate increased lymphocyte proliferation to either
mitogen or antigen stimulation after levamisole therapy. Although Lichtenfield et al. (6) reported an increase in the proliferative response to antigen,
mitogen, or allogenic cells when levamisole was added to lymphocyte cultures,
Copeland et al. (7) were unable to demonstrate such a response.

In this study, levamisole had no effect on the proliferative response of
human lymphocytes to either PHA or Con A using a wide range of concentrations of stimulating mitogens. In addition, over a wide range of concentrations, levamisole had no significant effect on the proliferative response of
lymphocytes stimulated by a peak concentration of Con A. Thus, this study
and the majority of previously published studies have failed to demonstrate
that levamisole affects the proliferative response of human lymphocytes
in vitro. These observations make it somewhat unlikely that levamisole

stimulates the immune response by increasing the proliferative response of human sensitized lymphocytes in vivo.

Our results demonstrate that levamisole augments mediator production of mitogen- and antigen-stimulated lymphocytes in vitro. A dose-dependent increase in MIF and MAF activity was present in the supernatants of mitogen-stimulated lymphocyte cultures containing levamisole. Since levamisole had no direct effect on lymphokine production, the increase in mediator production observed in the presence of mitogen or antigen would appear to be due to either an increase in the number of lymphocytes responding to the concentration of Con A or PPD used in these experiments or increased production of mediators per cell by the same population of responding cells. Our current data do not allow us to distinguish between these two alternatives.

The augmentation of mediator production by mitogen- and antigen-stimulated lymphocytes demonstrated in this study may well explain the increased delayed hypersensitivity reactions previously reported in patients treated with levamisole. Rocklin, Sheffer, and David (11) have reported that in vitro MIF production could be correlated with skin test reactivity in patients with sarcoidosis and Hodgkin's disease, whereas in vitro lymphocyte proliferative responses could not. Studies of the effect of levamisole on in vitro mediator production by lymphocytes obtained from anergic patients may help to substantiate the hypothesis that augmentation of defective mediator production is the mechanism by which levamisole stimulates the immune response in vivo.

SUMMARY

Levamisole has previously been demonstrated to increase delayed hypersensitivity reactions in anergic patients. In order to elucidate the mechanism by which levamisole stimulates the immune response in vivo, we have studied the in vitro effect of this substance on both human lymphocyte proliferation and lymphocyte mediator production. Our results indicate that in vitro levamisole augments the production of soluble mediators by mitogen stimulated lymphocytes, while having no effect on lymphocyte proliferation.

ACKNOWLEDGMENTS

Part of the data presented in this chapter has been accepted for publication in Cellular Immunology.

REFERENCES

1. Tripodi, D., Parks, L. C., and Brugmans, J. (1973): Drug-induced restoration of cutaneous delayed hypersensitivity in anergic patients with cancer. N. Engl. J. Med., 289:354-357.
2. Hirshaut, Y., Pinsky, C., and Marquardt, H. (1973): Effects of levamisole on delayed hypersensitivity reactions in cancer patients. Proc. Am. Assoc. Cancer Res., 14:109.

3. Verhaegen, H., DeCree, J., DeCock, W., and Verbruggen, F. (1973): Levamisole and the immune response. N. Engl. J. Med., 289:1148.

4. Churchill, W. H., and David, J. R. (1973): Levamisole and cell-mediated immunity. N. Engl. J. Med., 289:375-376.

5. Glogau, R., Spitler, L., O'Connor, R., Olson, J., Ostler, P., Silverman, S., and Smolin, G. (1975): Clinical and immunologic effects of levamisole. Clin. Res., 23:291A.

6. Lichtenfield, L. J., Desner, M., Mardiney, M. R., and Wiernik, P. H. (1974): Amplification of immunologically induced lymphocyte ^{3}H thymidine incorporation by levamisole. Fed. Proc., 33:790.

7. Copeland, D., Stewart, T., and Harris, J. (1974): Effect of levamisole on in vitro human lymphocyte transformation. Cancer Chemother. Rep., 58:167-170.

8. Rocklin, R. E., Meyers, O. L., and David, J. R. (1970): An in vitro assay for cellular hypersensitivity in man. J. Immunol., 104:95-102.

9. Nathan, C. F., Karnovsky, M. L., and David, J. R. (1971): Alterations of macrophage functions by mediators from lymphocytes. J. Exp. Med., 133:1356-1376.

10. Lowry, O. H., Rosebrough, N. J., Farr, A. L., and Randall, R. J. (1951): Protein measurement with the Folin-Phenol reagent. J. Biol. Chem., 193:265-275.

11. Rocklin, R. E., Sheffer, A., and David, J. R. (1972): Sarcoidosis: A clinical and in vitro immunologic study. In: Proceedings of the Sixth Leucocyte Culture Conference, edited by M. R. Schwarz, pp. 743-757. Academic Press, New York.

Control of Neoplasia by Modulation of the Immune System, edited by M. A. Chirigos. Raven Press, New York 1977.

EFFECT OF LEVAMISOLE ON THE CHEMOTAXIS OF NEUTROPHILS AND MONOCYTES

H. Lian Liauw and *Vera J. Stecher

Research Division, CIBA-GEIGY Corp., Ardsley, New York 10502

INTRODUCTION

Levamisole, an immunopotentiator, has been reported to have a wide range of stimulatory effects on several cell types in various species (1-4). It was, therefore, of interest to determine the influence of levamisole on the chemotactic response of both neutrophils and macrophages. Since the directional migration of leukocytes is a component of cell reactivity, the sensitization of cells with Bacillus Calmette Guerin (BCG) prior to stimulation with the drug was also investigated.

MATERIALS AND METHODS

A description of the methodology used in the Boyden chamber assay procedure has been published (5), as well as details of a recent miniaturization and modification developed by Jungi (6).

Cellulose nitrate 3-μm micropore filters were used in the neutrophil studies and 8-μm pore size filters were employed in the study of macrophage migration. In both cases the membrane filters were purchased from Sartorius Division, Brinkman Instruments, Inc.

Rat peritoneal exudates were induced with sterile 7% sodium caseinate and neutrophils were harvested 16 hr later. Rat macrophages were obtained from peritoneal exudates 96 hr after the injection of 2% rice starch.

---

*Adjunct Associate Professor, New York Medical College Department of Pathology, Valhalla, New York.

Human neutrophils were obtained by the method of Hulliger and Blazkovec (7) using density-gradient sedimentation of peripheral blood from healthy male donors. Cells were suspended in Gey's solution containing 2% HSA at a concentration of 2×10^6 cells/ml. The upper compartment of the chemotaxis chamber was filled with 1×10^6 cells. In the experiments where levamisole was used, equal volumes of cell suspension (4×10^6 cells/ml) and a sterile solution of the drug were mixed prior to distribution of 0.5 ml (1×10^6 cells) in the upper compartment of the test chamber. A standard chemotactic agent, E. coli lipopolysaccharide-activated rat serum (8), was used throughout these studies. The assay was carried out at pH 7.1 using sterile technique, and each sample was run in triplicate.

After 3 and 5 hr of incubation at $37°C$ in the case of neutrophils and macrophages, respectively, the filters were removed, fixed, and stained with Weigert iron hematoxylin. Four fields of the lowermost surface of the filter membrane were counted microscopically. The mean count of four fields (320X) on each of three individual filters was used as the index of chemotactic activity.

Sensitization was achieved by injecting 0.1 ml of BCG vaccine (Glaxo Labs., Ltd.) intradermally at the nuchal region of rats. These animals showed a positive tuberculin reaction when skin tested with 10 μg of PPD 11 days later. Induced peritoneal neutrophils and macrophages were therefore harvested 11 days after the initial BCG immunization and assayed for chemotactic activity.

Levamisole HCl was kindly supplied by American Cyanamid Company, Princeton, New Jersey.

RESULTS

The effect of levamisole on normal human peripheral blood neutrophils was tested in vitro by incubating the cells with the drug at different concentrations. The results, illustrated in Fig. 1, demonstrate that levamisole at concentrations ranging from 10^{-7} M to 10^{-3} M has an inhibitory effect on the migration of normal human neutrophils. A maximum effect of approximately 50% inhibition of the chemotactic response was observed from 10^{-4} M to 10^{-6} M levamisole.

In a repeat of earlier studies (9) it was confirmed that there is essentially no difference in the chemotactic activity of peritoneal neutrophils and macrophages from BCG-immunized and nonimmunized rats (Table 1). Using this baseline data, it was of interest to investigate the effect of levamisole on leukocyte chemotaxis, and to determine if the drug differentially influences cells obtained from normal and BCG-immunized animals.

Table 2 illustrates that the chemotactic activity of peritoneal neutrophils from sensitized as well as normal rats is markedly inhibited by levamisole at 10^{-3} M and 10^{-5} M. Indeed, at 10^{-5} M, levamisole was responsible for a 90% inhibition of migration of normal neutrophils. At this concentration, neutrophils from BCG-immunized animals were less sensitive to levamisole, showing a 39% inhibition of chemotaxis when compared with controls. Trypan

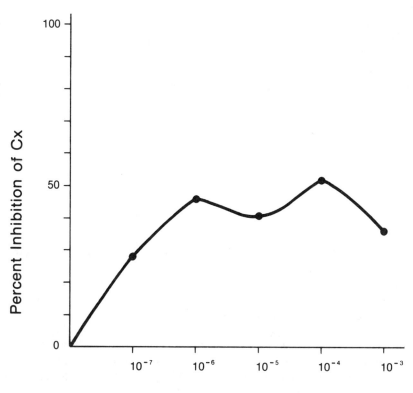

Levamisole Conc. (Mole)

FIG. 1. Effect of levamisole on chemotactic response (Cx) of normal human peripheral blood PMN leukocytes. The percent inhibition of chemotaxis was calculated on the basis of mean cell counts according to the following formula:

$$\frac{\text{Mean Cx activity of cells with levamisole} - \text{mean Cx activity of untreated cells}}{\text{mean Cx activity of untreated cells}}$$

Levamisole was diluted in Gey's balanced salt solution, adjusted to pH 7.1, and sterile-filtered prior to testing.

TABLE 1. Chemotactic activity of peritoneal neutrophils and macrophages from BCG-immunized and nonimmunized rats

| Cell type | Chemotactic activity (cells/field) | | Percent change |
| | Immunization | | |
	BCG	None	
PMN	281	324	−13
Macrophages	129	131	0

TABLE 2. Effect of levamisole on chemotactic response of BCG-sensitized
and normal rat peritoneal neutrophils

Levamisole (final conc.)	Percent inhibition of cell migration	
	BCG-sensitized	Nonsensitized control
1×10^{-3} M	-83	-83
1×10^{-5} M	-39	-90

blue studies performed on cells following a 3-hr incubation at 37° C with the drug indicated that levamisole did not influence leukocyte viability.

Finally, the effect of levamisole on the chemotactic response of peritoneal macrophages from BCG-immunized and nonimmunized rats was studied. At concentrations of 10^{-3} M and 10^{-4} M, levamisole produced a striking enhancement in the chemotactic response of macrophages from BCG-sensitized animals (Table 3). Although the effect of the drug on macrophages from nonimmunized animals was minimal, it was in clear contrast to the strong inhibitory effect found in the case of neutrophils. As was the case for neutrophils, a trypan blue assay indicated that levamisole was not influencing viability of the macrophages.

TABLE 3. Effect of levamisole on chemotactic response of rat
peritoneal macrophages

Levamisole (final conc.)	Percent change [a]	
	BCG-sensitized	Nonsensitized
1×10^{-3} M	+60	+15
1×10^{-4} M	+65	n.d.
1×10^{-5} M	+12	+23

[a] Percent change was expressed as (Mean Cx activity of cells with levamisole - mean Cx activity of untreated cells) ÷ mean Cx activity of untreated cells.

DISCUSSION

It is well established that the delayed hypersensitivity component of immunity is mediated predominantly by macrophages, and that BCG is responsible for an activating effect on macrophages (4). Furthermore, in its role as an immune-stimulating drug, levamisole has been shown to enhance the delayed hypersensitivity reaction (10). It is therefore not surprising that the BCG-activated macrophages treated with levamisole in our study were considerably more responsive to a chemotactic agent than were normal macrophages treated with the drug.

No difference was found between the chemotactic activity of peritoneal neutrophils and macrophages from BCG-immunized and nonimmunized rats. However, levamisole treatment of leukocytes in vitro distinguishes between macrophages from BCG-sensitized rats and those of normal animals. The enhancing effect of the drug on the chemotaxis of activated macrophages represents yet another change in the sensitivity of this cell after it has been stimulated with BCG.

As might be expected, BCG sensitization of the donor animal did not influence the chemotactic response of their neutrophils following in vitro treatment with levamisole. However, the strong inhibitory effect of levamisole on rat neutrophil migration was not anticipated and remains unexplained. Normal human peripheral blood neutrophil chemotaxis was likewise inhibited by levamisole over a broad concentration range. The bell-shaped pattern (Fig. 1) which emerges when inhibition of cell migration is plotted against concentration of the drug is typical of that found in previous chemotaxis studies (11).

In view of the potential extensive use of levamisole as an immunopotentiator, it is of importance to confirm the strong in vitro inhibitory effect of the drug on neutrophil chemotaxis by the use of in vivo models (12, 13).

SUMMARY

Levamisole was shown to be active in modulating the in vitro chemotactic activity of human peripheral blood neutrophils as well as rat peritoneal neutrophils and macrophages. At concentrations of 10^{-4} M to 10^{-6} M it was responsible for an approximately 50% inhibition of the chemotactic response of neutrophils from normal human peripheral blood. Levamisole enhanced the migration of macrophages from BCG-sensitized rats and inhibited migration of neutrophils from both normal and BCG-immunized animals.

REFERENCES

1. Hadden, J. W., Coffey, R. G., Hadden, E. M., Lopez-Corrales, E., and Sunshine, G. H. (1975): Effects of levamisole and imidazole on lymphocyte proliferation and cyclic nucleotide levels. Cell. Immunol., 20:98-103.

2. Renoux, G., and Renoux, M. (1972): Antigenic competition and non-specific immunity after a rickettsial infection in mice: Restoration of antibacterial immunity by phenyl-imidothiazole treatment. J. Immunol., 109:761-765.
3. Mitchell, M. S., Kirkpatrick, D., Mokyr, M. B., and Gery, I. (1973): On the mode of action of BCG. Nature (New Biol.), 243:216-217.
4. North, R. J. (1969): Cellular kinetics associated with the development of acquired cellular resistance. J. Exp. Med., 130:299-311.
5. Stecher, V. J. (1975): The chemotaxis of selected cell types to connective tissue degradation products. Ann. N. Y. Acad. Sci., 256:177-189.
6. Jungi, T. W. (1975): Assay of chemotaxis by a reversible Boyden chamber eliminating cell detachment. Int. Arch. Allergy Appl. Immunol., 48:341-352.
7. Hulliger, L., and Blazkovec, A. A. (1967): A simple and efficient method of separating peripheral-blood leucocytes for in vitro studies. Lancet, I:1304-1305.
8. Meltzer, M. S., Jones, E. E., and Boetcher, D. A. (1975): Increased chemotactic responses of macrophages from BCG-infected mice. Cell. Immunol., 17:268-276.
9. Perper, R. J., Oronsky, A. L., Stecher, V. J., and Sanda, M. (1976): The effect of BCG on extravascular mononuclear cell accumulation in vivo. (Submitted for publication.)
10. Tripodi, D., Parks, L. C., and Brugmans, J. (1973): Drug-induced restoration of cutaneous delayed hypersensitivity in anergic patients with cancer. N. Engl. J. Med., 289:354-357.
11. Stecher, V. J., and Sorkin, E. (1974): The chemotactic activity of leukocytes related to blood coagulation and fibrinolysis. In: Antibiotics and Chemotherapy, Vol. 19, edited by E. Sorkin, pp. 362-368. S. Karger, Basel.
12. Perper, R. J., Sanda, M., Stecher, V. J., and Oronsky, A. L. (1975): Physiologic and pharmacologic alterations of rat leukocyte chemotaxis (Cx) in vivo. Ann. N. Y. Acad. Sci., 256:190-209.
13. Wiener, S. L., Wiener, R., Urivetzky, M., Shafer, S., Isenberg, H. D., Janov, C., and Meilman, E. (1975): The mechanism of action of a single dose of methylprednisolone on acute inflammation in vivo. J. Clin. Invest., 56:679-689.

Control of Neoplasia by Modulation of the Immune System, edited by M. A. Chirigos. Raven Press, New York 1977.

LEVAMISOLE: ACTION ON PHAGOCYTOSIS AND COMPARTMENTAL DISTRIBUTION

*Américo J. Olivari, **Rosa M. Bergoc, *Oscar Burrone, **Ricardo A. Caro, *Julio N. Feierstein, *Horacio M. Glait, **Jorge E. Ihlo, *Oscar A. Varela, and *Alejandro F. Rojas

*Centro Oncológico de Medicina Nuclear, Facultad de Medicina, Universidad de Buenos Aires, Comisión Nacional de Energía Atómica, Buenos Aires, Argentina, and **Cátedra de Física, Facultad de Farmacia y Bioquímica, Universidad de Buenos Aires, Buenos Aires, Argentina

INTRODUCTION

The antihelminthic agent levamisole [L-(-)-2,3,5,6-tetrahydro-6-phenyl-imidazo-(2,1b)-thiazole hydrochloride] has variable effects on the immune system, such as the restoration of the delayed cutaneous hypersensitivity of anergic patients with cancer (1), the increase of the remission of murine leukemia induced by chemotherapy (2), the production of immunostimulation against the infection of Brucella Abortus in mice (3), as well as the increase of the clearance of carbon particles from the bloodstream, under certain conditions (4). Since the drug is actually utilized in the treatment of cancer as an immunostimulant (5), it is important to establish its mechanism of action.

Considering that phagocytosis is a fundamental phenomenon in the immunological process, either through a direct phagocytic activity or as an antigen-processing mechanism, we studied the immediate effect of the drug on the phagocytosis of radiogold particles.

With the same purpose, we also studied the compartmental distribution of the drug labeled with ^{35}S in rabbits.

MATERIALS AND METHODS

Studies on Phagocytosis

Fifty-four Wistar rats, weighing between 250 and 350 g, sterile apyreto-genic [198]Au colloids, with mean particle size ranging between 2.0 and 3.5 nm, stabilized with gelatin of isoelectric point 4.7, ionic gold content smaller than 1% and pH between 5 and 6 were utilized.

The mean particle size as well as the gold concentration were determined by spectrophotometric methods.

The animals were anesthetized with an intraperitoneal dose of 1 g/kg of body weight of urethane. After adequate dissection, the technique proposed by Cohen et al. (6) was utilized in order to obtain an efficient extracorporeal blood circulation. Each animal received, through a plastic canula inserted into the jugular vein, between 1.9 and 3.1 X 10^{16} particles of [198]Au colloid per kg of body weight, which was calculated according to previously described methods (7). The radioactivity remaining in the bloodstream was measured continuously by means of a well counter and plotted synchronically by a rate-meter and paper recorder.

The levamisole, in 0.1 ml of aqueous solution, was administered through the jugular vein immediately before the [198]Au colloid, at a dose of 2 mg/kg of body weight to 20 animals and at a dose of 20 mg/kg of body weight to 15 animals; 11 animals were utilized as controls. In 2 additional experiments, 20 mg/kg of body weight of levamisole were injected 30 min before the [198]Au colloid; in 6 other experiments, three with 2 and three with 20 mg/kg of body weight, the levamisole was administered 10 min after the injection of the radiogold colloid.

Studies with ^{35}S-Levamisole

The preparation of labeled levamisole with sulfur-35 (^{35}S) was obtained by the sequence of reactions shown in Fig. 1.

The radioatom was introduced by reaction of ^{35}S-thiourea (Amershan-Searle, 16.8 μCi/mM) and tetramisole was obtained. ^{35}S-levamisole was extracted by successive passages through aqueous and toluenic phases at different pH's. The specific activity obtained was 0.109 mCi/mM; it was tried in four different chromatographic systems and shown to be 99.0% pure.

Two rabbits were given an intracardiac injection of 25 mg of ^{35}S-levamisole (8.33 mg/kg) with a radioactive dose of 9.5 μCi/animal. Blood samples were obtained, using the same procedure after 5, 10, 20, 30, 45, 60, 90, and 120 min of the injection. The blood samples were centrifuged and 200-μl plasma aliquots were measured in a liquid scintillation spectrometer; chemical and color quenching corrections were made by standard external method ([133]Ba). Chromatographies were made on TLC plaque (aluminum sheets, silica gel-coated 60 F, 254-layer thickness-25-Merck) in a system with ethylic ether, methanol, ammonia (190:10:5) v/v, to discard the metabolites present in the plasma samples. In this system the levamisole

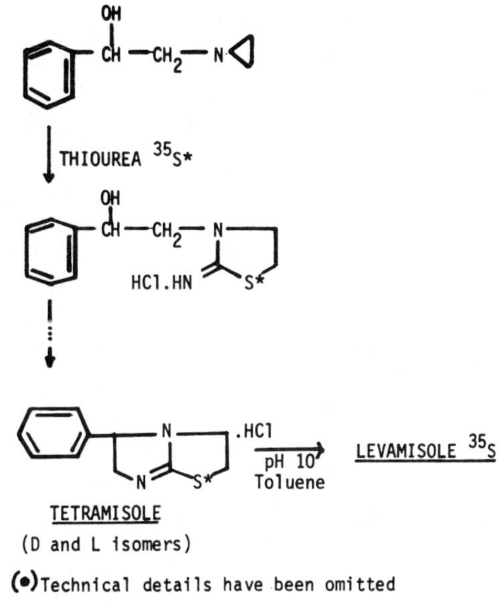

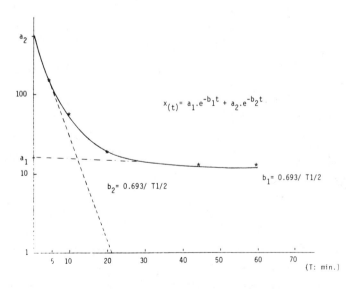

FIG. 1. General procedure for labeling levamisole-[35]S.

$$x_{(t)} = a_1 \cdot e^{-b_1 t} + a_2 \cdot e^{-b_2 t}$$

$b_2 = 0.693/ T1/2$

$b_1 = 0.693/ T1/2$

FIG. 2. Curve of plasma radioactivity vs. time, for levamisole-[35]S.

has an Rf of 0.826 at 20°C. This permitted the establishment of the percentage of pure levamisole from the total radioactivity in each plasma sample.

Analysis of data: A curve of plasma radioactivity against time was obtained (Fig. 2). These data were analyzed in terms of two exponential components:

$$X_{(t)} = a_1 \cdot e^{-b_1 \cdot t} + a_2 \cdot e^{-b_2 \cdot t}$$

where $X_{(t)}$ = concentration of radioactivity in plasma at time t.

That conforms a mammilary system of two compartments, using the method described by Matthews (8) and Rescigno (9).

The distribution volumes of the two compartments, N_1 and N_2, can be given by

$$N_1 = \frac{X}{a_1 + a_2}$$

$$N_2 = N_1 \frac{a_1 \cdot a_2 (b_2 - b_1)^2}{(a_1 \cdot b_2 + a_2 \cdot b_1)^2}$$

where X = total radioactivity injected.

The turnover rate F is given by

$$F = N \cdot R$$

$$F = R \cdot N_1$$

$$R = \frac{b_1 \cdot b_2}{a_1 \cdot b_2 + a_2 \cdot b_1}$$

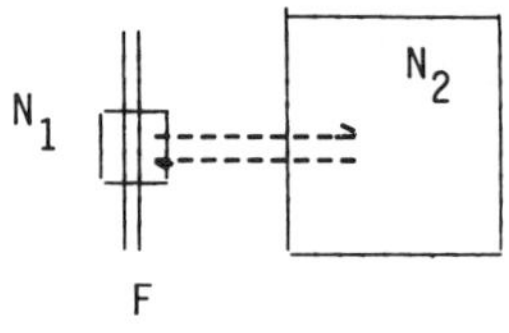

$$N_1 = \frac{X}{a_1 + a_2}$$

$$N_2 = N_1 \frac{a_1 \cdot a_2 (b_2 - b_1)^2}{(a_1 \cdot b_2 + a_2 \cdot b_1)^2}$$

N_1 = 4.26 % Body Weight

N_2 = 74.98 % Body Weight

F = 11.16 ml/min.

FIG. 3. Analysis of the distribution compartments of levamisole-^{35}S in rabbits.

where N is the total volume of the system and R (fractional turnover rate) is

$$R = \frac{b_1 \cdot b_2}{a_1 b_2 + a_2 b_1}$$

Using the values of a_1 and a_2 (intercept values at 0 time of each exponential) and b_1 and b_2 (exponential constant of each exponential function) determined from the plasma radioactivity data (Fig. 3), the magnitudes of the constants of the compartmental model may be calculated.

RESULTS

Phagocytosis

Figure 4 shows an actual control curve, where the exponential decrease of the blood radioactivity can be clearly observed; the rate of phagocytosis is equal to 4.32×10^{14} particles/kg of body weight/min.

Figure 5 shows the curves obtained with 2 and 20 mg of levamisole/kg of body weight as compared to a control experiment; the rates of phagocytosis are 1.53×10^{14} and 4.72×10^{12} particles/kg of body weight/min, respectively.

With the purpose of analyzing if the phenomenon found with levamisole can be somehow assimilated to the reticuloendothelial "blockade" process, provoked by the injection of a large excess of gelatin molecules, levamisole

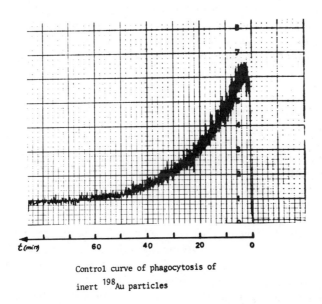

Control curve of phagocytosis of
inert ^{198}Au particles

FIG. 4. Actual control curve of blood radioactivity vs. time, for ^{198}Au.

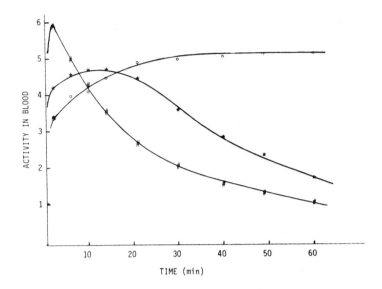

FIG. 5.   Comparison of blood radioactivity vs. time curves under two different levamisole dosage. #, control; *, levamisole 2 mg/kg; O, levamisole
20 mg/kg.

(20 mg/kg) was injected 30 min before radiogold; no difference was observed
between the control and levamisole curves.

In six experiments, the drug was injected 10 min after the administration
of the radiogold (three with 2 mg/kg and three with 20 mg/kg).   Figure 6
shows the curves obtained; the first parts of them are similar to the control,
but immediately after the levamisole injection, the slope is strongly modified,
and this modification is related to the dose of levamisole injected.

Compartmental Distribution of ^{35}S-Levamisole

The mathematical analysis of the curve of plasma radioactivity versus
time (see Methods) permitted us to obtain a biexponential curve that determines a mammillary system of two compartments (Figs. 2 and 3).   The first
compartment comprises 4.26% of the body weight, and is very similar to the
plasma volume; and the second is 74.98% of the body weight, that is, higher
than the total body water compartment.

The rates of interchanges between them is the other important constant
that characterizes the system.   Compartment 1, the central compartment,
has an exchange rate with compartment 2 (the peripheral compartment) that
comprises the 19.8% of its volume per minute.   Compartment 2 exchanges
0.989% of its volume per minute with compartment 1.   The turnover rate of
the total system is 11.16 ml/min.

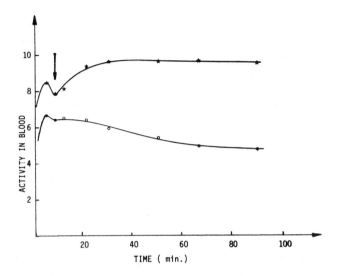

FIG. 6. Levamisole action when injected 10 min after ^{198}Au colloid. Arrow indicates i.v. administration of levamisole. O, 2 mg/kg; *, 20 mg/kg.

DISCUSSION

Phagocytosis

The described results show an effective and immediate action of levamisole on the phagocytosis of gelatin-protected radiogold colloids by the reticuloendo-thelial system, demonstrating a strong decrease of the rate of phagocytosis. The injection of levamisole immediately before the administration of the radiocolloid demonstrates a clear diminution of the rate of phagocytosis, which is proportional to the dose of the drug.

A very significant change in the disappearance of the ^{198}Au colloids from the bloodstream could be observed when levamisole was injected 10 min after the radiocolloid particles, with an increase of the blood radioactivity. This can be interpreted as a decrease of the adsorption of the particles on the reticuloendothelial cell's surface and even as a desorption of radiocolloidal particles into the bloodstream.

It was important to exclude the possibility of a mechanical resemblance between the phenomenon of the immediate decrease of the rate of phagocytosis induced by levamisole and the competitive inhibition produced by gelatin in the reticuloendothelial "blockade" (10). This is why we studied this problem by injecting the drug 30 min before the colloid's administration. Since the obtained curves showed no significant difference from the control patterns, this possibility can clearly be discarded.

Hoebeke and Franchi (4) studied the action of levamisole on the blood clearance of carbon particles in mice. They found an increase of the phago-cytic capacity 24 hr after the administration of the drug. These data do not contradict our results, owing to the different times utilized in their work, but they are consistent with other experiments on culture of lymphocytes with phytohemagglutinins (PHA), where an inhibition or a stimulation of growth was found according to the action time of the drug (11, 12).

It is quite certain that the described immediate action of levamisole should be attributed to an interaction of the drug with the active adsorption sites at the cell surface, because if the drug is injected immediately before the colloid, the binding of the radioactive particles to the reticuloendothelial system (RES) cells is strongly hindered; and if the drug is administered 10 min after the colloid, a desorption of the particles can be observed.

The analysis of the curves was based on the kinetic model of phagocytosis proposed by Caro et al. (13). According to this, which agrees with the previous supposition, levamisole influences the entrance of the particle into the cell's interior, and this action could be made through modifications on the levels of cyclic nucleotides (cyclic AMP or cyclic GMP) (14-16), or through divalent cations (16, 17) as demonstrated in other systems. Further studies will be undertaken in order to investigate these possibilities.

Compartmental Distribution of ^{35}S-Levamisole

The compartmental distribution of ^{35}S-levamisole, by the mathematical method applied, shows two compartments, one central whose size is similar to the plasmatic compartment comprising 4.26% of the body weight, that exchange very rapidly with the peripheral compartment that comprises 74.98% of the body weight of the animals studied.

The rate of exchange between the compartments points out the rapidity by which levamisole leaves the central compartment, and is in agreement with previous suppositions because of its low molecular weight; 19.8% of the volume of compartment 1 exchanges with compartment 2 per minute; and 0.989% of the volume of compartment 2 exchanges with compartment 1 per minute.

The second or peripheral compartment is larger than the water compartment; this could be related to the observation described by Boyd et al. that levamisole was found bound to cellular proteins (18). It is important to note that the peripheral compartment really could include a third compartment, but only with computer analysis could this be determined.

The turnover rate of the system, 11.16 ml/min, emphasizes the velocity of elimination of the drug in the animals studied, and this is in accord with Boyd et al. (18), who showed that 90% of levamisole is eliminated in less than 24 hr.

In conclusion: Levamisole decreases the velocity of phagocytosis in spite of a positive immunomodulatory effect seen clinically in cancer patients. In the experimental animal models we have studied, the rapid onset of action is consistent with the compartmental distribution found for levamisole. The relevance of these findings in our model to the clinical situation in man remains to be determined.

SUMMARY

The immediate action of Levamisole [L-(-)-2,3,5,6-tetrahydro-6-phenyl-imidazo-(2,1b)-thiazole hydrochloride] on the phagocytosis of [198]Au colloidal particles and its compartmental distribution has been analyzed with the purpose of establishing the mechanism of action of the drug.

An immediate and strong decrease of the rate of phagocytosis was observed, which was dose-dependent, and its action was on the mechanism of entrance of the particle into the reticuloendothelial cell's interior.

The compartmental distribution of labeled levamisole shows two compartments, one central and the other peripheral, with very rapid elimination of the drug.

ACKNOWLEDGMENTS

We gratefully acknowledge the skillful technical assistance of Mrs. Raquel Baldrich and Ms. Magdalena Racedo.

REFERENCES

1. Tripodi, D., Parks, L. C., and Brugmans, J. (1973): Drug-induced restoration of cutaneous delayed hypersensitivity in anergic patients with cancer. N. Engl. J. Med., 289:354-357.
2. Chirigos, M. A., Pearson, J. W., and Pryor, J. (1973): Augmentation of chemotherapeutically induced remission of a murine leukemia by a chemical immuno-adjuvant. Cancer Res., 33:2615-2618.
3. Renoux, G., and Renoux, M. (1971): Effet immunostimulant d'un imidothiazole dans l'immunisation des souris contre l'infection par Brucella Abortus. C. R. Acad. Sci., 272D:349-350.
4. Hoebeke, J., and Franchi, G. (1973): Influence of tetramisole and its optical isomers on the mononuclear phagocytic system. Effect on carbon clearance in mice. J. Reticuloendothel. Soc., 14:317-323.
5. Rojas, A. F., Mickiewicz, E., Feierstein, J. N., Glait, H., and Olivari, A. J. (1976): Levamisole in advanced human breast cancer. Lancet, 1:211-215.
6. Cohen, Y., Cousterousse, O., and Chivot, J. J. (1964): Pharmacodynamie des colloides radioactifs. Min. Nucl., 8:357-366.
7. Bergoc, R. M., Caro, R. A., Ciscato, V. A., and Radicella, R. (1969): Cinética de la desaparición del caudal sanguíneo de coloides de oro radioactivo protegidos con polivinilpirrolidona (PVP). Rev. Biol. Med. Nucl., 1:9-14.
8. Matthews, C. M. (1957): Phys. Med. Biol., 2:36-49.
9. Rescigno, A. (1956): Biochim. Biophys. Acta, 21:111-122.
10. Bergoc, R. M., and Caro, R. A. (1975): The competitive nature of reticuloendothelial "blockade." Int. J. Nucl. Biol. Med., 2:33-36.

11. Hadden, J. W., Coffey, R. G., Hadden, E. M., Lopez-Corrales, E., and Sunshine, G. H. (1975): Effects of levamisole and imidazole on lymphocyte proliferation and cyclic nucleotide levels. Cell. Immunol., 20:98-103.

12. Copeland, D., Stewart, T., and Harris, J. (1974): Effect of levamisole (NSC-177023) on in vitro human lymphocyte transformation. J. Cancer Chem. Rep., 58(Part I):167-170.

13. Caro, R. A., Ciscat, V. A., and Radicella, R. (1970): A theoretical analysis of the kinetic of the phagocytosis of radiogold in the rat. J. Appl. Radiat. Isotopes, 21:405-411.

14. Bourne, H. R., Lehrer, R. I., Cline, M. J., and Melmon, K. L. (1971): Cyclic 3'-5' adenosine monophosphate in the human leukocyte: Synthesis, degradation and effects on neutrophil candidacidal activity. J. Clin. Invest., 50:920.

15. Cox, J. P., and Karnovsky, M. L. (1973): The depression of phagocytosis by exogenous cyclic nucleotides, prostaglandins and theophylline. J. Cell Biol., 59:480-490.

16. Stossel, T. P., Mason, R. J., Hatwig, J., and Vaughan, M. (1972): Quantitative studies of phagocytosis by polymorphonuclear leukocytes: Use of emulsions to measure the initial rate of phagocytosis. J. Clin. Invest., 51: 615-624.

17. Janssen Pharmaceutica (1970): Basic Medical Information on Levamisole. II, January 1970.

18. Boyd, J. E., Bullock, M. W., Champagne, D. A., Gatterdam, P. E., Morici, I. J., Plaisted, P. H., Spicer, L. D., Wayne, R. S., and Zulalian, J. (1968): Metabolism of L-tetramisole in rats. American Cyanamid Co. May 1968.

Control of Neoplasia by Modulation of the Immune System, edited by M. A. Chirigos. Raven Press, New York 1977.

ROLES OF THE IMIDAZOLE OR THIOL MOIETY ON THE IMMUNO-STIMULANT ACTION OF LEVAMISOLE

*Gerard Renoux and Micheline Renoux

Laboratoire d'Immunologie, Faculté de Médecine, 37032 Tours, Cedex, France

INTRODUCTION

The immunostimulatory activity of levamisole has been well documented from a series of experimental or clinical studies since its first demonstration (1). However, negative or questionable findings have also been reported.

On the other hand, most experimental findings suggest that at least two different mechanisms of action are involved in the capacity of levamisole to modify the immune response. For example, a dose of 5 mg/kg of levamisole given 18 hr before, simultaneously to, or 6 hr after immunization of mice with sheep red blood cells (SRBC) induced a dispersing effect which inhibited one-third of the immune response, left unaffected the second third, and significantly increased the response in the last third of animals. This effect disappeared 24 hr after immunization in mice treated with levamisole, and was never found after the use of additional doses (2). Hadden et al. (3,4) demonstrated a biphasic effect of levamisole on phytohemagglutinin-induced proliferation of T-cell-enriched mouse spleen cells. We also evidenced the complex relationship of animal strain, age and sex, and dose or time of administration have in determining the effectiveness of levamisole on the immune response (5). Finally, it was found in current studies that the antigen employed played an important role in modulating the efficacy of levamisole. This role was independent of the magnitude of response induced by the antigen alone in normal untreated mice. For instance, levamisole-treated female C57BR/cd mice evidenced an enhanced antibody response to Brucella endotoxin, but no modification of their responsiveness to SRBC. In contrast,

---

*Associated Scientist, Memorial Sloan-Kettering Cancer Center, New York, New York 10021.

TABLE 1. Strain, sex, and antigen influences on IgG-antibody production
in 6- to 8-week-old mice treated with 25 mg/kg of levamisole

Strain and H-2	Males Modulation of		Females Responses to	
	SRBC	BRU	SRBC	BRU
A a	M+	H+	H0	H0
B6 b	L +	H0	L0	H0
C d	L ++++		M++	
D2 d	H ++	M-	M+	M0
BR k		M+	M0	M+
C3 k	M+++	N0	M+	L-

A: A/ORL; B6: C57BL/6; C: BALB/C; D2: DBA/2; BR: C57BR/cd; C3:
C3H/He. H, M, L, N = high, medium, low, or nonresponding mouse strain,
respectively. SRBC = 10^8 sheep red blood cells; BRU = 1 µg of the ABS
fraction of B. abortus. + to ++++ = 2- to 10-fold increase in responses, in
comparison with untreated control mice; 0 = not affected; - = inhibition of response by levamisole treatment.

levamisole increased the response of DBA/2 mice to SRBC and inhibited the
production of Brucella antibodies (Table 1).

Certainly, the effects of levamisole on cells of the immunological system
differ from that of adjuvants, or biological immunopotentiators. The role of
levamisole in modifying tumor growth could not be directly compared with the
effects of chemotherapeutic agents, supposedly active only on neoplastic
cells.

Progress in understanding the mode of action of levamisole and related
compounds would guide and improve its clinical and experimental use.

The apparent discrepancies might be a reflection of insufficient knowledge
on the mechanisms of action of that drug.

Since levamisole possesses a thiazole and an imidazole moiety, we decided to evaluate the respective role(s) of each part in triggering an increased
immune response. Tests were performed to determine a possible relationship between chemical structure and effectiveness on immunological events
(6, and current studies).

The bulk of results permits us to delineate in the main how this new group
of immunopotentiators may work. We summarize here the findings comparing the activities of imidazole (IMZ), levamisole (LMS), and sodium diethyldithiocarbamate (DTC). This latter compound was chosen from a series of
other thiol derivatives in order to exemplify the role of the sulfur moiety in

enhancing the immune response. We present data to indicate that the imidazole or the "thiol" moiety behave differently in the activation of immunocompetent cells in vitro or in vivo. The data presented point out the importance of hormonal mediation, evoked by the sulfur moiety, for T-cell recruitment and activation (5, 7).

MATERIALS AND METHODS

Mice

Female IOP (specific pathogen-free, IFFA-CREDO, Lyon, France) weighing 20 to 22 g were employed for studies of the modification of immune responsiveness under drug treatment. nu/nu mice (Centre de Sélection des Animaux de Laboratoire, CNRS, Orléans, France) were originated from a strain isolated at the Institute of Animal Genetics, Edinburg. Animals were kept in an air-conditioned room at 24° C, and fed antibiotic-free pellets and water ad libitum.

Reagents

Pyrogen-free sterile distilled water was employed to prepare all reagents that were injected with pyrogen-free sterile syringes to eliminate the well-known activation of antibody-forming cells by endotoxins from ubiquitous Gram-negative organisms.

Levamisole was a gift from Janssen Pharmaceutica; imidazole and sodium diethyldithiocarbamate were purchased from Sigma (St. Louis, Missouri, USA) and from Merck (Darmstadt, F.D.R.), respectively.

Detection of PFC

Direct (IgM) and indirect (IgG) spleen antibody-forming cells (PFC) were evidenced and counted according to techniques already described (2, 5). In vitro modification in the number of PFC that may be induced by incorporation of the drugs into the medium was tested by the technique summarized in Fig. 1.

Production and Assay of Serum-Enhancing Factor

Mice were treated with selected doses of the drugs, and bled 24 hr later. Blood was collected in pyrogen-free bottles and was allowed to clot for 1 to 2 hr at room temperature. Sera were harvested after centrifugation at 4° C and aliquoted in volumes adequate for administration to several mice and stored at -78° C. Samples were thawed just prior to use and were not refrozen. Limulus assays (Pyrotest, Difco) for endotoxin indicated that there was no measurable endotoxin present at the time of injection. Sera thus prepared were injected i.p. into groups of IOP mice at the time of

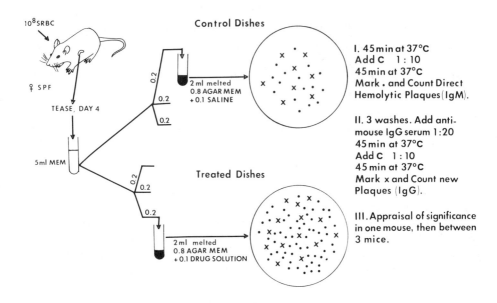

FIG. 1. A schematic diagram of experiments to evidence _in vitro_ effects of chemicals on antibody excretion by spleen cells.

immunization with 10^8 SRBC. Direct and indirect PFC were counted 48 hr after treatment of recipient mice and data recorded as mean PFC $\pm$ standard error (SE) viable nucleated cells. Adequate control groups were included.

Differentiation of T-Cells in _nude_ Mice

A second set of experiments used nu/nu mice of the Edinburg strain instead of the nu/nu mice bred on a BALB/c background (Memorial Sloan-Kettering Cancer Center, New York) previously employed. Healthy-looking nu/nu mice were injected intraperitoneally with the chosen drug at selected doses. Four days after treatment, cell suspensions were made separately from spleen and from pooled lymph nodes and tested for expression of TL and Thy antigens by the cytotoxicity assay using specific anti-TL (E/TL$^-$ A vs. ASL1) and anti-Thy 1.2 (θ/AKR^b vs. ASL1) sera kindly provided by E. A. Boyse (Memorial Sloan-Kettering Cancer Center).

RESULTS

Effects on Spleen PFC

The activities of DTC and LMS in inducing a modification of the number of antibody-forming cells were compared in mice immunized by intravenous injections of 10^8 SRBC. Both drugs were administed by the subcutaneous route, in doses that ranged from 0.6 to 25 mg/kg, at time intervals that varied from 18 hr before to 24 hr after injection of the antigen.

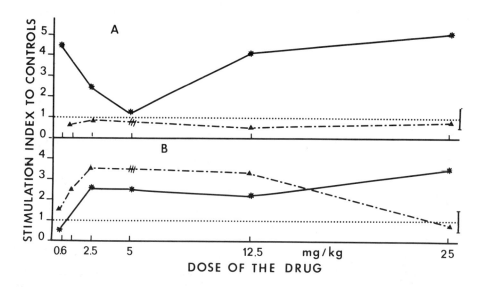

FIG. 2. Levamisole and diethyldithiocarbamate effects on mouse antibody-forming spleen cells. I. Treatments 18 hr before (A) or simultaneously (B) to immunization with 1 X 10^8 SRBC. $\triangle$——$\triangle$ levamisole; *——* sodium diethyldithiocarbamate.

$$\text{Stimulation index} = \frac{\text{PFC}/10^8 \text{ splenocytes in treated mice}}{\text{PFC}/10^8 \text{ splenocytes in controls}}$$

Simultaneously injecting SRBC and LMS, in the doses between 0.6 and 12.5 mg/kg, resulted in a higher increase of the number of PFC than after similar treatment with DTC. However, a 5-mg/kg dose of LMS evidenced a dispersing effect that has been previously described (2). In contrast, a 25-mg/kg dose of DTC induced a marked enhancement of the immune response, whereas LMS influence vanished at that dose (Fig. 2). Even more striking are the differences observed between the two drugs when they were administered at different time intervals in relation to the antigenic stimulus. In these situations, DTC demonstrated a potent stimulatory effect to increase the number of PFC, whereas LMS was inactive (Figs. 2,3).

The effect of IMZ in modifying spleen cell responsiveness was tested by administering the drug simultaneously with antigen (Tables 2,3). IMZ alone was unable to modify the magnitude of IgM or IgG spleen-cell responses to SRBC. A dose of 0.05 mg/kg (and of 1.25 mg/kg, not shown in the tables) would classify mice immunized with SRBC as nonresponders not affected by IMZ and as responders which evidenced a significant increase in the number of PFC when compared to untreated controls. The very similar finding observed in mice treated with a 25-mg/kg dose of LMS, could not be a haphazard coincidence, because LMS hydrochloride salt contains 27.8% imidazole (1.4 IMZ in 5 LMS).

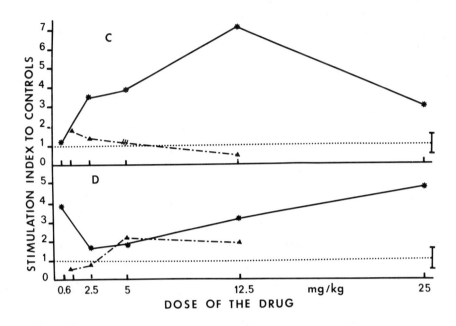

FIG. 3.   Levamisole and diethyldithiocarbamate effects on mouse antibody-forming spleen cells. II. Treatments 6 hr (C) or 24 hr (D) after immunization with 1 X 10[8] SRBC. For legend, see Fig. 2.

Synergy, inhibition, or addition between LMS or DTC and IMZ to modify immunologic reactivity were tested to verify earlier findings that theophylline inhibited LMS (8) and enhanced DTC-induced potentiation (6). Indeed, these data imply that these drugs may behave through different pathways, involving cyclic nucleotide activities, terminating in an increased antibody synthesis and excretion. In brief, one may show an additive effect on IgM-PFC production of the association of 25 mg/kg of DTC and 2.5 mg/kg of IMZ, whereas the same amounts of LMS and IMZ resulted in an inactive product (Table 2). Adjunction of IMZ inhibited the capacity of LMS to increase the number of specific IgG-PFC, whereas both doses of IMZ enhanced the effect of 25 mg/kg of DTC on IgG antibody-forming spleen cells (Table 3). These findings confirm that the mode of action of LMS, a cyclic sulfur-containing compound, is not identical to that of DTC, a noncyclic thio-derivative, although the end product, antibody production, might be obtained at similar levels.

In Vitro Modifications of the Number of PFC

Activities of the drugs were tested in vitro to show if an immediate dose effect might trigger changes in synthesizing and excreting specific antibodies by separated B lymphocytes, in an assay that reasonably excluded cooperation with other immunocompetent cells. Spleen lymphocytes obtained 4 days after mouse immunization with 10[8] SRBC were analyzed for their IgM and

TABLE 2. Effects of imidazole, levamisole, and sodium diethyldithiocarbamate on IgM plaque-forming spleen cells of mice immunized
with 1 X 10^8 SRBC

Treatment (mg/kg)	Imidazole		
	0	0.05	2.5
0	610 ± 68	1,164 ± 565 [a]	670 ± 118
LMS 2.5	2,440 ± 370	607 ± 87	550 ± 120
25	906 ± 120	1,678 ± 580 [a]	953 ± 225
DTC 2.5	1,480 ± 190	1,917 ± 160	2,150 ± 195
25	1,750 ± 84	2,515 ± 190	2,305 ± 200

LMS: levamisole; DTC: sodium diethyldithiocarbamate. Results expressed as PFC/10^8 nucleated spleen cells, 2 days after immunization and
treatment.

[a]Dispersing effect: administration of the drug classified mice as nonresponders, unaffected, or inhibited and as responder animals evidencing a
significant increase in the number of PFC.

TABLE 3. Effects of imidazole, levamisole, and sodium diethyldithiocarbamate on IgG plaque-forming spleen cells of mice immunized
with 1 X 10^8 SRBC

Treatment (mg/kg)	Imidazole		
	0	0.05	2.5
0	37 ± 8	42 ± 20	38 ± 11
LMS 2.5	178 ± 51	27 ± 3	24 ± 6
25	201 ± 97	65 ± 9	35 ± 1
DTC 2.5	112 ± 28	60 ± 1	74 ± 2
25	75 ± 10	147 ± 15	100 ± 12

See Table 2 for abbreviations.

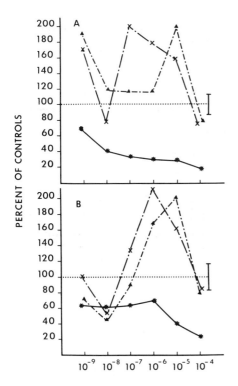

FIG. 4. Effects of levamisole, imidazole, and sodium diethyldithiocarbamate in modifying in vitro B-cell expression of IgG (A) or IgM (B) antibodies in splenocytes of mice 4 days after immunization with 1 X 10^8 SRBC. ▲——▲ levamisole; *——* sodium diethyldithiocarbamate; X——X imidazole.

IgG antibody responses in the presence of a range of LMS, DTC, or IMZ concentration added to the agar medium. Drug molarity was calculated for 1 X 10^6 lymphocytes/ml of medium. Figure 4 represents the mean of experiments conducted in triplicate for each drug concentration from spleen-cell suspensions of 10 mice. Both IgM and IgG antibody excretion was inhibited by all DTC concentrations. The effect of LMS on IgM-PFC parallels that of IMZ at all concentrations tested, with the peak stimulation at 10^{-6} M. In contrast, LMS gave rise to two peaks of stimulation in the number of IgG-PFC at 10^{-9} M and 10^{-5} M, whereas IMZ showed a complicated dose-response relationship with two peaks of stimulation at 10^{-9} M and 10^{-7} M to 10^{-5} M and inhibition at 10^{-8} M and 10^{-4} M. Present findings uncover as yet an undescribed aspect of sulfur derivatives on the cells of the immune system. LMS could directly stimulate B cells for an increased excretion of antibodies that depend on the activities of the imidazole moiety, and especially with regard to IgM antibody-producing cells. A compound devoid of imidazole ring, DTC, is inhibitory for B-cell antibody excretion under similar test conditions.

Production of Serum-Enhancing Factors

LMS was found to be capable of inducing in animals the production, or the increase, of serum factors which enhance the immune response of recipients

(5, 7). Similar experiments were conducted with the aim of delineating the respective role played by imidazole or sulfur in creating transferable enhancement of the immune response to SRBC.

In brief, IMZ was consistently unable to demonstrate any such activity in doses that ranged from 0.05 mg/kg to 25 mg/kg. In contrast, doses of 2.5 mg/kg or 25 mg/kg of DTC were potent inducers of serum-enhancing factors in mice. Indeed, 0.2 ml of serum from DTC-treated mice induced a threefold increase of the number of both IgM and IgG plaque-forming spleen cells when administered to normal mice immunized with SRBC.

Induction of In Vivo T-Cell Differentiation

A single treatment with 2.5 mg/kg or 25 mg/kg of LMS induced in nude mice the differentiation from prothymocyte to thymocyte (Thy-1 bearing cells) of spleen cells tested by the cytotoxic assay 4 days after treatment (5, and current studies). Similar assays have been repeated with DTC and IMZ. Four days after in vivo treatment with either LMS or DTC, spleens of nu/nu mice contained 15 to 38% of the TL^- $Thy-1^+$ phenotype, typical of later T-cell differentiation. IMZ was unable to promote in vivo prothymocyte differentiation under similar experimental conditions. In vitro induction assays according to the Komura and Boyse method (9) were consistently negative in doses of each of the drugs ranging from 10^{-6} M to 10^{-2} M.

In summary, neither LMS, DTC, or IMZ induced in vitro maturation steps in the T-cell development. However, LMS and DTC were able to trigger in vivo mechanisms that induced the acquisition of cytotopic T-cell surface markers in spleens of treated nu/nu mice. This capacity was not shared by IMZ.

DISCUSSION

Available data indicate that levamisole and imidazole have virtually identical in vitro effects on nonspecific cellular activities which intervene in triggering immune events. These effects were not shared by sodium diethyldithiocarbamate, a sulfur compound devoid of the imidazole nucleus. Furthermore, none of the three drugs induced in vitro differentiation from prothymocytes to thymocytes (Table 4).

The role of the imidazole moiety in inducing some of the activities of levamisole is still unclear. It increased in vitro PHA-induced DNA synthesis and cyclic GMP levels (3,4). However, the known in vivo activities of imidazole are disappointing and might partly account for questionable findings. A treatment with imidazole divided mice immunized with SRBC into nonresponders and responder animals. The dispersing effect on responses to SRBC was also observed after treatment with 5 mg/kg of levamisole (2). We evidenced that physiological parameters such as strain, sex, and age modulated the stimulatory effects of levamisole (5, and current studies). Time of administration of levamisole relative to antigen injection was also found to be important. For example, an 18-hr pretreatment or a 6-hr posttreatment

TABLE 4. A comparative summary: effects of levamisole, imidazole, and sodium diethyldithiocarbamate on in vivo or in vitro immune or related cellular events

Drug	In vivo				In vitro			
	PFC	DTH	ESF	Thy-1.2	DNA synthesis	Ig synthesis	cyclic GMP	KB test
LMS	+	+	+	+	+	+	+	0
IMZ	0	0	0	0	+	+	+	0
DTC	+	+	+	+	0	-	NT	0

PFC: Plaque-forming spleen cells to sheep red blood cells; DTH: delayed-type hypersensitivity to sheep red blood cells (10); ESF: production of serum-enhancing factors; Thy-1 induction: promotion of Thy-1.2 bearing cells in treated nu/nu mice. DNA synthesis and cyclic GMP levels for LMS and IMZ quoted from Hadden et al. (3, 4). Ig synthesis: in vitro effects of drugs added to the medium prior to adjunction of splenocytes in PFC assays for IgG or IgM antibody plaque-forming cells. KB test: the in vitro Komuro and Boyse (9) assay for thymocyte maturation from spleen cells of nu/nu mice.

in relation to the antigenic stimulus by SRBC inhibited the number of specific PFC in comparison to control mice (2, and present data). Repeated pre-treatments with levamisole induced in mice a tolerance-like effect to SRBC (2). These results are to be compared with the effects of levamisole on skin graft rejection, where similar findings were observed. Renoux et al. (10) obtained accelerated graft rejections in male to female C57BL/6 skin graft assays in 3 of 5 tests involving treatment with 20 to 25 mg/kg of levamisole at day 0, and in 2 of 4 tests in mice treated at day +7. Graft rejection time was not modified by pretreatment or by multiple doses of levamisole. It is tempting to correlate those observations with the inability of imidazole to increase the in vivo immune response.

On the other hand, the immunostimulatory activity of levamisole on tumor growth in rodents is, indeed, a variable one. A previous report (11) on the activity of levamisole in the treatment of Lewis lung carcinoma in syngeneic mice has never been confirmed. Johnson et al. (12) reported regression of Moloney sarcoma virus-induced tumors in mice treated with levamisole in 2 of 4 tests. These results could be explained in terms of (a) low antigenicity of syngeneic transplantable tumors and (b) influences of a series of variables, such as dose level, time of administration of levamisole relative to virus inoculation, immune status of the host, and strength of the virus challenge (12). Undoubtedly, each of these factors should play a role in modulating levamisole activities. The immune status of the host is, indeed, an import-ant parameter. In advanced cancer patients treated with levamisole, a pro-longed survival was associated with an increased T-cell response to phyto-hemagglutinin, regardless of the type of solid tumor, and levamisole was inactive below a certain level of responsiveness prior to treatment (10).

However, an important observation might give another point of considera-tion to account for published data on tumor experimentation. Kassel (personal communication) observed that under some dose conditions, levamisole ad-ministered to AKR mice induced regression of tumor size in many animals, whereas such doses of imidazole induced a tumor progression. It is tempting to hypothesize that a substance which can enhance the responses of lympho-cytes to proliferation-producing agents (e.g., PHA) may well enhance tumor proliferation in a sensitive tumor population, a parameter to be added to the other variables, as summarized above.

In contrast, levamisole and sodium diethyldithiocarbamate induce in vivo stimulation of immune events, including recruitment of T-cells from pre-committed cells, whereas imidazole will not enhance these responses (Table 4).

At this stage of information, in vivo enhancement of the immune response is linked to the availability of sulfur-containing compounds to produce serum factors which, in turn, recruit and activate immunocompetent cells for better responses to antigenic stimuli (5, 7, and current work). Since these factors are neither species-specific nor antigen-specific, and are produced by a variety of thiols and disulfides (but not in similar amounts), these find-ings are consistent with the interpretation that these agents produced, or liberated, a hormone-like product that combined with specific receptors in cell membranes of cells committed to thymocyte differentiation.

Present data confirm and extend the contention that levamisole acts through two different mechanisms. One type of action is associated with a direct effect of the imidazole moiety on lymphocytes, the second leads to an increased hormonal production to recruit more immunocompetent cells, particularly T-cells.

The activities of levamisole in modifying the immune response cannot be mistaken with those already described and so-called immunopotentiators. Levamisole, a synthetic low-molecular-weight pure crystalline white compound, is devoid of antigenicity and of the undesirable attributes of adjuvant containing live and potentially disease-causing organisms. In particular, levamisole does not induce spleno- or adeno-megalia. We are dealing here with a new class of drugs, that act by enhancing the number and the availability of immunocompetent cells, instead of modifying nonspecific immunity. It should be stressed that the effectiveness of these immunoinducers, and especially that of levamisole, could not be evaluated in terms of a linear dose effect, as their activities are modulated by parameters involving the physiologic and pathologic status of the host as well as the antigenicity and the invasive power of the parasite. Most of these parameters are still under evaluation. Progress in determining the molecular effects of levamisole and related compounds on cellular metabolism would help to unravel the complexities of immunological activation. They will, in turn, serve as a guide for clinical trials, including therapy of tumors in laboratory animals. These needs are emphasized by the encouraging results already observed in cancer patients and in patients affected with diseases where autoimmunity is involved.

SUMMARY

The biphasic effect of levamisole on immune responses suggests that two different mechanisms of action are involved. The activities of levamisole, of its imidazole moiety, and of sodium diethyldithiocarbamate (DTC), devoid of the imidazole nucleus, were compared in in vitro and in vivo tests, in an attempt to delineate these mechanisms.

In vitro, levamisole and imidazole shared virtually identical enhancing effects on DNA synthesis, cyclic GMP levels, or on antibody expression by separated B-cells. DTC was inactive in these assays. The three drugs were unable to promote in vitro induction of TL^+ or Thy^+ antigen-bearing cells.

On the contrary, levamisole or DTC treatment induced in vivo (a) maturation of thymocytes in nu/nu mice, (b) production of a transferable enhancing serum factor, (c) enhancement of delayed hypersensitivity, and (d) increase in the number of plaque-forming spleen cells. Imidazole was found to be inactive in these assays. However, a dispersing effect of imidazole, dividing mice into nonresponder and responder animals in the same group of treatment and immunization, may well account for nonstimulatory or inhibitory effects of levamisole observed in certain experimental situations.

Present findings favor the hypothesis that enhancing effects of thio-derivatives are due to the capacity of increasing or creating a hormonal stimulus acting on immunocompetent cells.

REFERENCES

1. Renoux, G., and Renoux, M. (1971): Effet immunostimulant d'un imidothiazole dans l'immunisation des souris contre l'infection par Brucella abortus. C. R. Acad. Sci., 272D:349-350.
2. Renoux, G., and Renoux, M. (1974): Modulation of immune reactivity by phenylimidothiazole salts in mice immunized by sheep red blood cells. J. Immunol., 113:779-790.
3. Hadden, J. W., Coffey, R. G., Hadden, E. M., Lopez-Corrales, E., and Sunshine, G. H. (1975): Effects of levamisole and imidazole on lymphocyte proliferation and cyclic nucleotide levels. Cell. Immunol. (in press).
4. Sunshine, G. H., Lopez-Corrales, E., Hadden, E. M., Coffey, R. G., Wanebo, H., and Hadden, J. W. (1976): Levamisole and imidazole: In vitro effects in mouse and man and their possible mediation by cyclic nucleotides. In: Modulation of Host Immune Resistance in the Prevention and Treatment of Induced Neoplasias, edited by M. A. Chirigos. Fogarthy International Center Proceedings, No. 28, U. S. Government Printing Office, Washington, D. C. (in press).
5. Renoux, G., Kassel, R. L., Renoux, M., Fiore, N. C., and Guillaumin, J. M. (1976): Immunomodulation by levamisole in normal and leukemic mice. Evidence for a serum transfer. In: Modulation of Host Immune Resistance in the Prevention and Treatment of Induced Neoplasias, edited by M. A. Chirigos. Fogarthy International Center Proceedings, No. 28, U. S. Government Printing Office, Washington, D. C. (in press).
6. Renoux, G., and Renoux, M. (1974): Immunopotentiation par les thiols et disulfures. C. R. Acad. Sci., 278D:1139-1141.
7. Renoux, G., Renoux, M., Guillaumin, J. M., Kassel, R. L., and Fiore, N. C. (1975): L'action antitumorale du levamisole sur la leucémie spontanée AKR et la stimulation des réponses aux hématies sont médiatisées par des facteurs sériques. Ann. Immunol., 126C:99.
8. Renoux, G., and Renoux, M. (1972): Inhibition par la theophylline de la stimulation immunologique induite par le phenylimidothiazole. C. R. Acad. Sci., 274D:3149-3151.
9. Komuro, K., and Boyse, E. A. (1973): In vitro demonstration of thymic hormone in the mouse by conversion of precursor cells into lymphocytes. Lancet, 740-743.
10. Renoux, G., Renoux, M., Teller, M. N., Mountain, I. M., McMahon, S., and Guillaumin, J. M. (1976): Potentiation of T-cell mediated immunity by levamisole. Clin. Exp. Immunol., 25 (in press).
11. Renoux, G., and Renoux, M. (1972): Levamisole inhibits and cures a solid malignant tumour and its pulmonary metastases in mice. Nature (New Biol.), 240:217-218.

12. Johnson, R. K., Houchens, D. P., Gaston, M. R., and Goldin, A. (1975): Effects of levamisole (NSC-177023) and tetramisole (NSC-102063) in experimental tumor systems. Cancer Chemother. Rep., 59:697-705.

13. Renoux, G., and Renoux, M. (1975): Influences de l'administration de levamisole sur la réactivité des lymphocytes T de cancéreux avancés. Nouv. Presse Med., 5:67-70.

Control of Neoplasia by Modulation of the Immune System, edited by M. A. Chirigos. Raven Press, New York 1977.

ANTITUMOR EFFECTS OF LEVAMISOLE ON AN ALLOGENEIC HAMSTER MELANOMA AND A SYNGENEIC RAT HEPATOMA

*, ** Ali Bin Ibrahim, † Richard Triglia, *, ‡ Peter C. Dau, and
*, ‡ Lynn E. Spitler

* Laboratory of Cellular Immunology, Children's Hospital of San Francisco, San Francisco, California 94118, and the ** Departments of Microbiology, †Immunology, and ‡Medicine, University of California School of Medicine, San Francisco, California 94143

INTRODUCTION

The drug tetramisole [2,3,5,6-tetrahydro-6-phenylimidazo-(2,1-b)-thiazole hydrochloride] and its levo-isomer, levamisole, have been widely used as anthelmintics in both man and animals (1-5). Renoux and Renoux (6,7) were the first to report the immunostimulating effects of these drugs. They found that, following immunization of mice with a living Brucella vaccine, administration of levamisole increased resistance to infection with B. abortus. They further demonstrated the production of increased numbers of IgM plaque-forming cells following the injection of sheep red blood cells in mice receiving levamisole therapy (8). Levamisole therapy also restored the depression of immunity following Brucella vaccination in Coxiella burnetii-infected mice, probably through a cellular mechanism because antibody titers against Brucella remained depressed (9). Administration of tetramisole to graft donors but not recipients increased the graft-versus-host (GVH) reactivity in F_1 hybrid mice. This increased GVH reactivity was attributed to stimulation of donor macrophages (10).

The effect of levamisole on malignancy has been examined in experimental animal models. Renoux and Renoux (11) have found a favorable effect of levamisole on primary tumors, whereas others have not (13-15). Chirigos et al. (12) observed the therapeutic effect of tetramisole in tumor-bearing mice only when it was given during drug-induced tumor remission. There is a general agreement, however, that whereas levamisole may not influence the growth of primary tumors, it does control the metastatic spread of tumor cells to the lungs and other organs (11,13-16).

81

In this chapter we present our preliminary observations on two solid transplantable tumors: Fortner's melanotic melanoma #1 of allogeneic Syrian golden hamsters (17) and the HTC cell line derived from Morris hepatoma 7288c of syngeneic Buffalo rats (18). We find that under the appropriate experimental conditions, levamisole can be shown to have an antitumor effect in both systems.

MATERIALS AND METHODS

Levamisole: Levamisole was a gift from the Janssen Pharmaceutica Company, Brussels, Belgium.

Animals: Eight- to 10-week-old female Syrian golden hamsters and male Buffalo rats weighing 160 to 180 g were obtained from the Simonsen Laboratories, Gilroy, California.

Melanoma: Fortner's melanotic melanoma #1 (17) used in these experiments has been maintained by serial subcutaneous (s.c.) transplantations in Syrian golden hamsters. The tumor cells used were taken from animals bearing tumor from the 170th to 180th tumor transplantation generations. The tumor was kindly provided by Dr. David Paslin.

Melanoma Tumor Cell Preparation and Inoculation

Peripheral tumor tissue was taken from one donor hamster, minced in Hank's balanced salt solution (HBSS), squeezed through gauze, and placed in a 0.25% trypsin shaker bath for 15 min. The single cell suspension so obtained was then washed twice in HBSS and spun at 2,000 rpm for 10 min. The cells were resuspended in Eagle's minimum essential medium, passed through 102 Nitex mesh, and concentrated to 4 X 10^6 cells/0.1 ml. The cell suspension consisted of 85% viable cells upon trypan blue (0.1%) exclusion tests. Eight- to 10-week-old female Syrian golden hamsters were inoculated with 0.1 ml of the tumor cell suspension in the right flank, which almost always gave rise to a palpable tumor at each inoculation site in about 2 weeks. The tumor size was recorded in millimeters as the average of three perpendicular measurements — length, width, and depth.

Hepatoma Cell Culture and Inoculation

The HTC cell line was kindly provided to us by Dr. Gordon Tomkins. It has been under continuous culture for several years in his laboratory and is mycoplasma-free. The HTC line was derived from the ascites form of the Morris hepatoma tumor 7288c, originally arising in a male Buffalo rat fed on a diet containing 0.04% N, N'-2, 7-fluorenylenebis-2, 2, 2-trifluoroacetamide (18).

HTC cells growing in Swim's 77 medium containing 10% calf serum and 50 U penicillin and 50 μg of streptomycin per milliliter were washed once in HBSS and adjusted to the desired cell concentration in HBSS. The tumor cells were generally 99% viable by the trypan blue exclusion test. The primary hepatoma tumors were induced in syngeneic male Buffalo rats weighing 160 to 180 g by injecting 1×10^5 to 1×10^6 HTC cells s.c. in the right flank. This almost always resulted in a palpable tumor at each inoculation site in about 6 weeks. Intradermal tumors were produced by injecting 2×10^5 HTC cells in a volume of 0.1 ml i.d. into the left flank. The tumor size was recorded in millimeters as the average of two perpendicular measurements — length and width.

Treatment of Primary Tumors with Levamisole

The effect of three doses, 2.5 mg, 10 mg, and 50 mg/kg of body weight, of levamisole was studied. The treatment was started one week after the s.c. implantation of melanoma tumor. Levamisole or water was given orally in 1-ml volumes by means of a syringe and a 21-gauge blunt needle to which a plastic tubing was attached. The plastic tube was introduced down the throat of a lightly anesthetized hamster and 1 ml of levamisole or water was injected. Involuntary swallowing was generally observed. The various doses as indicated were administered to each animal for 3 consecutive days each week. The same method was used for the oral administration of levamisole to hamsters and rats throughout this study.

Treatment of Recurrent Tumors with Levamisole

Two weeks after inoculation, melanomas were surgically removed. Just prior to surgery, the animals were shaved and anesthetized by injecting intraperitoneally 9 mg/100 g of body weight of pentobarbital. The dark, visible, superficial tumor was excised and the skin closed with nylon sutures. All animals survived the surgery. One week after surgery, levamisole therapy was started. Three doses were tested, 2.5 mg, 10 mg, and 50 mg/kg. Levamisole or water was given orally in 1-ml volumes for 3 consecutive days each week. Hamsters showing no recurrent tumors were excluded from the study. Rat hepatomas were excised in a similar fashion.

RESULTS

Toxicity of Levamisole

Table 1 summarizes the data on toxicity. Since the dilutions of levamisole were made in water, water was included as a control. The doses of 5 to 10 mg/kg of body weight appeared to be nontoxic to the hamsters. As the dose was increased to 50 mg/kg or more, the toxic effect of the drug represented by the death of animals was observed. Administration of 300 mg/kg or more of levamisole to hamsters resulted in 100% mortality; death in this case occurred rather dramatically, and the animals died within 15 min of the oral administration of the drug. Symptoms were usually violent seizures and

TABLE 1. Toxicity of levamisole for hamsters

Dosage [a]	Percent survival [b]
H_2O (1 ml)	100
5 mg/kg	100
10 mg/kg	100
50 mg/kg	80
100 mg/kg	63
200 mg/kg	45
≥300 mg/kg [c]	0

[a] mg/kg = mg of levamisole in 1 ml/kg of body weight.

[b] Survived for 3 weeks receiving three doses per week.

[c] Died within 15 min.

salivation. The LD_{50} for hamsters was between 100 and 200 mg/kg. Therefore, the doses selected for further study were 2.5, 10, and 50 mg/kg of body weight. The doses of 1.25, 2.5, and 5 mg/kg of body weight levamisole were found to be nontoxic to the rats.

Effect of Levamisole on the Growth of Primary Melanoma in Hamsters

Hamsters bearing primary melanoma tumors were treated with three doses of levamisole, 2.5, 10, and 50 mg/kg of body weight. Some beneficial effect of levamisole was observed when compared with the control animals receiving water. Normal hamsters inoculated s.c. with 4 X 10^6 melanoma cells generally die within 9 weeks. Some of the levamisole-treated animals, however, survived through the twelfth week, suggesting a favorable effect of levamisole. All control animals as well as levamisole-treated animals exhibited pulmonary metastases as well as other metastases at the time of death.

Effect of Levamisole on the Growth of Primary Hepatoma in Rats

The favorable effect of levamisole observed on the primary hamster melanoma tumors was not apparent on the growth of primary hepatoma in

TABLE 2. Effect of 2.5 mg/kg of levamisole injected subcutaneously 1 week after hepatoma tumor cell implantation in Buffalo rats

No. of rats	Concentration of HTC[a] injected	Treatment	Average survival after HTC injection (days)
6	2×10^5 s.c.	0.1 ml of levamisole (2.5 mg/kg) injected s.c. every alternate day	72
4	2×10^5 s.c.	0.1 ml of water injected s.c. every alternate day	78

[a] HTC = hepatoma tumor cells

syngeneic Buffalo rats. The levamisole-treated and control animals seemed to die more or less at the same time with progressive tumor growth. Tables 2, 3, and 4 summarize the data. Table 2 shows the effect of 2.5 mg/kg of levamisole injected s.c. every alternate day starting from 1 week after s.c. injection of HTC cells in Buffalo rats. The average survival of the levamisole-treated animals was 72 days when compared with 78 days for the untreated control animals. Table 3 similarly presents the effect of levamisole administered orally starting from 1 week after the s.c. transplantation of HTC cells in Buffalo rats. The levamisole was administered for 3 consecutive days each week. The animals receiving 1.25, 2.5, and 5 mg/kg of body weight of levamisole exhibited an average survival of 79, 72, and 79 days, respectively, when compared with the control animals, which lived for an average of 82 days. Table 4 shows the effect of 2.5 mg/kg of levamisole injected s.c. either once or every alternate day starting from 24 hr after s.c. injection of HTC cells in Buffalo rats. The average survival of animals receiving only one dose of levamisole was 78 days when compared with 79 days for the untreated control animals. Similarly, the animals receiving multiple doses of levamisole exhibited an average survival of 79 days when compared with the control animals, which lived for an average of 82 days.

Effect of Levamisole on the Growth of Recurrent Melanoma in Hamsters

Three different doses of levamisole, 2.5, 10, and 50 mg/kg of body weight, were tested. The levamisole was administered orally to each hamster for 3 consecutive days each week until the completion of the experiment. The control group received water. The groups receiving 50 mg/kg and 10 mg/kg of

TABLE 3. Effect of different concentrations of levamisole administered orally 1 week after hepatoma tumor cell implantation in Buffalo rats

No. of rats	Concentration of HTC[a] injected	Treatment	Average survival after HTC injection (days)
4	2×10^5 s.c.	1 ml of levamisole (1.25 mg/kg) given orally 3 days a week	79
4	2×10^5 s.c.	1 ml of levamisole (2.5 mg/kg) given orally 3 days a week	72
4	2×10^5 s.c.	1 ml of levamisole (5.0 mg/kg) given orally 3 days a week	79
4	2×10^5 s.c.	1 ml of water given orally 3 days a week	82

[a] HTC = hepatoma tumor cells

levamisole behaved similarly to the control group except that the group receiving 10 mg/kg of levamisole exhibited a slightly prolonged survival rate. The group receiving 2.5 mg/kg of levamisole gave the most encouraging results of all, and therefore this dose was subsequently used in all of our experiments.

Our data are represented in Figs. 1 and 2. Figure 1 shows the average rate of recurrent melanoma tumor growth in 12 control hamsters receiving water. It can be seen that none of the untreated animals survived beyond 9 weeks from the date of recurrence of the tumor. None of the animals exhibited any sign of regression of the tumor, and the average size reached in such animals was about 40 mm in diameter. In contrast, Fig. 2 shows the dramatic effect of 2.5 mg/kg of levamisole on the average growth of recurrent melanoma tumors in hamsters. Three patterns of tumor growth were observed. About a third (5 of 17) of the animals exhibited complete regression of the tumors by the end of the sixth week and remained free of tumors through the completion of the experiment. No evidence of metastases was observed in these animals upon autopsy. Another one-third (6 of 17) of the animals generally behaved like the controls for the first 4 to 6 weeks and then exhibited a delayed regression of the tumors which was generally incomplete. Four of these animals died with metastases before the termination

TABLE 4. Effect of 2.5 mg/kg of levamisole injected subcutaneously 24 hr after hepatoma tumor cell implantation in Buffalo rats

No. of rats	Concentration of HTC[a] injected	Treatment	Average survival after HTC injection (days)
4	2×10^5 s.c.	0.1 ml of levamisole (2.5 mg/kg) injected s.c. once	78
4	2×10^5 s.c.	0.1 ml of water injected s.c. once	79
4	2×10^5 s.c.	0.1 ml of levamisole (2.5 mg/kg) injected s.c. every alternate day	79
4	2×10^5 s.c.	0.1 ml of water in- jected s.c. every alternate day	83

[a] HTC = hepatoma tumor cells.

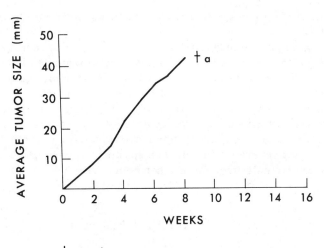

†=death
a=twelve animals

FIG. 1. Recurrent melanoma growth in control hamsters receiving water orally.

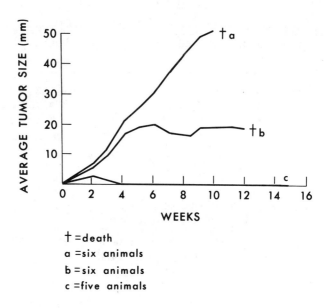

FIG. 2. Recurrent melanoma growth in hamsters receiving 2.5 mg/kg of levamisole orally.

of the experiment. The other two survived the full 15 weeks, but they too exhibited evidence of metastases upon autopsy. Levamisole had little effect on the remaining six animals except for a slightly extended survival.

Effect of Levamisole on the Growth of Recurrent Hepatoma in Buffalo Rats

In a preliminary experiment, two rats exhibiting recurrent hepatomas were treated orally with 2.5 mg/kg of levamisole. Both animals showed regression of the tumors within 6 weeks of treatment. In one animal, the tumor underwent complete regression by the end of the third month and did not recur. In the other animal, the tumor underwent only partial regression, and the animal survived the full 6 months of the experiment. In contrast, the untreated control animal died of progressive tumor growth within 3 months. Unfortunately, the rate of recurrence in rats was so low in comparison with hamsters that further experiments in recurrent hepatoma were not undertaken in this system.

The Growth of Intradermal Tumors in Rats

Intradermal injections of 2×10^5 HTC cells led to a variable incidence of i.d. tumors, averaging 42% of injected animals. In one experiment, eight out of eight untreated animals developed palpable tumors within 2 weeks which then regressed completely within 6 weeks of transplantation. Upon subsequent challenge with 1×10^5 HTC cells s.c., these rats did not develop s.c. tumors over an observation period of 6 weeks, although the same s.c. dose of HTC cells produced 100% tumors within 2 weeks in six control rats. In another experiment, 12 normal rats which had not developed i.d. tumors within 6 weeks of i.d. transplantation were also resistant to challenge with 1×10^5 HTC cells given s.c., although all six control animals developed progressively growing s.c. tumors within 2 weeks. These rats did not develop s.c. tumors over an observation period of 6 weeks, but prolonged observation revealed small tumors developing in all 12 animals during the seventh to eighth week. Whether the animals developed i.d. tumors after the first HTC cell injection or not, they never developed i.d. tumors following subsequent i.d. injection of HTC cells.

Combined Effect of Levamisole and Intradermal-Injections of HTC Cells on Hepatoma Tumors in Buffalo Rats

Since the i.d. injection of HTC cells in Buffalo rats resulted in resistance to a subsequent challenge with HTC cells given s.c. 6 weeks later, we decided to study the combined effect of levamisole and i.d. injections of HTC cells in syngeneic Buffalo rats. This was done in two separate experiments: (a) immunotherapy, and (b) immunoprophylaxis.

Immunotherapy

In this experiment 1×10^5 HTC cells were injected s.c. into each of 18 Buffalo rats in the right flank. They were then divided into three groups. The experimental animals (group 1) received three weekly i.d. injections of 2×10^5 HTC into the left flank beginning 3 days after s.c. injection and also received 2.5 mg/kg of body weight of levamisole orally beginning on the fifth day after the s.c. injection of HTC cells. Levamisole was administered for 3 consecutive days each week. The control animals received s.c. injections of HTC and either i.d. injections of HTC cells and water orally (group II) or levamisole alone (group III) in a schedule identical to that administered to the experimental animals. Figure 3 presents our preliminary data. The average size of hepatoma tumor growth in the experimental animals which received both levamisole and i.d. injection of HTC cells was less than the average size of tumors in control animals which received as therapy either i.d. injections of HTC cells alone or levamisole alone. Only one of 12 rats injected i.d. with HTC in this experiment developed an i.d. tumor. This rat, which belonged to group I, exhibited s.c. tumor like the others, but unfortunately it died during anesthesia.

Immunoprophylaxis

Three groups of seven Buffalo rats each were studied. The experimental animals (group I) received 2×10^5 HTC cells i.d. in the left flank. Two days later they were started on levamisole orally in a dose of 2.5 mg/kg of

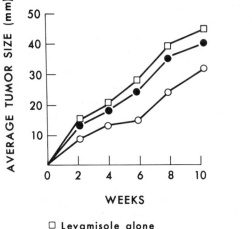

□ Levamisole alone
● Intradermal injections of HTC alone
○ Levamisole plus intradermal injections of HTC

FIG. 3. The combined effects of levamisole and i.d. injections of HTC cells on rat hepatoma. Immunotherapy experiment: subcutaneous transplantation of HTC cells preceded i.d. injection of HTC cells by 3 days.

body weight. Levamisole was administered for 3 consecutive days each week. On the day after the initiation of the levamisole therapy (3 days after the i.d. injection of HTC cells), they were injected s.c. with 1×10^5 HTC cells. They were then given two more i.d. injections of HTC cells at weekly intervals starting 1 week from the first i.d. injection. Control animals were given s.c. injections of HTC cells and i.d. injections of HTC cells and

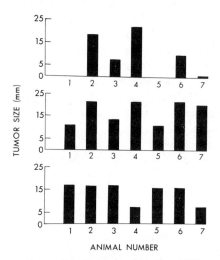

FIG. 4. The combined effects of levamisole and i.d. injections of HTC cells on rat hepatoma. Immunoprophylaxis experiment: subcutaneous transplantation of HTC cells followed i.d. injection of HTC cells by 3 days. Animal no. 7 in the experimental group completely rejected its tumor by the end of the fourth week.

TOP: Levamisole plus intradermal injections of HTC
MIDDLE: Intradermal injections of HTC
BOTTOM: No levamisole and no intradermal injections of HTC

water orally (group II) or s.c. injections of HTC cells and water (group III) in a schedule identical to that in the experimental animals. Two out of seven animals in the experimental group receiving a combination of i.d. injections of HTC cells and levamisole exhibited no s.c. tumors over an observation period of 6 weeks starting from the day of s.c. injection of tumor cells. One additional animal in the same group developed a small s.c. tumor of about 1 mm in diameter, which then regressed completely by the end of the fourth week. In contrast, the control animals which received neither i.d. injections of HTC cells nor levamisole and the animals which received therapy consisting of i.d. injections of HTC cells alone all developed progressively growing s.c. tumors. (See Fig. 4.)

Although we saw no correlation between i.d. tumor development and the rate of growth of s.c. tumor, it appeared that the s.c. tumor had some influence over the growth of the i.d. tumor because in earlier experiments normal animals receiving i.d. tumors alone rejected their tumors completely by the end of the sixth week.

The data presented in this report are strictly preliminary. The above-mentioned animals are still under observation, and a detailed report of our findings will be published elsewhere at a later date.

DISCUSSION

The therapeutic effect of levamisole was studied on the subcutaneous growth of two solid transplantable tumors: Fortner's melanotic melanoma #1 in allogeneic Syrian golden hamsters (17) and the HTC cell line derived from the Morris hepatoma 7288c in syngeneic Buffalo rats (18). The most effective dose of levamisole was found to be 2.5 mg/kg of body weight, and it was nontoxic in both hamsters and rats. Treatment of primary hamster melanomas with levamisole resulted in a beneficial effect in the sense that some of the levamisole-treated animals survived longer than the untreated control hamsters. Similar treatment of primary rat hepatomas with levamisole had no effect. The immune response toward allogeneic tumors is probably directed chiefly against histocompatibility antigens rather than the relatively weak tumor-associated antigens (19). A primary host immune response against relatively strong histocompatibility antigens in the hamster melanoma system may have provided an adequate basis for a therapeutically effective immunopotentiating effect by levamisole, whereas the primary host immune response toward relatively weak tumor-associated antigens in the syngeneic rat hepatoma system was inadequate to allow a therapeutic effect of levamisole to manifest itself. A favorable effect of levamisole in a primary tumor system has only been reported by Renoux and Renoux (11), whereas no therapeutic effect has been reported in most primary tumor models (12-16).

After local excision of the primary tumor, the effect of levamisole on both recurrent hamster melanoma and recurrent rat hepatoma was beneficial. Because the rate of recurrence in rats was much lower than in hamsters, we worked mainly with the recurrent hamster melanoma. About one-third of the levamisole-treated hamsters exhibited complete regression of their recurrent tumors within 6 weeks, without apparent metastases at autopsy; another one-third showed delayed regressions with pulmonary and other metastases; and the remainder showed only slightly prolonged survival in comparison to control animals receiving no levamisole therapy.

In total, 88% of the levamisole-treated hamsters lived longer than the untreated control animals. Sixty-five percent of the treated animals exhibited complete or partial regression of the local recurrence, and of these about 50% were completely free of tumor at autopsy. Reduction of tumor load by surgery may itself favor an immune response in both allogeneic and syngeneic systems (Chirigos et al., unpublished observations), which could then be stimulated further by levamisole. Chirigos et al. (12) have also obtained similar results by reducing the tumor mass with the help of 1,3 bis (2-chloroethyl)-2-nitrosourea (BCNU) and then treating with tetramisole. They have reported that administration of tetramisole alone did not affect the survival of the tumor-bearing animals, but when tetramisole was administered during the BCNU-induced remission, the long-term survival rate increased from 25% in control animals to over 60% in tetramisole-treated animals.

The i.d. injections of hepatoma tumor cells in Buffalo rats resulted in a variable incidence of i.d. tumors, averaging 42% of injected animals; palpable i.d. tumors always regressed completely within 6 weeks of transplantation. Subcutaneous tumor challenge at that time produced no tumor within a 6-week period of observation, regardless of whether the i.d. tumor transplant had produced palpable tumor or not. These animals were also completely resistant to repeated i.d. tumor challenge.

It has been known since 1937 that inoculation of tumor cells i.d. can result in immunization of the host (20,21). Recently, Churchill et al. (22) have observed that when normal syngeneic strain-2 guinea pigs were inoculated i.d. with 3×10^6 line-1 ascites tumor cells, a papule was formed which increased in size for a few days and then regressed. A second i.d. injection of tumor cells produced a papule which grew to a smaller size than the first injection and regressed more rapidly. The third injection of living tumor cells showed no papule growth. Animals that had received three i.d. injections of ascites line-2 tumor cells resisted intramuscular challenge with 4×10^6 tumor cells. McCoy et al. (23) have also reported that the optimum immunization against tumor-associated transplantation antigen in syngeneic BALB/c mice was obtained by immunizing the syngeneic hosts with an i.d. inoculation of viable plasmacytoma cells followed by therapeutic drug-induced tumor regression with aniline mustard.

The combined effect of levamisole and i.d. injections of HTC cells on the growth of s.c. transplanted HTC cells in syngeneic Buffalo rats was studied in two separate experiments. In an immunotherapy experiment we found treatment with a combination of three weekly i.d. injections of HTC cells and levamisole, started 3 days after the s.c. transplantation of HTC cells, resulted in an average decrease of tumor size when compared with the average tumor size of animals which received as therapy either i.d. injections of HTC cells alone or levamisole alone. Kronman et al. (24) have reported successful treatment of a solid hepatoma in strain-2 guinea pigs by repeated i.d. injections of living tumor cells alone, an effect not seen in our rat hepatoma model. The therapeutic effect of the i.d. immunization on the guinea pig hepatoma was dependent on the dose of the tumor cells inoculated intramuscularly; the use of a smaller s.c. tumor inoculum might have also improved the results of our immunotherapy with combined levamisole and i.d. tumor cell inoculations.

In an immunoprophylaxis experiment, we found that the treatment of syngeneic rats with a combination of three weekly i.d. injections of HTC cells and levamisole, started 3 days prior to the s.c. transplantation of IITC cells, resulted in a 44% reduction in tumor incidence compared to control animals which received i.d. HTC cell injections without levamisole therapy or animals which received neither therapeutic modality.

No effect of i.d. tumor development upon the growth of s.c. tumors was seen. On the other hand, the presence of s.c. tumor was found to delay the rejection of i.d. tumors beyond the 6-week period found in normal rats. Kronman et al. (26) have also noted in their syngeneic strain-2 guinea pig model that i.d. papules persisted longer in those animals which had intramuscular tumor than in those animals which did not have intramuscular tumor.

We conclude from both the immunotherapy and immunoprophylaxis experiments that levamisole can act therapeutically against a rat hepatoma when administered under favorable conditions. Following the creation of an immune response in the syngeneic rats toward tumor-associated antigens by injecting live tumor cells i.d., levamisole may have worked by boosting this response further to the point where its effect was clinically demonstrable.

Our results may help to clarify some of the conflicting data which have been reported concerning the efficacy of levamisole in animal tumor systems. Specifically, it appears that effective levamisole immunotherapy of malignancy requires a certain critical level of a preexisting antitumor immune response to be present, as well as a minimal tumor burden. Levamisole was thus effective against both melanoma and hepatoma recurrences following local excision, but only minimally effective against the melanoma and ineffective against the hepatoma when administered concurrently with primary tumor transplantation without subsequent excision. It was effective against primary s.c. tumor in the rat hepatoma model only when given concomitantly with distant i.d. injections of HTC cells, where tumor cells are more immunogenic than when given s.c.

These studies provide encouragement with regard to the potential usefulness of levamisole in human malignancy. For example, the drug was most effective in treating local recurrences following excision of the primary tumor transplants. Patients who are candidates for immunotherapy are in a similar situation: They have had excision of their primary tumor, and the goal of immunotherapy is to prevent local recurrence and distant metastases.

The results with the rat hepatoma model may have direct application to the situation in human malignant melanoma, where the location of the primary tumor is almost always i.d. Our observations suggest that the i.d. administration of rat hepatoma cells provides the necessary level of antitumor immune response for levamisole therapy to be effective against tumors growing s.c. at a distant site. By analogy in human melanoma, the initial period of intradermal tumor growth could sensitize the host sufficiently against the tumor to provide an adequate basis for a therapeutic effect of levamisole against melanoma metastatic to distant sites.

SUMMARY

Levamisole immunotherapy of primary transplants of the allogeneic Fortner's melanotic melanoma #1 in Syrian golden hamsters prolonged survival of Buffalo rats bearing transplants of the HTC cell line derived from syngeneic Morris hepatoma 7288c. When given orally to hamsters showing local melanoma recurrence following surgical excision of the primary transplant, levamisole produced tumor regression in 68% of the animals; about one-half of these were tumor-free at autopsy, whereas regression was never observed in control animals receiving water.

Subcutaneous (s.c.) inoculation of HTC cells was found always to give rise to a progressively growing malignancy which was fatal in about 12 weeks, whereas intradermal (i.d.) inoculation produced locally growing tumors which regressed in 6 weeks, leaving the rats immune to subsequent s.c. challenge. Although i.d. inoculations of hepatoma cells alone had no effect on the growth of a s.c. hepatoma inoculated either 3 days prior to i.d. injections of HTC cells or 3 days later, combination with levamisole therapy resulted in slowing of the s.c. tumor growth in the first instance and elimination of 43% of the s.c. tumors in the second instance. These observations have important implications regarding the potential of this agent in the immunotherapy of human malignancy.

REFERENCES

1. Thienpont, D., Vanparijs, O. F. J., Raeymaekers, A. H. M., Vandenberk, J., Demoen, P. J. A., Allewijn, F. T. N., Marsboom, R. P. H., Niemegeers, C. J. E., Schellekens, K. H. L., and Janssen, P. A. J. (1966): Tetramisole (R8299), a new, potent broad spectrum anthelmintic. Nature, 209:1084-1086.

2. Walley, J. K. (1966): Tetramisole (dl, 2, 3, 5, 6-tetra-hydro-6-phenyl-imidazo 12, 1-6) (thiazole hydrochloride — Nilverm) in the treatment of gastric-intestinal worms and lung worms in domestic animals. 1. Sheep and Goats. Vet. Rec., 78:406-414.

3. Lionel, N. D. W., Mirando, E. H., Nanayakkara, J. C., and Soysa, P. E. (1969): Levamisole in the treatment of ascariasis in children. Brit. Med. J., 4:340-341.

4. Thienpont, D., Brugmans, J., Abadi, K., and Tanamal, S. (1969): Tetramisole in the treatment of nematode infections in man. Am. J. Trop. Med., 18:520-525.

5. Gatti, F., Krubwa, F., Vandepitte, J., and Thienpont, D. (1972): Control of intestinal nematodes in African school-children by the trimestrial administration of levamisole. Ann. Soc. Belg. Med. Trop., 52:19-32.

6. Renoux, G., and Renoux, M. (1971): Immunostimulant effect of an imidothiazole in the immunization of mice infected with Brucella abortus. C. R. Acad. Sci., 272:349-350.

7. Renoux, G., and Renoux, M. (1972): Immunology — Immunostimulating action of derivatives of phenyl imidothiazole on splenic cell producing antibodies. C. R. Acad. Sci., 274:756-757.

8. Renoux, G., and Renoux, M. (1973): Stimulation of anti-Brucella vaccination in mice by tetramisole, a phenyl-imidothiazole. Infect. Immunol., 8:544-548.

9. Renoux, G., and Renoux, M. (1972): Antigenic competition and nonspecific immunity after a rickettsial infection in mice: Restoration of antibacterial immunity by phenyl-imidothiazole treatment. J. Immunol., 109:761-765.

10. Renoux, G., and Renoux, M. (1972): Immunology — Effect of phenylimidothiazole (tetramisole) on the graft-versus-host reaction. C. R. Acad. Sci., 274:3320-3323.

11. Renoux, G., and Renoux, M. (1972): Levamisole inhibits and cures a solid malignant tumor and its pulmonary metastases in mice. Nature (New Biol.), 240:217-218.

12. Chirigos, M. A., Pearson, J. W., and Prylor, J. (1973): Augmentation of chemotherapeutically induced remission of a murine leukemia by a chemical immunoadjuvant. Cancer Res., 33:2615-2618.

13. Potter, C. W., Carr, I., Jennings, R., Rees, R. C., McGinty, F., and Richardson, V. M. (1974): Levamisole inactive in treatment of four animal tumors. Nature, 249:567-569.

14. Renoux, G., Kassel, R. L., Renoux, M., Fiore, N. C., Guillaumin, J., and Palat, A. (1975): Immunomodulation by levamisole in normal and leukemic mice. Evidence for a serum transfer. In: Modulation of host immune resistance in the prevention or treatment of induced neoplasias, edited by M. A. Chirigos. Fogarty International Center Proceedings, No. 28, U.S. Government Printing Office, Washington, D.C.

15. Fidler, I. J., and Spitler, L. E. (1975): Effects of levamisole on in vivo and in vitro murine host response to syngeneic transplantable tumor. J. Natl. Cancer Inst., 55:1107-1112.

16. Sadowski, J. M., and Rapp, F. (1975): Inhibition by levamisole of metastases by cells transformed by herpes simplex virus type 1. Proc. Soc. Exp. Biol. Med., 149:219-222.

17. Fortner, J. G., Mahy, A. G., and Schrodt, G. R. (1961): Transplantable tumors of the Syrian (golden) hamster. 1. Tumors of the alimentary tract, endocrine glands and melanomas. Cancer Res., 21:161-198.

18. Thompson, E. B., Tomkins, G. M., and Curran, J. F. (1966): Induction of tyrosine α-ketoglutarate transaminase by steroid hormones in a newly established tissue culture cell line. Proc. Natl. Acad. Sci. U.S.A., 56:296-303.

19. Hersey, P. (1973): Thymus-dependent cytotoxic lymphocytes in the rat. Eur. J. Immunol., 3:748-754.

20. Andervont, H. B. (1937): Use of pure strain animals in studies on natural resistance to transplantable tumors. Public Health Rep., 52:1885-1895.

21. Gross, L. (1943): Intradermal immunization of C3H mice against sarcoma that originated in animal of same line. Cancer Res., 3:326-333.
22. Churchill, W. H., Jr., Rapp, H. J., Kronman, B. S., and Borsos, T. (1968): Detection of antigens of a new diethylnitrosamine-induced transplantable hepatoma by delayed hypersensitivity. J. Natl. Cancer Inst., 41:13-29.
23. McCoy, J. L., Dean, J. H., Law, L. W., Williams, J., McCoy, N. T., and Holiman, B. J. (1974): Immunogenicity, antigenicity and mechanisms of tumor rejection of mineral-oil-induced plasmacytomas in syngeneic BALB/c mice. Int. J. Cancer, 14:264-276.
24. Kronman, B. S., Wepsic, H. T., Churchill, W. H., Jr., Zbar, B., Borsos, T., and Rapp, H. J. (1970): Immunotherapy of cancer: An experimental model in syngeneic guinea pigs. Science, 168:257-259.

Control of Neoplasia by Modulation of the Immune System, edited by M. A. Chirigos. Raven Press, New York 1977.

EFFECT OF LEVAMISOLE ON METASTASES BY HERPESVIRUS-TRANSFORMED CELLS

Elizabeth W. Doller and Fred Rapp

Department of Microbiology, The M. S. Hershey Medical Center, The Pennsylvania State University, College of Medicine, Hershey, Pennsylvania 17033

INTRODUCTION

Oncogenic transformation of hamster embryo fibroblast (HEF) cells by ultraviolet (UV)-irradiated herpes simplex virus type 2 (HSV-2) was demonstrated by Duff and Rapp (1,2) in 1971. Two years later, it was also reported by Duff and Rapp (3) that herpes simplex virus type 1 (HSV-1) could oncogenically transform hamster embryo cells. Most properties of transformed cells were similar: They expressed HSV-specific antigens in the cytoplasm and on the surface; they produced tumors in newborn hamsters; HSV-specific neutralizing antibody was induced in tumor-bearing animals; transformed cells were resistant to superinfection by HSV (4,5). Neither the HSV-2-transformed cells (6) nor the HSV-1-transformed cells (3) exhibited C-type viruses. The tumors produced in hamsters by HSV-1- or HSV-2-transformed cells regularly metastasized to the lungs (3,7).

Levamisole, the L-isomer of tetramisole, a potent antihelminthic drug (8), has been shown to affect various limbs of the immune system. This drug stimulates phagocytosis by macrophages (9) and increases humoral (10) and cellular immunity (11,12). It has also been reported to increase the length of remission of murine leukemia (13) and to cure mice of solid tumors (14).

Since the HSV-1-transformed hamster cells metastasize, and since levamisole has been used to inhibit metastases in other animal model systems, Sadowski and Rapp (15) studied the effect of levamisole on metastases by HSV-1-transformed hamster cells. They found that levamisole, given weekly, reduced the incidence of metastases, even when administered after the primary tumors were palpable. This study was carried out to investigate further the effect of levamisole on metastases by HSV-1-transformed hamster cells.

MATERIALS AND METHODS

Cells

The origin of the HSV-1-transformed hamster cells (14-012-8-1) has previously been described by Duff and Rapp (3). These cells were oncogenic in newborn hamsters. The cells from one tumor (designated 14-012-8-1T#10) were oncogenic in weanling hamsters and were therefore used in these studies. Properties of the tumor cells were the same as those described earlier for the in vitro transformed cells. The 14-012-8-1T#10 cells were maintained in medium 199 supplemented with 10% fetal calf serum, 10% tryptose phosphate broth, 0.15% $NaHCO_3$, 100 units of penicillin per ml and 100 μg of streptomycin per ml in 250-ml plastic flasks (Corning, New York).

Levamisole Hydrochloride

Levamisole, the L-isomer of 2,3,5,6-tetrahydro-6-phenyl-imidazo-(2,1,-b)-thiazole, was obtained from Janssen R and D, Inc., New Brunswick, New Jersey. The drug was dissolved in phosphate-buffered saline (pH 7.2) to concentrations of 20, 10, or 5 mg/ml immediately prior to use.

Injection of Tumor Cells

HSV-1-transformed hamster cells (14-012-8-1T#10) at approximately passage 40 were dispersed with 0.5% trypsin, pelleted, and resuspended in medium 199 supplemented with 10% fetal calf serum, 10% tryptose phosphate broth, and 0.15% $NaHCO_3$, to a concentration of 10^6 cells/ml. Each hamster was inoculated subcutaneously in the upper back with 10^5 cells in 0.1 ml of medium.

Injection of Hamsters with Levamisole

Each weanling golden Syrian hamster (Lakeview Hamster Colony, Newfield, New Jersey) was injected intraperitoneally with 0.5, 1, or 2 mg of levamisole in 0.1 ml of saline. Experimental protocol and drug regimens are depicted in Fig. 1. The animals received tumor cells on day 0 and were sacrificed 10 weeks later. During the 10-week period, groups of animals began receiving levamisole at different intervals as explained in the figure. There were 10 animals per group.

To determine the effect of levamisole on primary tumors, the following three regimens were used: (a) One group received drug on the same day as the tumor cells; (b) another group received drug on the day of tumor cell injection and 1 week later; and (c) a third group received drug 2, 4, 6, 8, and 10 days after inoculation of the tumor cells.

DRUG TREATMENT REGIMEN

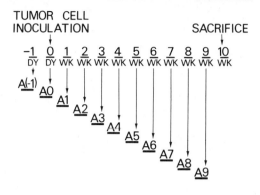

FIG. 1. A(-1): hamsters received drug the day before tumor cells, the day of tumor cells, and once a week for 9 weeks; A0: hamsters received drug the day of tumor cells and once a week for 9 weeks; A1: hamsters received drug 1 week after tumor cells and once a week for 8 weeks; A2: hamsters received drug 2 weeks after tumor cells and once a week for 7 weeks; A3: hamsters received drug 3 weeks after tumor cells and once a week for 6 weeks; A4: hamsters received drug 4 weeks after tumor cells and once a week for 5 weeks; A5: hamsters received drug 5 weeks after tumor cells and once a week for 4 weeks; A6: hamsters received drug 6 weeks after tumor cells and once a week for 3 weeks; A7: hamsters received drug 7 weeks after tumor cells and once a week for 2 weeks; A8: hamsters received drug 8 weeks after tumor cells and at 9 weeks; A9: hamsters received one injection 9 weeks after tumor cells.

Code for symbols: DY = day, WK = week.

Detection of Metastases

Ten weeks after inoculation of the tumor cells, the hamsters were sacrificed and autopsied. Internal organs were examined for gross metastases; the lungs were removed and examined more closely for visible pulmonary metastases. The number of animals with metastases was recorded, and the percentage of metastases was calculated.

RESULTS

Effect of Levamisole on Primary Tumors

The effect of levamisole on primary tumors was examined in two ways. In one experiment, hamsters were inoculated with 10^5 14-012-8-1T#10 cells. Levamisole was given to one group of 10 animals at the same time as the cells. A second group received one dose of levamisole with the cells and a second dose 1 week later. A third group received five doses of drug 2, 4, 6,

TABLE 1. Incidence of primary tumors in hamsters during the first 28 days
after inoculation of HSV-1-transformed cells

	6-7 days	10 days	14 days	28 days
No drug	0/10 [a]	4/8	5/8	7/8
Levamisole [b] given with cells	3/10	5/10	9/10	10/10
Levamisole given with cells and 1 week later	2/10	5/9	8/9	8/9
Levamisole given 2, 4, 6, 8 and 10 days after cells	0/10	5/9	6/9	9/9

Animals were palpated for tumors at 6-7, 10, 14, and 28 days after inoculation of tumor cells.

[a] Animals with tumors over total animals in the group.

[b] Two milligrams of levamisole was given with each injection.

8, and 10 days after the tumor cells. The controls received no drug. These regimens were chosen to determine whether early and rigorous treatment would reduce the incidence of tumors during a 28-day period, since these cells usually produce tumors in all injected animals within 28 days. This procedure was carried out with doses of 0.5, 1, and 2 mg of levamisole. Results given in Table 1 for 2-mg doses were similar to those obtained with 0.5 mg and 1 mg. Tumors began to appear 6 to 7 days after injection of the cells. Approximately 50% of the animals in all groups developed tumors within 10 days. The incidence continued to increase, and essentially all hamsters had primary tumors 28 days after initiation of the experiment. The Fisher exact test for 2 X 2 tables failed to reveal any statistical difference among the groups for incidence of primary tumors; it would appear that levamisole does not alter the rate of induction of primary tumors.

The effect of levamisole on primary tumors was examined in another manner. The diameter of the tumors was measured 3 and 5 weeks after inoculation of tumor cells. At these time points, all animals had tumors. Animals were injected according to the protocol listed in Materials and Methods and Fig. 1, but only 2 mg per injection was used. The results from representative groups are presented in Table 2. The sizes of tumors at 3 and 5 weeks did not differ from those of tumors in the control group. No

TABLE 2.   Size of tumors induced by HSV-1-transformed cells in hamsters
receiving 2 mg of levamisole

Group [a]	Tumor size (cm) after 3 weeks	Tumor size (cm) after 5 weeks	Animals per group
A(-1)	0.71 + 0.10	1.2 + 0.12	8-10
A1	0.68 + 0.07	1.1 + 0.07	8-10
A3	0.53 + 0.08	1.0 + 0.17	8-10
A5	0.58 + 0.07	0.94 + 0.13	8-10
Control	0.65 + 0.05	1.2 + 0.08	8-10

[a] Code for groups is explained in Fig. 1.

statistical difference was observed among the groups using the Student's t-test. It can thus be concluded that levamisole did not affect the size of the primary tumors.

Effect of Levamisole on Pulmonary Metastases

Since levamisole has been used to reduce metastases in other animal tumor systems, and since 14-012-8-1T#10 tumors usually metastasize to the lungs of the hamsters, the effect of levamisole on pulmonary metastases was examined. The experimental protocol is described in Materials and Methods and Fig. 1. The rationale for this protocol is as follows. Sadowski and Rapp (15) showed that levamisole inhibited metastases to the lungs when 2 mg of drug was given weekly upon tumor palpability. However, they did not determine whether the drug was more effective when started before the tumor cells were inoculated or before the tumor was palpable.

When animals received 1 mg per injection starting the day of inoculation of cells (group A0), or 1 week (group A1), 2 weeks (A2), or 3 weeks (A3) later, the incidence of metastases was reduced compared to the controls (Fig. 2). When drug was started 4 weeks after the inoculation of tumor cells (A4), levamisole was ineffective in reducing metastases. It is interesting to note that when levamisole treatment was begun the day before tumor cell inoculation (A-1), the incidence of metastases was not significantly reduced.

Almost identical results were obtained in animals receiving 2 mg per injection (Fig. 3). However, this higher dosage of the drug was still effective when given as late as 4 weeks after injection of tumor cells.

The incidence of metastases in animals receiving 0.5 mg with each injection was the same as the controls, regardless of when drug treatment was begun.

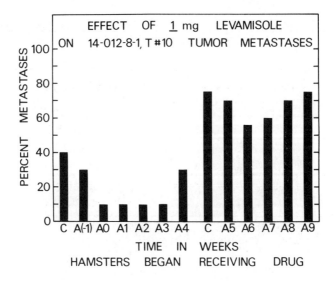

FIG. 2. The effect on metastases of 1 mg of levamisole injected intraperitoneally in hamsters receiving 10^5 HSV-1-transformed cells (14-012-8-1T#10) subcutaneously.

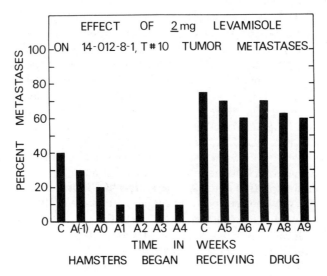

FIG. 3. The effect on metastases of 2 mg of levamisole injected intraperitoneally in hamsters receiving 10^5 HSV-1-transformed cells (14-012-8-1T#10) subcutaneously.

The Fisher exact test was used to determine whether the incidence of metastases in the drug-treated groups differed from that in controls. The incidence for groups A(-1), A5, A6, A7, A8, and A9 was not statistically different than the controls. Although the reductions were not statistically significant for groups A0, A1, A2, A3 and A4 (p value = 0.1), the observation that almost identical results were obtained for two doses (1 mg and 2 mg) suggests a reproducible effect.

DISCUSSION

The type of tumor which is frequently detrimental to humans is the adeno-carcinoma. An animal model for adenocarcinoma could be very useful in understanding human disease. The HSV-1 transformation system could serve in this role since the 14-012-8-1T#10 cells cause adenocarcinomas in hamsters. These tumors also mimic human disease in that they are invasive and frequently metastasize to the lungs. Since levamisole has been shown to be an antitumor agent in other animal systems (presumably by altering the immune response) (13,14), and since metastases by HSV-transformed ham-ster cells can be inhibited by immunological manipulation (16), attempts were made to determine the effect of levamisole on 14-012-8-1T#10 tumors. Sadowski and Rapp (15) reported that levamisole inhibited metastases by 14-012-8-1T#10 tumors when the drug was given weekly from the time the tumor was palpable. This suggested either that metastases were not yet present when drug treatment was begun, or that the drug was effective in helping the host eliminate a small tumor load. The possibility that levamisole is directly toxic to metastasizing cells cannot, therefore, be ruled out.

If one assumes that levamisole acts by stimulating immunity, the data in Figs. 2 and 3 can best be explained as follows. In the groups in which the incidence of metastases is depressed (A0, A1, A2, and A3 with 1 mg of drug and A0, A1, A2, A3, and A4 with 2 mg of drug), drug treatment is begun when there is sufficient antigen in the host to elicit an immune response, presumably aided by levamisole. This response is strong enough to destroy cells that have metastasized and to prevent new metastases. However, if drug treatment is not begun until later, the level of antigen is so high that any immune response, even with levamisole, is no longer effective. Alter-natively, metastases which had formed may be too large to be destroyed by the immune mechanism.

Ironically, if levamisole is given the day before tumor cell inoculation, at the time of tumor cell implantation, and then weekly [group A(-1)], metastases are not markedly reduced. It is possible that giving the drug before tumor implantation actually inhibits the immune response, and that by the time the response recovers, the tumor load is too great to be eliminated. Renoux and Renoux (17) have shown that levamisole depresses the immune response to sheep red blood cells when the drug is given prior to the antigen. These re-sults suggest that (a) levamisole is not directly toxic to metastasizing cells since the animals in this group received the largest dosage and yet had an incidence of metastases similar to the controls; and (b) metastasizing cells must be present quite early in the host if they can take hold before a stimulated host can mount a specific response.

It is important to note that the time of drug treatment is critical. If levamisole is given too early or too late, the effect on incidence of metastases is lost. Extrapolating to humans, levamisole treatment would have to commence while metastases are either undetectable or very small. Chirigos et al. (13) have also demonstrated this in a mouse system in which levamisole was effective in extending remission of leukemia induced by a chemotherapeutic agent.

Regardless of drug regimen, levamisole did not alter the rate of primary tumor formation during a 28-day observation period, nor did the drug alter the size of tumors during a 21- or 35-day period. It is possible that inoculation of 10^5 tumor cells exceeds the ability of the host to control growth, even with the help of levamisole.

In conclusion, levamisole appears to be somewhat effective in controlling small tumor loads, such as metastasizing cells. Continuous treatment with drug beginning approximately 1 week after tumor cell inoculation is most effective, but treatment can be delayed for some weeks without detriment to the host. However, levamisole proved ineffective in preventing primary tumors in this experimental system.

SUMMARY

Levamisole, a potent antihelminthic drug, was studied for activity against primary tumors and metastases caused by herpes simplex virus type 1-transformed hamster cells (14-012-8-T#10). This drug had no effect on the incidence of primary tumors during the first 28 days after inoculation of tumor cells regardless of the dose (0.5, 1, or 2 mg per injection) or drug regimen. The diameters of primary tumors were measured 3 and 5 weeks after tumor cell inoculation; sizes were the same for drug-treated and control animals, regardless of drug regimen. Thus, levamisole appears to offer no protection against these primary tumors.

Levamisole did reduce the incidence of metastases by the transplanted cells. Animals receiving 1 mg per injection within 3 weeks or 2 mg per injection within 4 weeks demonstrated a reduced incidence of metastases to the lungs. The results suggest that the compound can support the host in controlling spread of cells to distant sites, perhaps by increasing the strength of the immunologic response to the tumor cells.

ACKNOWLEDGMENTS

This study was conducted under Contract N01 CP 53516 within the Virus Cancer Program of the National Cancer Institute, NIH, PHS.

REFERENCES

1. Duff, R., and Rapp, F. (1971): Oncogenic transformation of hamster cells after exposure to herpes simplex virus type 2. Nature (New Biol.), 233:48-50.

2. Duff, R., and Rapp, F. (1971): Properties of hamster embryo fibroblasts transformed in vitro after exposure to ultraviolet-irradiated herpes simplex virus type 2. J. Virol., 8:469-477.

3. Duff, R., and Rapp, F. (1973): Oncogenic transformation of hamster embryo cells after exposure to inactivated herpes simplex virus type 1. J. Virol., 12:209-217.

4. Doller, E., Duff, R., and Rapp, F. (1973): Resistance of hamster cells transformed by herpes simplex virus type 2 to superinfection by herpes simplex viruses. Intervirology, 1:154-167.

5. Duff, R., and Doller, E. (1973): Cellular transformation by herpes simplex virus. In: Virus Research, edited by C. Fred Fox and William S. Robinson, pp. 353-372. Academic Press, New York.

6. Rapp, F., Conner, R., Glaser, R., and Duff, R. (1972): Absence of leukosis virus markers in hamster cells transformed by herpes simplex virus type 2. J. Virol., 9:1059-1063.

7. Rapp, F., and Duff, R. (1972): In vitro cell transformation by herpesviruses. Fed. Proc., 31:1660-1668.

8. Thienpont, D., Vanpaijs, O., Raeymakers, A., Vandenberk, J., Demoen, P., Allewijn, F., Marsboom, R., Niemegeers, C., Schellekens, K., and Janssen, P. (1966): Tetramisole (R8299), a new, potent broad spectrum antihelminthic. Nature, 209:1084-1086.

9. Hoebeke, J., and Franchi, G. (1973): Influence of tetramisole and its optical isomers on the mononuclear phagocytic system — effect on carbon clearance in mice. J. Reticuloendothel. Soc., 14:317-323.

10. Lods, J. C., Dujardin, P., and Halpern, G. (1975): Action of levamisole on antibody protection after vaccination with anti-typhoid and para-typhoid A and B. Ann. Allergy, 34:210-212.

11. Woods, W., Fleigelman, M., and Chirigos, M. (1975): Effect of levamisole on the in vitro immune response of spleen lymphocytes. Proc. Soc. Exp. Biol. Med., 148:1048-1050.

12. Tripodi, D., Parks, L., and Brugmans, J. (1973): Drug-induced restoration of cutaneous delayed hypersensitivity in anergic patients with cancer. New Engl. J. Med., 289:354-357.

13. Chirigos, M., Pearson, J., and Pryor, J. (1973): Augmentation of chemotherapeutically induced remission of a murine leukemia by a chemical immunoadjuvant. Cancer Res., 33:2615-2618.

14. Renoux, G., and Renoux, M. (1972): Levamisole inhibits and cures a solid malignant tumor and its pulmonary metastases. Nature (New Biol.), 240:217-218.

15. Sadowski, J., and Rapp, F. (1975): Inhibition by levamisole of metastases by cells transformed by herpes simplex virus type 1 (38776). Proc. Soc. Exp. Biol. Med., 149:219-222.

16. Duff, R., Doller, E., and Rapp, F. (1973): Immunologic manipulation of metastases due to herpesvirus transformed cells. Science, 180:79-81.
17. Renoux, G., and Renoux, M. (1974): Modulation of immune reactivity by phenylimidothiazole salts in mice immunized by sheep red blood cells. J. Immunol., 113:779-790.

Control of Neoplasia by Modulation of the Immune System, edited by M. A. Chirigos. Raven Press, New York 1977.

IMMUNOPOTENTIATION IN A HERPESVIRUS MODEL: AN OVERVIEW

*,**Gerald W. Fischer, *Martin H. Crumrine, *,**Melvin W. Balk, **Sandra P. Chang, and **Yoshitsugi Hokama

*Department of Pediatrics and Clinical Investigation Service, Tripler Army Medical Center, Honolulu, Hawaii 96819, and **Department of Pathology, John A. Burns School of Medicine, University of Hawaii, Honolulu, Hawaii 96822

INTRODUCTION

Levamisole[1] (LMS) is a synthetic anthelmintic demonstrated in 1971 by Renoux and Renoux (1) to alter immunologic responses of mice. Since that initial report, many studies of the immunologic action of this drug have been conducted (2-5). We have previously reported the effect of LMS in suckling rats challenged with bacterial pathogens (6). During the past 2 years we have been studying the effect of LMS in a model of herpes simplex type 2 (HSV2) encephalitis in suckling rats.

A viral model was chosen for study because viruses not only cause morbidity and mortality from acute infections (7), but also produce chronic or latent infections that may be either recurrent or slowly progressive (8). Current evidence suggests that some viruses may be the etiologic agent producing certain neoplastic diseases such as Burkitt's lymphoma and cervical carcinoma. Viruses are also considered to play a role in auto-immune disease such as systemic lupus erythematosus (SLE) (9). The herpes virus group is currently among those viruses reported to produce several different disease forms (7,10) and was therefore chosen as an ideal organism to study.

Suckling rats instead of adult animals were used in these studies because of their immature immune status (11,12). Since some viral diseases often occur as the result of immunologic impairment or suppression (13), the naturally deficient immune system of neonatal animals seemed suitable for

---

[1] Levamisole for purposes of this chapter will be used synonymously with tetramisole.

these studies. Normal immunologic maturation and the effectiveness of LMS could be studied in this model without adding extrinsic agents to suppress the immune system.

This report is an overview of several studies conducted by the authors on the effect of LMS in a suckling rat model of HSV2 encephalitis (14-16).

MATERIAL AND METHODS

Animals

Ten-day-old Wistar rats were utilized in these studies. All animals were either obtained from a commercial breeder or were from our own animal colony. With the exception of treatment regimens, all animals were handled in a similar manner and housed in polycarbonate solid-bottom cages with commercial hardwood bedding. Standard laboratory chow and water were provided ad libitum.

Virus

Herpes simplex type 2 was obtained from the Center for Disease Control, Atlanta, Georgia. The virus was passed twice in RK-13 cells, pooled, and then aliquoted into smaller volumes prior to freezing at -70° C for storage (titer, 10^3 to 10^4 $TCID^{50}$/ml). Eagles minimal essential media, containing 2% fetal bovine serum, 100 units of penicillin/ml, and 50 µg of streptomycin/ml was used for propagation and maintenance of all viral tissue cultures. Infection was induced by intraperitoneal injection of 0.02 ml of HSV2 on the tenth day of life.

Drug

Levamisole (Janssen R & D, Inc.), 1 mg/ml, was given subcutaneously at a dose of approximately 3.0 mg/kg per dose.

Systemic Infection and LMS

Suckling Wistar rats were challenged with HSV2 on the tenth day of life. LMS was given either the day before, simultaneous with, or the day after viral challenge. All LMS-treated animals received a second dose 24 hr after the initial LMS injection. Littermate controls received normal saline as a placebo. All animals were observed two months for survival.

Combined LMS and Adenine Arabinoside

Seventy-seven suckling rats received HSV2 on the tenth day of life. With the exception of 11 controls, all animals received a subcutaneous injection of adenine arabinoside (Ara-A), 500 mg/kg per dose, 48 and 72 hr after viral inoculation and placed in either an early or late LMS treatment group. The first group of animals were given LMS 4 and 24 hr after viral challenge. In this group, Ara-A was given following LMS in an attempt to eradicate any virus remaining after immunotherapy. The second group of animals received the drugs by the same routes, but Ara-A was given first to reduce the viral load, and then followed by LMS 4 and 24 hr after the last Ara-A dose. The two drugs were injected at separate anatomical sites to reduce the possibility of any direct effect that the drugs might have on each other. Eleven control animals were given HSV2 and normal saline as a placebo. Since in the previous studies all deaths occurred 8 to 10 days after viral challenge, animals were observed for 2 weeks to determine survival in all subsequent studies.

Antibody Response with LMS and Ara-A

A third study was conducted comparing placebo treatment to LMS alone, Ara-A alone, and Ara-A combined with LMS. All animals, including controls, received HSV2 on day 10, and all dosage and routes of injection were given exactly as before. Serum was taken 14 days after challenge from all animals surviving and pooled with littermate's serum to determine if LMS enhanced the antibody response to HSV2.

Splenectomy and LMS

Five-day-old rats were divided into three groups: splenectomized; sham surgery; or no surgery, these animals being controls. Levamisole treatment and viral challenge were given on the tenth day of life as before. One group of eight animals was also splenectomized, but did not receive virus or levamisole to determine the effect of splenectomy alone on survival.

RESULTS

Systemic Infection and LMS

Fifty-nine of 146, or 40%, of LMS-treated animals survived compared with only 3/136, or 2%, of placebo-treated rats (Table 1). Treatment delayed 24 hr after HSV2 injection was not significantly different from simultaneous or pretreatment with LMS. Survivors demonstrated no signs of herpes infection, while the rats that died developed a hunched posture and generalized seizures 5 to 6 days after viral challenge. LMS did not show any antiviral or cytotoxic activity in vitro against the study organism at a concentration of 100 µg/ml.

Combined LMS and Ara-A

The combination of Ara-A and LMS was not beneficial. There was no significant difference between the treatment regimens, and only 5/66, or 8%, of the animals were alive when the study was terminated at 14 days (Table 1). Using the combined therapy of levamisole and Ara-A, increased survival was not attained, thus suggesting antagonism. In the third study, utilizing both LMS and Ara-A, 11 of 36, or 31%, of LMS-treated animals survived, compared to 1/22, or 4% of controls (Table 1). No other group had significant survival, but the addition of Ara-A to LMS therapy dropped the survival to only 4/36, or 11%, again demonstrating apparent antagonism.

TABLE 1. Survival of suckling rats challenged with HSV2

Regimen	Treated		Placebo	
LMS alone				
Pretreatment	26/63	(41%)	0/62	(0%)
Simultaneous	11/20	(55%)	0/19	(0%)
Posttreatment	22/63	(35%)	3/55	(5%)
Combined total	59/146	(40%)	3/136	(2%)
LMS plus Ara-A				
LMS pretreatment	2/29	(7%)	0/11	(0%)
LMS posttreatment	3/37	(8%)	0/11	(0%)
Combined total	5/66	(8%)	0/11	(0%)
LMS and Ara-A				
LMS alone	11/36	(31%)	1/22	(4%)
Ara-A alone	7/34	(21%)	1/22	(4%)
LMS plus Ara-A	4/36	(11%)	1/22	(4%)
LMS and splenectomy				
LMS and no surgery	4/9	(44%)	—	
LMS and sham	12/22	(54%)	—	
LMS and splenectomy	2/29	(7%)	—	
Placebo and splenectomy	—		2/11	(18%)
Splenectomy alone [a]	7/8	(88%)	—	

[a] These animals were splenectomized, but received no viral challenge or therapy.

Antibody Response with LMS Ara-A

Antibody, as measured by the complement fixation test, was detected in all treatment groups except for the animals receiving LMS alone. Although LMS-treated animals had significantly increased survival, antiherpes complement fixation antibody was not demonstrated at a level of 1:8 in any of the three littermate groups. Antiherpes neutralizing antibody was not found in any of the groups.

Splenectomy and LMS

Levamisole therapy was ineffective in splenectomized animals. There was a distinct difference between the onset of clinical disease in the splenectomized rats when compared to the sham and control animals. Seizure activity was noted as early as 2 days after viral challenge in the splenectomized animals, but did not occur before 4 days in animals with intact spleens.

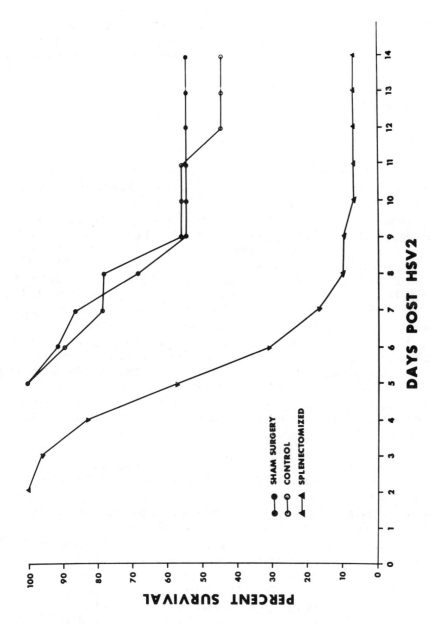

FIG. 1. Effect of splenectomy on LMS therapy in suckling rats challenged with herpes simplex virus.

Mean survival time was significantly less in splenectomized rats when compared to normal or sham animals ($p < 0.01$; using Student's t-test). Deaths were first noted on the fourth day following viral challenge in splenectomized animals, but did not occur until the sixth day in control or sham animals (Fig. 1). At 14 days, survival of control animals was not significantly different from animals that received sham surgery, 44% and 54%, respectively, but there was a significant difference between sham and splenectomized animals ($p < 0.05$) (Table 1). Of the eight animals that were splenectomized but did not receive virus, one died within 24 hr following surgery. This was considered a technical failure. The remaining seven animals were healthy throughout the study period.

DISCUSSION

Immunopotentiation therapy with LMS significantly increased survival in this suckling rat model of HSV2 encephalitis. Antiherpes antibody was not detected in animals receiving LMS alone, but was present in the other treatment groups. This might indicate that LMS decreased antibody formation or B-lymphocyte activity. This may be mediated through T-lymphocytes in the spleen. If LMS stimulates splenic regulator T-cells to repress B-cell activity and enhances antiviral T-cell activity to eradicate the virus, then all of the present data in this model are compatible. The fact that Ara-A inhibited the protective effect of LMS and that animals treated with Ara-A and LMS had antiherpes antibody indicates that B-cell repression is blocked by Ara-A. To test this hypothesis, spleens were removed from normal 10-day-old rats and the spleen cells studied in vitro. The effects of LMS, Ara-A, the combination of Ara-A and LMS, and control conditions on tritiated thymidine uptake were observed in cell cultures. In the 24-hr cultures LMS significantly increased tritiated thymidine uptake, whereas Ara-A suppressed it. This enhanced DNA synthesis by LMS has been repeated several times by our laboratory and did not occur with liver, thymus, or peripheral blood cells. It also did not occur in animals that had reached 30 days of age, thus it may represent, in part, accelerated immunologic maturation. Immature spleen cells appear to be the target cells for LMS activity in this model.

More recent information obtained by adding tritiated LMS to suckling rat spleen cell cultures, before and after exposure to a glass surface, indicates that labeled LMS is detected in both adherent and nonadherent cells. Adherent cells (considered macrophages) become rapidly labeled in 6 to 12 hr, while the nonadherent cells (lymphocytes) slowly increase incorporation of radioactivity over 24 hr. These data suggest that in this model LMS provides enhanced protection by stimulating antiviral (killer) T-cells and suppressor T-cells that inhibit B-cell activity. This hypothesis is summarized in Fig. 2. Splenic macrophages also appear to be involved in LMS protection of suckling rats. This action may be either by direct antiviral activity or by mediating the lymphocyte response.

Levamisole appears to have an effect on splenic lymphoid cells and in this manner regulates immunologic activity in viral diseases. It may also be of

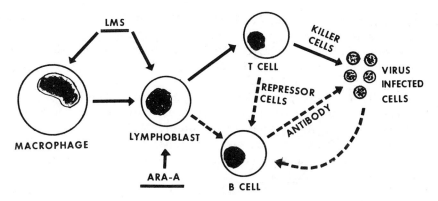

FIG. 2. Proposed mechanisms of LMS protection and Ara-A inhibition.

benefit in treating a variety of immunologic disease processes. In this model, the decrease in antibody formation may be beneficial if the antibody produced a blocking phenomenon and inhibited antiviral T-cells from effectively
destroying the virus. Levamisole inhibition of "blocking" antibodies in neoplasia therapy or antibodies directed against "self" in autoimmune diseases,
such as a systemic lupus erythematosus, would also be advantageous. Stimulation of T-cells and macrophages might also provide effective therapy in a
broad number of diseases such as acute and chronic viral infections and
immunodeficiency states.

A precautionary statement, however, should not be neglected. One must
not move too rapidly from animal studies to human application, without care-
fully controlled trials. Drug actions may be different and detrimental.
Evidence from our laboratory indicates that LMS may accentuate experimental
allergic encephalitis.

SUMMARY

Immunopotentiation therapy with levamisole significantly increased survival in this experimental model of neonatal herpes simplex type 2 encephalitis. The protective effect of levamisole, however, was inhibited by adenine
arabinoside and splenectomy. Present data suggest that levamisole may
initially act on macrophages followed by proliferation of T-lymphocyte
populations, i.e., antiviral T-lymphocytes and regulator T-lymphocytes that
repress B-cell function. Levamisole may be a valuable immunopotentiating
agent for treating diseases of viral origin and other diseases in which cell-
mediated immunity plays a vital role.

REFERENCES

1. Renoux, G., and Renoux, M. (1971): Immunostimulant effect of an
    imidothiazole in the immunization of mice infected with Brucella abortus.
    C. R. Acad. Sci., 272:349.

2. Verhaegen, H., DeCree, J., DeCock, W., and Verbruggen, F. (1973): Levamisole and the immune response. N. Engl. J. Med., 289:1148.

3. Hoebeke, J., and Franchi, G. (1973): Influence of tetramisole and its optical isomers on the mononuclear phagocytic system. J. Reticuloendothel. Soc., 14:317-323.

4. Hirshant, Y., Pinsky, C., Marquardt, H., and Oettgen, H. F. (1973): Effects of levamisole on delayed hypersensitivity reactions in cancer patients. Proc. Am. Assoc. Cancer Res., 14:109.

5. Tripodi, O., Parks, L. C., and Brugmans, J. (1973): Drug-induced restoration of cutaneous delayed hypersensitivity in allergic patients with cancer. N. Engl. J. Med., 289:354.

6. Fischer, G. W., Oi, V. T., Kelley, J. L., Podgore, J. K., Bass, J. W., Wagner, F. S., and Gordon, B. L. (1974): Enhancement of host defense mechanisms against Gram-positive infections with levo-tetramisole (levamisole) in neonatal rats. Ann. Allergy, 33:193-198.

7. Oxbury, J. M., and MacCallum, F. O. (1973): Herpes simplex virus encephalitis: Clinical features and residual damage. Postgrad. Med. J., 49:387-389.

8. Bellanti, J. A. (1971): Immunology, chap. 11, pp. 269-291. W. B. Saunders Co., Philadelphia.

9. Schwartz, R. S. (1975): Virus and systemic lupus erythematosus. N. Engl. J. Med., 293:132-136.

10. Rawls, W. E., Tompkins, W. A. F., and Melnick, J. L. (1970): The association of herpesvirus type 2 and carcinoma of the uterine cervix. Am. J. Epidemiol., 91:547.

11. Argyris, B. F. (1968): Role of macrophages in immunologic maturation. J. Exp. Med., 128:459.

12. Braun, W., and Lasky, L. J. (1967): Antibody formation in newborn mice instituted through adult macrophages. Fed. Proc., 26:642.

13. Ch'ien, L. T., Cannon, N. J., Charamella, L. J., Dismukes, W. E., Whitley, R. J., Buchanan, R. A., and Alford, C. A. (1973): Effect of adenine arabinoside on severe herpesvirus hominus infections in man. J. Infect. Dis., 128:658-663.

14. Fischer, G. W., Podgore, J. K., Bass, J. W., Kelley, J. L., and Kobayashi, G. Y. (1975): Enhanced host defense mechanism with levamisole in suckling rats. J. Infect. Dis., 132:578-581.

15. Fischer, G. W., Balk, M. W., Crumrine, M. H., and Bass, J. W. (1976): Immunopotentiation and antiviral chemotherapy in a suckling rat model of herpesvirus encephalitis. Suppl. J. Infect. Dis., June.

16. Fischer, G. W., Balk, M. W., and Crumrine, M. H. (1976): In preparation.

Control of Neoplasia by Modulation of the Immune System, edited by M. A. Chirigos. Raven Press, New York 1977.

EFFECT OF LEVAMISOLE ON A LETHAL PSEUDOMONAS INFECTION MODEL IN THE RAT

Andrew M. Munster

Department of Surgery, Medical University of South Carolina, and the Veterans Administration Hospital, Charleston, South Carolina 29403

INTRODUCTION

Patients with thermal burns are uniquely susceptible to potentially lethal sepsis by Pseudomonas aeruginosa. These patients also manifest suppression of several immunological defense mechanisms, of which impairment of cell-mediated immunity and of neutrophil function are the best documented (1,2). The advent of a potentially immunostimulatory agent such as levamisole is therefore of great interest in this area.

Our laboratory has for several years been working with a standardized mortality model using the burned rat inoculated with Pseudomonas aeruginosa (3). We evaluated the effects of treatment with levamisole on this model.

MATERIALS AND METHODS

Basic Model

Sprague-Dawley rats weighing 180 to 220 g were inflicted a standard scald burn to a precalculated area of the total body surface according to the method of Walker and Mason (5). They were then inoculated on the burn surface with varying doses of Pseudomonas aeruginosa strain 8283 or 1244. These strains, originally obtained from the U.S. Army Institute of Surgical Research, are now carried in our laboratory. This model yields a mortality rate precisely related both to dose and to the interval between burn and inoculation (3).

Levamisole

Powdered levamisole was obtained through the courtesy of Janssen R&D, Inc., New Brunswick, New Jersey. The powder was dissolved in

115

pyrogen-free distilled water and administered intraperitoneally in doses of 1 to 4 mg daily, according to the experiment.

Supernatants from Cultured Spleen Cells

The technique for the preparation of this material has been detailed elsewhere (4). Briefly, Sprague-Dawley rats were immunized by several weekly injections of phenol-killed Pseudomonas, then the spleens were harvested. Spleen cells were cultured in the presence of killed Pseudomonas, and the 24-hr supernatants of culture used for injection in doses of 1 to 2 ml i.p. daily. These supernatants, which have been exhaustively investigated by us previously, are felt to contain soluble products of thymic-dependent splenic lymphocytes.

Phagocytosis

The technique for determining phagocytic indices was a modification of the method of Sbarra et al. (6). Briefly, leucocytes were harvested from the peritoneal cavity of Sprague-Dawley rats injected 18 hr previously with 10 ml of 12% sodium caseinate. This preparation yields greater than 90% granulocytes. After washing and estimation of viability, 5×10^6 leucocytes were incubated with 10^5 bacteria, autologous serum, and media for 90 min. Control cultures contained bacteria, serum, and media without leucocytes. The phagocytic index was expressed as the percentage of viable bacteria remaining in the medium of experimental compared with control cultures.

Experimental Groups and Statistical Analysis

Each group consisted of 8 to 12 animals and an equal number of controls. Mean day of death was compared by Student's t-test where the experiment consisted of one experimental and one control group, or analysis of variance where it consisted of several groups. The absolute number of surviving rats was compared between groups by χ^2 analysis.

RESULTS

Results are shown in Tables 1-4. The mortality rate for all groups was between 60 and 100%. The shortest mean survival was in the control group inoculated immediately postburn with 10^8 Pseudomonas 8283 (3.8 ± 0.3 days, Table 1). The longest survival was in the control group inoculated 18 hr postburn with Pseudomonas 1244 (18.1 ± 1.4 days, Table 3). None of the experimental groups, however, when matched with their appropriate controls, showed either significant reduction in mortality or significant delay in the mean day of death. The generally longer survival times in the groups shown in Table 2 can be attributed to a somewhat smaller burn size in this group. The prolonged survival rates of the groups in Table 3 are due to the

TABLE 1. The effect of treatment begun 4 hr after infection (burn size: 20%)

Organism and dose		Treatment	Day of death $\pm$ SE	Percent mortality
8283	10^8	Levamisole 1 mg X 6	3.8 $\pm$ 0.3	100
		Control	4.1 $\pm$ 0.4	100
1244	10^8	Levamisole 1 mg X 6	6.2 $\pm$ 0.4	100
		Levamisole 1 mg X 6		
		+ supernate 2 ml X 6	7.3 $\pm$ 0.4	70
		Supernate 2 ml X 6	5.9 $\pm$ 0.3	100
		Control	6.2 $\pm$ 0.4	100
1244	10^7	Levamisole 1 mg X 10	9.3 $\pm$ 0.8	80
		Levamisole 1 mg X 10		
		+ supernate 2 ml X 10	8.0 $\pm$ 0.9	90
		Supernate 2 ml X 10	7.7 $\pm$ 0.4	100
		Control	7.6 $\pm$ 0.5	100

TABLE 2. The effect of treatment begun 1 hr before infection
(burn size: 15%)

Organism and dose		Treatment	Day of death $\pm$ SE	Percent mortality
1244	10^7	Levamisole 1 mg X 5	10.9 $\pm$ 0.7	100
		Levamisole 2 mg X 5	11.6 $\pm$ 0.8	100
		Levamisole 4 mg X 5	11.6 $\pm$ 1.3	100
		Control	13.0 $\pm$ 1.0	90

TABLE 3. The effect of treatment begun 18 hr before infection
(burn size: 20%)

Organism and dose	Treatment	Day of death $\pm$ SE	Percent mortality
1244 10^7	Levamisole 1 mg X 5	17.6 ± 1.4	60
	Levamisole 2 mg X 5	17.9 ± 1.2	100
	Control	18.1 ± 1.4	70

TABLE 4. Phagocytic indices (Pseudomonas 1244 only — Experimental
Groups correspond to Table 1)

Group	Index (%)
Control — no treatment	100
Control — burn only	90
Control — burn, infected with 10^8 organisms	90
Levamisole plus supernate	98
Levamisole alone	94
Supernate alone	76

prolongation of the burn-inoculation interval to 18 hr, which is in accordance with the basic model.

The phagocytic indices are shown in Table 4. Indices from rats which had undergone various modalities of treatment did not differ statistically from one another or from untreated controls. This was not unexpected, however, since the basic model had a phagocytic index of 90% — the particular strain of Pseudomonas used for this experiment, namely 1244, is well phagocytized in the burned rat. The other strain, 8283, which is phagocytized only to the extent of about 50% in the burned rat, was not tested in these particular studies.

DISCUSSION

The failure of levamisole to alter the mortality of Pseudomonas-infected, burned rats is difficult to interpret, since the precise mechanism of host defense against Pseudomonas is not known. Initially, it is probable that activation of the alternate complement pathway occurs. This is followed by complexing with IgM antibody early in the course of infection; later, under the influence of helper T-cells, IgG production increases and complexing occurs with IgG antibody. The bacterium-complement-antibody complex is phago-cytosed by the granulocyte, where final disposition of the infecting agent occurs. Of these steps, the effect of levamisole has been best studied in cell-mediated immunity (7,8), but the relevance of cell-mediated immunity in host defense against Pseudomonas is uncertain. Even in the case of cell-mediated immunity, there are reports indicating that levamisole may have little effect (9). There is some evidence that levamisole is most effective when used as pretreatment after the immunosuppressive event but prior to infection. We attempted to reproduce this situation in our experiments with little benefit.

In conclusion, using a model of Pseudomonas infection in the burned rat, no reduction of mortality could be demonstrated with levamisole therapy.

SUMMARY

The effect of levamisole [L-2,3,5,6-tetrahydro-6-phenylimidazo-(2,1-6)-thiazole, NSC-177023] on the mortality of burned rats infected with Pseudomonas aeruginosa was studied. Levamisole was administered in three separate dose schedules with treatment beginning either before or after infection. In two groups, levamisole was combined with supernatants from cultured immune spleen cells. In a further group, phagocytic indices of granulocytes from levamisole-treated animals were studied. No significant differences from controls could be demonstrated in any group.

ACKNOWLEDGMENT

I am indebted to Dr. Karl Eurenius for the determination of phagocytic indices.

REFERENCES

1. Munster, A. M., Eurenius, K., Katz, R. M., Canales, L., Foley, F. D., and Mortensen, R. F. (1973): Cell-mediated immunity after thermal injury. Ann. Surg., 177:139-143.
2. Alexander, J. W., and Wixon, D. (1970): Neutrophil dysfunction and sepsis in burn injury. Surg. Gynacol. Obstet., 130:431-438.
3. Munster, A. M., Leary, A. G., Spicer, S. S., and Fisher, M. W. (1974): Effect of lymphocytotherapy on the course of experimental Pseudomonas sepsis. Ann. Surg., 179:482-488.
4. Munster, A. M., and Leary, A. G. (1974): Lymphocyte culture products in the treatment of Pseudomonas sepsis in the rat. Surg. Forum, 25:33-34.

5. Walker, H. L., and Mason, A. D. (1968): A standard animal burn. J. Trauma, 8:1049-1051.

6. Sbarra, A. J., Shirley, W., Selvaraji, R. J., Ouchi, E., and Rosenbaum, E. (1964): The role of the phagocyte in host-parasite interactions. I. The phagocytic capabilities of leucocytes from lymphoproliferative disorders. Cancer Res., 24:1958-1968.

7. Woods, W. A., Fliegelman, M. J., and Chirigos, M. A. (1975): Effect of levamisole (NSC-177023) on DNA synthesis by lymphocytes from immunosuppressed C57BL mice. Cancer Chemother. Rep., 59:531-536.

8. Woods, W. A., Siegel, M. J., and Chirigos, M. A. (1974): In vitro stimulation of spleen cell cultures by Poly I, Poly C, and levamisole. Cell. Immunol., 14:327-331.

9. Copeland, D., Stewart, T., and Harris, J. (1974): Effect of levamisole (NSC-177023) on in vitro human lymphocyte transformation. Cancer Chemother. Rep., 58:167-170.

Control of Neoplasia by Modulation of the Immune System, edited by M. A. Chirigos. Raven Press, New York 1977.

LEVAMISOLE AND CYTOXAN IN A MURINE TUMOR MODEL: IN VIVO AND IN VITRO STUDIES

David S. Gordon, Linda S. Hall, and J. Steven McDougal

Clinical Immunology Laboratory, Parasitology Division, Center for Disease Control, Public Health Service, U.S. Department of Health, Education, and Welfare, Atlanta, Georgia 30333

INTRODUCTION

The drug levamisole (LMS) has been under careful scrutiny as an immunomodulatory agent. In animal models LMS has protected newborn rats against bacterial pathogens (1) and a usually lethal dose of herpes virus (2). The drug reportedly can restore antibacterial immunity in animals immunosuppressed by concurrent rickettsial infections (3). In a clinical setting LMS is efficacious in herpes infections (4), aphthous stomatitis (5), and recurrent warts (6).

Metastases from neoplasms induced in weanling hamsters by herpes virus are reduced by LMS treatment (7), and LMS appears synergistic with chemotherapy in a murine leukemia system (8). Of particular interest is the extension of the studies to clinical oncology with preliminary but encouraging results in carcinoma of the breast (9) and lung (10).

This study was designed (a) to evaluate the efficacy of levamisole in chemoimmunotherapy of a murine tumor model in vivo and (b) to evaluate the deviations in the immune system induced by such therapy in the tumor-bearing (TB) animal.

Use of trade names is for identification only and does not constitute endorsement by the Public Health Service or by the U.S. Department of Health, Education, and Welfare.

MATERIALS AND METHODS

Animals

Mice were 6- to 10-week-old F_1 (B10D2/New X Balb/C) hybrids bred in our own facility. Within any given experiment all mice used were of the same sex (usually females). The breeders were purchased from Jackson Laboratories, Bar Harbor, Maine.

Tumor

The tumor used was a methylcholanthrene-induced fibrosarcoma (Meth-A) of the Balb/C mouse originally obtained from the Sloan-Kettering Institute (11). The same "generation" of cells was used for all experiments, and frozen aliquots were thawed and passed once through F_1 hybrids. Tumor cells were harvested at 6 to 9 days, washed, and counted, and 3 to 4 X 10^5 were injected intraperitoneally (i.p.) into each mouse. This dose routinely kills 90% of test animals.

Drugs

Cyclophosphamide (Cytoxan) (Mead-Johnson, Evansville, Indiana) was reconstituted according to the manufacturer's instructions and given at 150 mg/kg per mouse intraperitoneally. Levamisole (LMS) was supplied as a 5% solution by Janssen R&D, Inc. (New Brunswick, New Jersey), diluted in a buffered balanced salt solution (BSS) and given at 10 mg/kg, i.p.

Spleen Cell Suspensions (SCS)

Spleens were harvested from animals killed by cervical dislocation, extensively washed with a pH 7.2 BSS, finely minced with iris scissors over stainless steel screens (60 mesh) in Petri dishes, and washed again with BSS. Remaining clumps were forced through the screen with the plunger of a 5 cm^3 syringe, washed with BSS, harvested from the dishes with a #19 needle on a syringe, and passed through smaller needles to achieve a better suspension. Mononuclear cell counts were done in Turk's solution (1 to 3 X 10^8 cells/spleen) and 0.5% trypan blue (50 to 80% viable). Sterile technique was used throughout for suspensions destined for tissue culture.

Cell Markers — Preparation

SCS were treated with buffered NH_4Cl to lyse red blood cells (RBC), washed three times, incubated with latex (1.1 μm Dow, Inc., Indianapolis, Indiana) at $37^{\circ}C$ for 30 min (final concentration, 0.1%), layered over 100% fetal calf serum, spun at 400 X g, washed, and resuspended to 5 X 10^7/ml.

Rosetting Assays

Erythrocyte-antibody-complement (EAC) cells were prepared by adding the IgM fraction of rabbit antisheep RBC (Cordis Labs, Miami, Florida) to sheep erythrocytes (SRBC) at a subagglutinating dose (1:120), washing and then adding fresh frozen mouse serum as a source complement (1:5 dilution). This reagent was prepared fresh for each experiment, and the EAC cells were added at a 50:1 ratio to the spleen cells (SC) at 37°C for 30 min. After gentle resuspension and addition of a drop of methylene blue (1% in PBS, pH 7.2) to facilitate counting, latex negative SC with three or more attached SRBC were counted as positive.

Erythrocyte-antibody-IgG (EAg) cells were prepared by adding rabbit IgG anti-SRBC (Cordis Labs) to freshly washed 5% SRBC at a subagglutinating dilution (1:600) for 30 min at 37°C. Cells were centrifuged, washed twice, and resuspended to a 2.5% solution. The EAg was added to the SC (60:1), centrifuged at 100 X g for 1 min in the cold, incubated at room temperature for 30 min, and gently resuspended (with the addition of methylene blue). At least 200 latex-negative cells were examined for the presence of three or more attached SRBC. "E" and EA-IgM controls were always included with the rosetting assays.

Fluorescent Assays

Fluorescein isothiocyanate (FITC)-horse antirat thymocyte (HART) anti-serum was supplied by C. Balch (12) and used at 0.02 ml (undiluted/2 X 10^6 SC) in the cold and in the presence of 0.1% sodium azide. This reagent has been absorbed twice with rat kidney, twice with fetal rat liver, and once with nude mouse SC, each time with three parts reagent to one part cells. It stains 100% of mouse thymocytes, and it does not stain mouse bone marrow, nude mouse SC, or rhodamine antimouse immunoglobulin positive normal mouse spleen cells. The FITC-Fc receptor test was an indirect assay using human IgG from Cohn fraction II (Pentex, Miles Lab., Kankakee, Illinois) aggregated according to Dickler (13) and monospecific FITC goat antihuman γ chain (GAHγ) kindly supplied by C. Reimer (CDC). The FITC GAHγ is totally negative with mouse spleen cells when used alone. Cell surface im-munoglobulin (SmIg) was estimated in an indirect assay by using a thymocyte-absorbed rabbit antisera to precipitated mouse immunoglobulin and FITC goat antirabbit Ig (supplied by C. Reimer).

In all fluorescent assays only latex-negative cells were counted. All as-says were carried out on a Leitz epi-illuminated Orthoplan phase-contrast fluorescent microscope equipped with a 100-W HBO mercury lamp and K515 and BG38 suppression filters, a KP500 interference filter, and a K480 edge filter.

Lymphocyte Transformations

Spleen cells were cultured in 1-ml aliquots which contained 2 to 3 X 10^6 spleen cells, 1% human serum or 10^{-4} M 2-mercaptoethanol, RPMI 1640 (HCO_3 buffer), penicillin 100 μm/ml, streptomycin 50 μg/ml, and amphotericin B 2 μg/ml.

Phytohemagglutinin (PHA, 1:4,000 final concentration, Difco, Detroit, Michigan), Concanavalin A (Con A, 1 to 5 μg/culture, Pharmacia, Piscataway, New Jersey), and Pokeweed mitogen (PWM, 1:50 final concentration, Grand Island Biological, Grand Island, New York) were used as mitogens when appropriate. All cultures were pulsed with 1 μCi of tritiated thymidine (6.7 Ci/mole, New England Nuclear, Boston, Massachusetts) after 60 hr incubation (5% CO_2, 37°C) and harvested at 72 hr, with 5% TCA and absolute methanol washes. The pellets were solubized in NCS (Amersham Searle, Arlington Heights, Illinois) at 50°C for 30 min and counted in a toluene-based fluor on a Beckman 350 LS scintillation counter.

Antibody Responsiveness

Primary SRBC antibody responses were obtained by immunizing animals with 5 X 10^8 SRBC IP 4 days before spleen cell harvesting. Secondary SRBC responses were obtained by immunizing 25 days before harvest and again 4 days before harvest.

Direct (IgM) anti-SRBC plaque-forming cells (PFC) were assayed by the Cunningham-Szenberg modification of the Jerne technique (14). Indirect (IgG) PFC were assayed by inhibiting direct PFC with rabbit antimouse μ chain antisera and developing IgG plaques with rabbit antimouse γ chain antisera (15).

Overall Schema

The day of tumor transplantation was designated as day 0. Some control animals did not receive Cytoxan or LMS, other control animals received only Cytoxan on day 2. All test animals received Cytoxan on day 2 and LMS. All test animals were given LMS on day 4, 6, or 9, or on days 4, 5, and 6. Additional controls included animals bearing the transplanted tumor that did not receive Cytoxan but were given LMS on the same days as the test animals. Primary PFC responses were obtained by immunizing on day 10. Secondary PFC responses were obtained by immunizing 10 days before tumor transplantation and again on day 10. Spleens were always harvested on day 14 for all in vitro assays. The in vitro assays were done on the spleens of test animals given Cytoxan on day 2 and LMS on day 9 as well as the spleens of the corresponding controls.

RESULTS

In Vivo

In six repeated experiments, an increase in the duration of survival of TB animals has been observed. In three separate experiments we have also seen synergistic effects when levamisole (LMS) is used in concert with Cytoxan. A typical example is shown in Fig. 1.

Multiple doses of LMS (days 4 to 6) after Cytoxan treatment have been equally effective but not more effective than single doses. In no instance has LMS alone affected the mean survival time.

Cell Markers

Cell marker studies have not been particularly helpful. Spleens of animals harvested 12 days after Cytoxan treatment are larger than those of controls without tumors or of controls with untreated tumors. This is shown by an increase in weight as well as an increase in cell numbers recovered from the suspensions. In general the percent of $SmIg^+$ cells is less, and the percent of $HART^+$ cells is greater in the Cytoxan-treated animals than in the other groups. No other trends are apparent in the Cytoxan-treated animals.

The size of the spleens and cell recovery from them was lower in Cytoxan- and LMS-treated animals or in animals treated with LMS alone than in the corresponding controls. As with Cytoxan there are no apparent differences in the distribution of EAC^+, EAg^+, or FITC-Fc+ cells in the spleens of animals treated with LMS.

Mitogens

Cytoxan-treated animals appear to have an increase in splenocyte spontaneous DNA synthesis. This is true whether animals do or do not have tumors (Table 1). We have frequently seen decreased response to all mitogens 12 days after Cytoxan treatment. The further addition of LMS has had little effect on the PHA response but may help restore the Con A response. The results of one experiment are noted in Table 2.

Antibody Responsiveness

Treatment of normal animals with Cytoxan 8 days before primary immunization with SRBC and evaluation of the spleen cell suspensions 4 days after immunization reveals inhibition of the direct plaque (IgM) response (Table 3). This inhibition is partially corrected by LMS. The secondary IgM response is also depressed by Cytoxan treatment, but we have not consistently seen restoration by the addition of LMS to the treatment regime. The effect of these manipulations on indirect plaque formation (IgG) is less clear.

The more interesting observations, however, relate to TB animals. The primary IgM SRBC response of the TB mouse is markedly inhibited when

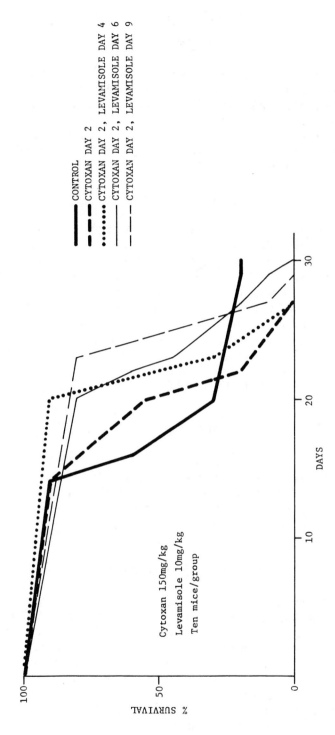

FIG. 1. Survival chemotherapy model of Cytoxan- and/or LMS-treated mice bearing the Meth-A tumor.

TABLE 1. Effects of therapy on the spontaneous DNA synthesis of spleens from tumor-bearing mice and nontumor-bearing untreated littermates

Experiment	Treatment groups				
	I	II	III	IV	V
1	8.1 $\pm$ 0.8	4.5 $\pm$ 1.6	16.6 $\pm$ 1.8	8.6 $\pm$ 0.9	14.3 $\pm$ 2.5
2	5.4 $\pm$ 0.5	12.0 $\pm$ 0.4	11.8 $\pm$ 1.0	—	12.0 $\pm$ 1.1
3	5.5 $\pm$ 0.3	4.5 $\pm$ 0.2	13.1 $\pm$ 1.2	7.6 $\pm$ 0.7	13.9 $\pm$ 0.3
4	6.0 $\pm$ 1.0	—	19.3 $\pm$ 0.7	—	28.0 $\pm$ 0.7

Experiments 1-3: tumor-bearing mice.

Experiment 4: nontumor-bearing mice.

Treatment groups:

> I = non-TB littermates
> II = TB not treated
> III = Cytoxan treated day 2
> IV = LMS treated, day 9
> V = Cytoxan treated day 2, and LMS treated day 9

All cultures carried out with 1% human serum.

Results are means and standard deviations of triplicates in cpm X 10^{-3}.

compared with that of littermates without tumors (Fig. 2). The effects of Cytoxan treatment of the TB mouse have been variable, but Cytoxan-LMS treatment has consistently improved the primary IgM-SRBC response. We have not adequately evaluated the response to LMS alone; therefore the results in Fig. 2 for LMS treatment require confirmation.

The secondary IgM response is also depressed by the tumor-bearing state, as is the secondary IgG response. The response of the Cytoxan-treated TB mouse has always been less than that of the untreated controls without tumors, but the response has been variable when compared with that of untreated TB mouse. The addition of LMS, however, has always partially restored both the IgM and the IgG response (Fig. 3).

TABLE 2. Mitogen responsiveness of tumor-bearing mice and nontumor-bearing littermates — effects of therapy

Group	PHA	Con A (5 µg)	Con A (1 µg)	PWM
Non-TB control	187 ± 11	189 ± 34	330 ± 59	98 ± 30
TB not treated	161 ± 39	174 ± 33	271 ± 15	76 ± 14
TB + Cytoxan day 2	44 ± 7	66 ± 14	209 ± 21	32 ± 6
TB + Cytoxan day 2, LMS day 9	47 ± 4	132 ± 13	222 ± 11	36 ± 3

All cultures carried out with 1% human serum.

Results are means and standard deviations of triplicate samples in cpm X 10^{-3}.

Mitogen concentration noted in text.

TABLE 3. Direct plaque-forming response of nontumor-bearing mice — effects of therapy

Immunization schedule	Treatment groups			
	I	II	III	IV
A	4 ± 7	4 ± 6	4 ± 8	8 ± 7
B	52 ± 23	31 ± 7	47 ± 6	58 ± 5
C	1,831 ± 143	698 ± 81	1,631 ± 78	1,004 ± 92
D	484 ± 33	204 ± 57	342 ± 18	331 ± 162

Treatment groups:

I = no therapy
II = Cytoxan treated, day 2
III = LMS treated, day 9
IV = Cytoxan treated day 2, and LMS treated day 9

Immunization schedule (methods in text):

A = no SRBC control
B = SRBC 10 days before tumor transplant
C = SRBC 10 days after tumor transplant
D = SRBC 10 days before and 10 days after tumor transplant

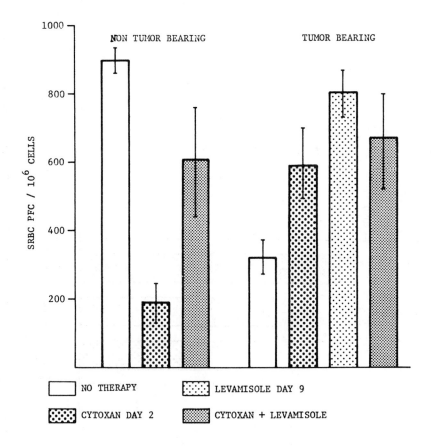

FIG. 2. Primary IgM direct plaque-forming response of tumor-bearing mice and nontumor-bearing littermates (spleen cells) — effects of therapy.

DISCUSSION

We have been able to document the previously reported findings (8, 16) of synergy between LMS and an active antineoplastic agent (Cytoxan) in a murine tumor model, and the lack of effect of LMS when used alone. It is important to recall that these findings are valid only within the rather narrow confines of the experimental design.

We have clearly not delineated the beginning and the end of the effective times to give LMS as adjuvant therapy with the effective chemotherapy. We have also not induced cures, only increases in duration of survival. It is possible that optimization of chemotherapy (dosage, time) and optimization of LMS (time) would lead to a significant number of cures. Furthermore, the response of the host to an i.p. tumor (which grows in suspension) may be quite different from the response to a solid tumor, both in terms of survival and immunologic aberrations. Nonetheless, an adjuvant effect of LMS has been clearly demonstrated and is quite encouraging.

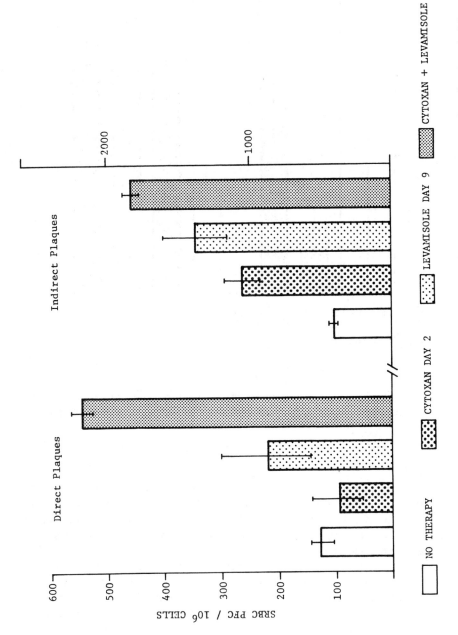

FIG. 3. Secondary IgM (direct) and IgG (indirect) plaque-forming response of treated and untreated tumor-bearing mice (spleen cells).

As functionally documented by Stockman et al. (17), the T-cell compartment in murine spleens recovers more quickly than the B-cell compartment after high-dose Cytoxan treatment. We have observed, using cell marker methodology, an influx of T-antigen positive lymphocytes 12 days after Cytoxan treatment. Unfortunately, we were unable to delineate whether or not the Fc+ subset of T-cells (18,19) was also increased.

We have preliminary data obtained in both the normal and TB animal that suggests increases in splenocyte spontaneous DNA synthesis occurring 5 days after LMS treatment. These results are consistent with the observations of Merluzzi et al. (20) and Woods et al. (21), who studied the blastogenic activity of LMS in vitro, and with other observations (22) of elevated spontaneous DNA synthesis in the spleens of animals treated in vivo with LMS. These results could be explained by recent data which suggest that the effects of LMS on cells may be mediated through modulation of cyclic nucleotides (23).

Perhaps the most remarkable findings relate to the alterations induced in antibody responsiveness by the TB state and to the subsequent changes found after Cytoxan and/or LMS therapy. There can be no question that in our model the presence of tumors is markedly immunosuppressive to the development of a primary or secondary antibody response to a T-dependent antigen and alleviated to some extent by the therapeutic modalities we used.

SUMMARY

Levamisole has an adjuvant effect when used in combination with Cytoxan in a methylcholanthrene-induced transplantable murine sarcoma. In vivo studies have shown an increase in the mean survival time of tumor-bearing mice treated with Cytoxan and an even better survival in mice treated with Cytoxan and levamisole, whereas levamisole without Cytoxan has not increased survival.

Primary and secondary antibody responses to a T-dependent antigen are markedly suppressed by the tumor-bearing state, and significant correction of this deficit is achieved by levamisole therapy. Furthermore, the Cytoxan-induced depression of the spleen cell concanavalin A response is also improved by levamisole. Thus, direct evidence of immunostimulation of a suppressed immune system was obtained with levamisole.

REFERENCES

1. Fischer, G. W., Oi, V. T., Kelley, J. L., Podgore, J. K., Bass, J. W., Wagner, F. S., and Gordon, B. L. (1974): Enhancement of host defense mechanisms against Gram-positive pyogenic coccal infections with levo-tetramisole (levamisole) in neonatal rats. Ann. Allergy, 33:193-198.
2. Fischer, G. W., Podgore, J. K., Bass, J. W., Kelley, J. L., and Kobayashi, G. Y. (1975): Enhanced host defense mechanisms with levamisole in suckling rats. J. Infect. Dis., 132:578-581.

3. Renoux, G., and Renoux, M. (1972): Antigenic competition and non-specific immunity after a rickettsial infection in mice: Restoration of antibacterial immunity by phenyl-imidothiazole treatment. J. Immunol., 109:761-765.

4. Kint, A., and Verlinden, L. (1974): Levamisole for recurrent herpes labialis. N. Engl. J. Med., 291:308.

5. Symoens, J., and Brugmans, J. (1974): Treatment of recurrent aphthous stomatitis and herpes with levamisole. Br. Med. J., 4:592.

6. Helin, P., and Bergh, M. (1974): Levamisole for warts. New Engl. J. Med., 291:1311.

7. Sadowski, J. M., and Rapp, F. (1975): Inhibition by levamisole of metastases by cells transformed by herpes simplex virus type 1. Proc. Soc. Exp. Biol. Med., 149:219-222.

8. Perk, K., Chirigos, M. A., Fuhrman, F., and Perrigrew, H. (1975): Brief communication: Some aspects of host response to levamisole after chemotherapy in a murine leukemia. J. Natl. Cancer Inst., 54:253-255.

9. Debois, J. M. (1975): Trends in survival of patients with breast cancer treated with levamisole. Preliminary communication.

10. Amery, W., Chairman, Study group for bronchogenic carcinoma (1975): Immunopotentiation with levamisole in resectable bronchogenic carcinoma: A double blind controlled trial. Br. Med. J., 3:461-464.

11. Old, L. J., Boyse, E. A., Clarke, D. A., and Carswell, E. A. (1962): Antigenic properties of chemically induced tumors. Ann. N.Y. Acad. Sci., 101:80-106.

12. Balch, C. M., and Feldman, J. D. (1974): Thymus dependent (T) lymphocytes in the rat. J. Immunol., 112:79-86.

13. Dickler, H. (1974): Studies of the human lymphocyte receptor for heat-aggregated or antigen-complexed immunoglobulin. J. Exp. Med., 140:508-522.

14. Cunningham, A. J., and Szenberg, A. (1968): Further improvements on the plaque technique for detecting single antibody forming cells. Immunology, 14:599-600.

15. Pierce, C. W., Johnson, B. M., Gershon, H. E., and Asofsky, R. (1971): Immune responses in vitro. III. Development of primary γM, γG and γA plaque-forming cell responses in mouse spleen cell cultures stimulated with heterologous erythrocytes. J. Exp. Med., 134:395-416.

16. Chirigos, M. A., Fuhrman, F., and Pryor, J. (1975): Prolongation of a chemotherapeutically induced remission of a syngeneic murine leukemia by L-2,3,5,6-tetrahydro-6-phenylmididazo [2,1-b] thiazole hydrochloride. Cancer Res., 35:927-931.

17. Stockman, G. D., Heim, L. R., South, M. A., and Trentin, J. J. (1973): Differential effects of cyclophosphamide on the B and T cell compartments of adult mice. J. Immunol., 110:277-282.

18. Stout, R. D., and Herzenberg, L. A. (1975): The Fc receptor on thymus-derived lymphocytes. II. Mitogen responsiveness of T lymphocytes bearing the Fc receptor. J. Exp. Med., 142:1041-1051.

19. Anderson, C. L., and Grey, H. M. (1974): Receptors for aggregated IgG on mouse lymphocytes. Their presence on thymocytes, thymus-derived and bone marrow-derived lymphocytes. J. Exp. Med., 139: 1175-1188.

20. Merluzzi, V. J., Badger, A. M., Kaiser, C. W., and Cooperband, S. R. (1975): In vitro stimulation of murine lymphoid cell cultures by levamisole. J. Clin. Exp. Immunol. (in press).

21. Woods, W. A., Fliegelman, M. J., and Chirigos, M. A. (1975): Effect of levamisole on the in vitro immune response of spleen lymphocytes. Proc. Soc. Exp. Biol. Med., 148:1048-1050.

22. Woods, W. A., Fliegelman, M. J., and Chirigos, M. A. (1975): Effect of levamisole (NSC-177023) on DNA synthesis by lymphocytes from immunosuppressed C57 BL mice. Cancer Chemother. Rep., 59:531-536.

23. Hadden, J. W., Coffey, R. G., Hadden, E. M., Lopez-Corrales, E., and Sunshine, G. H. (1975): Effects of levamisole and imidazole on lymphocyte proliferation and cyclic nucleotide levels. Cell. Immunol., 20:908.

Control of Neoplasia by Modulation of the Immune System, edited by M. A. Chirigos. Raven Press, New York 1977.

PHASE I TRIAL OF LEVAMISOLE IN PATIENTS WITH NONRESECTABLE BRONCHOGENIC CARCINOMA

J. Leonard Lichtenfeld, Peter H. Wiernik, and Deborah G. Shortridge

Section of Medical Oncology, National Cancer Institute, Baltimore Cancer Research Center, Baltimore, Maryland 21201

INTRODUCTION

Reports that levamisole improved the immune response in animals (1-5) and extension of these observations to human studies in vivo and in vitro (6-10) have prompted considerable interest in this drug as a potentially valuable immune modulating agent, particularly in the treatment of cancer.

Since little information was generally available regarding the clinical toxicities of levamisole, the Baltimore Cancer Research Center performed a modified phase I trial in an effort to define further these toxicities and to investigate the effects of levamisole on a limited number of immunologic parameters in vivo. We also sought to determine whether levamisole had any salutory effect on the natural course of advanced bronchogenic carcinoma, since there were indications that the drug had a beneficial effect when employed as adjuvant therapy in the treatment of resectable lung cancer (11) and advanced breast cancer treated with radiation (12).

The preliminary analysis of this data through October 20, 1975, is presented in this chapter.

METHODS

Twenty-eight patients were entered into this study from June 15, 1974, through October 2, 1975. Twenty-five patients initially had nonresectable primary disease, and 3 additional patients had developed documented recurrent bronchogenic carcinoma following previous surgical resection. No patient had received chemotherapy prior to entering the study, although several had received palliative radiation therapy for symptomatic complications of their disease.

Pertinent characteristics of the patient population are summarized in Table 1. There was a greater than expected number of patients with

TABLE 1. Characteristics of patients with nonresectable bronchogenic carcinoma evaluated in a phase I trial of levamisole

	Intermittent	Continuous	Total
Male/female	10/5	12/1	22/6
Median age (years)	53	60	57.5
(range)	(43-61)	(39-71)	(39-71)
Histology:			
Squamous	5	6	11
Adenocarcinoma	8	4	12
Large cell	2	3	5
Small cell	0	0	0
Disease extent:			
Lung primary			
+/- ipsilateral hilar nodes	2	3	5
Mediastinal nodes,			
supraclavicular nodes or			
pleura/diaphragm	6	2	8
Other organ involvement	7	8	15

adenocarcinoma, with a predominance of this cell type in the intermittent treatment group. Twenty-three of the patients were classified as stage III, with disease extension to the mediastinal nodes or beyond (13).

Pretreatment and serial studies are summarized in Table 2. All patients had a complete history and physical examination prior to beginning levamisole therapy. Routine laboratory studies as listed were performed, including a chemistry profile which consisted of calcium, phosphorus, total protein, albumin, cholesterol, glucose, blood urea nitrogen, total bilirubin, uric acid, alkaline phosphatase, SGOT, and LDH.

Delayed hypersensitivity was measured with five intradermal recall antigens, including dermatophytin "0" (1:100; Hollister-Stier Laboratories, Spokane, Washington), histoplasmin (Parke, Davis and Co., Detroit, Michigan), mumps (2 CFU; Eli Lilly and Co., Indianapolis, Indiana), purified protein derivative (5 TU; PPD; Parke, Davis and Co., Detroit, Michigan), and streptokinase-streptodornase (40 U; SKSD; Lederle Laboratories, Pearl River, New York). All tests were administered across the back in a volume of 0.1 cm^3, and read at 48 hr by measuring induration in two perpendicular diameters. All patients were sensitized de novo with dinitrochlorobenzene (DNCB; Eastman Kodak, Rochester, New York) using a modification of the technique previously described by Catalona et al. (14). Doses of 2,000 and 100 μg of DNCB were sprayed on the medial aspect of contralateral upper extremities in a 2-cm diameter. Patients were observed for 14 days to monitor for the development of spontaneous induration. Those failing to

TABLE 2. Study design of a phase I trial of levamisole

Pretreatment	During treatment		Monthly
	Weekly		
History and physical	X4	then	X
CBC, differential, platelets	X4	then	X
Chemistry profile	X4	then	X
Electrolytes			X
Creatinine			X
Sedimentation rate			X
Reticulocyte count			X
Urinalysis			X
Clotting parameters			X
Chest film			X
Electrocardiogram			X
Immunologic studies			X
Metastatic evaluation	(repeated as indicated)		

develop a spontaneous flare reaction were rechallenged on day 14 with 100 μg of DNCB. This test was read at 48 hr with greater than 50% induration with erythema considered a positive response.

Additional immunologic parameters included serum protein electrophoresis, quantitative immunoglobulins G, A, M, and D measured by standard immuno-diffusion techniques (Kallestad Radial Diffusion Plate, Kallestad Laboratories, Minneapolis, Minnesota), and determination of antibody titers for mumps, rubella, rubeola, tetanus, diphtheria, and blood group antigens.

Metastatic evaluation, which was performed within 2 weeks prior to levamisole treatment, included metastatic bone survey, bone scan, brain scan, liver/spleen scan, and iliac crest bone marrow aspiration and biopsy.

Any patient with grossly abnormal baseline hematologic or biochemical studies or positive marrow biopsy was excluded from study. Patients were evaluated weekly for the first 4 weeks following the initiation of levamisole treatment and then at least monthly until completing levamisole therapy.

Following the completion of pretreatment evaluation, patients were entered consecutively into five progressive dose increments: 15, 45, 90, 120, and 150 mg/m^2 every 12 hr. Six patients were treated at each dose level. Three patients received the drug for 3 consecutive days weekly (intermittent schedule), and the next 3 patients received levamisole on a

TABLE 3.   Total levamisole dose

Dose [a]	N [b]	Intermittent [c]	Continuous [c]
15	3/3	2,600 (600 - 5,550)	7,283 (2,950- 9,900)
45	3/3	17,600+ (4,200-28,800+)	3,908 (3,400 - 4,275)
90	3/3	10,650 (4,200-22,050)	7,966 (3,600-12,600)
120	3/3	19,933+ (17,800-24,000+)	25,200+ (15,300-43,500+)
150	3/1	4,116 (2,100- 6,325)	2,550 (2,550)

[a] Mg/m^2 q 12 hr.

[b] Number of patients intermittent/continuous schedule.

[c] Mean milligrams (range).

daily (continuous) schedule. Levamisole was continued until intolerable toxicity occurred or there was gross evidence of disease progression. The study was discontinued at 150 mg/m^2 when it became evident that dose-limiting toxicity had been achieved.

RESULTS

The total quantity of levamisole administered at each dose level is summarized in Table 3 and ranged from 600 mg total dose to 43,500+ mg.

All 28 patients were evaluated for subjective and objective toxicities of levamisole. These data are shown in Table 4. These toxicities appeared independent of intermittent or continuous administration, except that the 4 days off therapy for the former group did permit some degree of recovery from the subjective effects of the drug.

The most prominent toxicity was gastrointestinal, including anorexia, nausea, and emesis. These effects were observed to some degree with all dose regimens but were particularly severe at 90 mg/m^2 and above. Lethargy and weakness were likewise observed in several patients and were more dose-related than gastrointestinal effects, with extreme debilitation occurring in 3 of 4 patients at the 150 mg/m^2 level. Other less frequent effects included diaphoresis without associated temperature abnormalities, mild metallic taste, dysosmia (absent or aberrant sense of smell), and skin

TABLE 4. Levamisole toxicity

Toxicity	Dose [a]				
	15 (6 pts)	45 (6 pts)	90 (6 pts)	120 (6 pts)	150 (4 pts)
Gastrointestinal (anorexia, nausea, emesis)	3/1/0[b]	0/2/3	0/2/4	2/1/3	0/0/4
Lethargy/weakness	1/0/0	1/0/0	0/1/2	0/2/1	0/0/3
Diaphoresis	0/0/0	0/0/0	0/1/0	1/1/0	1/0/1
Metallic taste	1/0/0	0/0/0	1/0/0	3/1/0	0/0/0
Dysosmia	0/0/0	0/0/1	0/0/0	0/0/2	0/0/0
Rash	1/0/1	0/1/0	0/0/0	2/0/0	0/0/0

[a] Mg/m^2 q 12 hr.

[b] Mild/moderate/severe toxicity.

rash which tended to be mild and nonprogressing despite uninterrupted levamisole therapy. A severe urticarial eruption requiring discontinuation of levamisole occurred in one patient on the 15 mg/m^2 intermittent schedule.

Weight loss was also observed in many patients, apparently due in part to the gastrointestinal effects of levamisole, although the contribution of disease activity cannot be overlooked. Weight loss was greatest in those patients receiving levamisole on the 150 mg/m^2 intermittent schedule and all continuous schedules above 15 mg/m^2.

Hematologic toxicity was observed in 2 patients who developed selective granulocytopenia (Fig. 1). Both received levamisole at the 90 mg/m^2 dose level, with one patient treated intermittently and the other continuously. One patient had recurrent granulocytopenia with resumption of levamisole treatment. Both have subsequently maintained normal white counts since discontinuing levamisole.

No other hematologic, biochemical, clotting, or electrocardiographic changes have been observed which can be directly attributed to levamisole treatment. Many patients developed mild to moderate proteinuria without associated abnormalities in BUN or creatinine.

Twenty-three patients were evaluated for the effects of levamisole on recall and de novo antigen response. Five patients were not included, 1 because of early death and 4 because they failed to complete 1 month of therapy due to drug toxicity.

Levamisole failed to improve recall antigen responses as shown in Table 5. When 10 mm of induration was used as the standard for a positive test, analysis by paired t-test actually showed a significant decrease in the number

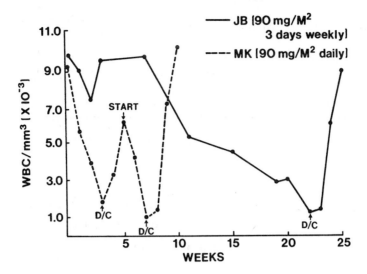

FIG. 1. Granulocytopenia in 2 patients receiving high dose levamisole. WBC returned to normal after drug was discontinued ("D/C") and recurred promptly in the patient who resumed therapy ("START").

of positive tests per patient when evaluated after completing 1 month of treatment. This was observed in patients on each of the dose schedules. When a similar analysis was performed using 5 mm of induration as the criterion for a positive test, no significant increase or decrease in the number of positive tests per patient was observed.

Subsequent serial monthly testing performed while the patient remained on levamisole failed to demonstrate any positive effect of levamisole on recall antigen response when evaluated in the present manner or by mean diameter, median diameter, or maximum diameter.

DNCB responses are reviewed in Table 6. These responses were graded according to the criteria described by Catalona et al. (14). Six of 10 patients who were DNCB-negative (grade 0) before levamisole treatment responded to a 100-μg DNCB challenge following 1 month of levamisole, whereas 4 of these patients remained DNCB-negative. Two of 9 patients who failed to develop spontaneous induration with DNCB but did respond to DNCB challenge before levamisole treatment (grade 2) failed to respond when tested after 1 month of levamisole. Four patients developed spontaneous induration to DNCB at the sites where sensitizing doses were applied (grades 3 and 4), and all of these patients retained their positive response with subsequent testing. Again, no dose or schedule relationship was evident.

No consistent effect on antibody titers, serum immunoglobulin concentrations, or serum proteins has been observed.

Patients who converted their DNCB responses from negative to positive had a significantly longer period of stable disease when compared to those patients who failed to develop reactivity to DNCB as shown in Table 7. No significant effect on survival has been demonstrated.

TABLE 5. Responses to recall antigens in patients treated with levamisole

No. of positive[a] tests	Pre-levamisole[b]	Post-levamisole[b]
0	4	5
1	4	6
2	6	5
3	2	4
4	5	2
5	2	1

[a] ≥ 10 mm induration.

[b] Number of patients.

$p = < 0.05$

For positive test ≥ 5 mm induration: $p = 0.20$

TABLE 6. Responses to DNCB in patients treated with levamisole

Pre-levamisole response[a]	Post-levamisole response to 100 μg DNCB challenge		
	Positive[b]	Negative	p
0	6	4	< 0.01
1	0	0	—
2	7	2	$0.2 > p > 0.1$
3	1	0	—
4	3	0	—

[a] As defined by Catalona et al. (14).

[b] Greater than 50% induration and erythema.

Although the number of patients in each treatment group was small, analysis of the interval to progression for the 3 patients receiving levamisole on the 150 mg/m^2 every 12 hr intermittent schedule revealed a significantly decreased interval (median 9 days; range 9 to 9 days; $p = 0.04$) compared to all other patients receiving levamisole on the intermittent schedule (median 46 days; range 7 to 105+ days) but at lower doses.

Levamisole has had no discernible effect ($p = 0.23$; Gehan modification of the Wilcoxin test) on the survival of patients with nonresectable bronchogenic carcinoma as shown in Fig. 2 when comparing a group of 10 patients whose

TABLE 7. DNCB conversion and disease stability/survival in patients
treated with levamisole

DNCB response						
Pre	Post		Days to			
Levamisole		N[a]	progression[b]	p	Survival[b]	p
(–)	(+)	6	80.5 (31–356+)	0.01	192.5+ (87+–376+)	0.34
(–)	(–)	4	14 (7–23)		93.5+ (42–205)	

[a] Number of patients.

[b] Median days (range).

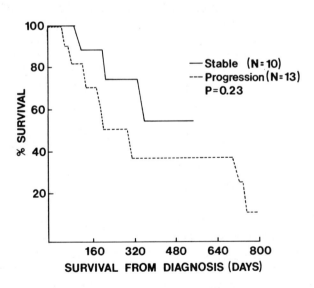

FIG. 2. Effect of levamisole on survival from diagnosis in patients with
nonresectable bronchogenic carcinoma. Levamisole had no effect on
survival for patients with stable disease compared to those with progression
(see text).

disease progressed (i.e., an increase of more than 25% in the sum of the products of two perpendicular diameters of all measured lesions) within the initial 35 days of treatment. No objective disease regression was observed in any patient receiving levamisole.

DISCUSSION

Previous experience with levamisole indicated that this drug could improve DNCB responses in some patients with advanced malignancy (6,7). The potential value of such an agent, which has little serious toxicity and can be administered orally, as an immune modulator in malignancy or other disease states is obvious, particularly when compared to other biologic preparations such as bacillus Calmette-Guerin which have been associated with a moderate degree of morbidity and occasional mortality (15,16).

The present study confirms that levamisole is reasonably well tolerated at a dose of 45 mg/m^2 every 12 hr and at a lower dose schedule of 15 mg/m^2 every 12 hr. Higher doses produced severe weakness and lethargy and, at 150 mg/m^2 every 12 hr, may have influenced the rate of disease progression adversely. It should be noted, however, that these doses are considerably higher than the standard dose of 2.5 mg/kg daily.

Although in vitro evidence has indicated that levamisole can modify the immune response (8-10), no similar effect was observed with the limited measures evaluated in vivo as part of this trial. Although 6 patients did convert their DNCB response from negative to positive, it must be emphasized that this observation did not result from a controlled, double-blind trial and therefore does not permit a firm conclusion that levamisole alone was responsible for this phenomenon. Converters did, however, have a longer interval to progression than nonconverters. Similar effects on survival have not yet been demonstrated.

The toxicities associated with this drug appear to be relatively mild, particularly at the 15 and 45 mg/m^2 dose levels. Gastrointestinal effects were the most prominent, whereas severe debilitation from lethargy and weakness occurred primarily with the higher dose schedules. There was an increase in subjective toxicity with prolonged administration, but this was not limiting at the recommended dose of 45 mg/m^2 every 12 hr. No severe biochemical effects were observed, even in patients who received levamisole in high doses for prolonged periods of time. Hematologic toxicity was limited to selective granulocytopenia in 2 patients as described, and therefore close attention must be given to this parameter when treating patients with levamisole, particularly if used in combination with other known cytotoxic agents.

Results suggesting that levamisole may prolong the disease-free interval following resection of bronchogenic carcinoma have been reported (11). More recent review of the data, however, has not supported this observation, as described elsewhere in this volume (17). Our own experience in patients with advanced nonresectable bronchogenic carcinoma other than small cell treated with levamisole has failed to yield any evidence that levamisole has a meaningful effect on survival in these patients. Numerous studies with available chemotherapeutic agents in this disease have likewise been unrewarding in producing improvement in the quality or duration of survival in treated patients (18).

Classically, immunotherapy has worked best in systems where tumor burden has been maximally reduced either by surgery or chemotherapy, and similar results have been found in at least one animal model treated with combination chemotherapy and levamisole (4). Obviously, the patients in the present toxicity study had evidence of gross disease and there was no possibility of reducing disease burden. It is interesting to note, however, that the patients who apparently benefited most in the previously cited clinical trial (11) were those who had the largest primary tumors which were resectable.

Whether levamisole has activity in the management of malignant disease as adjunctive or primary therapy in combination with cytotoxic agents awaits further controlled clinical trials and evaluation of its activity both in vitro and in animal systems.

SUMMARY

Twenty-eight patients with nonresectable or recurrent bronchogenic carcinoma other than small cell were treated as part of a phase I trial of levamisole. Doses ranged from 15 to 150 mg/m^2 every 12 hr for 3 consecutive days weekly (intermittent) or daily (continuous). Gastrointestinal side effects including nausea, emesis, and anorexia were encountered most frequently, and lethargy and weakness were prominent in patients receiving large doses of levamisole. Additional frequent toxicities included dysosmia, metallic taste, skin rash, and weight loss. Granulocytopenia occurred in 2 patients, with prompt recovery following discontinuation of levamisole. No other major hematologic or biochemical effects were observed. No effect was noted on several measures of in vivo immune response, including recall antigen skin tests, immunoglobulins, or antibody titers. Six of 10 patients who failed to respond to DNCB challenge before levamisole did respond after 1 month of drug treatment, while 2 of 13 DNCB-positive patients became negative to challenge with DNCB after 1 month of levamisole. No effect on the natural course of the disease was observed.

REFERENCES

1. Renoux, G., and Renoux, M. (1971): Immunologie: Effect immunostimulant d'un imidothiazole dans l'immunisation des souris contre l'infection par Brucella abortus. C.R. Acad. Sci. (D), 272:349–350.
2. Renoux, G., and Renoux, M. (1972): Immunologie: action immunostimulante de derives du phenylimidothiazole sur les cellules spleniques formatrices d'anticorps. C.R. Acad. Sci. (D), 274:756–757.
3. Renoux, G., and Renoux, M. (1972): Action du phenylimidothiazole (tetramisole) sur la reaction du greffon centre l'hote. Role des macrophages. C.R. Acad. Sci. (D), 274:3320–3323.

4. Chirigos, M. A., Pearson, J. W., and Pryor, J. (1974): Augmentation of chemotherapeutically induced remission of a murine leukemia by a chemical immunoadjuvant. Cancer Res., 33:2615-2618.

5. Perk, K., Chirigos, M. A., Fuhrman, F., and Perrigrew, H. (1975): Some aspects of host response to levamisole after chemotherapy in a murine leukemia. J. Natl. Cancer Inst., 54:253-256.

6. Tripodi, D., Parks, L. C., and Brugmans, J. (1973): Drug induced restoration of cutaneous delayed hypersensitivity in anergic patients with cancer. N. Engl. J. Med., 289:354-357.

7. Hirshaut, Y., Pinsky, C., Marquardt, H., and Oettgen, H. F. (1973): Effects of levamisole on delayed hypersensitivity reactions in cancer patients (abstr.) Proc. Am. Assoc. Cancer Res., 14:109.

8. Lichtenfeld, J. L., Desner, M. R., Wiernik, P. H., and Mardiney, M. R., Jr. (1976): The modulating effects of levamisole on human lymphocyte response in vitro. Cancer Treat. Rep., 60:571-574.

9. Pabst, H. F., and Crawford, J. A. (1974): Enhancement of in vitro cellular immune response by L-tetramisole (abstr). Pediatr. Res., 8:416.

10. Biniaminov, M., and Ramot, B. (1975): In-vitro restoration by levamisole of thymus-derived lymphocyte function in Hodgkin's disease. Lancet, 1:464.

11. Study Group for Bronchogenic Carcinoma (1975): Immunopotentiation with levamisole in resectable bronchogenic carcinoma: A double blind controlled trial. Br. Med. J., 3:461-464.

12. Rojas, A. F., Mickiewicz, E., Feierstein, J. N., Glait, H., and Olivari, A. J. (1976): Levamisole in advanced human breast cancer. Lancet, 1:211-215.

13. Mountain, C. F., Carr, D. T., and Anderson, W. A. D. (1974): A system for the clinical staging of lung cancer. Am. J. Roentgenol., 120:130-138.

14. Catalona, W. J., Taylor, P. T., Rabson, A. S., and Chretien, P. B. (1972): A method for DNCB contact sensitization: A clinicopathologic study. N. Engl. J. Med., 286:399-402.

15. Sparks, F. C., Silverstein, M. J., Hunt, J. S., Haskell, C. M., Pilch, Y. H., and Morton, D. L. (1973): Complications of BCG immunotherapy in patients with cancer. N. Engl. J. Med., 289:827-830.

16. Aungst, C. W., Sokal, J. E., and Jager, B. V. (1975): Complications of BCG vaccination in neoplastic disease. Ann. Intern. Med., 82:666-669.

17. Amery, W. (1976): Double-Blind Placebo-Controlled Clinical Trials of Levamisole in Resectable Bronchogenic Carcinoma. This Volume.

18. Selawry, O. S. (1974): The role of chemotherapy in the treatment of lung cancer. Semin. Oncol., 1:259-272.

Control of Neoplasia by Modulation of the Immune System, edited by M. A. Chirigos. Raven Press, New York   1977.

PHASE I EVALUATION OF IMMUNE EFFECTS OF LEVAMISOLE

Yashar Hirshaut, Carl M. Pinsky, Susan E. Krown, Harold Wanebo, and Herbert F. Oettgen

Memorial Sloan-Kettering Cancer Center, New York, New York 10021

INTRODUCTION

Levamisole is an agent which is capable of augmenting immune responses and producing tumor regression in experimental animals (1). In man, levamisole has been reported to increase the response to vaccines (2,3), enhance delayed hypersensitivity (4), increase total hemolytic complement (5), and produce a beneficial effect in patients with a variety of non-neoplastic diseases. Among the conditions said to respond to levamisole are aphthous stomatitis (6), recurrent herpes labialis and genitalis (7,8), warts (9), Crohn's disease (10), rheumatoid arthritis (11), and hepatitis (12). Given an agent which is thought to have such a broad spectrum of activity, it is no surprise that levamisole is undergoing clinical trials to determine its effectiveness as an anticancer agent as well. These trials are generally based on the assumption that the optimal dose of the new drug is 150 mg on 3 consecutive days every 2 weeks, and that levamisole has been demonstrated to act as an immunopotentiator in man. In fact, however, the relationships of levamisole dose to toxicity and immune augmentation need to be explored further. To obtain such information, which is necessary for the design of sound clinical studies of levamisole, a phase I investigation has been undertaken. The nature of this study and early results are presented here.

MATERIALS AND METHODS

Study Design

As shown in Fig. 1, there are two phases, acute and chronic. In the acute phase, administration of a single dose of levamisole is preceded and followed by 2 weeks of observation. At three points marked E, extent of disease is

FLOW SEQUENCE FOR PHASE I TRIAL OF LEVAMISOLE

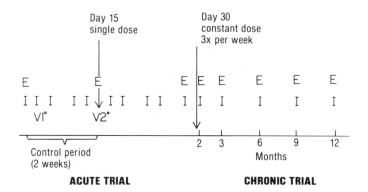

FIG. 1.

evaluated and toxicologic tests are performed. Immune parameters are measured twice weekly. Vaccines are given at the beginning of the control period and 1 hr after the acute drug dose. This initial phase of the study is intended to permit observation of the effects of a single dose, without the superimposed effects of closely spaced subsequent doses. During the chronic trial, levamisole is given 3 times a week. Testing is done regularly but less frequently. Doses are kept constant for each patient throughout the trial but are increased after 3 patients have been entered at a given dose level.

Immune Parameters

The immune parameters followed are shown in Table 1. Humoral immunity is assessed by measuring immunoglobulin levels and B-cells in the peripheral blood. In addition, responses to vaccination and fluctuations in complement levels are noted. The vaccines employed are bivalent influenza virus (purified subvirion) and typhoid (S. typhosa vaccine, U.S.P.), both supplied by Wyeth Laboratories, Inc. Each vaccination is given subcutaneously with a volume of 0.5 ml of vaccine. Patients alternate in the sequence in which they receive these two vaccines, so that each patient serves as a control for the next patient and vice versa. Cell-mediated immunity is evaluated by lymphocyte counts, T-cell enumeration, skin tests for delayed hypersensitivity, and measurements of the proliferative response of lymphocytes in vitro. Quantitation of serum immunoglobulins (IgG, IgA, and IgM) is performed by single radial immunodiffusion using commercial plates.

TABLE 1. Phase I immunotherapy trial: immune parameters

Humoral immunity
  Immunoglobulins: IgA, IgG, IgM
  B-cells (%)
  Response to vaccinations
    S. typhi
    Influenza
  Complement

Cell-mediated immunity
  Lymphocyte count
  T-cells (%)
  Delayed cutaneous hypersensitivity, primary and secondary response
    DNCB
    Mumps, SK/SD
    PPD, Candida
  In vitro mitogen response, nonspecific and specific stimuli
    PHA, concanavalin A, pokeweed, C. Albicans, E. coli, S. aureus,
    tuberculin, SK/SD, mumps, mixed bacterial vaccine

Reticuloendothelial
  Nitroblue tetrazolium
    Resting
    LPS-stimulated

B-lymphocytes are differentiated by a direct immunofluorescence test using a fluoresceinated polyvalent anti-immunoglobulin antiserum (13) to determine the number of lymphocytes positive for surface immunoglobulins. The method for performing EAC rosettes is a modification of the technique of Biando et al. (14) with human A erythrocytes and fresh mouse serum as a source of complement. Ingestion of latex particles is used as a marker for phagocytic monocytes (15). Antibody titers are performed by the Bacteriology Laboratory of Memorial Hospital. The influenza levels are measured by a complement-fixation test using reagents supplied by Microbiological Associates, Inc. Antibody titers to S. typhosa antigens A, B, C, D, and H are determined with an agglutination assay using Lederle, Inc., reagents. Complement and C-complement assays are determined as previously described (16).

    T-rosettes in blood are enumerated by the method of Jondal (17) with minor modifications. Twenty percent human AB serum, absorbed three times with sheep red blood cells, is included in the lymphocyte suspension for the determination of the number of spontaneous rosette-forming lymphocytes with sheep erythrocytes. Skin testing methods used have been described elsewhere (18). Sensitization and challenge with dinitrochlorobenzene (DNCB) is carried out according to the method of Eilber and Morton (19). Patients are tested for preexisting delayed hypersensitivity to common antigens, including dermatophyton-O (1:100, a Candida antigen; Hollister-Stier Laboratories, Yeadon, Pennsylvania), mumps skin test antigen (Eli Lilly and Co., Indianapolis, Indiana), intermediate strength tuberculin (Parke-Davis Co., Detroit, Michigan), and streptokinase/streptodornase (Lederle Laboratories, Pearl River, New York). These antigens are injected interdermally in volumes of 0.1 ml. The tests are read at 48 hr, and considered positive if the diameter of induration is 5 mm or more.

To observe the stimulation of isolated lymphocytes by mitogens and specific antigens, lymphocytes are isolated from heparinized blood on Ficoll-Isopaque density gradients. After washing and resuspension in RPMI 1640 supplemented with glutamine, penicillin, streptomycin, and 15% pooled normal human serum, 0.2 cc of mononuclear cell suspension containing 1×10^5 lymphocytes is incubated in microtiter plates. Transformation of lymphocytes is measured by incorporation of ^{14}C-thymidine. All individual cultures are performed in triplicate. Stimulation with nonspecific mitogens is performed in such a way as to derive a dose-response curve using six different concentrations of PHA-P, four different concentrations of conconavalin A, and three different concentrations of pokeweed mitogen. The standard panel of microbial antigens includes <u>Staph. aureus</u>, <u>Candida albicans</u>, <u>E. coli</u>, Streptokinase-Streptodornase (SK/SD), two highly purified protein derivatives of mycobacterium (PPD), and mumps virus. A dose-response curve using three different concentrations is performed for each antigen. Only the data for PHA-P and pokeweed mitogen are summarized in this chapter.

RESULTS

So far 14 patients have been entered. Doses employed have ranged from 150 to 750 mg or about 90 to 450 mg/M^2. The toxicity observed in this patient group is shown in Table 2. Side effects are clearly more common in patients receiving higher doses. Various manifestations of gastric distress are the most frequent limiting toxicity requiring a decrease in dose. This point is reemphasized in Table 3. It shows the toxic results of levamisole ingestion in 30 patients participating in other protocols. Most of these had received no more than 150 mg per dose. The five most common side effects relate to the gastrointestinal tract.

Measurements made over the period of 1 year in a 17-year-old girl who had a bronchial carcinoid surgically removed are presented graphically in Fig. 2. She has remained free of disease. There was considerable fluctuation in values during the control period. For example, counts per minute following PHA stimulation rose just before the first dose of levamisole was given. After 1 year on a putative immunopotentiator, no dramatic changes are seen except perhaps for the rise in the mitogenic response produced by PHA.

Data concerning the humoral immune responsa are given in Table 4. At 2 weeks following an acute dose of levamisole, 55% (6/11) of patients demonstrated a 10% or greater increase in IgM level. The increase persisted beyond the first month of chronic treatment. Most patients showed only

TABLE 2. Levamisole phase I trials: side effects at doses indicated

	Dose and number of patients affected									
No. of patients:	4		3		3		3	2	2	1
Dose:	150 mg		300 mg		450 mg		600 mg		750 mg	
Side effect	Acute	Chronic	Acute	Chronic	Acute	Chronic	Acute	Chronic	Acute	Chronic
Nausea	—	—	—	—	—	1	1	1	—	1
Vomiting	—	—	—	—	1	—	1	1	—	1
Cramps — abdominal pain	—	—	—	—	—	—	1	1	—	—
Headache	—	—	—	—	—	—	1	—	—	—
Insomnia	—	—	—	—	—	1	—	—	—	—
Lightheadedness	—	—	—	—	—	—	—	1	—	—
Dizziness	—	—	—	—	—	1	—	1	—	—
Weakness	—	—	—	—	—	1	—	1	1	1
Queasiness	—	—	—	—	—	1	—	—	—	—

D.B. PHASE I LEVAMISOLE STUDY

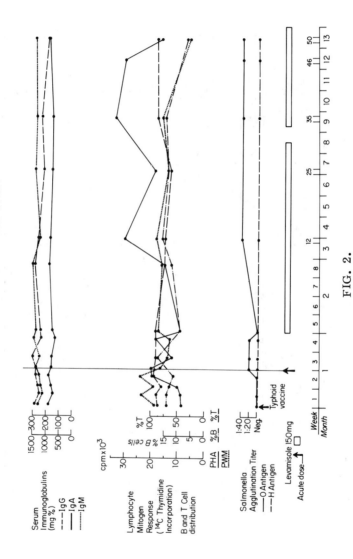

FIG. 2.

TABLE 3. Levamisole trials: side effects

Symptom	Patients		Percent	
	Acute	Chronic	Acute	Chronic
Bitter taste	13	12	43	40
Queasiness	9	11	30	37
Nausea	7	11	23	37
Abdominal cramps	6	5	20	17
Diarrhea	5	5	17	17
Tiredness	5	5	17	17
Vomiting	4	7	13	23
Insomnia	4	5	13	17
Lightheadedness	4	4	13	13
Headache	4	3	13	10
Eructation	3	3	10	10
Dizziness	3	1	10	3
Pruritis	1	1	3	3

Patient number = 30.

minor changes in IgG or IgA levels. There was no correlation between increase in quantity of immunoglobulins and dose size. The response evoked
by the influenza vaccination was poor with or without levamisole. Total
complement, C1q and C3 levels were not affected by levamisole ingestion.
The two most interesting changes following treatment were (a) a rise in the
proportion of circulating B-cells, and (b) a rise in Salmonella "0" antibody
titers. Vaccination with typhoid vaccine appears to be more effective when
levamisole is given at the same time as the vaccine. The respective geometric
anti-"0" titers at 14 days for (a) 5 patients vaccinated 2 weeks prior to treatment and (b) an equal number vaccinated shortly after levamisole ingestion is
27.9 versus 69.2. However, the number of patients is still too small, and
the standard deviations too large, to permit firm conclusions. Little change
was observed in cell-mediated immune reactions, as shown in Table 5.
Lymphocyte counts and T-cell counts were generally stable. No patients
have, so far, converted from DNCB-negative to -positive status. Increased
skin reactivity has also not been observed for common antigens. The response of lymphocytes to mitogens in vitro was unaffected.

TABLE 4. Levamisole phase I trial: humoral immunity

Parameter	Pre-Rx[a]	1 hr	48–72 hr	7 days	14 days	2 months	3 months
IgM, mg%	155	165	194	150	172	157	110
IgG, mg%	1,259	1,320	1,200	1,223	1,393	1,396	1,392
IgA, mg%	377	379	561	400	243	514	289
Percent B-cells	10	11.6	15.8	13.4	17.7	14	12.7
Influenza antibody[b]							
A	3.94	1.70	1.41	4.26	4.83	2.97	8
B	1.88	1.60	1.20	1.45	1.78	1.66	1.41
C	2.88	3.98	1.70	5.37	3.98	2.51	1
Salmonella antibody[b]							
0	11.0	14.7	16.8	34.8	40.0	44.3	14.2
H	11.2	10.0	11.5	21.4	15.2	18.1	16.8
Complement							
Total	114	114	113	117	113	128	109
Clq	24	25	22	24	27	25	24
C3	144	137	177	115	137	118	117

[a] Mean values at indicated intervals.

[b] Geometric mean titer.

TABLE 5. Levamisole phase I trial: cell-mediated immunity

Parameter	Pre-Rx[a]	1 hr	48-72 hr	7 days	14 days	2 months	3 months
Lymphocyte count	1,438	1,477	1,545	1,282	1,290	1,301	1,247
Percent T-cells	76	79	74	71	74	82	90
Delayed hypersensitivity							
DNCB (- to +), %				None			
PPD (- to +), %				None			
Candida (- to +), %	—	8	None	8	8	None	None
Lymphocyte response, in vitro							
PHA (cpm X 10^3)	13.5	13.7	10.8	13.4	12.8	14.7	20.7
Pokeweed (cpm X 10^3)	6.5	5.2	7.8	5.0	6.5	6.3	9.4

[a] Mean values at indicated intervals.

DISCUSSION

Since levamisole produces convulsions in animals at high doses followed by death (20), we have proceeded cautiously in escalating dose levels. So far it is established that 600 mg are tolerated for periods as long as 3 months without serious toxicity. The side effects that appear at this time most likely to limit the tolerated dose are those related to the gastrointestinal tract.

The immunostimulatory effects of levamisole in man remain to be firmly established. Previous findings concerning its effects on augmentation of antibody responses are not consistent (21). Potentiation of delayed hypersensitivity has been described but not confirmed (22). Total complement levels are said to increase in some conditions but decrease in others (23). The current study has not been underway long enough to provide definitive answers. Several observations can be made, however, on the basis of the available data. First, immunopotentiating effects of levamisole vary considerably from individual to individual. This is particularly true in cancer patients, whose immune system may be affected in varying degree by their disease. Second, in those instances where an increase in immune responsiveness has been observed, it was not dose-dependent for any of the measured parameters. Finally, most immunologic changes seen have been subtle. As this phase I study continues it is hoped that careful analysis will reveal components of the human immune system which are affected by levamisole, and that rational trials of levamisole in cancer therapy can be designed on that basis.

ACKNOWLEDGMENTS

This work was supported in part by National Cancer Institute contract no. 1-CB-53970 and grant CA 05826 as well as a grant from the American Cancer Society.

REFERENCES

1. Oettgen, H. F., Pinsky, C. M., and Delmonte, L. (1976): Treatment of cancer with immunomodulators: Corynebacterium parvum and levamisole. Med. Clin. North Am. (in press).
2. Renoux, G., Renoux, M., Morand, P. H., and Dartigues, P. (1973): Action immunostimulante du levamisole sur les personnes agees. Rev. Med. Tours, 7:797-801.
3. Brugmans, J., Schuermans, V., De Cock, W., Thienpont, D., Janssen, P., Verhaegen, H., Van Nimmen, L., Louwagie, A. C., and Stevens, E. (1973): Restoration of host defense mechanisms in man by levamisole. Life Sci., 13:1499-1504.
4. Tripodi, D., Parks, L. C., and Brugmans, J. (1973): Drug-induced restoration of cutaneous delayed hypersensitivity in anergic patients with cancer. N. Engl. J. Med., 289:354-357.

5. Verhaegen, H., De Cree, J., De Cock, W., and Verbruggen, F. (1973): Levamisole and the immune response. N. Engl. J. Med., 289:1148-1149.

6. Verhaegen, H., De Cree, J., and Brugmans, J. (1973): Treatment of aphthous stomatitis. Lancet, 2:842.

7. Kint, A., and Verlinden, L. (1974): Levamisole for recurrent herpes labialis. N. Engl. J. Med., 291:308.

8. Symoens, J., and Brugmans, J. (1974): Treatment of recurrent aphthous stomatitis and herpes infections with levamisole. Br. Med. J., Dec. 1974.

9. Helin, P., and Bergh, M. (1976): Clinical use of levamisole in the treatment of common warts. N. Engl. J. Med. (in press).

10. Bertrand, J., Renoux, G., Renoux, M., and Palat, A. (1976): Maladie de Crohn et levamisole. Unpublished data.

11. Schuermans, Y. (1976): Levamisole in the treatment of rheumatoid arthritis. Unpublished data.

12. Symoens, J. (1974): The effects of levamisole on host defense mechanisms. Physician's handbook. Janssen R & D, Inc. New Brunswick, New Jersey.

13. Pernis, B., Ferrarini, M., Forni, L., and Amante, L. (1971): Immunoglobulins on lymphocyte membranes. In: Progress in Immunology, edited by B. Amos. Academic Press, New York.

14. Biando, C., Patrick, R., and Nussenzweig, V. (1970): A population of lymphocytes bearing a membrane receptor for antigen-antibody-complement complexes. J. Exp. Med., 132:702.

15. Cline, M. J., and Lehrer, R. I. (1968): Phagocytosis by human monocytes. Blood, 32:423.

16. Day, N. K., Geiger, H., Mc Lean, R., Resnick, J., Michael, A., and Good, R. A. (1973): The association of respiratory infection, recurrent hematuria and local glomerulonephritis with activation of the complement system in the cold. J. Clin. Invest., 52:1698-1706.

17. Jondal, M., Holm, G., and Wigzell, H. (1972): Surface markers on human T and B lymphocytes: A large population of lymphocytes forming non-immune rosettes with sheep red blood cells. J. Exp. Med., 136:207.

18. Pinsky, C. M., Hirshaut, Y., and Oettgen, H. F. (1973): Treatment of malignant melanoma by intra-tumoral injection of BCG. National Cancer Monograph 39, pp. 225-228.

19. Eilber, A. R., and Morton, D. L. (1970): Impaired immunologic reactivity and recurrence following cancer surgery. Cancer, 25:362-367.

20. Janssen Pharmaceutica (1974): Safety evaluation of levamisole. Clinical research report on levamisole, no. 15. Janssen Pharmaceutica, Beerse, Belgium.

21. Vertenten, L. (1974): The effect of levamisole on antibody production after primary vaccination against tetatus. Clinical research report on levamisole, no. 29. Janssen Pharmaceutica, Beerse, Belgium.

22. Hirshaut, Y., Pinsky, C. M., Fried, J., and Oettgen, H. F. (1974): Trial of levamisole as immunopotentiator in cancer patients. <u>Proc. Am. Assoc. Cancer Res.</u>, 15:(503)126.

23. Verhaegen, H., De Cock, W., and De Cree, J. (1974): The effect of levamisole on serum complement in patients with neoplastic disease. Clinical research report on levamisole, no. 16. Janssen Pharmaceutica, Beerse, Belgium.

Control of Neoplasia by Modulation of the Immune System, edited by M. A. Chirigos. Raven Press, New York 1977.

CLINICAL ACTION OF LEVAMISOLE AND EFFECTS OF RADIOTHERAPY ON IMMUNE RESPONSE

*Alejandro F. Rojas, *Julio N. Feierstein, *Horacio M. Glait, *Oscar A. Varela, **Roberto Pradier, and *Américo J. Olivari

*Centro Oncológico de Medicina Nuclear, Facultad de Medicina, Universidad de Buenos Aires, Comisión Nacional de Energía Atómica, Buenos Aires, Argentina, and **Servicio de Cabeza y Cuello, Instituto de Oncología "Angel H. Roffo," Universidad de Buenos Aires, Buenos Aires, Argentina

INTRODUCTION

The prognosis in cancer patients has been found to be related to immune competence. This relationship has been used for therapeutic attempts. About 50 years ago, Rénaud observed impaired tuberculin sensitivity in cancer patients (1). The increase in the incidence of lymphoma and other types of tumors in immune-suppressed renal-grafted patients further points to the importance of immunological factors in malignant disease.

Eilber and Morton (2) in 1970 reactivated the interest in the study of the immune system through the use of nonspecific antigens such as dinitro-chlorobenzene (DNCB) as well as recall antigens. They found an important immune defect in patients with either inoperable, recurrent, or metastasic tumors as opposed to those showing long survival, spontaneous regression, or who remained free of disease for more than 6 months. Normal population reacted strongly to DNCB in 95% of cases.

Attenuated or killed bacteria and a variety of microbial products have traditionally been used as immunomodulators; recent studies have shown that synthetic low-molecular-weight compounds, including thiazole derivates (3) and polynucleotides (4), may have an effect on the immune system as well.

Levamisole [L-(-)-2,3,5,6-tetrahydro-6-phenylimidazo-(2,1b)-thiazole hydrochloride], a thiazole derivate, is an agent which has had wide clinical use as antihelmintic (5) with few untoward side effects. In animal studies Renoux and Renoux (6) demonstrated that levamisole increased resistance to infections and stimulated cell-mediated immune reactions. Based on these findings, a clinical trial of levamisole was begun in 1972 in patients with inoperable breast cancer (stage III UICC classification). We report here that treatment with levamisole following radiation therapy increases reactivity to DNCB, prolongs the disease-free interval, and increases survival time.

In addition to the effects of radiation therapy on skin tests, blastic transformation to PHA in whole blood cultures, and peripheral lymphocyte count in a group of head and neck cancer patients, the first results on DNCB responsiveness to two schedules of levamisole administration, 450 and 900 mg/week, are presented.

MATERIALS AND METHODS

Patients

1. Breast cancer: at this Institution, stage III (UICC classification) breast cancer is treated primarily by radiation therapy. No further treatment is given until recurrence of metastasis occurs.

After completion of radiation therapy, alternative patients were assigned either to the control group or to the levamisole-treated group. Forty-three patients were evaluated, 20 in the treated group and 23 in the control group. The treated group received levamisole in one dose of 150 mg orally per day on 3 consecutive days, every other week, until there was evidence of progressing disease. The distribution of the patients in each group according to age, menopausal status, and parity is shown in Table 1, and their distribution according to TNM classification is shown in Table 2.

2. Head and neck cancer: One hundred head and neck cancer patients were studied, 82 males and 18 females, about the effect of radiation therapy on immune reactivity.

3. One hundred ninety-eight patients with different kind of tumors were compared in three groups: 96 in a control group, 64 patients in a classical dosage of levamisole (plan II) — 150 mg in one dose per day for 3 consecutive days every other week — and 42 patients in another plan that we named plan IV — 150 mg in one dose orally per day on 6 consecutive days every other week.

TABLE 1. Age, menopausal status, and parity of patients prior to radiotherapy

	Control	Levamisole
Average age	58.3	60.0
	(39–80)	(34–82)
Average age at menopause	49.1	49.5
	(41–57)	(42–56)
Number of premenopausal patients	3	2
Average number of children	2.2	1.8

(☒) = range.

TABLE 2. Distribution of patients according to TNM classification (UICC)

	Control	Levamisole
T3N1M0	34.8% (8)	30.0% (6)
T3N2M0	26.1% (6)	35.0% (7)
T3N3M0	13.0% (3)	10.0% (2)
T4N1M0	4.3% (1)	5.0% (1)
T4N2M0	17.4% (4)	5.0% (1)
T4N3M0	4.3% (1)	15.0% (3)
Total no. of patients	23	20

($\boxtimes$) = no. of patients.

Skin Tests

1. DNCB: Sensitization with DNCB and challenge was performed after the completion of radiotherapy. Challenge doses of 50 and 100 μg were applied and the reactions were read at 48 hr according to the following scale:

Negative reactions	{ 0 No response
	1 Erythema (E)
Weak positive reactions	2 (E) + induration more than 5 mm (I)
Strong positive reactions	{ 3 (E) + (I) + vesicle
	4 (E) + (I) + bulla

2. Intradermal skin tests: Intradermal skin tests were performed with 0.1 ml of Candida albicans antigen (1:1000) (Lab. Rivero and Co.) and 0.1 ml of PPD (2UT) (Doerr). Reactions were read at 48 hr and graded as follows: Negative (< 5 mm induration), 1+($> 5 < 10$ mm induration), 2+($> 10 < 20$ mm induration), 3+(> 20 mm induration), and 4+ (> 25 mm induration with central necrosis).

Lymphocyte Culture

In vitro lymphocyte reactivity was determined by phytohemagglutinin induction using a modified Park and Good technique (7). Cultures were prepared in triplicate with three different concentrations of PHA: 50, 100, and 150 μg/ml (Bacto-Phytohemagglutinin P, Difco Lab), and controls. Each individual culture contained 50 μl of blood and 50 μl of RPMI 1640. After

TABLE 3.   Comparison of skin test reactivity at completion of
radiotherapy (before) and after 20 months of follow-up

	Control	Levamisole
DNCB		
Before	60.9% (14/23)	60.0% (12/20)
After	42.9% (3/7)	83.3% (15/18)
Candida		
Before	52.2% (12/23)	55.0% (11/20)
After	41.9% (3/7)	77.8% (14/18)
PPD		
Before	21.7% (5/23)	20.0% (4/20)
After	28.6% (2/7)	33.3% (6/18)

(⧄) = (no. of patients with positive tests)/(total no. of patients tested).

% = percent of patients with positive tests.

incubation at 37° C for 24 hr, 0.5 uCi of tritiated thymidine was added
(Amersham Searle, 20 Ci/mM).   Twenty hours later cultures were filtrated
through glass fiber paper (Reeve-Angel) and the incorporated thymidine
quantified in a scintillation counter.

Lymphocyte reactivity was defined as the best average of the three cultures
prepared with any of the concentrations of PHA employed. Values between
control and 4,000 dpm were considered "poor"; "fair" between 4,000 and
9,000 dpm; and "good" over 9,000 dpm.   Non-cancer-bearing control patients
all had values over 9,000 dpm.

RESULTS

Breast Cancer

Table 3 compares the skin reactions to DNCB, C. Albicans, and PPD in
both groups before treatment and after 20 months of follow-up. Levamisole
treatment was associated with an increase in positive DNCB tests as compared with pretreatment reactivity in the same group ($p < 0.01$ by the
McNemar test) or with untreated controls ($p = 0.05$ Fisher's exact test).

In Fig. 1 is shown that levamisole treatment was associated with an increase in the number of strong positive reactions to DNCB 100 µg.

The effects of radiation therapy and levamisole treatment on the absolute
lymphocyte count are shown in Fig. 2. Both groups showed depression of
absolute lymphocyte counts after radiation therapy, although the control
group had a higher mean value prior to therapy. Six months after radiation

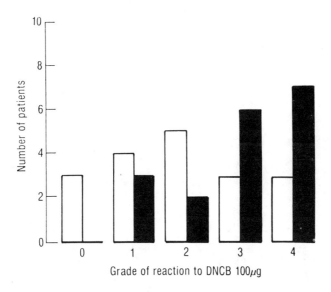

FIG. 1. Grade of reaction to DNCB before (□) and after (■) 20 months of levamisole treatment.

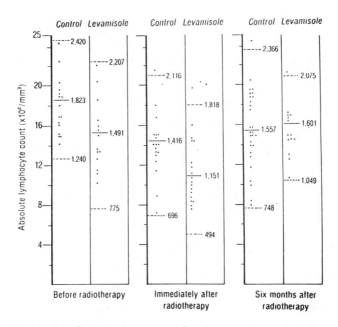

FIG. 2. Effect of radiation therapy and subsequent treatment on absolute lymphocyte count.

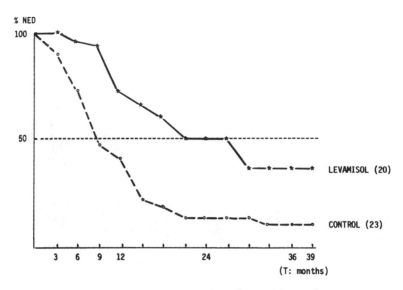

FIG. 3. Disease-free interval by life table analysis.

therapy, the levamisole-treated group had a mean lymphocyte count that exceeded the postradiation mean by 35.6% (p < 0.02 Student's t-test) and was higher than the pretreatment mean; the control patients' count had increased only by 10% and was lower than the pretreatment value for the group.

Figure 3 shows how long patients in either group remained free of disease. Twenty-four months after radiotherapy, 9% of the control patients and 50% of the treated patients showed no signs of recurrence. The median disease-free interval was 8 months for the control group and 21 months for the treated group (p < 0.01, generalized Wilcoxon test). At 39 months, 6.8% of the control patients and 36% of the levamisole-treated patients were free of disease.

Table 4 summarizes the sites and frequency of metastasis in both groups. No difference was found between the two groups except in the case of lung metastasis, which were more frequent in the levamisole-treated group.

Figure 4 shows the disease-free interval of patients who developed metastasis. The median was 9 months in the control group and 12 months in the treated group. No statistical difference was found with the generalized Wilcoxon test (p < 0.06).

Table 5 compares skin test conversion after 20 months of levamisole treatment in patients who developed recurrence and in patients who remained free of disease. An increase in reactivity to DNCB and Candida Albicans was seen in patients who remained free of disease. It can also be seen that those patients who remained with no evidence of disease had no negative reactions and had more than 90% of strong positive reactions.

Figure 5 shows the actuarial curves for the two groups. At 39 months, 55% of the patients treated with levamisole and 18.8% of control patients were alive (p < 0.01 by generalized Wilcoxon test).

TABLE 4.   Comparison of sites of metastasis

Site of metastasis	Control	Levamisole
Local recurrence	28.6% (6/21)	18.2% (2/11)
Skin	14.3% (3/21)	9.1% (1/11)
Nodes	23.8% (5/21)	18.2% (2/11)
Lungs	19.0% (4/21)	72.7% (8/11) [a]
Bones	38.1% (8/21)	27.3% (3/11)
Liver	19.0% (4/21)	0% (0/11)
Other	14.3% (3/21)	9.1% (1/11)

(▨) = (no. of patients with metastases at specific site)/(total no. of patients with metastases).

[a] = Fisher's exact test: p = 0.03.

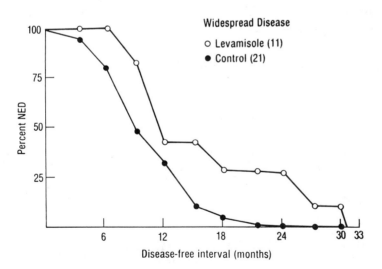

FIG. 4. Disease-free interval for those patients who developed recurrent disease.

TABLE 5. Changes in skin reactivity after levamisole in disease-free (NED) patients and in those with recurrent disease (REC) at 20 months

Antigen	Group	No. of patients with increased reaction[a]
DNCB	NED	11/12
	REC	4/6
Candida	NED	9/12
	REC	0/6
PPD	NED	0/12
	REC	0/6

[a] Conversions from negative to positive and from weakly to strongly positive included.

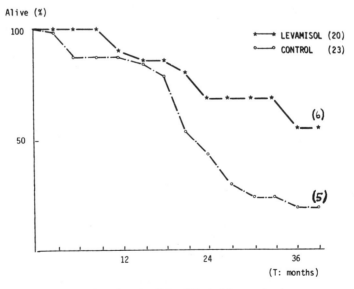

FIG. 5. Survival by life table analysis.

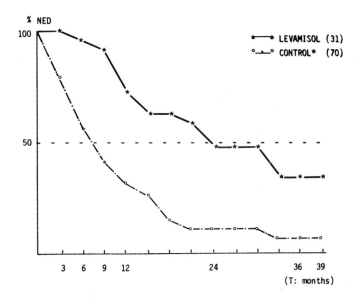

FIG. 6. Disease-free interval for historical controls and levamisole-treated (see text).

To confirm the validity of these results, a historical control group was analyzed; 70 patients who presented stage III breast cancer and were irradiated between the second semester of 1971 and the second semester of 1974. Figure 6 shows the disease-free interval for the historical controls and 31 patients treated with levamisole (this includes 11 patients entered in the last 12 months in the levamisole group). The median disease-free interval was 7.8 months for the historical controls and 24 months for the treated group. At 39 months, 7% of the historical control patients and 34.8% of the levamisole-treated patients were free of disease.

Figure 7 shows the actuarial curves for the historical controls and levamisole groups. At 39 months, 58% of the levamisole-treated patients and 15% of the historical controls were alive (p < 0.01 by generalized Wilcoxon test).

Figure 8 shows the clinical course of the patients between recurrence and death in both groups. No differences could be demonstrated between them.

Head and Neck Cancer

In a group of head and neck cancer patients we studied the effect of radiation therapy on the skin tests, blastic transformation to PHA in whole blood cultures, and peripheral lymphocyte count. Figure 9 shows the effect of radiation therapy on all positive tests. During the first trimester a decrease of the reactions was observed. A subsequent increase of these tests can be

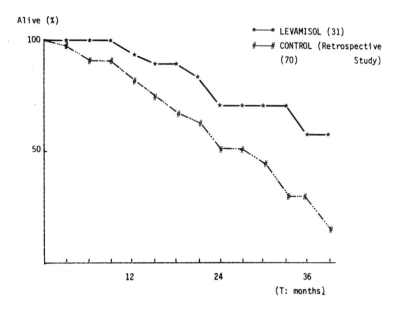

FIG. 7. Survival for historical controls and levamisole-treated (see text).

observed up to 1 year later. On the other hand, this recovery is not observed if we consider only the strong positive responses, which decreased progressively after radiation therapy (Fig. 10).

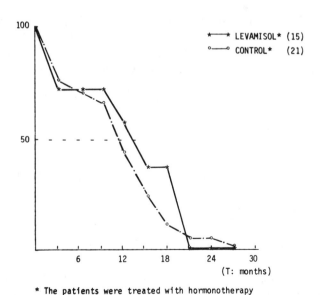

* The patients were treated with hormonotherapy
  and chemotherapy

FIG. 8. Time lapse from recurrence to death in both groups.

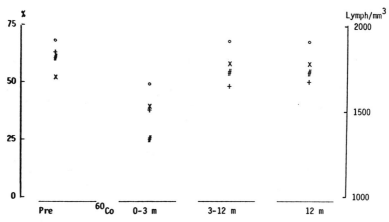

x DNCB
+ Candidine
# Blastic Transformation
° Lymphocyte Count

FIG. 9. Evolution of immune response after radiation therapy in head and neck cancer patients.

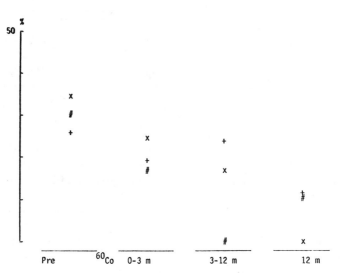

x DNCB
+ Candidine
# Blastic Transformation

FIG. 10. Evolution of strong skin reactivity and "good" blastic transformation after radiation therapy in head and neck cancer patients.

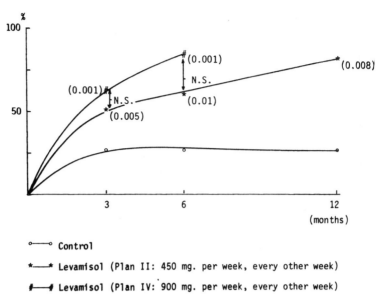

○———○ Control

——— Levamisol (Plan II: 450 mg. per week, every other week)

⌿———⌿ Levamisol (Plan IV: 900 mg. per week, every other week)

FIG. 11. DNCB 100 μg increase responsiveness between controls and levamisole-treated with the two plans (see text).

Two Schedules with Levamisole in 198 Cancer Patients

1. Plan II: 150 mg in a single dose, orally per day, on 3 consecutive days, every other week.

2. Plan IV: 150 mg in a single dose, orally per day, on 6 consecutive days, every other week.

Figure 11 shows the increase in DNCB responsiveness (negative to positive or weakly to strongly positive) in a group of cancer patients treated with the two plans. Levamisole given according to plan II significantly increased the response to DNCB 100 μg in comparison to the control. Plan IV increased reactions in a higher percentage and in a shorter time than with the so-called classic plan. In head and neck cancer patients no more than 15% of strong reactions can be observed after radiotherapy; after 6 months of treatment with levamisole according to plan IV, 50% of strong positive reactions were observed.

Table 6 shows the side effects found in the first 106 patients treated. A small percentage of side effects was found more in plan IV than in plan II, but with no statistical difference. In reference to PHA response in levamisole-treated patients, we observed an increase in the spontaneous responses and a decrease in the PHA response with whole blood cultures. This discordance between skin tests and PHA-P response was found in another group of patients without levamisole treatment: patients with prostatic carcinoma and melanoma. The significance of these results is unclear and is being studied further.

TABLE 6. Side effects found in the two schedules applied

		None	Mild	Severe
Levamisole, plan II	No.	58	4	2
(450 mg/week)	(%)	(90.6)	(6.3)	(3.1)
Levamisole, plan IV	No.	36	4	2
(900 mg/week)	(%)	(85.7)	(9.5)	(4.8)

χ^2: N.S.

No. = number of patients.

DISCUSSION

As shown in Tables 1 and 2, both groups were clinically comparable at the onset of therapy. We observed a significantly longer disease-free interval in levamisole-treated patients than in the control group (median 25 months vs. 9 months, respectively). This observation is consistent with the finding of Chirigos et al. (8,9) that levamisole prolongs remissions of a transplantable murine leukemia induced by chemotherapy.

The relative increase in frequency of pulmonary and pleural metastasis in levamisole-treated patients may be interpreted as a differential effect of immunomodulation on pulmonary tissue or merely as a reflection of the decreased number of patients with metastatic disease in this group.

Figures 4 and 5 suggest that levamisole lowers the progression of disease in patients who develop recurrence and that the drug takes time to be effective. In patients with rapidly progressive disease, where metastases appear in less than 9 to 12 months, levamisole may have had insufficient time to alter the course of the disease.

Administration of levamisole was associated with an increase in reactivity to DNCB. Patients who developed recurrence before 20 months showed no significant increase in skin reactivity, as opposed to patients who remained free of disease after 30 months of treatment. Similar results have been reported by Tripodi et al. (10), Brugmans et al. (11), and Fisher et al. (12), but were not confirmed by Hirshaut and associates (13). In some patients DNCB responsiveness increased gradually after long treatment periods, with negative tests converting to weakly positive tests and then to strongly positive tests over periods as long as 9 months. This pattern was associated with long disease-free intervals. Changes in skin reactivity to common antigens were not so striking and were, in general, poorly correlated with response to treatment.

The side effects that we have seen were dizziness, nausea, and vomiting. The most common side effect was alteration in the sense of smell. Less than 10% of patients had side effects, and in only 3 to 4% was it necessary to stop the treatment. Two patients who are free of disease have received over 30 gr without evidence of toxicity.

We do not know how levamisole affects tumors and cell-mediated immune response. This drug also has antiviral activity (14) and stimulates phagocytosis (15) or not (16). Since nonsteroideal drugs may have antiestrogenic activity and thereby influence the behavior of hormone-dependent breast cancer (17), our colleague Dr. R. E. Garola has investigated the possibility that levamisole and its dextroisomer, dextromisole, have antiestrogenic activity. Using competitive binding with estradiol in the uteri of prepubescent Sprague-Dawley rats, he has not found such effects. This investigation is now being extended to tumor tissue.

In reference to the action of radiotherapy on immune reactions, it is important to point out the diminished immune response after this type of treatment. All the reactions employed showed a lowering in reactivity between the end of radiotherapy and the 3 ensuing months, with a recuperation between 4 and 12 months that continued after a year, even though preirradiated levels were not reached.

When only strong reactivity is analyzed, it can be seen (Fig. 10) that it continues to decrease after 12 months postirradiation. This was more evident with DNCB (p:0.001) and blastic transformation (p:0.03) although the latter recuperated somewhat after 12 months. Candida Albicans reactivity diminishes to a slight degree. It is interesting to note the remarkable coincidence of the tendencies evidenced by the three tests. A similar depression of cellular immunity was reported (18) in patients averaging 9 years after irradiation for head and neck tumors. No clear cause for this effect could be invoked, since neither thymic nor extensive bone marrow irradiation were carried out.

Another important point is the significant difference in DNCB 100 μg reactivity between plan II and plan IV after 6 months of treatment. With the new plan the positive skin response is reached in shorter time and therefore it is possible to obtain better results with it.

CONCLUSIONS

1. Levamisole can improve the clinical course in patients with stage III breast cancer.
2. Levamisole can restore depressed skin test reactivity after radiotherapy in patients with breast cancer.
3. Levamisole has minimal toxicity.
4. The clinical effects may be dose related.

SUMMARY

Levamisole was employed in a clinical trial in breast cancer stage III UICC classification. In 43 evaluable patients, 23 control and 20 treated, there was a significant prolongation of the median disease-free interval

(8 vs. 21 months) and an increase in survival (18.8% vs. 55% alive) at 39 months, respectively. Skin reactivity and absolute lymphocyte counts were increased after levamisole treatment.

In a group of head and neck cancer patients, the effects of radiotherapy on skin tests and blastic transformation of lymphocytes to PHA-P were studied. It was demonstrated that the strong skin responses and "good" blastic trans- formation decreased progressively after radiation therapy up to 1 year later.

The first results on DNCB 100-μg reactivity with two schedules of levamisole treatment are presented.

ACKNOWLEDGMENT

We gratefully acknowledge the skillful technical assistance of Mrs. Raquel Bladrich and Ms. Magdalena Racedo.

REFERENCES

1. Rénaud, M. (1926): La cuti-reaction a la tuberculine chez les cancereux. Bull. Soc. Med. Paris, 50:1441-1442.
2. Eilber, F. R., and Morton, D. L. (1970): Impaired immunological reactivity and recurrence following cancer surgery. Cancer, 25:362-367.
3. Renoux, G., and Renoux, M. (1974): Modulation of immune reactivity by phenylimidothiazole salts in mice immunized by sheep red blood cells. J. Immunol., 113:779-790.
4. Braun, W., Ishizuka, M., Yajima, Y., Webb, D., and Winchurch, R. (1971): In: Biological Effects of Polynucleotides, edited by R. F. Beers and W. Braun, p. 139. Springer-Verlag, New York.
5. Thienpoint, D., Brugmans, J., Abadi, K., and Tanamal, S. (1969): Evaluation of tetramisole in the treatment of nematode infections in man. Am. J. Trop. Med. Hyg., 18:520-525.
6. Renoux, G., and Renoux, M. (1971): Effet immunostimulant d'un imidothiazole dans l'immunisation des souris contre l'infection par Brucella abortus. C.R. Acad. Sci. (D), 272:349-350.
7. Park, B. H., and Good, R. A. (1972): A new micromethod for evaluat- ing lymphocyte response to phytohemagglutinin: a quantitative analysis of the function of thymus-dependent cells. Proc. Natl. Acad. Sci. U.S.A., 69:371-374.
8. Chirigos, M. A., Pearson, J. W., and Fuhrman, F. S. (1974): Effect of tumor load reduction on successful immunostimulation. Proc. Am. Assoc. Cancer Res., 15:116.
9. Chirigos, M. A., Pearson, J. W., and Pryor, J. (1973): Augmentation of chemotherapeutically induced remission of a murine leukemia by a chemical immunoadjuvant. Cancer Res., 33:2615-2618.
10. Tripodi, D., Parks, L. C., and Brugmans, J. (1973): Drug-induced restoration of cutaneous delayed hypersensitivity in anergic patients with cancer. N. Engl. J. Med., 289:354-357.

11. Brugmans, J., Schuermans, V., De Cocr, W., Thienpoint, D., Janssen, D., Verhaegen, H., Van Nimmen, L., Louwagie, A. C., and Stevens, E. (1973): Restoration of host defense mechanisms in man by levamisole. Life Sci., 13:1499-1504.

12. Fischer, G. W., Oi, U. T., Ampaya, E. P., Kelley, J. L., and Bass, J. W. (1974): Enhanced host defense mechanism with phenyl-imidothiazole (abstr.). Pediatr. Res., 8:138.

13. Hirshaut, Y., Pinsky, C., Marquardt, H., and Oettgen, H. F. (1973): Effects of levamisole on delayed hypersensitivity reactions in cancer patients. Proc. Am. Assoc. Cancer Res., 14:109.

14. Kint, A., and Verlinden, L. (1974): Levamisole for recurrent herpes labialis. N. Engl. J. Med., 291:308.

15. Hoebeke, J., and Franchi, G. (1973): Influence of tetramisole and its optical isomers on the mononuclear phagocytic system. Effect on carbon clearance in mice. J. Reticuloendothel. Soc., 14:317-323.

16. Bergoc, R. M., Caro, R. A., Feierstein, J. N., Ihlo, J. E., Olivari, A. J., and Rojas, A. F. (1975): Levamisole. I. Immediate action on the phagocytosis of inert radiocolloidal particles. (In press.)

17. Hecker, E., Vegh, I., Levy, C. M., Magin, C. A., Martinez, J. C., Loureiro, J., and Garola, R. E. (1974): Clinical trial of Clomiphene in advanced breast cancer. Eur. J. Cancer, 10:747-749.

18. Tarpley, J. L., Potvin, C., and Chretien, P. B. (1975): Prolonged depression of cellular immunity in cured laryngopharyngeal cancer patients treated with radiation therapy. Cancer, 35:638-644.

Control of Neoplasia by Modulation of the Immune System, edited by M. A. Chirigos. Raven Press, New York 1977.

PRELIMINARY EXPERIENCE WITH LEVAMISOLE IN CANCER PATIENTS, AND PARTICULARLY IN BREAST CANCER

J. M. Debois

Head of the Department of Radiotherapy, St.-Norbertushospital, B-2570 Duffel, Belgium

In 1971, Renoux and Renoux (1) discovered that levamisole enhanced host defense mechanisms. In the same year (1971) Verhaegen found that a 3-day treatment course of levamisole could restore skin reactivity to PPD in patients with cancer and other debilitating diseases. This was confirmed in 1973 by Tripodi et al. (2) for PPD and DNCB in cancer patients, and the hypothesis that levamisole might be of benefit to cancer patients was born. In 1973 also, Chirigos et al. (3) published results indicating that levamisole prolonged chemotherapeutically induced tumor remission, i.e., that the additive effect provided by levamisole was evident during the immunosuppressed period induced by antitumoral therapy and when tumor load was minimal (Table 1).

Since 1973 much more has become known about levamisole (4). The significance of, for instance, an appropriate dose and dosage regimen in relation to disease, stage of disease, body weight, and, possibly, other factors can no longer be overlooked (5-7). The importance of laboratory investigations such as E-rosette, serum-blocking factors, and lymphocyte stimulation by suboptimal antigen concentrations is now clear (8,9) and should be considered when new studies of levamisole in cancer are contemplated.

It should be realized, however, that much of this was not known when, in 1972, it was suggested that the life expectancy of cancer patients could be improved by adding levamisole to the appropriate tumor-reductive therapy. A simple study was designed in which consecutive cancer patients referred to our department of radiotherapy were alternately allocated to levamisole therapy, the other patients constituting the reference group. The first results are now available for 375 patients with various tumors who have been followed up for a median period of 2 years.

Although the design of our study may appear naive and although some patients would today no longer be considered candidates for treatment with

175

TABLE 1. Landmarks in levamisole and immunotherapy of cancer

1971	Renoux	Augmentation of protective effect of a Brucella vaccine in mice
1971	Verhaegen	Restoration of delayed skin hypersensitivity reactions to PPD in debilitated patients
1973	Tripodi	Restoration of delayed skin hypersensitivity reactions to PPD and DNCB in cancer patients
1973	Chirigos	Augmentation of chemotherapeutically induced tumor remission

levamisole, we believe (a) that our results indicate that there is some reason for enthusiasm but (b) that this enthusiasm should obviously be guarded and (c) that our results might suggest some hypotheses for more definitive studies.

Table 2 presents a general description of the patients. All patients were referred to the radiotherapy department between October 1972 and June 1974. No particular selection was made. Alternate patients received levamisole (150 mg/day) for 3 days every other week in addition to the appropriate radiotherapy. The other patients received no levamisole and constituted the reference group. The patients are seen periodically for routine check-up and laboratory examinations. At present they have been followed for up to 3 years (median: 2 years). Survival rates are calculated by the actuarial method (10) from the day of admission to the study.

Figure 1 shows the 2-year survival rate in the total group and indicates that there is a small difference in survival between the levamisole-treated patients and the reference group. The greatest difference is 10% of patients at 17 months, the maximum difference in survival time being 8 months; i.e., 68% of the patients in the reference group were still alive after 12 months as compared with 68% at 20 months in the levamisole group.

Table 3 shows that death from cancer cannot be prevented in any of the groups, and that, with the exception of lung cancer, there is a small difference in survival in all groups at 6, 12, and 24 months. The difference is most pronounced in the patients with breast cancer, which actually turned out to be the largest group.

If patients with all stages of breast tumor are combined, the death rate is 20% (10 patients) in the levamisole group and 23% (14 patients) in the reference group (Table 4). However, the survival rate varies with the stage of disease from 100% for stages I and II down to less than 20% for stage IV in the reference group (Fig. 2). The median survival time for stage IV breast cancer is about 6 months in the reference patients and 20 months in the levamisole-treated patients, a difference of 14 months. At one-and-a-half years, 70% of the levamisole-treated patients were still alive as compared with only 20% of the reference patients. The results beyond one-and-a-half

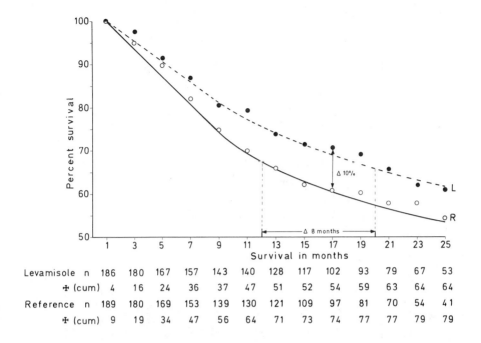

Levamisole n	186	180	167	157	143	140	128	117	102	93	79	67	53
✚ (cum)	4	16	24	36	37	47	51	52	54	59	63	64	64
Reference n	189	180	169	153	139	130	121	109	97	81	70	54	41
✚ (cum)	9	19	34	47	56	64	71	73	74	77	77	79	79

FIG. 1. Twenty-five-month survival rate in total group of 375 patients.

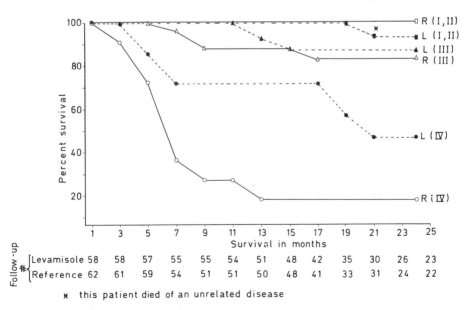

| Follow-up ✚ { | Levamisole | 58 | 58 | 57 | 55 | 55 | 54 | 51 | 48 | 42 | 35 | 30 | 26 | 23 |
| | Reference | 62 | 61 | 59 | 54 | 51 | 51 | 50 | 48 | 41 | 33 | 31 | 24 | 22 |

x this patient died of an unrelated disease

FIG. 2. Twenty-five-month survival rate by stage of disease in patients with breast cancer.

TABLE 2. Characteristics of the study population

Tumor site	Sex		Age (years) median (range)	Follow-up (months) median (range)	Immunotherapy	
	Male	Female			L	R
Breast	0	120	53 (26–82)	25 (5–37)	58	62
Head and neck	54	10	64 (19–91)	24 (1–36)	37	27
Lung	44	1	65 (39–84)	24 (9–37)	21	24
Ovaries and corpus uteri	0	41	61 (39–88)	24 (4–37)	19	22
Skin, rectosigmoid, G. U.	26	13	63 (27–79)	27 (5–37)	17	22
Blood-forming organs	11	6	57 (15–84)	23 (7–37)	11	6
Cervix uteri	0	36	61 (38–77)	22 (2–36)	20	16
Musculoskeletal	8	5	61 (37–83)	31 (8–35)	3	10
Total	143	232	61 (15–91)	24 (1–37)	186	189

L = levamisole; R = reference.

TABLE 3. Death rates (calculated by the actuarial method)

Tumor site	No. of patients included in study		Percent death					
			≤ 6 months		≤ 12 months		≤ 24 months	
	R	L	R	L	R	L	R	L
Breast	62	58	13	3	19	7	23	20
Head and neck	27	37	7	3	19	17	43	25
Lung	24	21	42	48	75	78	88	92
Ovaries and corpus uteri	22	19	14	11	28	27	49	43
Skin, rectosigmoid, G. U.	22	17	32	30	61	50	71	67
Blood-forming organs	6	11	17	18	38	27	38	37
Cervix uteri	16	20	13	5	29	21	37	29
Musculo-skeletal	10	3	—	—	—	—	—	—
Total	189	186	18	13	34	26	44	39

R = reference; L = levamisole.

TABLE 4. Number of deaths — breast cancer

Study group	Stages				
	I	II	III	IV	Total
Reference n	23	3	25	11	62
+	0	0	5	9	14
Levamisole n	23	4	24	7	58
+	1[a]	0	5	4	10

[a] This patient died of an unrelated disease.

TABLE 5. Radiotherapy for breast cancer

Telecobalt	R	L
Pre- and postmastectomy	19	18
Postmastectomy	20	23
+ Curietherapy	11	7
Posttumorectomy	12	10

R = reference group; L = levamisole group.

years should be interpreted with some caution, as there are too few patients within each subcategory. We would like to mention, moreover, that the various modes of radiotherapy applied are equally distributed in the two groups of patients (Table 5).

The design of our study is poor from a statistical standpoint. Our results, however, indicate that levamisole may be a helpful element in our efforts to prolong life, and at least the disease-free interval. But, as the overall reduction in the death rate is not more than 10% and the overall prolongation of survival time not more than 8 months, our enthusiasm should be guarded.

As suggested by the differential results obtained in our patients with breast cancer, special attention should be given in further studies to such factors as (Table 6) the following:

Selection of patient characteristics, diagnosis, and stage of disease; properly stratified and randomized studies will be required.

Levamisole dose, dosage regimen, and timing in relation to radiotherapy, surgery, and chemotherapy; body weight; and other factors.

Combination therapy with conventional antitumoral therapy and immunotherapy.

Cellular immune surveillance as a guide to appropriate treatment so that treatment can be continuously and appropriately monitored and modified.

Duration of disease-free interval and incidence of complete tumor remission and control of local and/or metastatic spread of disease are only a few of possible therapeutic criteria that must be assessed.

More than ever we now feel that the treatment of cancer will have to be individualized and that surgery, radiotherapy, hormonal therapy, chemotherapy, and immunotherapy must be used judiciously and need to be modified according to the development of the disease.

This will obviously make any ethically and medically justified study design exceedingly complicated and will be possible only if all existing clinical and laboratory techniques are regularly and skillfully used so that early diagnosis as well as adequate monitoring of the spread of the disease and of the immunological status of the patient are assured.

TABLE 6. Recommendations for further studies

Selection	Of patient characteristics, diagnostic categories
Dosage	Dose, schedule, and timing
Stringency	Properly stratified and randomized double-blind study
Combination	With conventional therapy With immunotherapy
Cellular immune surveillance	Individualized treatment
Quality of life	Disease-free interval Complete tumor remission Control of local and metastatic spread of the disease

ACKNOWLEDGMENT

Our special thanks go to Mrs. C. Van Dam-Wauters for her continuous interest in the study and dedication to the patients.

REFERENCES

1. Renoux, G., and Renoux, M. (1971): Effet immunostimulant d'un imido-thiazole dans l'immunisation des souris contre l'infection par Brucella abortus. C. R. Acad. Sci. (D), 272:349-350.
2. Tripodi, D., Parks, L. C., and Brugmans, J. (1973): Drug-induced restoration of cutaneous delayed hypersensitivity in anergic patients with cancer. N. Engl. J. Med., 289:345-357.
3. Chirigos, M. A., Pearson, J. W., and Pryor, J. (1973): Augmentation of chemotherapeutically induced remission of a murine leukemia by a chemical immuno-adjuvant. Cancer Res., 33:2615-2618.
4. Symoens, J. (1976): Levamisole: An antianergic chemotherapeutic agent. This Volume.
5. Amery, W. (1976): Double-blind placebo-controlled chemical trials of levamisole in resectable bronchogenic carcinoma. This Volume.
6. Amery, W. (1976): Double-blind levamisole trial in resectable lung cancer. Ann. N.Y. Acad. Sci. (in press).
7. Rojas, A., Mickiewicz, E., Olivari, A., Carugatti, A., and Lebenstejn, M. (1974): Levamisole: A preliminary report on toxicity, clinical action and effect on cell mediated sensitivity in cancer patients with 22 months of treatment. (unpublished data).
8. Ramot, B., Biniaminov, M., Schoham, C., and Rosenthal, E. (1976): The effect of levamisole on E-rosette-forming cells in vivo and in vitro in Hodgkin's disease patients. N. Engl. J. Med. (in press).

9. Renoux, G., Renoux, M., and Palat, A. (1974): Influences of levamisole on T-cell reactivity and on survival of untractable cancer patients. First Conference on Modulation of Host Resistance in the Prevention or Treatment of Induced Neoplasias. National Institutes of Health. The John E. Fogarty International Center and National Cancer Institute, Bethesda, Md., December 1974.

10. Berkson, J., and Gage, R. P. (1950): Calculation of survival rates for cancer. Proc. Mayo Clin., 25:270.

Control of Neoplasia by Modulation of the Immune System, edited by M. A. Chirigos. Raven Press, New York 1977.

ADMINISTRATION OF A SINGLE DOSE OF LEVAMISOLE TO CARCINOMA PATIENTS: IN VIVO AND IN VITRO ENHANCEMENT OF CELLULAR IMMUNE RESPONSE

Uri H. Lewinski, Giora M. Mavligit, Jordan U. Gutterman, and Evan M. Hersh

Department of Developmental Therapeutics, M. D. Anderson Hospital and Tumor Institute, The University of Texas System Cancer Center and The University of Texas Medical School at Houston, Texas 77025

INTRODUCTION

Impaired general immunocompetence in cancer patients is associated with advanced disease and poor prognosis (1-3). Administration of immunotherapy is intended to correct or reverse the immunological deficiencies in these patients (4-7). A variety of bacterial and nonbacterial biological products are currently used as immunopotentiating agents (8,9). Because of the nature of these agents, and especially their preparation, a great deal of variability in potency is anticipated from batch to batch. It is therefore difficult to assess their optimal dosage and to control many of the side effects associated with their administration. In this respect the use of synthetic chemical compounds as immune modulators may have a number of advantages. Initial studies showed that levamisole (2,3,5,6-tetrahydro-6-phenylimidazo-(2,1-b)-thiazole hydrochloride) can restore delayed-type hypersensitivity (DTH) skin reactions to DNCB and PPD (10-12). Furthermore, preliminary clinical results showed a beneficial effect in patients with resectable bronchogenic carcinoma (13). Therefore, we undertook the current study, which was designed to determine: (a) the maximum tolerated single dose, (b) the duration of its immunologic effect assessed by in vivo and in vitro immune parameters.

MATERIALS AND METHODS

Patients

Patients with histologically proven carcinoma were studied during their evaluation in the clinic (Table 1). After stratification according to previous

183

TABLE 1. Randomization plan, sex, age, and carcinoma site

	Levamisole			No levamisole		
	Previously			Previously		
	Treated [a]	Untreated	All patients	Treated	Untreated	All patients
Patients	13	13	26	11	13	24
Males	7	8	15	5	7	12
Females	6	5	11	6	6	12
Median age	48	54	51	53	49	53
Age range	36-67	25-67	25-67	36-67	32-67	32-67
Carcinoma site						
Colon	6	10	16	7	8	15
Breast	3	—	3	1	4	5
Lung	3	1	4	2	—	2
Miscellaneous [b]	1	2	3	1	1	2

[a] Chemotherapy; radiotherapy.
[b] Stomach (2), small bowel (1), pancreas (1), and head and neck (1).

treatment, 26 patients were randomized to receive levamisole while 24 patients served as controls. Patients who were previously treated with immunotherapy were excluded from the study. The distribution of sex, age, and primary tumor site was similar in both groups.

Levamisole (R12564, kindly provided by Janssen R&D, Inc., New Brunswick, New Jersey), was given orally after an informed consent was obtained from all the patients. Based on animal toxicity data, 265 mg/M^2 were administered as an initial single dose. Later on, because of excessive toxicity the dose was reduced to 200 mg/M^2.

Sequential immunological studies in vitro and in vivo were performed in relation to levamisole administration following seven time points: -24, 0, 4, 8, 24, 48, and 144 hr. At each time point, skin tests in vivo and lymphocyte blastogenesis in vitro were performed. Patients in both groups were studied in the same sequence, but only those in the levamisole group received the drug at the second study point (time 0).

Skin Tests

Initially, 44 patients were skin-tested with a battery of recall antigens, including dermatophytin, streptokinase-streptodornase, mumps antigen, Candida antigen, and PPD. Dermatophytin was the only antigen used for sequential studies in all the patients. Positive DTH reactions were taken as ≥ 2 mm of induration. The data were analyzed in two ways: first, in terms of significant changes in the size of induration between two study points. A positive change was defined as a conversion of skin-test reaction from negative to positive or $\geq 100\%$ increase in size. A negative change was defined as conversion from positive to negative or $\geq 50\%$ decrease in size. No change was defined as $<100\%$ increase or $<50\%$ decrease in size as well as total anergy. The overall sequential changes within each group as compared to the first study point were evaluated by the chi-square test. In a second analysis, skin-test reactions expressed in millimeters of induration were compared between the two groups of patients at each study point by the Wilcoxon-Mann-Whitney test for unpaired observations (14).

Lymphocyte Blastogenesis

Venous blood was defibrinated and lymphocytes separated on the Ficoll-Hypaque gradient as previously described (15). Lymphocytes were resuspended in RPMI-1640[1] supplemented with 100 units/ml of penicillin, 100 µg/ml of streptomycin, 2 mM/ml of L-glutamine, and 10% pre-levamisole autologous serum. The cell concentration was adjusted to 7.5 X 10^5/ml. 1.5 X 10^5 lymphocytes (0.2 ml) were distributed with a Hamilton repeating

---

[1] Grand Island Biological Company, Grand Island, New York.

dispenser[2] into each well of microplates.[3] In addition to 12 replicates of un-stimulated controls, 6 replicates of lymphocyte cultures were stimulated with each of the following: phytohemagglutinin[4] diluted 1:10, concanavalin A[5] diluted 1:10, pokeweed mitogen[1] diluted 1:20, streptolysin-O[4] in full strength, and mixed lymphocyte cultures (MLC). For the latter, the same stimulator cells were used throughout the study for each patient. For stim-ulator cells, donor lymphocytes were resuspended in RPMI-1640 supplemented with 20% heat-inactivated fetal calf serum antibiotics and L-glutamine. Ali-quot doses were frozen (Linde BF4 biological freezing system) with 10% DMSO and stored in liquid nitrogen. For use in MLC, cells were rapidly thawed, washed in RPMI-1640, irradiated with 4,000 r and mixed with the same number of responder cells. One microcurie of tritiated thymidine[6] was added for the last 8 hr of a 7-day incubation in a humidified incubator. The blastogenesis was terminated by cooling in a refrigerator and the cells were harvested with the MASH device.[7] The blastogenesis was estimated by thymidine uptake as measured by liquid scintillation counting and expressed as counts per minute (cpm)/1.5×10^5 lymphocytes. For the analysis, the mean cpm value of replicate experimental observations was used. The over-all net blastogenic responses (experimental cpm minus control cpm) were compared between the first and subsequent study points separately for both groups of patients by the Wilcoxon-Mann-Whitney test. These comparisons were based on differences in cpm between two individual measurements. A significant difference of cpm $\geq 25\%$ between two individual measurements was defined as $\geq 25\%$ increase or $\geq 20\%$ decrease in cpm. For differences in cpm of $\geq 50\%$; $\geq 100\%$, the corresponding values were $\geq 50\%$; $\geq 100\%$ increase or $\geq 33\%$; $\geq 50\%$ decrease in cpm.

RESULTS

Maximum Tolerated Single Dose of Levamisole

Fifteen of 26 patients who received the drug experienced one or more side effects (Table 2). One of 3 patients who were receiving 265 mg/m[2] of leva-misole experienced severe abdominal cramps, and another patient suffered

---

[2] Hamilton Company, Reno, Nevada.

[3] Microtest II Culture Plates, Falcon Plastics, Oxnard, California.

[4] Difco, Detroit, Michigan.

[5] Nutritional Pharmaceuticals Company, Cleveland, Ohio.

[6] Spec. Act. 1.9 Ci/mM, Schwartz-Mann, Orangeburg, New York.

[7] Microbiological Associates, Bethesda, Maryland.

TABLE 2.   Side effects from levamisole in 26 carcinoma patients

Side effect	Degree of toxicity (no. of patients)			
	Mild	Moderate	Severe	Overall
Nausea	8	2	3	13
Fatigue	1	3	2	6
Tremor	3	2		5
Vomiting	1	2		3
Dizziness	2	1		3
Abdominal pain	1	1	1	3
Mental depression	1	1		2
Hyperhydrosis	2			2
Nervousness	1			1
Polyuria	1			1
Hyperventilation	1			1
Facial flush	1			1

from recurrent vomiting and extreme weakness. Two patients receiving 200 mg/m^2 of levamisole, who suffered severe nausea, had impaired liver function. Overall, nausea, fatigue, and tremor were the most frequent side effects. These appeared within 90 min after ingestion of the drug and disappeared usually within 2 hr thereafter. It is noteworthy that the majority of side effects were mild and of short duration.

Delayed-type Hypersensitivity Reaction

In the levamisole-treated group there were more positive than negative changes in the size of induration when subsequent study points were compared to the first one. An inverse trend was observed in the control group. For the separate study points, these opposing trends did not reach statistical significance because of the large number of individual differences without a significant change in induration. In Table 3, the observations made on all the subsequent study points were lumped together and compared with the initial observation. Positive changes in the levamisole-treated group were significantly more frequent than negative changes (p = 0.008). In contrast, negative changes were more frequent in the control group, but this did not reach statistical significance. The ratio of positive to negative changes was significantly greater in the levamisole-treated as compared to controls

TABLE 3.   Dermatophytin skin test reactions (24 hr reading):
levamisole vs. control

Skin-test evaluation	Number of skin tests	
	Levamisole	Control
Positive change	31[a]	13[b]
Negative change	11[c]	23[d]
No change	57	55
All	99	91

p value (χ^2): a vs. c, 0.008; b vs. d, 0.18; a/c vs. b/d,
0.0018.

TABLE 4.   Kinetics of dermatophytin skin test reactions

Skin test applied   Skin test in millimeters of induration (mean values) read at

Study point	Time (hr)	24 hr			48 hr		
		Lev.	Cont.	p [a]	Lev.	Cont.	p
1	-24	3.1 N = 26	3.1 N = 24	0.1	5.0 N = 25	3.5 N = 23	0.4
2	0	5.7 N = 25	2.2 N = 23	0.2	5.4 N = 24	2.8 N = 22	0.16
3	4	5.6 N = 25	2.4 N = 23	0.09	5.3 N = 24	2.7 N = 22	0.2
4	8	4.9 N = 25	2.6 N = 23	0.36	4.8 N = 24	2.9 N = 22	0.03
5	24	6.1 N = 24	2.1 N = 22	0.012			

[a] Wilcoxon-Mann-Whitney test.

(p = 0.001).   These statistically significant changes were noted only when
24-hr skin-test readings were considered.   No significant differences between
the two groups of patients were observed when the 48-hr skin-test readings
were compared.

TABLE 5. Lymphocyte blastogenesis (cpm) induced by phytohemagglutinin 1:10

Treatment group	Hours study points	-24 (1)	0 ↓ (2)	4 (3)	8 (4)	24 (5)	48 (6)
Levamisole							
Mean		25,176	29,946	31,132	28,238	22,131	21,926
Median		20,434	28,866	23,461	20,430	18,983	17,574
p$_{\Delta cpm \geq 25\%}$[a]			0.2	0.2	<0.01	0.2	0.2
$\Delta cpm \geq 50\%$					0.07		
Control							
Mean		27,282	29,448	31,058	32,006	27,704	26,199
Median		24,154	24,172	27,059	29,101	21,194	21,945
p$_{\Delta cpm \geq 25\%}$			0.2	0.2	0.2	0.2	0.2

[a] Wilcoxon-Mann-Whitney test.

$\Delta cpm \geq 25\% = \geq 25\%$ ↑; $\geq 20\%$ ↓ between two individual measurements.
$\Delta cpm \geq 50\% = \geq 50\%$ ↑; $\geq 33\%$ ↓ between two individual measurements.
$\Delta cpm \geq 100\% = \geq 100\%$ ↑; $\geq 50\%$ ↓ between two individual measurements.

The size of induration was initially the same in both groups (Table 4). However, there were significant differences between the two groups when the skin tests were applied 8 hr after drug administration and read 48 hr later. Furthermore, when the skin-test application was delayed for 24 hr after drug administration, a significant difference in the size of induration was seen already at the 24-hr reading. There were no significant differences in the 24- and 48-hr readings of skin tests applied earlier than 8 hr after drug administration.

Lymphocyte Blastogenesis

In the controls, mean and median cpm values for spontaneous lymphocyte DNA synthesis declined on all the subsequent study points when compared with the first one. In the levamisole-treated group an opposite trend was observed on all the study points, but none of these differences reached statistical significance (therefore they are not shown in a table). The effect of levamisole administration on in vitro lymphocyte blastogenesis induced by phytohemagglutinin (PHA) is shown in Table 5. Lymphocyte blastogenesis was

TABLE 6. Lymphocyte blastogenesis (cpm) induced by concanavalin-A 1:10

Treatment group	Hours study points	-24 (1)	0↓ (2)	4 (3)	8 (4)	24 (5)	48 (6)
Levamisole							
Mean		8,227	9,698	9,338	9,046	7,936	8,921
Median		6,121	6,969	6,349	7,834	8,150	8,361
P Δcpm ≥ 25%[a]			>0.2	>0.2	<0.01	0.2	0.03
Δcpm ≥ 50%					0.01		0.01
Δcpm ≥ 100%					0.04		>0.2
Control							
Mean		7,700	9,238	9,036	9,699	8,196	10,487
Median		6,031	8,166	6,317	8,556	5,783	10,752
P Δcpm ≥ 25%			>0.2	>0.2	0.04	0.2	>0.2
Δcpm ≥ 50%					0.2		

[a] See footnote to Table 5.

significantly enhanced at the fourth compared to the first study point of the levamisole group only (p < 0.01). In lymphocyte blastogenesis induced by concanavalin A (Con A), the results are similar (Table 6), showing that levamisole significantly enhanced blastogenesis on the fourth and sixth study points. On both study points the difference remained significant upon upgrading the analysis using a difference of ≥ 50% between two individual measurements. Moreover, on the fourth study point the difference remained significant upon further upgrading of the analysis, whereas in the controls, significance was achieved only for a difference of ≥ 25% between two individual measurements.

Different results were obtained in lymphocyte blastogenesis induced by pokeweed mitogens (PWM) (Table 7). In the controls, lymphocyte blastogenesis was depressed on the fourth and sixth study points with statistical significance on the latter. This phenomenon was apparently minimized or completely aborted in the levamisole group. Studies of lymphocyte blastogenesis induced by streptolysin-O (SLO) also showed significant enhancing effect by levamisole on the fifth study point (Table 8). This enhancement still remained significant upon upgrading the analysis utilizing a difference of 100% in cpm between two individual measurements. What appears to be

TABLE 7. Lymphocyte blastogenesis (cpm) induced by pokeweed mitogen 1:20

Treatment group	Hours study point	-24 (1)	0 (2)	4 (3)	8 (4)	24 (5)	48 (6)
Control							
Mean		21,276	21,686	19,129	17,805	20,478	15,242
Median		22,069	19,581	16,469	15,608	17,112	13,873
p $\triangle$cpm $\geq 25\%$[a]			0.08	0.2	0.1[b]	0.2	<0.01[b]
$\triangle$cpm $\geq 50\%$			0.16		0.1		0.01
$\triangle$cpm $\geq 100\%$					0.15		0.01
Levamisole							
Mean		20,896	27,172	23,962	23,852	20,462	19,241
Median		19,065	22,038	21,465	20,848	18,373	16,410
p $\triangle$cpm $\geq 25\%$			>0.01	>0.2	>0.2	0.12	>0.2
$\triangle$cpm $\geq 50\%$			0.15				

[a] See footnote to Table 5.

[b] $1 > 4; 1 > 6$.

TABLE 8. Lymphocyte blastogenesis (cpm) induced by streptolysin–O 1:1

Treatment group	Hours study point	-24 (1)	0↓ (2)	4 (3)	8 (4)	24 (5)	48 (6)
Levamisole							
Mean		25,338	27,954	28,744	29,100	28,529	26,093
Median		16,723	19,401	24,961	26,916	20,773	17,949
p Δ cpm $\geq$ 25%[a]			0.04	0.2	0.2	0.03	0.2
Δ cpm $\geq$ 50%			0.06			0.01	
Δ cpm $\geq$ 100%			0.2			0.01	
Control							
Mean		21,111	22,933	23,159	24,888	17,499	22,673
Median		4,678	12,316	10,747	15,740	12,268	4,230
p Δ cpm $\geq$ 25%			0.2	0.2	0.2	0.2	0.2

[a] See footnote to Table 5.

an enhanced blastogenesis in the second study point is unrelated to levamisole administration and may be associated with the effect of skin testing on lymphocyte blastogenesis. The same evaluations carried out with MLC data did not show any effect by levamisole.

DISCUSSION

Administration of a single dose of levamisole to cancer patients enhanced delayed-type hypersensitivity reactions (DTH) to dermatophytin in vivo as well as lymphocyte blastogenesis to mitogens and antigens in vitro. The enhancing effect of levamisole on DTH to dermatophytin in the present study is in agreement with its previously reported enhancing effect on DTH to PPD and DNCB (10-12). The enhancing effect was demonstrated early (8 hr after drug administration), which is in agreement with reports showing rapid conversion of DNCB reaction from negative to positive after drug administration (16). It is noteworthy that the enhancing effect of levamisole on DTH was still present 48 hr after drug administration.

The enhancing effect by levamisole on lymphocyte blastogenesis is parallel to its effect on DTH; i.e., it begins as early as 8 hr after drug administration and is still present 48 hr later. These findings are in complete agreement with the studies of Verhaegen et al. (11) and Sunshine et al. (17). A significant enhancing effect by levamisole on spontaneous DNA synthesis in cancer patients' lymphocytes was not demonstrated in our study. This is at variance with other studies which did show enhancement but where levamisole was added to the cultures in vitro (18).

The mechanism of action of levamisole as an immunopotentiating agent is unclear. A growing body of evidence suggests that it stimulates mainly thymus-dependent lymphocytes (19,20). However, its effect on blastogenesis has been shown with T- and to a lesser extent with B-cell mitogens and antigens (21-23). This was also true in our study. It is noteworthy that controversy still exists as to the specificity of PWM and PHA being B- or T-cell mitogens, respectively (24,25). Levamisole may occasionally fail to enhance blastogenesis (26), but this could be due to the use of a narrow range of mitogen and/or antigen concentrations whereas most studies emphasize the complex combinations between optimal mitogen concentration and time of incubation which are necessary to achieve the enhancing effect (21,22).

The association between the cyclic nucleotides and the stimulatory effect of levamisole on lymphocytes and macrophages has been recently reported. Levamisole can induce a rise in intracellular concentration of 3',5'-cyclic guanosine monophosphate (cyclic GMP) in lymphocytes (17,27) and reduce the concentration of 3',5'-cyclic adenosine monophosphate (cyclic AMP) in both lymphocytes (17) and macrophages (28). The latter, apparently activated, became more phagocytic. Therefore, it is conceivable that the immunostimulatory effect of levamisole in vivo is mediated through changes in cyclic nucleotides in various cellular components of the immune system.

Clinical trials using levamisole as an immunopotentiator are now underway, and preliminary results appear to be rather promising (13). The results of the present study contribute information related to the toxicity, the maximum tolerated single dose, and the duration of levamisole-induced immune stimulation. Since its effect is of no less than 48 hr duration, the drug should be administered at intervals greater than 48 hr. No evidence is available to suggest that more frequent administration may result in a cumulative and favorable effect, whereas daily administration may be detrimental (10).

SUMMARY

A single maximum tolerated dose of levamisole was administered to 26 carcinoma patients who were subjected to serial immunological studies. Delayed-type hypersensitivity reaction to dermatophytin was more pronounced in this group of patients as compared to 24 controls. In vitro lymphocyte blastogenesis induced by mitogens and antigens was also enhanced in the levamisole-treated group. The enhancing effect by levamisole was measurable in both in vivo and in vitro studies as early as 8 hr after drug administration, and the effect was still present 48 hr thereafter. These results may help to improve the schedule of levamisole administration in clinical trials.

ACKNOWLEDGMENTS

This work was supported by Janssen R&D, Inc., New Brunswick, New Jersey. Drs. Mavligit and Gutterman are the recipients of Public Health Service Career Development Awards No. 1-104-CA-00130 and No. 1-K04-CA-71007-02, respectively.
We wish to thank Mrs. June Williams for secretarial assistance.

REFERENCES

1. Hersh, E. M., Whitecar, J. P., Jr., McCredie, K. B., Bodey, G. P., Sr., and Freireich, E. J. (1971): Chemotherapy, immunocompetence, immunosuppression and prognosis in acute leukemia. New Engl. J. Med., 285:1211-1216.
2. Catalona, W. J., and Chretien, P. B. (1973): Abnormalities of quantitative dinitrochlorobenzene sensitization in cancer patients: Correlation with tumor stage and histology. Cancer, 31:353-356.
3. Lee, Y. T. N., Sparks, F. C., Eilber, F. R., and Morton, D. L. (1975): Delayed cutaneous hypersensitivity and peripheral lymphocyte counts in patients with advanced cancer. Cancer, 35:748-755.
4. Gutterman, J. U., Mavligit, G., Gottlieb, J. A., Burgess, M. A., McBride, C. E., Einhorn, L., Freireich, E. J., and Hersh, E. M. (1974): Chemoimmunotherapy of disseminated malignant melanoma with dimethyl triazeno imidazole carboxamide and bacillus Calmette-Guérin. New Engl. J. Med., 291:592-597.

5. Gutterman, J. U., Rodriguez, V., Mavligit, G., Burgess, M. A., Gehan, E., Hersh, E. M., McCredie, K. B., Reed, R., Smith, T., Bodey, G. P., Sr., and Freireich, E. J. (1974): Chemoimmunotherapy of adult acute leukemia. Prolongation of remission in myeloblastic leukemia with BCG. Lancet, 2:1405-1410.

6. Morton, D. L., Eilber, F. R., Holmes, E. C., Hunt, J. S., Ketcham, A. S., Silverstein, M. J., and Sparks, F. C. (1974): BCG immunotherapy of malignant melanoma: Summary of a seven-year experience. Ann. Surg., 180:635-641.

7. Mathé, G., Schwarzenberg, L., Amiel, J. L., Pouillart, P., Hayat, M., de Vassal, F., Rosenfeld, C., and Jasmin, C. (1975): Immunotherapy of leukemia. Proc. Roy. Soc. Med., 68:211-217.

8. Robinson, E., Bartal, A., Cohen, Y., and Haasz, R. (1975): A preliminary report on the effects of methanol extraction residue of BCG (MER) on cancer patients. Br. J. Cancer, 32:1-4.

9. Morton, D. L. (1975): Cancer immunotherapy: An overview. Semin. Oncol., 1:297-310.

10. Verhaegen, H., Verbruggen, F., Verhaegen-Declercq, M. L., and De Cree, J. (1974): Effects du lévamisole sur les réactions cutanées d'hypersensibilité retardée. Nouv. Presse Med., 3:2483-2485.

11. Verhaegen, H., De Cree, J., Verbruggen, F., Hoebeke, J., De Brabander, M., and Brugmans, J. (1973): Immune responses in elderly cuti-negative subjects and the effect of levamisole. Verh. Dtsch. Ges. Inn. Med., 79:623-628.

12. Tripodi, D., Parks, L. C., Oettgen, H., Mavligit, G. M., and Levitch, P. (1974): Restoration of delayed hypersensitivity in anergic cancer patients by levamisole. J. Reticuloendothel. Soc., 15:77a.

13. Amery, W., for Study Group for Bronchogenic Carcinoma (1975): Immunopotentiation with resectable bronchogenic carcinoma: A double-blind controlled trial. Br. Med. J., 3:461-464.

14. Snedecor, G. W., and Cochran, W. G. (1967): Statistical Methods. The Iowa State University Press, Ames, Iowa.

15. Mavligit, G. M., Gutterman, J. U., McBride, C. M., and Hersh, E. M. (1972): Multifacetal evaluation of human tumor immunity using a salt extracted colon carcinoma antigen. Proc. Soc. Exp. Biol. Med., 140:1240-1245.

16. Tripodi, D., Parks, L. C., and Brugmans, J. (1973): Drug-induced restoration of cutaneous delayed hypersensitivity in anergic patients with cancer. New Engl. J. Med., 289:354-357.

17. Sunshine, G., Lopez-Corrales, E., Hadden, E. M., Coffey, R. G., Wanebo, H., and Hadden, J. W. (1976): Levamisole and imidazole: In vitro effects in mouse and man and their possible mediation by cyclic nucleotides. NCI Monograph (in press).

18. Woods, W. A., Fliegelman, M. J., and Chirigos, M. A. (1975): Effect of levamisole on the in vitro immune response of spleen lymphocytes (38686). Proc. Soc. Exp. Biol. Med., 148:1048-1050.

19. Renoux, G., and Renoux, M. (1974): Modulation of immune reactivity by phenylimidothiazole salts in mice immunized by sheep red blood cells. J. Immunol., 113:779-790.

20. Verhaegen, H., De Cock, W., De Cree, J., Verbruggen, F., Verhaegen-Declercq, M., and Brugmans, J. (1975): In vitro restoration by levamisole of thymus-derived lymphocyte function in Hodgkin's disease. Lancet, 1:978.

21. Pabst, H. F., and Crowford, J. (1975): L-Tetramisole: Enhancement of human lymphocyte response to antigen. Clin. Exp. Immunol., 21:468-473.

22. Lichtenfeld, J. L., Desner, M., Wiernik, P. M., Moore, S., and Mardiney, M. R., Jr. (1975): Amplification of human lymphocyte responsiveness to immunologic stimuli in vitro by levamisole. Fogarty International Center Proceedings No. 28. U.S. Government Printing Office, Washington, D.C.

23. Merluzzi, V. J., Kaiser, C. W., Moolten, F. L., Cooperband, S. R., and Levinsky, N. G. (1975): Stimulation of mouse spleen cells in vitro by levamisole. Fed. Proc., 34:1004.

24. Mellstedt, H. (1975): In vitro activation of human T and B lymphocytes by pokeweed mitogen. Clin. Exp. Immunol., 19:75-82.

25. Chess, L., MacDermott, R. P., and Schlossman, S. F. (1974): Immunologic functions of isolated human lymphocyte subpopulations. I. Quantitative isolation of human T and B cells and response to mitogens. J. Immunol., 113:1113-1121.

26. Copeland, D., Stewart, T., and Harris, J. (1974): Effect of levamisole (NSC-177023) on in vitro human lymphocyte transformation. Cancer Chemother. Rep., 58:167-170.

27. Hadden, J. W., Coffey, R. G., Hadden, E. M., Lopez-Corrales, E., and Sunshine, G. H. (1975): Effects of levamisole and imidazole on lymphocyte proliferation and cyclic nucleotide levels. Cell. Immunol., 20:98-103.

28. Lima, A. O., Javierre, M. Q., Da Silva, W. D., and Camara, D. S. (1974): Immunological phagocytosis: Effect of drugs on phosphodiesterase activity. Experientia, 30:945-946.

Control of Neoplasia by Modulation of the Immune System, edited by M. A. Chirigos. Raven Press, New York   1977.

DOUBLE-BLIND PLACEBO-CONTROLLED CLINICAL TRIAL OF LEVAMISOLE IN RESECTABLE BRONCHOGENIC CARCINOMA

Willem K. Amery*

Janssen Pharmaceutica, Research Laboratories, B-2340 Beerse, Belgium

INTRODUCTION

The chemical structure and the immunological properties of levamisole have already been presented by several speakers at this conference. I should like to confine myself to reminding you of the fact that levamisole behaves as an antianergic chemotherapeutic agent which restores host defense mechanisms when these are deficient.

This chapter reports the results from a third interim analysis of the data obtained so far in a double-blind study with levamisole in operable lung cancer. The first patient was selected for this trial in the first half of 1972 and the whole program is expected to be completed by the end of 1977. The first (1) and the second (2) analyses have been reported elsewhere, and most aspects of the present third analysis were presented one month ago at the New York Academy of Sciences (3). The present chapter, therefore, will summarize the most important features of this latter presentation and supplement it with a few as yet unreported items.

---

*On behalf of the Study Group for Bronchogenic Carcinoma whose composition is as follows: Prof. J. Cosemans, Dr. H. C. Gooszen, Prof. E. Lopes Cardozo, Dr. A. Louwagie, Dr. J. Stam, Prof. J. Swierenga, Dr. R. G. Vanderschueren, Dr. R. W. Veldhuizen (investigators); Eng. G. De Ceuster, Dr. L. Desplenter, J. Dony, Prof. A. Drochmans, Dr. P. A. J. Janssen, Dr. W. Tanghe (consultants); E. Denissen (coordinator); Dr. W. Amery (chairman).

PATIENTS AND METHODS

The criteria for the selection of the patients and the design of the trial have been published elsewhere (1,3). This report concerns the data from the first 148 patients who have been in the study for at least 1 year after surgery.

One tablet, containing either 50 mg of levamisole or a placebo, is given 3 times daily for 3 consecutive days every other week and these 3-day courses are started on the third day before surgery. The medication is individually coded, given according to a strictly double-blind design, and is separately randomized for each participating center. The concomitant use of cytostatics, corticosteroids, and irradiation is prohibited for the entire duration of the trial unless relapse is evident.

The end points of the study are the first sound suspicion of recurrence, the first proof of relapse, and death from the disease, or, if none of these end points has occurred, a disease-free follow-up of at least 2 years.

The patients are skin-tested with several doses of DNCB and with 10 I. U. of PPD before, shortly after, and 2 months after surgery. The histological appearance of the tumor is classified by means of the WHO criteria. The largest tumor diameter is measured after its fixation by the pathologist, its regional extent is estimated by means of a slightly modified (1) classification system, first described by Slack (4) and the tumor diameter and the regional extent category are, eventually, combined into a two-grade system (1) providing a rough assessment of the total preoperative tumor burden.

The statistical analysis is performed by means of the Fisher exact probability test, two-tailed, using a Wang 2200 computer and all data are stored in an IBM 370/135 computer.

RESULTS

Of the 148 patients, 69 have been taking levamisole and 79 have served as placebo controls. More than half of the patients in each treatment group had been operated upon at least 2 years before the start of this analysis.

The incidence of side effects reported by the patients in the two treatment groups is shown in Table 1. Apparently, there are no striking differences between levamisole and placebo.

For the three end points, there is a statistically nonsignificant trend in favor of levamisole. This is illustrated by Fig. 1, which shows the disease-free interval in the patients with proven relapse. Twelve patients on levamisole died from their cancer, and so did 16 placebo patients. The other causes of mortality were equally frequent in the two series and included 7 patients from each treatment group (Table 2).

Since the levamisole dose had been rather arbitrarily fixed at the start of the trial, we could not exclude the possibility that some patients might have been taking an inadequate dose of the drug. Therefore, the data were analyzed as related to the patients' weight. The details of this analysis are presented elsewhere (3). Essentially, it was found that levamisole had no

TABLE 1. Incidence of side effects in the two treatment groups

Type of side effect	Percent of patients on levamisole (N = 69)	Percent of patients on placebo (N = 79)
Gastroenterological		
Siallorrhoea	1.5	0.0
Nausea	18.8[a]	10.1
Lack of appetite	7.3	5.1
Gastric complaints	2.9	3.8
Pyrosis	2.9	0.0
Vomiting	1.5	3.8
Diarrhoea	2.9	2.5
Anomalies in hepatic tests	1.5	2.5
Loss of weight	4.4	6.3
Weight gain	1.5	1.3
CNS phenomena		
Fatigue	7.3[a]	6.3[a]
Apathy	2.9	1.3
Inertia	1.5	0.0
Adynamia	1.5	8.9
Nervousness	1.5	2.5
Sleep disorders	4.4	0.0
Subfebrility	4.4	5.1
Shiverings	2.9	0.0
General malaise	5.8[b]	2.5
Dizziness, vertigo	4.4	1.3
Migraine	1.5	0.0
Headache	1.5	2.5
Miscellaneous		
Aching joints	2.9	2.5
Excessive perspiration	2.9	0.0
Skin rash	1.5	2.5[a]
Backache	1.5	2.5
Abdominal pain	0.0	2.5

[a] In one patient, the side effect persisted after discontinuation of the double-blind treatment.

[b] Interruption of treatment did not prevent continuation in one patient.

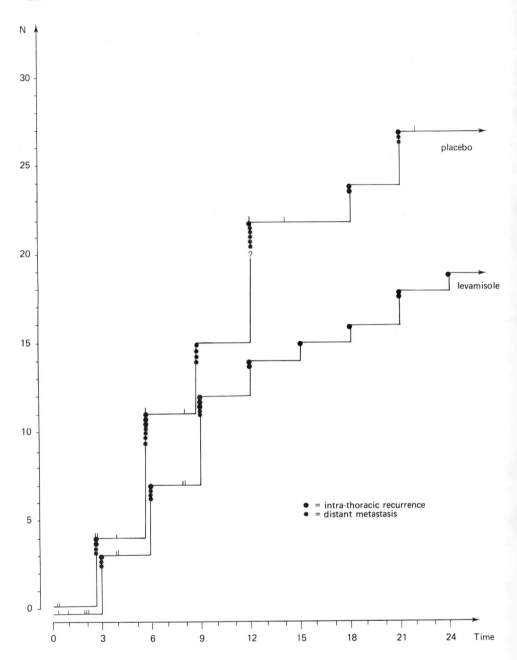

FIG. 1. Disease-free interval in patients with proven relapse: total population.

beneficial effect at all in patients weighing more than 70 kg. The disease-free interval in patients with proven relapse in the lower weight categories (i.e., ≤ 70 kg) is shown in Fig. 2.

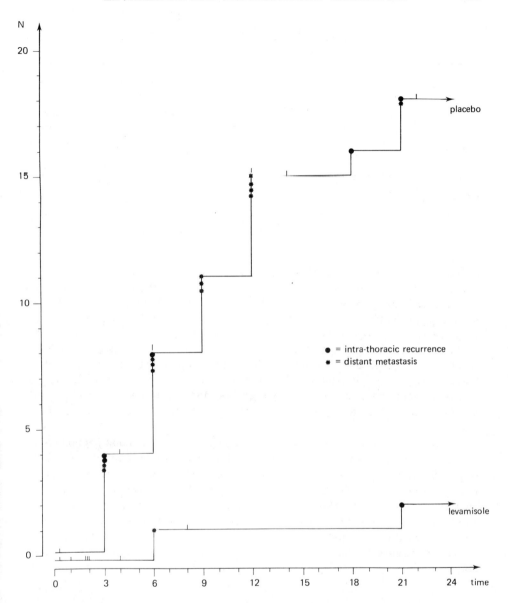

FIG. 2. Disease-free interval in patients with proven relapse and weighing ≤ 70 kg at the start.

The question remained as to whether other factors are helpful in predicting the levamisole effect in the patients belonging to these lower weight categories. From the analysis, it appeared that the initial degree of skin reactivity of the patients seemed to be unrelated to the beneficial effect of levamisole, although far more patients need to be studied before valid conclusions can be drawn as regards this aspect.

TABLE 2. Cause of death other than cancer

	Levamisole group (N = 69)	Placebo group (N = 79)
Surgical mortality	3	3
Other documented cause of death	3	3
Unknown cause of death	1	1
Total	7	7

Levamisole-treated patients with epidermoid carcinoma had fewer proven relapses than their placebo congeners ($p < 0.05$), but the number of patients showing another type of tumor is still too limited to allow a meaningful analysis although the trend in this more heterogenous population is also in favor of levamisole.

Levamisole patients with larger primaries (i.e., ≥ 4 cm largest diameter), those with more extensive tumors (i.e., the grouping categories in which there is evidence that tumor cells might have left or have already left the primary neoplasia), and those with a greater tumor load (i.e., grade II) all had fewer proven relapses ($p < 0.05$) than the placebo controls belonging to the same subgroups.

Lastly, proven relapses were subdivided into hematogenous secondaries and intrathoracic relapses in order to find out whether levamisole preferentially inhibited one of these two relapse types. Out of the 25 lower-weight levamisole patients, one had developed an intrathoracic recurrence and another one had a hematogenous secondary; the corresponding figures in the 35 placebo controls were 5 and 13. Therefore, levamisole caused an almost complete elimination ($p < 0.01$) of distant metastases, whereas the favorable trend with regard to the intrathoracic recurrences is not significant at this stage.

DISCUSSION

The major finding from this trial up to now is that levamisole in the dosage used is apparently effective only in patients weighing 70 kg or less. It is of interest that these patients have been taking about 2.5 mg/kg of levamisole per day, divided into three oral intakes, while the optimal dose for a single i.v. injection ranges from 1.25 to 2.5 mg/kg in several animal experiments. Therefore, we strongly recommend adapting the levamisole dose to the patients' weight or to their body surface in future trials.

Other important findings are that the effectiveness of levamisole seems to be established in epidermoid carcinoma, that patients with larger and/or more extensive tumors seem to be preferentially helped by levamisole, and that levamisole strikingly inhibits the formation of blood-borne metastases. It might be of interest in the latter context to note that the only adequately treated levamisole patient who developed a distant recurrence had interrupted his treatment for 1 month, 3 months after surgery; he developed liver metastases and died 2 months after this interruption.

SUMMARY

The present analysis reveals that the dose of levamisole should be adapted to the weight of the patients, according to a dosage scheme of 2.5 mg/kg/day. Adequately treated patients show markedly fewer recurrences during the first 2 years after surgery. Epidermoid carcinoma emerges as an established indication for levamisole treatment as an adjunct to surgery. Patients with larger and/or more extensive preoperative tumors seem to be preferentially helped by this type of immunotherapy. Levamisole treatment causes an almost complete elimination of hematogenous metastases.

REFERENCES

1. Study Group for Bronchogenic Carcinoma (1975): Immunopotentiation with levamisole in resectable bronchogenic carcinoma: A double-blind controlled trial. Br. Med. J., 3:461-464.
2. Amery, W. (1975): Double-blind trial with levamisole in resectable lung cancer. 9th International Congress of Chemotherapy, London, 13-18 July 1975.
3. Amery, W. K. (1976): Double-blind levamisole trial in resectable lung cancer. Ann. N.Y. Acad. Sci. (in press).
4. Slack, N. H. (1970): Bronchogenic carcinoma: Nitrogen mustard as a surgical adjuvant and factors influencing survival. Cancer, 25:987-1002.

Control of Neoplasia by Modulation of the Immune System, edited by M. A. Chirigos. Raven Press, New York 1977.

USE OF LEVAMISOLE IN THE THERAPY OF SYSTEMIC LUPUS ERYTHEMATOSUS: A CASE REPORT

*Benjamin L. Gordon, II and **John P. Keenan

*Kuakini Medical Center, 347 North Kuakini Street, Honolulu, Hawaii 96817, and John A. Burns School of Medicine, University of Hawaii, Leahi Campus, 3675 Kilauea Ave., Honolulu, Hawaii 96816; and

**John A. Burns School of Medicine, University of Hawaii, and Queen's Medical Center, 1301 Punchbowl Street, Honolulu, Hawaii 96813

INTRODUCTION

Systemic lupus erythematosus (SLE) is a diffuse multisystem vasculitic disease of connective tissue with a characteristic deficiency or absence of T-cell activity coupled with a hyperactivity in the B-cell system, produced in consequence of the lack of regulatory activity normally provided by the T-cell system (1). The excessive B-cell activity is expressed as numerous types of autoantibodies and other types of peculiar antibodies as well (1-6). Accompanying the presence of these antibodies is a polydispersed hyperglobulinemia accompanied by a consumptive hypocomplementemia (usually measured as a low C3 by radial immunodiffusion) due to the binding of complement by autoantibodies of appropriate classes and their antigens (4-6). Antibodies to most (if not all) antigens are produced in excessive amounts in SLE, and the immunologic tolerance developed during embryogenesis to antigens marked as "self" is readily broken, resulting in the production of autoantibodies (1-6). However, all of the latter effects are secondary to the loss of regulatory T-cell activity which characterizes SLE; ordinarily the T-cell system serves as an important regulator of B-cell function (1), preventing hyperactivity of the B-cell system, including the breaking of immune tolerance. It can thus be seen that if one were to restore regulatory activity to the T-cell system, the B-cell system would again be expected to come under its control.

The drug levamisole, originally developed in 1966 as a broad-spectrum anthelminthic agent (7), possesses marked immunostimulatory activity on the T-cell system (8-10) as well as on some of the nonspecific elements involved in immune responses, such as phagocytic cells (11, 12). Its effects on T-cells are particularly marked, and, for that reason, it was attempted to employ this agent in order to restore T-cell regulatory activity in patients with SLE, thus reversing their primary immunologic deficit.

Hopefully, reversal of their clinical disease would accompany this reversal of the T-cell defect. As will be seen, in the first patient in whom this therapy was attempted, the clinical results dovetailed perfectly with the predicted response.

CASE HISTORY

Patient IR-020675-1 is a 23-year-old American girl of Filipino ancestry, initially seen by the first author on June 2, 1975, with a presumptive diagnosis of collagen vascular disease, specific type undetermined. At that time her principal complaints were severe facial and periorbital edema (not steroid-induced, since both had been present prior to the patient having received any steroid), resulting in her right eye being swollen entirely shut for a period of 4.5 months. In addition, her left eye was swollen three-fourths shut, she had a severe skin rash which proved to be erythema nodosum over her entire body, she had increasingly large areas of patchy alopecia on the scalp, with the erythema nodosum skin rash also involving the scalp. A "lupoid" skin rash was seen spreading over her face, most marked in the pre-auricular areas, but rapidly coalescing to form a classic "butterfly" pattern. She had developed a high fever with a quotidian pattern, her temperature usually being normal on awakening and throughout the morning, but rising to a maximum of 101 to 103° F in the afternoon and early evening and often accompanied by rigors. She had constant arthralgias, particularly in the metacarpo-phalangeal joints and proximal interphalangeal joints of both hands, and in both ankles. Involvement of other joints was variable, but those aforementioned were nearly constant. Pain and stiffness were worse upon arising in the morning, and tended to improve somewhat throughout the day, although they did not disappear altogether. She displayed continual weakness and loss of strength, with malaise and cervical, inguinal, and femoral lymphadenopathy. She displayed mild to moderate hepatomegaly and anemia as well. She had been hospitalized twice for this problem prior to her first visit to the first author on June 2, 1965.

Prior to the onset of her illness in September 1974, she had remained in good health throughout her life. The initial manifestation in September 1974 was inguino-femoral lymphadenopathy, which did not yield to antibiotic treatment, and, in fact, spread to other locations during antibiotic therapy. Multiple laboratory tests were run on this young lady, but were not helpful in reaching diagnosis. One interesting finding was a positive Widal agglutination, maximal to S. paratyphoid B. But conformation of Salmonellosis was never bacteriologically achieved, and it is likely that this positive Widal was, in fact, a manifestation of the patient's lupus. A serum electropherogram revealed polydispersed hyperglobulinemia. Erythema nodosum developed shortly thereafter. Pyrexia continued until the patient was placed on prednisone, 40 mg/day, when the skin lesions and fever decreased. She was discharged from hospital on prednisone and tetracycline, which were discontinued a week after discharge from hospital. A month later, she developed polyarthralgias, which were not specifically treated, and were said to improve spontaneously over the next 2 months. A month later, she developed severe periorbital and facial edema, with alopecia and return of the erythema nodosum rash, as well as a "lupoid" facial rash. Her pyrexia also returned. All symptoms worsened, and about that time, the patient consulted another physician (the second author of this paper).

RESULTS

It was decided to admit the patient to Queen's Hospital in Honolulu for reassessment of her condition. By this time, she had developed a positive rheumatoid factor (RF); trace albuminuria, and hematuria, although her LE test remained negative. Her quotidian pyrexia had returned, with daily spikes as high as 104° F. She was admitted to Queen's on March 3, 1975, and remained in hospital for nearly a month, being discharged on March 31, 1975. She was treated initially with cyclophosphamide, then switched to prednisone, and kept on the latter drug at a dose of 80 mg/day. Her fever was brought under control, and was normal by time of discharge. During the 4 weeks of her hospitalization, she lost 8 lb. Skin and muscle biopsies showed marked vasculitis; liver biopsy showed mild steatosis only. She was found to be markedly anemic, and oral iron supplementation was employed. Transfusion was refused by the patient for religious reasons. Her alkaline phosphatase and bilirubin rose while on cyclophosphamide, but returned to normal when this drug was replaced by prednisone. Her hemoglobin reached a low point of 6.8 g-% on March 25, 1975, but a good reticulocyte response developed, and it had risen to 8.7 g-% by March 31, her date of discharge from hospital. Her discharge medications consisted of supplemental iron, folic acid, multivitamins, prednisone (80 mg/day), and a 1-week course of erythromycin to treat a Staph. infection in her throat.

The facial and periorbital edema, as well as the erythema nodosum and alopecia, continued to worsen, despite some subjective improvement; accordingly, her prednisone dosage was raised from 80 to 100 mg q.d. in May. Objective improvements were still not noted, though further subjective relief was obtained. She was referred to the first author of this paper for immunologic workup on June 2. At that time, her T-cell studies showed marked depression in a variety of parameters; her E-rosette count was 12% (normal = 60 to 80%), her lymphocyte stimulation tests to mitogens and antigens were extremely depressed, and her skin tests to a variety of recall T-antigens were extremely low. By contrast, her serum electropherograms and quantitative immunoglobulins showed polydispersed hyperglobulinemia, and her immunoelectropherogram was normal. The above combination, together with the primary vasculitic lesions seen in various tissues, indicated a diagnosis of SLE, despite the negativity of the LE-cell test.

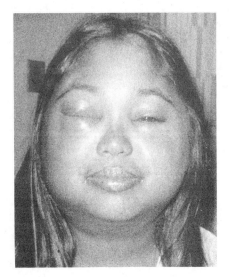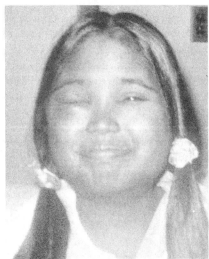

FIGS. 1,2. Taken March 1975 at Queen's Medical Center showing periorbital and facial edema and alopecia at central area of front hairline and behind this region.

For the reasons considered above, relating T-cell hypofunction to B-cell hyperfunction and clinical symptomatology in SLE, and because high doses of steroids had failed to control her disease, it was decided to try a course of levamisole in attempt to break the vicious cycle of T-cell hypofunction and B-cell hyperfunction encountered. The first course was administered on June 9. Within 2 weeks, subjective and objective improvements were noted; her edema was greatly diminished and she was able to see out of her right eye for the first time since February. Her strength was markedly improved. Her arthralgias were much reduced. By August, all areas of alopecia showed regrowth of hair. All signs and symptoms of disease had undergone significant reversal. Her lymphocyte stimulation tests to mitogens and antigens improved dramatically. By the 45th day following initiation of levamisole treatment, the patient stated that she felt entirely well. Her steroid dosage was accordingly reduced and was discontinued by early September. No ill effects, either from reduction of steroid or from the levamisole therapy were noted.

The improvement of this patient on levamisole and the elimination of steroid can only be described as spectacular, as is attested to in the accompanying series of photographs (Figs. 1-10 by permission of Annals of Allergy).

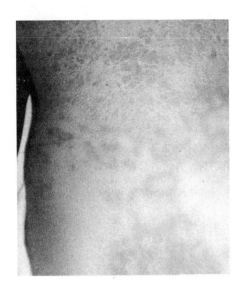

FIG. 3. Taken at Queen's Medical
Center, March 1975, showing
erythema nodosum type of rash over
back.

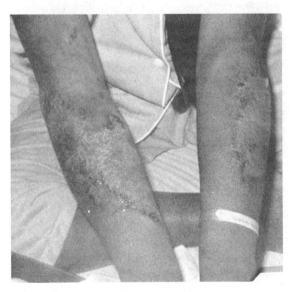

FIG. 4. Photograph taken at Queen's Medical Center, March 1975, showing
rash on arms of patient.

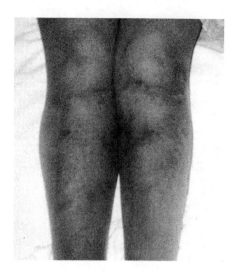

FIG. 5. Photograph taken at Queen's Medical Center, March 1975, showing rash over legs of patient prior to levamisole therapy.

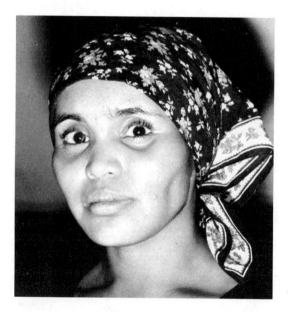

FIG. 6. Photograph taken August 29, 1975. (Treatment with levamisole began June 9, 1975). Note complete disappearance of facial and periorbital edema following levamisole therapy and drastic reduction in steroid dose.

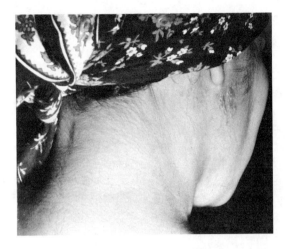

FIG. 7. Photograph taken August 29, 1975. Note small remnant of lupoid rash in area just below and in front of right ear, following levamisole treatment and despite drastic reduction in steroid dose. This rash is undergoing rapid clearing.

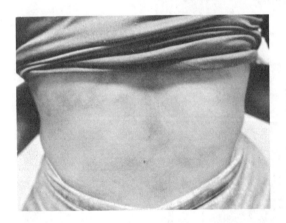

FIG. 8. Photograph taken August 29, 1975. Note clearance of rash from back on levamisole therapy and despite reduction of steroid dose. Compare with Fig. 3.

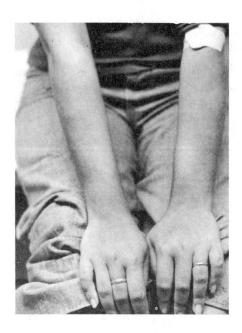

FIG. 9. Note clearance of rash from arms on levamisole treatment, despite reduction of steroid. Photograph taken August 29, 1975. Compare with Fig. 4.

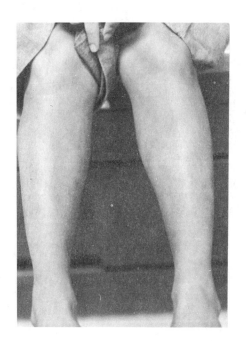

FIG. 10. Photograph taken August 29, 1975. Note disappearance of rash from legs, compared with Fig. 5, despite reduction of steroid dose, while on levamisole therapy.

DISCUSSION

In the human disease, SLE, and its experimental model in the New Zealand hybrid mouse (NZB/NZW mouse), a combination of genetic, immunologic, and extrinsic factors appear to be involved in initiating the lupus disease process (4-6). Generally, individuals developing the disease appear to develop primary T-cell immunodeficiency with consequent (secondary) loss of regulatory activity on the B-cell division, which then responds to the lack of regulation with a polydispersed hyperglobulinemia and loss of tolerance to antigens ordinarily marked as "self," thus providing the basal requirements for the development of the symptoms of SLE.

If it were possible to manipulate conditions in order to restore absent or defective T-cell responsiveness, the normal regulatory mechanisms which control the level of B-cell activity would once again become operative, and the secondary polydispersed hyperactivity of the B-cell division would disappear. Along with its disappearance, the signs and symptoms caused by B-cell hyperactivity would be expected either to diminish or to disappear altogether. The immunostimulant drug levamisole appeared to be able to exert this type of effect on the deficient T-cells of a patient with SLE, thus enabling the disease to be brought under control. In this way, the theoretical prediction dovetailed perfectly with the observed clinical status of a levamisole-treated patient suffering from SLE. Should further clinical studies bear these initial observations out, it would appear that the situation described herein provides an excellent example of how understanding the pathogenetic mechanisms of a disease enables the disease to be brought under control by appropriate manipulation of the basic defect — in this case, by use of the pharmacologic T-cell immunostimulant levamisole. This agent brought a variety of the T-cell parameters of a patient with SLE back to normal, and with their return to normal, enabled the disease to be brought under control, while at the same time allowing her steroid to be eliminated without ill effects of any kind. The clinical improvement observed, coupled with the improvement in immunologic laboratory investigations, appear to be so spectacular in this case as to justify its immediate publication as a single case report. Since theoretical considerations justifying the use of levamisole in SLE dovetail precisely with clinical and laboratory observations in this patient, and since levamisole is a relatively innocuous drug compared with the alternative forms of therapy available for SLE, we are presenting these data for the consideration of physicians treating this disease to be confirmed or refuted.

SUMMARY

The T-cell immunostimulant levamisole has been employed in the therapy of a 23-year-old woman previously on high doses of corticosteroids but controlled poorly with these agents. A single course of levamisole (150 mg/day for 3 days) was observed to cause significant improvement of her clinical disease and her laboratory parameters as well. She has received continuous 3-day courses of levamisole at 2-week intervals and has been doing consistently well on this regimen. Her steroids have been dropped from 100 mg of prednisone q.d. to total discontinuance of this drug. She is on no other medications of any type except for occasional aspirin, which she does not take regularly. Her clinical course on levamisole could appropriately be termed "spectacular." Moreover, the theoretical reasons behind its use in SLE fit perfectly with the observed response to the drug. Although it is far too early to tell, levamisole may be able to be discontinued altogether, and, in fact, the drug may be actually curative in SLE. Only the accumulation of further data will answer questions such as these. Thus, we offer the drug to other physicians to be employed in the treatment of SLE, in order that these results may be confirmed or refuted at the earliest possible time. It is well to note that this drug is far less toxic than any of the other agents available currently for the treatment of SLE, and apparently second to none in clinical efficacy. Therefore, there is little danger to the patient in treating him or her with a course of levamisole, whereas the potential value is extremely high, despite expected lack of clinical toxicity.

REFERENCES

1. Williams, H., Vaughan, J. H., Talal, N., and Zvaifler, N. J. (1975): Regulatory T-cells said to play major role in SLE. A précis of a symposium on SLE held at the 1975 Annual Meeting of the American College of Physicians. Skin and Allergy News, 44, July 1975.
2. Boonpucknavig, S., Vuttirojana, A., Ruangjirachuporn, W., and Siripont, J. (1975): B- and T-lymphocytes in autoimmune disease. Lancet, 2:414.
3. Harvey, A. M., Johns, R. J., Owens, A. H., and Ross, R. S. (1972): The Principles and Practice of Medicine. 18th ed., pp. 1236-1245. Appleton-Century-Crofts, New York.
4. Gordon, B. L. (1974): Essentials of Immunology, 2nd ed., pp. 207-210. F. A. Davis Co., Philadelphia.
5. Rodnan, G. P., McEwen, C., and Wallace, S. L. (1973): Primer on the Rheumatic Diseases, 7th ed. The Arthritis Foundation, New York.
6. Bellanti, J. A. (1971): Immunology, pp. 397-404. W. B. Saunders Co., Philadelphia.
7. Thienpont, D., Vanporijs, O. F. J., Raeymaekers, A. H. M., Vandenberk, J., Allewijn, F. T. N., Marsboom, R. P. H., Niemegeers, C. J. E., Schellekens, K. H. L., and Janssen, P. A. J. (1966): Tetramisole (R 8299), A new potent, broad spectrum anthelminthic. Nature, 209:1084.
8. Symoens, J. (1974): The effects of levamisole on host defense mechanisms: A review. Bulletin of Janssen Pharmaceutica Research Laboratories, B-2340, pp. 1-59. Beerse, Belgium.
9. Janssen R&D (1970): Basic Medical Information Brochure on Levamisole (R12,564). Janssen R&D, New Brunswick, N. J.
10. Renoux, G., and Renoux, M. (1971): Effet immunostimulant d'un imidothiazole dans l'immunisation des souris contre l'infection par Brucella abortus. C. R. Acad. Sci. (D), 272:349-350.

11. Fisher, G. W., Podgore, J. K., Bass, J. W., Wagner, F. S., and
     Kelley, J. L. (1974): Enhanced host defense mechanism with
     levamisole in newborn rats. Unpublished data, September 1974.
12. Fisher, G. W., Oi, V. T., Kelley, J. L., Podgore, J. K., Bass, J. W.,
     Wagner, F. S., and Gordon, B. L. (1974): Enhancement of host de-
     fense mechanisms against Gram-positive pyogenic coccal infections
     with levo-tetramisole (levamisole) in neonatal rats. Ann. Allergy,
     33:193-198.

Control of Neoplasia by Modulation of the Immune System. edited by M. A. Chirigos. Raven Press, New York 1977.

CLINICAL AND IMMUNOLOGIC EFFECTS OF LEVAMISOLE

*,**Lynn E. Spitler, **Richard G. Glogau, [†]Donald C. Nelms, **Christa M. Basch, [†]James A. Olson, [†]Sol Silverman, Jr., and **Ephraim P. Engleman

*Laboratory of Cellular Immunology, Children's Hospital of San Francisco, San Francisco, California 94118; and **Department of Medicine, University of California, San Francisco, and [†]School of Dentistry, San Francisco, California 94143

INTRODUCTION

Levamisole, a drug which has been widely used as an antihelminthic, has been shown to increase both humoral and cellular immune responses in animals (1,2) and cellular immune responses in man (3-5). In uncontrolled studies, levamisole has been reported to cure or decrease the frequency and severity of lesions in patients with recurrent aphthous stomatitis (6,7) or recurrent herpes labialis (8) and to cause clinical improvement in patients with rheumatoid arthritis.

In view of the above, we undertook a preliminary study to evaluate the clinical and immunologic effects of levamisole in selected patients.

MATERIALS AND METHODS

Patients (Table 1): Various patient groups were studied. The largest group consisted of patients with recurrent aphthous stomatitis. This included 50 subjects, 31 females and 19 males, ranging in age from 9 to 66.

Sixteen patients with classical or definite rheumatoid arthritis were treated: 4 males and 12 females with an average age of 43 years. The group of patients with recurrent herpes simplex infections included 26 subjects, 2 with labial herpes, 12 with genital herpes, and 9 with ocular involvement. Also studied were 2 patients with the Wiskott-Aldrich syndrome and 2 patients with chronic mucocutaneous candidiasis.

TABLE 1. Diseases treated with levamisole

	Number of subjects
Recurrent aphthous stomatitis	50
Rheumatoid arthritis	18
Recurrent herpes simplex	26
Labial	2
Genital	12
Ocular	9
Wiskott-Aldrich syndrome	2
Chronic mucocutaneous candidiasis	2
Familial trichophytin infection	1
Toxoplasmic chorioretinitis	2
Acne conglobata	2
Verruca vulgaris	1
Behcet's disease	2

Protocol of therapy: A panel of immunologic tests including skin tests (10), lymphocyte stimulation with antigen and PHA (11), leukocyte migration inhibition (12), rosette-forming cells (13), and chemotaxis (14) were performed before the initiation of therapy and 1 week after the first course of therapy (Table 2). Not all patients had every test performed.

The therapy protocols were varied, depending on the disease treated. Most patients received 150 mg/day for 3 days in a row every fortnight. Some patients received 150 mg for 2 days in a row every week. Some patients were treated with abortive therapy, taking medication only when they noted the onset of lesions. Children received a dose of 2.5 mg/kg at time intervals similar to those described above.

RESULTS

Skin test reactivity: A significant increase in skin test reactivity was considered to be an increase of more than 5 mm induration. Over 95% of the patients with recurrent aphthous stomatitis showed an increase in skin reactivity to one or more antigens (15). When individual test antigens were considered, there was a significant increase in reactivity to candida and PPD after levamisole therapy as determined by Student's t-test (Fig. 1). The results

TABLE 2. Immunologic tests performed before and after levamisole therapy

Skin tests:
  Candida
  Coccidioidin
  Mumps
  PPD
  Streptokinase–streptodornase
  Trichophytin
Lymphocyte stimulation with antigen and PHA
Leukocyte migration inhibition
Rosette–forming cells: short and long incubation
Chemotaxis

in patients with other diseases generally paralleled these results. The changes in skin test reactivity during levamisole therapy were at times very dramatic. Biopsy of one skin test site revealed a histologic picture of a typical delayed hypersensitivity reaction. It is of considerable interest that

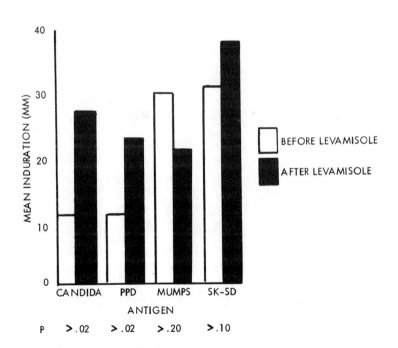

FIG. 1. Results of skin test reactivity in patients with recurrent aphthous stomatitis before and after levamisole therapy.

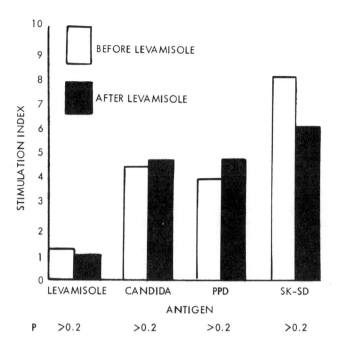

FIG. 2.   Results of lymphocyte stimulation in patients with recurrent aphthous stomatitis before and after levamisole therapy.

some patients experienced a flare at the DNCB test site following ingestion of levamisole.

Lymphocyte stimulation: Baseline radioactive thymidine incorporation was not significantly different after levamisole therapy as compared to before. In the patients with recurrent aphthous stomatitis, the stimulation indices to three antigens (PPD, SK-SD, and candida) were not significantly changed after therapy (15), even though skin test reactivity to the same antigens were markedly increased (Fig. 2). Addition of levamisole to the cultures with or without specific antigens did not alter the thymidine incorporation. Similar results were observed in patients with other diseases. In patients with rheumatoid arthritis, the PHA dose-response curve was low and did not increase after therapy. The one exception to the general observation that lymphocyte reactivity did not change occurred in patients with recurrent herpes simplex infections in whom lymphocyte stimulation by herpes simplex antigens consistently significantly decreased following levamisole therapy (16).

Leukocyte migration inhibition: Migration in control wells without antigen was unchanged after levamisole therapy. With three test antigens (candida, PPD, and SK-SD), there was no significant change in the migration after levamisole therapy (15) (Fig. 3). Addition of levamisole to the cultures did not affect the migration.

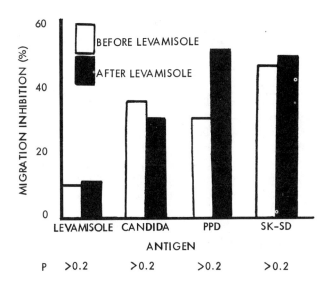

FIG. 3. Results of leukocyte migration inhibition in patients with recurrent aphthous stomatitis before and after levamisole therapy.

Rosette-forming cells: In the patients with rheumatoid arthritis, the mean total lymphocyte count and the number of long-incubation rosette-forming cells were significantly lower in the patient group than in the normal population and increased slightly, but not significantly, after therapy (9). The number of short-incubation rosette-forming cells, thought by some to represent a subpopulation of T-cells, was normal and did not change after therapy.

Chemotaxis: There was a statistically significant increase in chemotaxis after levamisole therapy when the test was performed using homologous, but not autologous, serum.

Clinical: Levamisole therapy caused a reduction in the number, frequency, and severity of recurrent aphthous stomatitis attacks in 62% of the patients tested. Six percent of these patients underwent permanent remission, 56% were improved, and 38% showed no response.

Of the 16 patients with rheumatoid arthritis, overall self-appraisal indicated subjective improvement in 10 patients, no change in 4, and increase in symptoms in 2. The subjective and objective changes noted in some patients included decrease in morning stiffness, faster timing on the 50-yard walk, increased grip strength, and decrease in the number of painful joints. Subcutaneous nodules disappeared or were much smaller in 5 of 6 patients who had nodules prior to the initiation of therapy. In 2 patients the latex titer for rheumatoid factor, which had been 1:160 or higher, fell to less than 1:40.

In the patients with herpes simplex infections, the results in the patients with herpes simplex of the cornea were most consistent. Healing usually began after the first course of therapy, and in 8 of the 9 patients treated, complete healing of the active infection occurred with only residual scarring.

Most patients were treated for 3 to 6 months. In only 1 of the 8 responding patients was there relapse following the cessation of therapy, and this patient responded to a second course.

Two patients who were referred by dermatologists with the diagnosis of herpes were found to have no antibody to herpes and their lymphocytes did not respond in vitro to herpes antigens. It was thus concluded that they did not in fact have herpes infections.

Two patients with the Wiskott–Aldrich syndrome appeared to have improved. One patient had improvement in his eczema, and he also had molluscum contagiosum and verruca vulgaris, which improved. A second patient with the Wiskott–Aldrich syndrome had persistent cat scratch fever which did not respond to nonspecific or to specific transfer factor but which did respond to levamisole.

Two patients with mucocutaneous candidiasis were treated and did not show a response. Similarly, 1 patient with familial trichophytin infection failed to respond.

Two patients with toxoplasmic chorioretinitis showed a good response. One of these patients subsequently underwent relapse despite continued therapy. The other one had lesions which appeared to be healed, so therapy was stopped. She underwent relapse and responded well to the reinitiation of therapy.

Two patients with acne conglobata were treated because they were found to be anergic. Both experienced improvement. A patient with persistent verruca vulgaris experienced itching but no objective change in the lesions during 3 months of levamisole therapy. The lesions subsequently underwent complete regression following administration of one dose of transfer factor. Two patients with Behcet's disease appeared to have clinical benefit.

Side effects were observed in the majority of patients but for the most part were not severe. Dysgeusia, irritability, and/or drowsiness occurred most frequently but necessitated termination of therapy in only 1 patient. Skin rash occurred in a few patients and required termination of therapy. Occasionally, patients complained of headache and/or gastrointestinal distress. Two patients developed marked tender lymphadenopathy during the course of therapy which regressed with continued therapy. One patient with rheumatoid arthritis developed a peripheral neutropenia which necessitated termination of therapy.

DISCUSSION

The results presented herein indicate that levamisole has a definite effect on immunologic responses; specifically, it increases skin test reactivity. The observation that the DNCB test site flared following ingestion of levamisole provides striking confirmation of the enhancing effect of levamisole on delayed sensitivity.

Although the changes in skin test reactivity were quite striking, we did not observe a parallel change in the in vitro parameters of cellular immunity, lymphocyte stimulation, and leukocyte migration inhibition in response to the

same antigens. Moreover, we did not see a change in the nonspecific parameters of cellular immunity — the PHA response, lymphocyte count, or
rosette-forming cells. It is possible that changes in lymphocyte reactivity
did, in fact, occur but that we failed to detect these changes due to the timing
of performance of the in vitro studies. These studies were done, however,
at the same time that the changes in skin test reactivity were observed.

A second explanation for these observations could be that levamisole does
not affect the central immune response but rather acts on some other aspect
of immune reactivity, perhaps on the polymorphonuclear leukocytes or the
macrophages. Increased reactivity of these cells could account for an increase in skin test reactivity by causing an increase in the local inflammatory
response without a change in lymphocyte reactivity. That levamisole may be
affecting the polys is supported by the observation of increased chemotactic
response following levamisole therapy.

Transfer factor, a dialyzable extract of sensitized leukocytes, also increases skin test reactivity and has been used in the therapy of a variety of
conditions associated with primary or acquired cellular immune deficiency
(11). In normal subjects, transfer factor causes parallel conversion of
lymphocyte stimulation and migration inhibition. In patients with immunodeficiency diseases, conversion of migration inhibition usually occurs in
parallel with conversion of skin test reactivity, whereas conversion of lymphocyte stimulation may or may not occur. It would seem, therefore, that the
mechanism of action of levamisole differs from that of transfer factor. This
is further supported by the observation that the 2 patients with mucocutaneous
candidiasis did not respond to levamisole, whereas this disease is one which
may respond most dramatically to transfer factor.

The clinical effects of levamisole appear encouraging in a number of
diseases. Since these diseases are all conditions which have a varied course
and in which spontaneous remissions may occur, it is necessary to perform
appropriate controlled randomized double-blind studies to analyze clearly
the clinical efficacy of levamisole. Such studies are currently underway.

SUMMARY

The clinical and immunologic effects of levamisole were evaluated in over
100 patients with a variety of diseases including aphthous stomatitis,
rheumatoid arthritis, herpes simplex, toxoplasmic retinochoroiditis, the
Wiskott-Aldrich syndrome, and chronic mucocutaneous candidiasis. The
clinical results were sufficiently encouraging to warrant the design of controlled randomized double-blind trials, which have now been initiated. There
was a consistent and dramatic increase in skin test reactivity without a concomitant increase in lymphocyte stimulation or leukocyte migration inhibition.
In patients with recurrent herpes simplex infections, there was a consistent
decrease in the lymphocyte stimulation by herpes antigens in vitro during the
course of therapy.

ACKNOWLEDGMENTS

This work was supported by Research Career Development Award A1 43012, National Institutes of Health grant A1 13399, and a gift from the Janssen Pharmaceutical Co.

We thank Mrs. Christine von Muller, Miss Jennifer Brunn, Mrs. Elizabeth Harsh, Mrs. Nenita Arias, and Mr. Anicito Gonzaga for excellent technical assistance.

REFERENCES

1. Renoux, G., and Renoux, M. (1971): Effet immunostimulant d'un imidothiazole dans l'immunisation des souris contre l'infection par Brucella abortus. C. R. Acad. Sci. (D), 272:349-354.
2. Renoux, G., and Renoux, M. (1973): Stimulation of anti-Brucella vaccination in mice by tetramisole, a phenyl-imidothiazole salt. Infect. Immun., 8:544-548.
3. Tripodi, D., Parks, L. C., and Brugmans, J. (1973): Drug-induced restoration of cutaneous delayed hypersensitivity in anergic patients with cancer. New Engl. J. Med., 289:354-357.
4. Verhaegen, H., De Cree, J., De Cock, W., and Verbruggen, F. (1973): Levamisole and the immune response. New Engl. J. Med., 289:1148-1149.
5. Verhaegen, H., De Cree, J., Verbruggen, H., Hoebeke, J., de Brabander, M., and Brugmans, J. (1973): Immune responses in elderly cuti-negative subjects and the effect of levamisole. Verh. Dtsch. Ges. Inn. Med., 79:623-8.
6. Verhaegen, H., De Cree, J., and Brugmans, J. (1973): Treatment of aphthous stomatitis. Lancet, II:842.
7. Symoens, J., and Brugmans, J. (1974): Treatment of recurrent aphthous stomatitis and herpes with levamisole. Br. Med. J., 4:592.
8. Kint, A., and Verlinden, L. (1974): Levamisole for recurrent herpes labialis. New Engl. J. Med., 291:308.
9. Basch, C. M., Spitler, L. E., and Engleman, E. P. (1975): The effects of levamisole in rheumatoid arthritis. Arthritis Rheum., 18:385.
10. Spitler, L. E. (1976): Delayed hypersensitivity skin testing. In: Manual of Clinical Immunology (in press).
11. Spitler, L. E., Levin, A. S., and Fudenberg, H. H. (1973): Human lymphocyte transfer factor. In Methods in Cancer Research, Vol. 8, edited by H. Busch, pp. 59-106. Academic Press, New York.
12. Astor, S. H., Spitler, L. E., Frick, O. L., and Fudenberg, H. H. (1973): Human leukocyte migration inhibition in agarose using four antigens: Correlation with skin reactivity. J. Immunol., 110:1174-1179.
13. Wybran, J. (1973): Thymus-derived rosette-forming cells in various human disease states: Cancer, lymphoma, bacterial and viral infections, and other diseases. J. Clin. Invest., 52:1026-1032.

14. DeMeo, A. N., and Anderson, B. R. (1972): Defective chemotaxis associated with a serum inhibitor in cirrhotic patients. New Engl. J. Med., 286:735-740.

15. Olson, J. A., Nelms, D. C., Silverman, S., and Spitler, L. E. (1976): Levamisole, a new treatment for recurrent aphthous stomatitis. Oral Surg., 41:588-600.

16. Glogau, R., Spitler, L., Nelms, D., O'Connor, R., Olson, J., Ostler, P., Silverman, S., and Smolin, G. (1973): Clinical and immunologic effects of levamisole. Clin. Res., 23:291A.

Control of Neoplasia by Modulation of the Immune System, edited by M. A. Chirigos. Raven Press, New York 1977.

EFFECTS OF LEVAMISOLE ON NEUTROPHILS AND MONONUCLEAR CELLS FROM NORMAL INDIVIDUALS AND FROM PATIENTS WITH ABNORMAL LEUKOCYTE CHEMOTAXIS

Daniel G. Wright, *Charles H. Kirkpatrick, and John I. Gallin

Clinical Physiology and *Clinical Allergy and Hypersensitivity Sections, Laboratory of Clinical Investigation, National Institute of Allergy and Infectious Diseases, Bethesda, Maryland 20014

INTRODUCTION

The directed migration or chemotaxis of leukocytes has long been considered an important aspect of inflammatory responses and host defense. It has been only recently, however, that widely available and reproducible techniques have been developed to measure this leukocyte function in vitro. Only in the past few years has the identification of defective leukocyte chemotaxis in patients with syndromes of recurrent infection been described (1).

We have investigated the effects of levamisole on in vitro chemotactic responses of leukocytes from normal, healthy individuals and from two groups of patients in whom recurrent infection has been associated with defective leukocyte chemotaxis. These include patients with the Chediak-Higashi syndrome (2,3) and patients with the syndrome characterized by recurrent pyogenic infections and hyperimmunoglobulin E (4-6). Our observations are the subject of this report.

MATERIALS AND METHODS

In these studies human neutrophils and mononuclear cells were separated from heparinized blood by techniques that involve dextran sedimentation (2) and hypaque-ficoll gradients (7). In vitro leukocyte chemotaxis was evaluated with modified Boyden chambers in which leukocyte suspensions, in an upper compartment, are separated from a chemotactic stimulus in a lower compartment by micropore filters. The filters act as a barrier through which the cells migrate in response to the chemotactic stimulus. Neutrophil chemotaxis was measured using a radioassay employing ^{51}Cr-labeled leukocytes

227

obtained by dextran sedimentation and a double micropore filter system developed in our laboratory (8). For this assay chemotaxis was expressed as corrected counts per minute in the lower micropore filter (cor cpm LF). Mononuclear cell chemotaxis was measured using the morphologic technique of Snyderman et al. (9) utilizing one micropore filter. Mononuclear cell chemotaxis was expressed as cells per high power field (cells/hpf) migrating to the under surface of the filters.

Neutrophil oxidative metabolism, as reflected by hexose monophosphate shunt activity (10), and cellular cyclic nucleotide levels (11) were measured by standard methods. In these studies leukocytes were exposed to levamisole or to control solutions during the functional assays and without preincubation with drug.

RESULTS AND DISCUSSION

Table 1 represents the results of experiments with normal human neutrophils and mononuclear cells in which the chemotactic responsiveness of the leukocytes to endotoxin-activated serum (2) is compared with and without levamisole. Enhancement of neutrophil chemotaxis was consistently observed at a high concentration, 5×10^{-3} M, and a lower concentration, 10^{-7} M. Enhanced mononuclear cell chemotaxis was also consistently observed with 10^{-7} M levamisole; enhancement was observed as well at 5×10^{-3} M levamisole in individual experiments, but this result was variable.

Enhanced neutrophil chemotaxis with 5×10^{-3} M levamisole was found to be related at least in part to stimulation of random migration of the cells. When buffer alone was used in the lower compartment of the chemotactic chambers, a small number of cells migrate through to the lower micropore filter; this migration response to buffer is an indicator of spontaneous or random migration of the cells (12). As is shown in Table 2, 5×10^{-3} M levamisole markedly augmented random migration of neutrophils, whereas lower concentrations of drug lacked this effect.

Of particular interest was the possibility that levamisole might also enhance the chemotactic responsiveness of leukocytes from patients with abnormal leukocyte chemotaxis, and we have been able to study two groups of such patients. Humans and animals with the Chediak-Higashi (C-H) syndrome typically suffer from recurrent pyogenic infections, sometimes fatal (13). Leukocytes from patients with the C-H syndrome are characterized by giant granules, and among other leukocyte functional abnormalities, both their neutrophils (2) and mononuclear cells (3) have been shown to have markedly impaired chemotactic responses in vitro.

Recently, another clinical syndrome has been recognized, associated with abnormal leukocyte chemotaxis. In this syndrome of children and teenagers, patients suffer from recurrent abscesses and pneumonia, have marked elevations of IgE, defective in vitro lymphocyte proliferation, and defective leukocyte chemotaxis (6). This syndrome lacks a widely accepted eponym. Here we have referred to it as the hyperimmunoglobulin E (HIE) syndrome. The chemotactic responsiveness of leukocytes from C-H patients and from HIE patients is typically less than 25% and less than 50% of normal, respectively

TABLE 1. Effects of levamisole on normal human leukocyte chemotaxis

Levamisole [a]	Chemotaxis [b]	
	Neutrophils [b]	Mononuclear cells [b]
10^{-8} M	-1 ± 24 (5)	-7 ± 9 (4)
10^{-7} M	$+49 \pm 12$ (6) $p < 0.05$	$+34 \pm 18$ (4) $p < 0.05$
10^{-6} M	-3 ± 2 (5)	$+25 \pm 20$ (4)
10^{-4} M	$+7 \pm 7$ (6)	-13 ± 26 (4)
5×10^{-3} M	$+87 \pm 15$ (8) $p < 0.01$	$+5 \pm 10$ (5)

[a] Concentration of drug to which cells are exposed during chemotaxis measurements.

[b] Chemotactic response to 2.5% serum activated with E. coli endotoxin; percent difference from chemotactic response of control leukocytes not treated with levamisole. Standard errors of the means, numbers of experiments, and statistically significant differences from cells without levamisole are indicated (paired sample t-test).

In studies with leukocytes from 2 C-H patients and from 4 HIE patients, we found that levamisole at 10^{-7} M significantly improved the abnormal in vitro chemotactic response of HIE neutrophils and mononuclear cells (Table 3). Moreover, the leukocytes from these patients appeared relatively more sensitive to the stimulatory effects of levamisole than did normal leukocytes. In contrast, the abnormal function of C-H leukocytes was not altered by levamisole at this concentration.

In related studies, we found that the enhanced chemotactic response of normal neutrophils exposed to 10^{-7} M levamisole was associated with enhancement of neutrophil oxidative metabolism by the drug at this concentration (Table 4). In these studies, the hexose monophosphate shunt activity of phagocytizing neutrophils was significantly increased when the cells were in the presence of 10^{-7} M levamisole. On the other hand, 5×10^{-3} M levamisole decreased the oxidative metabolism of the cells. This result is additional evidence that this high concentration acts on the cells in a manner different from the effect seen at lower concentrations (10^{-7} M).

When cyclic nucleotide levels were measured in normal leukocytes exposed to levamisole, we found that the drug at 10^{-7} M caused significant elevations of mononuclear cell cyclic GMP (Table 5). Small increments in cyclic GMP were also observed in neutrophils exposed to 10^{-7} M levamisole, but these changes were small and not statistically significant. Significant

TABLE 2. Effects of levamisole on neutrophil random migration

Levamisole[a]	Random migration[b]
10^{-8} M	-11 ± 9 (5)
10^{-7} M	$+11 \pm 11$ (5)
10^{-6} M	$+7 \pm 3$ (5)
10^{-4} M	$+24 \pm 1$ (5)
5×10^{-3} M	$+127 \pm 40$ (5) $p < 0.01$

[a] Concentration of drug to which cells are exposed during random migration measurements.

[b] Migratory response to buffer alone as stimulus in chemotactic chambers; percent difference from response of control neutrophils not treated with levamisole. Standard errors of the means, numbers of experiments, and statistically significant differences from cells without levamisole are indicated (paired sample t-test).

TABLE 3. Effects of 10^{-7} M levamisole on chemotaxis of leukocytes from patients with the Chediak-Higashi (C-H) and hyperimmunoglobulin E (HIE) syndromes

	C-H syndrome[a]		HIE syndrome[a]	
	Neutrophils	Mononuclear cells	Neutrophils	Mononuclear cells
Untreated cell	$11\% \pm 2$ (5)	$45\% \pm 10$ (2)	$41\% \pm 5$ (9)	$54\% \pm 4$ (4)
Cells with 10^{-7} M levamisole	$9\% \pm 3$ (4)	$40\% \pm 8$ (2)	$77\% \pm 4$ (6)[b]	$83\% \pm 2$ (2)[b]

[a] Chemotactic response of patients' leukocytes to endotoxin activated serum: percent of chemotactic response of leukocytes from normal volunteers. Standard errors of the means and numbers of experiments are indicated.

[b] Statistically significant improvement of chemotactic response of patients' leukocytes by treatment with levamisole (10^{-7} M), $p < 0.05$ (paired sample t-test).

TABLE 4. Effects of levamisole on hexose monophosphate shunt activity
of normal human neutrophils

Levamisole [a]	HMP shunt activity [b]
10^{-8} M	+12 ± 25 (4)
10^{-7} M	+35 ± 4 (4) p < 0.05
10^{-6} M	+36 ± 19 (4)
10^{-4} M	−15 ± 17 (4)
5 X 10^{-3} M	−64 ± 11 (4) p < 0.05

[a] Concentration of drug to which cells are exposed during HMP shunt
measurements.

[b] Hexose monophosphate shunt activity of neutrophils phagocytizing latex
particles, 30 min: percent difference from HMP shunt activity of control
cells not treated with levamisole. Standard errors of the means, numbers
of experiments, and statistically significant differences are indicated (paired
sample t-test).

TABLE 5. Effects of levamisole on cyclic GMP levels in normal human
mononuclear cells

Levamisole [a]	Cyclic GMP [b]
10^{-8} M	+123 ± 103 (3)
10^{-7} M	+263 ± 62 (3) p < 0.05
10^{-6} M	+136 ± 121 (3)
10^{-4} M	+47 ± 20 (3)
5 X 10^{-3} M	+13 ± 8 (3)

[a] Concentration of drug to which cells are exposed during cyclic GMP
assay.

[b] Cyclic GMP: percent difference from cyclic GMP levels of control cells
not treated with levamisole. Standard errors of the means, numbers of experiments, and statistically significant differences are indicated (paired
sample t-test).

TABLE 6. Chemotaxis of neutrophils from patients with HIE syndrome before and after oral levamisole

Experiments [a]	Neutrophil chemotaxis [b]	
	Before Drug	After Drug
A	37%	61%
B_1	30%	42%
B_2	50%	53%
C_1	25%	63%
C_2	58%	72%
D	70%	103%

[a] Six experiments with HIE patients designated A, B, C, and D; patients B and C were each studied before and after two separate courses of levamisole.

[b] Neutrophil chemotactic response to sodium caseinate (5 mg/ml); percent of the chemotactic response of neutrophils from normal volunteers studied concurrently with the patients. Results indicate statistically significant improvement in the abnormal chemotaxis of patients' cells after levamisole: $p < 0.01$ (paired sample t-test).

changes in cyclic AMP were not observed in the leukocytes. These results are consistent with recent reports by others who found that levamisole in the range of 10^{-8} to 10^{-6} M raised cyclic GMP levels in murine lymphocytes (14).

The activity of levamisole at 10^{-7} M was of particular interest because this concentration of drug has been shown to be attained in blood after oral administration in humans. Under an NIAID-approved protocol, 4 HIE syndrome patients were given 150 mg of levamisole by mouth on each of 2 successive days. The chemotactic response of their neutrophils to sodium caseinate (5 mg/ml) was studied before and 2 hr after this 2-day course of drug. In each case, leukocyte chemotaxis was improved after ingestion of the drug (Table 6).

In summary, these studies demonstrate that levamisole in vitro enhances the chemotactic response of normal leukocytes and of leukocytes from certain patients with abnormal leukocyte chemotaxis at a concentration (10^{-7} M) that may be attained in vivo. This concentration of drug in vitro also was found to enhance neutrophil oxidative metabolism and to raise cyclic GMP levels in mononuclear cells. In addition, abnormal neutrophil chemotaxis in patients with the HIE syndrome was found to be improved after the leukocytes had been exposed to levamisole in vivo. It should be emphasized, finally, that these in vitro studies do not demonstrate in any way that levamisole is clinically beneficial in patients with syndromes of recurrent infection. Any clinical use of levamisole must be evaluated by careful and properly controlled, randomized trials.

SUMMARY

Levamisole enhances the in vitro chemotactic responsiveness of normal human neutrophils and mononuclear cells at a concentration (10^{-7} M) that may be attained in vivo. This concentration of drug in vitro also improves the abnormal chemotaxis of leukocytes from patients with a syndrome of recurrent pyogenic infection and hyperimmunoglobulin E (HIE syndrome). This concentration of levamisole (10^{-7} M) may also be shown to enhance neutrophil oxidative metabolism and to elevate cyclic GMP in mononuclear cells. Leukocytes from patients with the HIE syndrome demonstrate improved in vitro chemotaxis after exposure to levamisole in vivo.

REFERENCES

1. Gallin, J. I., and Wolff, S. M. (1975): Leukocyte chemotaxis: Physiological considerations and abnormalities. Clin. Haematol., 4:567-607.
2. Clark, R. A., and Kimball, H. R. (1971): Defective granulocyte chemotaxis in the Chediak-Higashi syndrome. J. Clin. Invest., 50:2645-2652.
3. Gallin, J. I., Klimerman, J. A., Padgett, G. A., and Wolff, S. M. (1975): Defective mononuclear cell hemotaxis in the Chediak-Higashi syndrome of humans, mink and cattle. Blood, 45:863-870.
4. Clark, R. A., Root, R. K., Kimball, H. R., and Kirkpatrick, C. H. (1973): Defective neutrophil chemotaxis and cellular immunity in a child with recurrent infections. Ann. Intern. Med., 78:515-519.
5. Gallin, J. I. (1975): Abnormal chemotaxis: Cellular and humoral components. In: The Phagocytic Cell in Host Resistance, edited by J. A. Bellanti and D. H. Dayton, pp. 227-249. Raven Press, New York.
6. Van Scoy, R. E., Hill, H. R., Ritts, R. E., and Quie, P. G. (1975): Familial neutrophil chemotaxis defect, recurrent bacterial infections, mucocutaneous candidiasis and hyperimmunoglobulinemia E. Ann. Intern. Med., 82:766-771.
7. Boyum, A. (1968): Isolation of mononuclear cells and granulocytes from human blood. Scand. J. Clin. Lab. Invest., (Suppl.), 77:96-100.
8. Gallin, J. I., Clark, R. A., and Kimball, H. R. (1973): Granulocyte chemotaxis: An improved in vitro assay employing ^{51}Cr labeled granulocytes. J. Immunol., 110:233-240.
9. Snyderman, R., Altman, L. C., Hausman, M. S., and Mergenhagen, S. E. (1975): J. Immunol., 108:857-860.

10. Mickenberg, I. D., Root, R. K., and Wolff, S. M. (1970): Leukocyte function in acquired hypogammaglobulinemia. J. Clin. Invest., 49: 1528-1538.

11. Sandler, J. A., Gallin, J. I., and Vaughan, M. A. (1975): Effects of serotonin, carbamylcholine and ascorbic acid on leukocyte cyclic GMP and chemotaxis. J. Cell. Biol., 67:476-479.

12. Gallin, J. I., and Rosenthal, A. S. (1974): The regulatory role of divalent cations in human granulocyte chemotaxis: Evidence for an association between calcium exchanges and microtubule assembly. J. Cell Biol., 62:594-609.

13. Blume, R. S., and Wolff, S. M. (1972): The Chediak-Higashi syndrome, studies in four patients and a review of the literature. Medicine, 51:247-280.

14. Hadden, J. W., Coffey, R. G., Hadden, E. M., Lopez-Corrales, E., and Sunshine, G. H. (1975): Effects of levamisole and imidazole on lymphocyte proliferation and cyclic nucleotide levels. Cell. Immunol., 20:98-103.

Control of Neoplasia by Modulation
of the Immune System, edited by
M. A. Chirigos. Raven Press, New
York   1977.

LEVAMISOLE THERAPY IN ADVANCED CANCER PATIENTS.
A PROGNOSTIC TEST?

*Gerard Renoux and Micheline Renoux

Laboratoire d'Immunologie, Faculté de Médecine, 37032 Tours, Cedex,
France

This study was undertaken on 56 advanced cancer patients with solid
tumors which could no longer be controlled by chemo- and or radiation ther-
apies. These patients were separated into two groups on the basis of vol-
unteering. Nine female and 16 male cases entered the control group; 14
women and 17 men were treated by oral administration of 150 mg of levamisole, 3 days a week.

Evaluations of their immune status were performed before initiating the
treatment, 2 months after, and repeated approximately each 6 months.

A series of findings emerge from this first series of cancer patients
treated with levamisole. First is a significant difference in survival time
between the control and the treated groups (Table 1). Actually survived
among male patients: 1/5 pulmonary cancers, 1/2 osteosarcoma, 3/3 cancers of the tongue, 3/3 larynx neoplasias, and 1/1 colon carcinoma; and
among female patients: 1/3 breast cancer, 1/1 intrajugal epithelioma, 2/3
disseminated epitheliomas, and 1/2 rhabdomyosarcomas.

A second finding is the prognostic value of the level of T-cell responsiveness to a suboptimal dose of phytohemagglutinin, observed in the course of
levamisole therapy (Table 2). These tests were performed with a dose of
2.5 µg of protein content of PHA-M Difco per ml of RPMI-Hepes medium
and 10^6 lymphocytes. Such a dose of PHA induced blastogenesis of $45 \pm 5\%$
of total lymphocytes, that is, about 65% blastogenesis of the T-cell

---

*Associated Scientist, Memorial Sloan-Kettering Cancer Center, New
York, New York 10021.

TABLE 1. Survival in advanced cancers treated with levamisole

| | Surviving | Deceased | |
		Number	MST
Treated			
Men	9	14	124 (21-320)
Women	5	9	254 (33-742)
Controls			
Men	0	16	65 (12-142)
Women	0	9	48 (10-110)

MST: mean survival time in days after the first immunologic tests of 15 treated and of 25 untreated patients.

Surviving: 14 of 31 treated patients who are actually living 12 to 38 months from initiation of levamisole therapy.

population evaluated by rosetting, in control tests on samples from 200 healthy subjects of both sexes. In these first series, blast cells were counted on 1,000 lymphocytes on May-Grunwald-Giemsa-stained smears.

At the first examination, the mean value of suboptimal PHA-induced blastogenesis was found at $13 \pm 10\%$ of the total lymphocyte population for the 56 patients under study. These figures were independent of age and sex, and of the type of malignant neoplasia. They confirmed the well-known immuno-depression that accompanies cancers.

For the sake of clarity, we report here only the data that were obtained in evaluations made 2 months after initiating levamisole treatment. If the immune system of a patient under levamisole therapy was able to mount an enhanced response to a suboptimal dose of PHA-M, then at least a 6-month survival could be predicted. On the contrary, a standing-in response, or a depressed response, correlated with a poor short-term prognosis (Table 2). Identical findings were found in a 12- to 38-month survey of the treated patients, that is, a clear-cut relationship between the level of T-cell responsiveness and the survival time of cancer patients.

This test is now in use in our hospital for the surveillance of cancers, whatever the therapy employed. Similar relationships were also found in Crohn's disease and in sarcoidosis. Present findings confirm that levamisole-induced recruitment and activation of T-cells is a fact in man as in laboratory

TABLE 2. Prognosticative value of levamisole-induced T-cell responsiveness to 2.5 µg protein of PHA-M

| | Survival time | | | | |
| | < 6 months | | | > 6 months | |
Number [a]	1st test	2nd test [b]	Number [a]	1st test	2nd test [b]
4	8 ± 1	6 ± 1.2	7	5.5 ± 1.2	16.6 ± 1.5
			8	13.5 ± 1.0	25.3 ± 1.4
3	25.6 ± 3	12.6 ± 4	6	23 ± 2.1	32.1 ± 4.2
1	35	3	2	33 ± 0	46 ± 1.0

[a] Number: number of patients evidencing a level of blastogenesis in response to a suboptimal dose of PHA-M, which induced $45 \pm 5\%$ blast cells in normal healthy controls.

[b] A 2-month interval between 1st and 2nd test.

animals. Of course, such activities will be possible only if enough precursor cells are present together with persisting adequate cell membrane receptors. An evaluation of the availability of the immune system to be activated by levamisole and related compounds should be a prerequisite in studies attempting an evaluation of their usefulness in cancers or in autoimmune diseases.

Control of Neoplasia by Modulation of the Immune System, edited by M. A. Chirigos. Raven Press, New York 1977.

EFFECT OF LEVAMISOLE ON LYMPHOCYTES OF HODGKIN'S DISEASE PATIENTS IN VIVO AND IN VITRO

B. Ramot and M. Biniaminov

Institute of Hematology, Chaim Sheba Medical Center and Sackler Medical School, Tel Aviv University, Tel Aviv, Israel

Levamisole, a known antihelmintic drug, has lately attracted attention as an immunomodulator. Since it is well known that the cellular immune functions are compromised in Hodgkin's disease patients, the effect of this drug on Hodgkin's disease was studied.

Preliminary data on the in vivo effect of the drug on 10 patients with Hodgkin's disease has been published (1). It was found that, after 150 mg of levamisole had been administered for 3 days, skin test-negative individuals converted to positive, mainly in response to mumps and candida. Furthermore, the low peripheral blood E-rosette-forming cell number rose to normal levels.

As a result of these observations it was important to determine the length of time the in vivo levamisole effect persists. Furthermore, does levamisole affect lymphocytes in vitro, and is there any relationship between the in vivo and in vitro effects of the drug? It was observed that $40\,\mu g/ml$ of levamisole added to 10^6 ficoll isolated lymphocytes and incubated for half an hour raised the E-rosette number from a mean of $33.6 \pm 12.5\%$ to $56.7 \pm 14.6\%$. The drug had no effect on normal lymphocytes, where the mean rosette number was $52.4 \pm 12.5\%$ prior to incubation, and $54.6 \pm 10.8\%$ after incubation.

The 10 Hodgkin's disease patients who had received levamisole 6 months previously were restudied. It was found that the skin tests that improved after the first levamisole trial (2) had not changed as compared to the results obtained at the first study. On the other hand, the E-rosette number was again low. These patients were again given 150 mg of levamisole a day for 3 days, and their E-rosette numbers were determined 7 days, 1 month, and 2 months later.

It was found that the E-rosette number continued to be normal for about 2 months. During this period, levamisole had no effect in vitro.

239

These results would suggest that small doses of levamisole have an effect on the immunological handicap of Hodgkin's disease patients. As a result of these observations, a study was initiated on patients with Hodgkin's disease stage IIIB and IVB. Only patients in complete clinical remission are included in the study. The patients receive levamisole or placebo for 6 months. The incidence of infections and length of remission will be determined. One observation of interest is that one Hodgkin's disease patient under levamisole therapy developed varicella. The number of eruptions was very small, and the disease subsided in a few days.

These in vitro and in vivo results have encouraged us to study the effect of levamisole in poor-risk cases of acute lymphatic leukemia, acute myeloid leukemia, and other lymphomas. This study has just begun.

In summary, we would like to point out that since immune modulators can stimulate as well as overstimulate or suppress cellular immunity, it appears to us that any clinical trials at this stage of knowledge should be performed only in patients in remission, and the dose of the drug given should correlate to the amount needed to normalize the E-rosette-forming cell number. The dose of 150 mg of the drug for 3 days, or 150 mg a day for 2 days, every 2 weeks or every month, appears to us, therefore, to be a reasonable dose for a clinical trial in immunosuppressed patients.

REFERENCES

1. Levo, Y., Rotter, V., and Ramot, B. (1975): Restoration of cellular immune response by levamisole in patients with Hodgkin's disease. Biomedicine, 23:198.
2. Ramot, B., Biniaminov, M., Shoham, C., and Rosenthal, E. (1976): The effect of levamisole on E-rosette forming cells in vivo and in vitro in Hodgkin's disease patients. New Engl. J. Med., 294:809-811.

Control of Neoplasia by Modulation of the Immune System, edited by M. A. Chirigos. Raven Press, New York 1977.

POTENTIAL ROLE FOR THYMOSIN IN THE TREATMENT OF PRIMARY IMMUNODEFICIENCY DISEASES AND CANCER

Allan L. Goldstein, Geraldine H. Cohen, and Gary B. Thurman

Division of Biochemistry, The University of Texas Medical Branch, Galveston, Texas 77550

INTRODUCTION

Historical accounts of the development, characterization, production, and properties of thymic hormones, especially thymosin, are available in several review articles (1-4). Based on 10 years of experimental studies in animal models and extensive toxicity studies in animals, clinical trials with thymosin fraction 5 were initiated in April 1974. The patient population included individuals with primary immunodeficiency diseases and those with far advanced cancer. Some preliminary results from these clinical studies have been reported previously (5-11) or are being presented at this conference by Schafer et al. (12) and Ammann and Wara (13). In this report we discuss procedures for preparation and bioassay of thymosin suitable for use in humans and data on the first 59 patients treated with thymosin.

PREPARATION OF THYMOSIN

Bovine thymosin fraction 5 is a partially purified calf thymus preparation extracted as previously described (14,15) and recently modified (4). Thymosin fraction 5 was administered subcutaneously or intramuscularly in a 0.9% sodium chloride solution, pH 7.0. Clinical lots met FDA-approved standards for nonpyrogenicity, sterility, and lack of acute toxicity. Recent chemical and biological studies indicate that there may be several biologically active peptides within the thymosin fraction 5 preparation (4). We are presently attempting to purify and characterize all of the biologically active peptides. These peptides may act individually or in concert to influence the various T-cell functions in the mammalian immune system.

BIOLOGICAL TESTING OF THYMOSIN

The bioassays used routinely to screen thymosin preparations for clinical use include two in vitro tests and a third which combines in vivo and in vitro procedures.

MLR bioassay: The mixed lymphocyte reaction (MLR) bioassay (16,17) for thymosin fraction 5 (Fig. 1) is based on the observation that bovine thymosin fraction 5 enhances the capacity of CBA/J thymocytes to respond against allogeneic mitomycin C-treated C57B1/6J spleen cells but not against syngeneic mitomycin C-treated spleen cells. In our hands, endotoxin-free fractions prepared from other bovine tissues, such as spleen, did not contain MLR-enhancing activity.

IN VITRO THYMOSIN MLR ASSAY

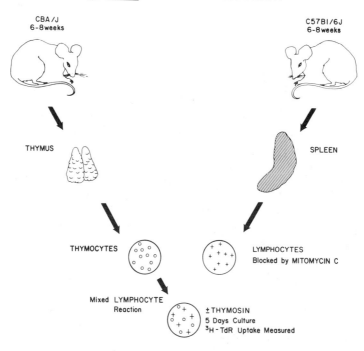

FIG. 1. Method for detection and quantitation of thymosin in vitro. Thymocytes from CBA/J mice are cultured with mitomycin C-blocked spleen cells from CBA/J or from C57B1/6J mice in the presence or absence of thymosin. ^{3}H-thymidine is added to the cultures during the last 8 hr of the 5-day incubation period. Thymosin bioactivity is measured as the lowest concentration at which the ratio of the stimulation index (cpm of allogeneic cultures divided by cpm of the syngeneic cultures) of the thymosin-supplemented cultures to the stimulation index of the control cultures (no thymosin) is 2 or greater. [See Cohen and Goldstein (16) for further details.]

IN VIVO – IN VITRO THYMOSIN MITOGEN ASSAY

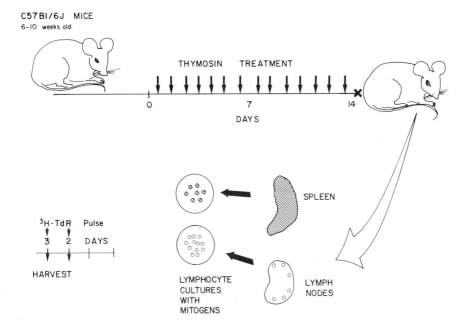

FIG. 2. In vivo-in vitro method to assay thymosin. C57B1/6J mice are treated daily for 14 days with thymosin by intraperitoneal injection. One day after the final injection, spleen and lymph node lymphocyte microcultures are prepared. The cells are either unstimulated, or stimulated with PHA-P, Con A, or LPS. Eight hours before harvesting, ^{3}H-thymidine is added to the cultures. Lymphocyte stimulation is then measured by determining the amount of ^{3}H-thymidine uptake by the various cultures. [See Thurman and Goldstein (17) for further details.]

Mitogen bioassay: The mitogen bioassay (18, 19), as diagramed in Fig. 2, is based on the observation that there is an increased spleen and lymph node lymphocyte response to mitogens, particularly to concanavalin A (Con A), following in vivo treatment with thymosin. Recent experiments indicate that in vivo treatment can markedly enhance blastogenesis of lymph node cells from C57B1/6J mice, B6AF$_1$ mice, normal mice, aged mice, as well as NZB and nude mice caused by Con A and, to a lesser extent, by phytohemagglutinin (PHA-P) and pokeweed mitogen (PWM). We think that thymosin supplement in normal (nonthymectomized) mice accelerates the rate of T-cell maturation and consequently causes shifts in the proportions of lymphocyte subpopulations in the various lymphoid tissue.

Human E-rosette bioassay: In collaborative studies with Wara et al. (5, 6) and others (7, 20-23), we found that thymosin increases both the percent and the absolute number of E-rosettes formed in vitro by peripheral blood

WARA– AMMANN E–ROSETTE BIOASSAY

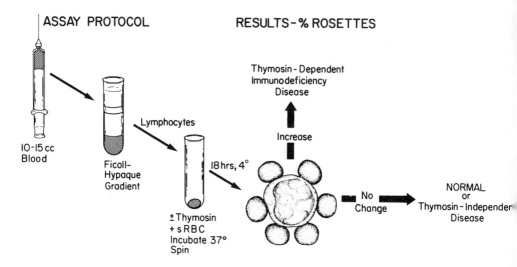

FIG. 3. Peripheral blood lymphocytes are isolated using a ficoll-Hypaque gradient. The lymphocytes are adjusted to a concentration of 5 X 10^6 cells/ ml of HRPMI-1640. Sheep red blood cells (SRBC) are washed and resuspended at 80 X 10^6 cells/ml. Lymphocytes in a volume of 0.1 ml are incubated with 0.1 ml of thymosin at concentrations of 50 to 500 µg/ml, or with control media. The suspensions are incubated for 10 min at 37° C following which 0.2 ml of SRBC's are added and the cell suspension is centrifuged for 5 min at 200 X g. Following incubation overnight (18 hr) at 4°C, triplicate wet cell preparations are examined by phase microscopy and the percentage of lymphocytes binding 3 or more SRBC is determined.

lymphocytes obtained from most patients with thymic-dependent immunodeficiency diseases. Thymosin does not increase E-rosettes of most normal individuals. These observations led to the development of a simple E-rosette-thymosin assay for the identification of patients with possible thymosin-dependent immune disorders (Fig. 3).

E-ROSETTES AND THYMOSIN IN VITRO

As shown in Table 1, in vitro incubation of peripheral blood lymphocytes with thymosin increased the number of rosette-forming cells in patients with a variety of clinical disorders including most primary immunodeficiency diseases, several types of autoimmune diseases, and cancer. Thymosin does not appear to influence in vitro the number of rosette-forming cells of most normal individuals or patients with severe combined immunodeficiency diseases, some types of cancer, and some types of autoimmune diseases such as rheumatoid arthritis and myasthenia gravis. The E-rosette-thymosin assay has been particularly helpful in identifying immunodeficient patients

TABLE 1. In vitro effect of thymosin on human E-rosettes

Disease category	Typical ranges of thymosin-induced increases in % E-rosettes
Primary cell-mediated immunodeficiencies	16-33
Severe combined immunodeficiencies	0- 3
Thymosin-responsive cancer patients	9-31
Thymosin-responsive allergy patients	10-19
Active systemic lupus erythematosus	12-25
Sjögren's syndrome	15-30
Influenza virus infection (24 hr postinoculation)	10-20
Normals	0- 5

most likely to benefit from thymosin administration. Patients whose E-rosette numbers were elevated by incubation with thymosin in vitro were usually those who initially had a subnormal percentage of E-rosettes. Of interest is the observation that the blood lymphocytes of many normal individuals with a history of allergy (24), as well as those from individuals with influenza virus infections (25), also respond to thymosin in vitro in this assay. Major findings using this E-rosette assay are summarized in Table 2.

CLINICAL STUDIES WITH THYMOSIN

To date, more than 70 patients have been or are presently under treatment with thymosin. The data compiled in this chapter were acquired under the direction of cooperating investigators at the University of Texas Medical Branch in Galveston and the other clinical centers listed in the acknowledgments at the end of this chapter. Informed consent was obtained in writing from all patients in these studies. Tables 3 and 4 summarize data on the first 59 patients treated with thymosin according to phase I protocols for which case reports are complete. Eighteen patients were children with primary immunodeficiency diseases and 41 patients had far advanced cancer.

Phase I Studies with Cancer Patients

In the cancer studies (Table 3), patients received daily doses ranging from 1 to 250 mg/M^2. Generally, a "course" of thymosin therapy consisted of

TABLE 2. Summary of major in vitro findings using the E-rosette assay
with thymosin

---

1. Thymosin increases E-rosettes in a dose-related manner in thymus-
dependent primary immunodeficiency diseases.

2. Thymosin increases the number of E-rosettes (T-cells) to normal levels
in patients with many secondary immunodeficiency diseases.

3. "Null cells"[a] appear to be targets of thymosin action with respect to E-
rosette increases.

4. In general, the number of PBL E-rosettes from normal individuals does
not increase when incubated with thymosin.

5. Increased E-rosettes after incubation with thymosin in vitro correlates
well with beneficial responses to thymosin in vivo.

---

[a] Lymphocytes bearing none of the usual T- or B-cell markers.

daily injections for 7 to 21 days. Many of the patients received multiple
courses over a period of a few weeks to several months. A few patients
were placed on "maintenance courses" consisting of one, two, or three injections of thymosin per week from one to several months. To date, there
are no indications of liver, kidney, heart, bone marrow, or CNS toxicity
attributable to thymosin at any dose studied. No side effects were reported
for 66% of the patients treated with thymosin. About 24% of the treated patients developed skin reactions at the injection site, which were usually mild
and intermittent during the course of treatment. About 12% of the patients
developed skin reactions or systemic reactions of an allergic nature which
warranted removal from the study.

The majority of cancer patients who responded in vitro to thymosin showed
a significant increase in percentage of T-cells in the blood following a short
course (7 days) of thymosin treatment, and/or showed negative-to-positive
conversion when skin-tested with recall antigens. The E-rosette enhancement effect by thymosin is most pronounced when the endogenous E-rosette
levels were below 50% initially. The majority of patients who initially
showed some depression of delayed-type skin hypersensitivity exhibited increased responsivity to recall antigens (dermatophytin, candida, mumps,
SK-SD, and PPD) and to KLH after thymosin administration. Although clinical improvements have been noted in a few of the cancer patients treated
with several courses of thymosin, we do not presently know if these observations are a result of thymosin activity.

TABLE 3. Summary of thymosin clinical trials in cancer patients
(phase I study)

Patients:	
17 leukemia or lymphoma	2 pancreatic cancer
4 multiple myeloma	2 leiomyosarcoma
4 disseminated melanoma	1 oral cancer
1 gall bladder cancer	1 glioma
1 stomach and esophageal cancer	1 mycosis fungoides
1 choriocarcinoma	2 lung cancer
2 breast cancer	1 hypernephroma
	1 dysgerminoma

Dose of thymosin:	1 to 250 mg/M^2 per injection
Length of treatment:	7 days to 18 months
Side effects:	None (66%), mild local skin reactions (24%), severe skin reactions or systemic reactions (12%), no evidence of liver, CNS, kidney, or bone marrow toxicity
% E-rosettes:	Increased in > 50% of patients
Delayed hypersensitivity:	Increased in > 50% of patients initially exhibiting some depression
Clinical response:	Cellular immune functions increased; clinical improvement noted in a few of the cancer patients, but it is not known whether these findings are a result of thymosin activity

Phase I Studies of Patients with Primary Immunodeficiency Diseases

A positive response of these patients' PBL to thymosin in vitro in the E-rosette bioassay (Fig. 3) appears to be a good indicator of potential in vivo efficacy. About 90% of the children with primary immunodeficiency diseases who responded in vitro to thymosin, as measured by an increase in E-rosettes, responded similarly in vivo.

As summarized in Table 4, there were significant increases in cellular immune functions and improved clinical courses noted during thymosin treatment of several of the 18 immunodeficient patients. Most frequently reported were increased percentage of E-rosettes in 8 patients (44%), skin test

TABLE 4. Summary of clinical trials in primary immunodeficiency
(phase I studies)

Patients:	1 unspecified T-cell disorder
	3 Nezelof
	1 DiGeorge
	3 thymic hypoplasia
	1 Wiscott-Aldrich
	6 severe combined immunodeficiency
	3 ataxia telangiectasia
Dose of thymosin:	1 to 400 mg/M^2 per injection
Length of treatment:	7 days to 21 months
Side effects:	None (50%), mild skin reactions (33%), severe skin reactions and/or systemic reaction (17%), no evidence of CNS, liver, kidney, or bone marrow toxicity
E-rosettes:	Increased in 44%[a] of patients
Absolute PBL:	Increased in 22% of patients
Delayed hypersensitivity:	Increased in 44% of patients
Lymphocyte blastogenesis:	Mitogen response increased in 28%, MLR in 17%
Clinical status:	Significant clinical improvements such as decreased infections in 39% of patients

[a] Percent changes include the 6 cases of severe combined immunodeficiency.

conversion in 8 patients (44%), increased in vitro reactivity to mitogens by peripheral blood lymphocytes (PBL) in vitro in 5 patients (22%), and increased MLR of PBL in 3 patients (17%). One patient has now received thymosin on a weekly basis for 21 months and has not developed any reactions or apparent resistance to this agent. It should be noted that the changes in T-cell numbers and functions reported include the 6 patients with severe combined immunodeficiencies who seem to lack stem cells responsive to thymosin in vitro, and if these are excluded, the percentages in all categories scored above would be significantly higher.

Based on these preliminary encouraging findings, expanded clinical studies have been initiated in cooperation with Hoffmann-LaRoche, Inc., and clinical investigators here at UTMB and at other major medical centers. It is hoped that these trials will further delineate the effective dose levels and pharmacologic effects of thymosin, as well as determine the usefulness of thymosin as an immunotherapeutic agent, either alone or in combination with other therapeutic agents.

DISCUSSION

The phase I studies with thymosin point to a potential role for thymosin in the treatment of primary immunodeficiency diseases and possibly of cancer in conjunction with the more conventional modalities of therapy. Increased percentages of PBL E-rosettes and skin test conversions following thymosin administration were the most frequently noted changes in patients with both classes of diseases. Although a few of the cancer patients receiving thymosin improved clinically, it is not yet known whether such findings are merely coincidental or a result of thymosin activity. It is clear, however, that several patients with primary immunodeficiency disorders exhibited significant improvements and partial correction of their immunodeficiencies during thymosin treatments. The promising results using thymosin in children with thymic-dependent primary immunodeficiency disease suggest that thymosin be tried before implementation of the more aggressive approaches such as thymus transplants.

The most frequently reported side effects were skin reactions at the injection site. There were occasional systemic reactions, which appeared to be of an allergic nature. The side effects noted thus far are considered to be mild in comparison to those precipitated by other forms of immunotherapy such as BCG, Corynebacterium parvum, or polynucleotides. Except as described above, there were no indications of toxicity in any of the major organ systems attributable to treatment with thymosin fraction 5.

The consensus of opinion among physicians collaborating in this clinical study is that the potential benefits of thymosin treatment far outweigh the identified and potential risks to the human subjects involved, and that there is a need to continue trials with this experimental immunotherapeutic agent.

Although the basic mechanisms of thymosin action are not yet well defined, data from several laboratories suggest that thymosin influences precursor T-cells and very rapidly induces their maturation into more mature T-cells (26-28). This maturation into immunologically competent T-lymphocytes may occur as a result of derepression or activation of genetically programmed lymphoid stem cells. In vitro studies by Cohen et al. (16,17) indicate that thymosin can also act on immature thymocytes (T_1-cells) to facilitate differentiation into more immunologically competent lymphocytes (T_2-cells) in the presence of antigen. It is not clear at this time whether a single molecular species in thymosin fraction 5 is responsible for the described effects.

A major thrust in our present research program is to determine if and how the various immune disorders are related to production and/or secretion of thymosin by the thymus gland. We are assessing the potential therapeutic value of thymosin in a number of different viral diseases and autoimmune diseases in animals and in vitro models (29). We hope that these studies will yield new insight that will lead to better management of similar disorders in humans. Our early clinical experiences suggest that thymosin will have a role in boosting the immune responses of patients with specific thymic malfunctions by stimulating the production and regulation of T-cell subpopulations.

SUMMARY

Preliminary data from phase I clinical trials with thymosin point to a potential role for thymosin in the treatment of thymic-dependent primary immunodeficiency diseases and possibly of cancer in conjunction with conventional modalities of therapy. Significant improvements were observed in T-cell numbers and T-cell functions in several children with primary immunodeficiency diseases and in some patients with cancer following thymosin administration. A simple in vitro E-rosette assay using PBL and thymosin has been developed which appears to be predictive for identifying patients who will benefit by thymosin administration. Ongoing experimental studies suggest that thymosin is involved in maintaining control over the production of specialized subpopulations of T-cells which regulate immune balance. Decreased production and/or secretion of thymosin may be related to the development of a number of thymic-dependent disorders including some autoimmune diseases and cancer.

ACKNOWLEDGMENTS

This study was supported in part by grants from the National Cancer Institute CA 14108, CA 15419, and CA 16964, and The John A. Hartford Foundation, Inc.

The phase I clinical findings summarized in the text were based on data (published and unpublished) obtained by the following collaborating investigators: John J. Costanzi, M. D., and Armond S. Goldman, M. D., University of Texas Medical Branch at Galveston; Evan M. Hersh, M. D., Lawrence A. Schafer, M. D., and Jordan U. Gutterman, M. D., M. D. Anderson Hospital and Tumor Institute, Houston, Texas; Arthur J. Ammann, M. D., and Diane W. Wara, M. D., University of California Medical Center, San Francisco, California; Thomas A. Waldmann, M. D., National Cancer Institute, Bethesda, Maryland; Charles S. August, M. D., University of Colorado Medical Center, Denver, Colorado; Robert C. Seeger, M. D., University of California School of Medicine, Los Angeles, California; Harry R. Hill, M. D., University of Utah School of Medicine, Salt Lake City, Utah; Robert H. Reid, M. D., Henry Ford Hospital, Detroit, Michigan; J. Einhorn, M. D., Karolinska Institute, Stockholm, Sweden; Claude Griscelli, M. D., Groupe Hospitalier Necker Enfants Malades, Paris, France; Lars A. Hanson, M. D., Institute of Medical Microbiology, University of Goteborg, Goteborg, Sweden.

REFERENCES

1. Goldstein, A. L., Thurman, G. B., Cohen, G. H., and Hooper, J. A. (1975): Thymosin: Chemistry, biology and clinical applications. In: The Biological Activity of Thymic Hormones, edited by D. W. van Bekkum, pp. 173-197. Kooyker Scientific Publications, Rotterdam, The Netherlands.

2. White, A., and Goldstein, A. L. (1975): The endocrine role of the thymus, and its hormone thymosin, in the regulation of the growth and maturation of host immunological competence. Adv. Metab. Disord., 8:361-376.

3. Goldstein, A. L., Thurman, G. B., Cohen, G. H., and Hooper, J. A. (1975): The role of thymosin and the endocrine thymus in the ontogenesis and function of T-cells. In: Molecular Approaches to Immunology, pp. 243-265. Academic Press, New York.

4. Hooper, J. A., McDaniel, M. C., Thurman, G. B., Cohen, G. H., Schulof, R. S., and Goldstein, A. L. (1975): The purification and properties of bovine thymosin. Ann. N.Y. Acad. Sci., 249:125-144.

5. Wara, D. W., Goldstein, A. L., Doyle, W., and Ammann, A. J. (1975): Thymosin activity in patients with cellular immunodeficiency. New Engl. J. Med., 292:70-74.

6. Goldstein, A. L., Wara, D. W., Ammann, A. J., Sakai, H., Harris, N. S., Thurman, G. B., Hooper, J. A., Cohen, G. H., Goldman, A. S., Costanzi, J. J., and McDaniel, M. C. (1975): First clinical trial with thymosin: Reconstitution of T-cells in patients with cellular immunodeficiency diseases. Transplant. Proc., 7(1):681-686.

7. Sakai, H., Costanzi, J. J., Loukas, D. F., Gagliano, R. G., Ritzmann, S. E., and Goldstein, A. L. (1975): Thymosin induced increase in E-rosette forming capacity of lymphocytes in patients with malignant neoplasms. Cancer, 36:974-976.

8. Costanzi, J. J., Gagliano, R., Loukas, D., Sakai, H., Thurman, G. B., Harris, N. S., and Goldstein, A. L. (1975): Use of thymosin in patients with disseminated neoplasia-toxicity and immunological correlation (Abstr.). Proc. Am. Assoc. Cancer Res., 16:135.

9. Schafer, L. A., Washington, M. L., and Goldstein, A. L. (1975): Thymosin immunotherapy — Phase I study (Abstr.). Proc. Am. Assoc. Cancer Res., 16:1233.

10. Goldstein, A. L., Thurman, G. B., Cohen, G. H., Costanzi, J. J., Goldman, A., Hersh, E., Schafer, L. A., Ammann, A., Wara, D., and Waldmann, T. (1975): Clinical studies with thymosin: Phase I trials in patients with primary and secondary immunodeficiency diseases (Abstr.). Eur. Immunol. Soc. Meetings.

11. Schafer, L. A., Goldstein, A. L., Gutterman, J. U., and Hersh, E. M. (1976): In vitro and in vivo studies with thymosin in cancer patients. Ann. N.Y. Acad. Sci. (in press).

12. Schafer, L. A., Getterman, J. U., Hersh, E. M., Mavligit, G. M., and Goldstein, A. L. (1976): In vitro and in vivo studies of thymosin activity in cancer patients. This Volume.

13. Ammann, A., and Wara, D. (1976): The in vitro and in vivo effect of thymosin versus fetal thymus transplantation on cellular function in primary immunodeficiency disease. This Volume.

14. Goldstein, A. L., Slater, F. D., and White, A. (1966): Preparation, assay and partial purification of a thymic lymphocytopoietic factor (thymosin). Proc. Natl. Acad. Sci. (U.S.A.), 56:1010-1017.

15. Goldstein, A. L., Guha, A., Hardy, M. A., and White, A. (1972): Purification and biological activity of thymosin, a hormone of the thymus gland. Proc. Natl. Acad. Sci. (U.S.A.), 69:1800-1803.

16. Cohen, G. H., Hooper, J. A., and Goldstein, A. L. (1975): Thymosin induced differentiation of murine thymocytes in allegeneic mixed lymphocyte cultures. Ann. N.Y. Acad. Sci., 249:145-153.

17. Cohen, G. H., and Goldstein, A. L. (1975): Mixed lymphocyte reaction bioassay for thymosin. In: The Biological Activity of Thymic Hormones, edited by D. W. van Bekkum, pp. 257-259. Kooyker Scientific Publications, Rotterdam, The Netherlands.

18. Thurman, G. B., and Goldstein, A. L. (1975): Mitogen bioassay for thymosin: Increased mitogenic responsiveness of murine lymphocytes in vitro following in vivo treatment with thymosin. In: The Biological Activity of Thymic Hormones, edited by D. W. van Bekkum, pp. 261-264. Kooyker Scientific Publications, Rotterdam, The Netherlands.

19. Thurman, G. B., Ahmed, A., Strong, D. M., Gershwin, M. E., Steinberg, A. P., and Goldstein, A. L. (1975): Thymosin induced increase in mitogenic responsivity of lymphocytes of normal, NZB and nude mice. Transplant. Proc., 7(1):299-303.

20. Wybran, J., Levin, A. S., Fudenberg, A. A., and Goldstein, A. L. (1975): Thymosin: Effects in normal human blood T-cells. Ann. N.Y. Acad. Sci., 249:300-307.

21. Touraine, J., Touraine, F., Incefy, G. F., Goldstein, A. L., and Good, R. A. (1975): Thymic factors and human T-lymphocyte differentiation. In: The Biological Activity of Thymic Hormones, edited by D. W. van Bekkum, pp. 31-35. Kooyker Scientific Publications, Rotterdam, The Netherlands.

22. Harris, J., Sengar, D., Hyslop, D., Green, L., and Goldstein, A. L. (1975): Immunodeficiency in chronic uremia: Preliminary evidence for thymosin deficiency. Transplantation, 20:176-178.

23. Scheinberg, M. A., Cathcart, E. S., and Goldstein, A. L. (1975): Thymosin-induced reduction of "null cells" in peripheral-blood lymphocytes of patients with systemic lupus erythematosus. Lancet, i:424.

24. Thurman, G. B., and Goldstein, A. L. (1975): Unpublished data.

25. Scheinberg, M. A., Blacklow, H. R., Goldstein, A. L., Parrino, T. A., Ross, F. B., and Cathcart, E. S. (1976): Influenza: Response of T cell lymphopenia to thymosin. New Engl. J. Med., 294:1208-1211.

26. Goldstein, A. L., Guha, A., Howe, M. L., and White, A. (1971): Ontogenesis of cell-mediated immunity in murine thymocytes and spleen cells and its acceleration of thymosin, a thymic hormone. J. Immunol., 106:773-780.

27. Bach, J. F., Dardeene, M., Goldstein, A. L., Guha, A., and White, A. (1971): Appearance of T-cell markers in bone marrow rosette forming cells after incubation with thymosin, a thymic hormone. Proc. Natl. Acad. Sci. (U.S.A.), 68:2734-2738.

28. Scheid, M. P., Hoffman, M. K., Komuro, K., Hammerling, U., Boyse, E. A., Cohen, G. H., Hooper, J. A., Schulof, R. S., and Goldstein, A. L. (1973): Differentiation of T-lymphocytes induced by preparations from thymus and by non-thymic agents. The determined state of the precursor cell. J. Exp. Med., 138:1027-1032.

29. Goldstein, A. L., Thurman, G. B., Cohen, G. H., and Rossio, J. L. (1976): The endocrine thymus: Potential role for thymosin in the treatment of autoimmune disease. Ann. N.Y. Acad. Sci., 274:390-401.

Control of Neoplasia by Modulation of the Immune System, edited by M. A. Chirigos. Raven Press, New York 1977.

EFFECTS OF THYMUS EXTRACTS ON THE IMMUNE RESPONSIVENESS OF LEUKEMIC MICE

Herman Friedman

Department of Microbiology, Albert Einstein Medical Center, Philadelphia, Pennsylvania 19141

INTRODUCTION

It is now widely accepted that the thymus serves an important role in development and maintenance of immunocompetence. Although much effort is being devoted to assessment of cellular components of the thymus in immunity, it is evident that various subcellular factors derived from the thymus gland may serve an important function in immune competence (1-3). For example, a variety of soluble extracts derived from thymus glands are now known to exert a marked influence on immune responses. Purified protein-rich extracts from the calf thymus, when administered directly to immuno-deficient animals such as mice or when added to cultures of lymphocytes from immunologically impaired individuals, often result in restored immune responsiveness (1-3). Most of these studies have dealt with restoration of immune competence of lymphocytes derived from individuals with congenital immunodeficiencies or with malignancies. In this laboratory much effort has been devoted to studying the mechanisms of leukemia virus-induced immunosuppression (4-6). In such studies it was found that lymphoid cells from mice infected with Friend leukemia virus (FLV) show marked immuno-logic deficiency when tested for immune responsiveness to a wide variety of antigens. Impaired antibody formation to antigens such as sheep erythrocytes (a T-dependent immunogen) and to bacterial lipopolysaccharides (LPS), generally considered T-independent antigens, becomes evident in FLV-infected mice at the cellular level, both in vivo and in vitro, using appropriate immunoplaque assays for enumerating antibody forming cells. Such studies suggested that immune impairment associated with FLV infection was due to an effect on antibody precursor cells rather than antibody forming cells per se. Furthermore B-lymphocytes, rather than helper T-cells, appeared to be preferentially suppressed early in FLV infection, at least in terms of

255

immune responsiveness to sheep erythrocytes. Various substances have been studied which can alter immunoresponsiveness of splenocytes from FLV-infected animals, including bacterial endotoxins, other mitogens, adjuvants, etc. (7). In the present study the effects of calf thymus extracts capable of influencing immune responses were examined with regard to their ability to affect antibody formation in vivo in FLV-infected animals and, more recently, in vitro using splenocytes from infected animals.

GENERAL EXPERIMENTAL METHODS AND PROCEDURES

Inbred Balb/c mice were used for these studies; they were obtained from Cumberland View Farms, Clinton, Tennessee, or Jackson Memorial Laboratories, Bar Harbor, Maine, and were 18 to 20 g at the initiation of each experiment. The mice were infected by intraperitoneal (i.p.) inoculation with FLV which has been propagated in this laboratory for approximately 10 years by passage through Balb/c mice (5-8). The virus preparation consisted of both the spleen focus forming and lymphatic leukemia virus components of the Friend complex and had no detectable contamination with lactic dehydrogenase virus. For infection, mice were injected i.p. with 0.2 ml of a clarified FLV homogenate containing approximately 10^2 ID_{50} doses. Development of splenomegaly was used as an indicator of infection. In some instances the number of infectious virus units was determined by the in vitro culture assay using D_{56} indicator cells. In addition, the development of splenic macrofoci in infected mice was also used as an assay for virus activity. To determine immunocompetence, both noninfected control and FLV-infected mice were injected i.p. with 0.2 ml of a 10% suspension of washed sheep RBCs and the numbers of individual antibody plaque-forming cells (PFC) to the red blood cells were determined 4 or 5 days later by the direct hemolysis in agar assay for 19 IgM PFCs exactly as described earlier. For in vitro experiments the Dutton-Mishell or Marbrook culture systems were used, usually with 5×10^6 spleen cells per culture (8). In all cases at least 3 to 4 duplicate culture vessels were used in each experiment. For immunization 2×10^6 washed sheep erythrocytes were added at the time of culture initiation. PFCs were determined per million viable spleen cells or per culture. A purified calf thymus extract prepared from pooled thymus glands using the method initially described by Hand et al. (8) was utilized for in vivo studies. Thymosin prepared by Dr. Allan Goldstein was utilized for the in vitro studies. In both cases 10 to 100 μg of lyophilized thymus extract was dissolved in sterile, pyrogen-free saline and either injected directly into mice by the intravenous (i.v.) route or added to cultures of splenocytes.

EXPERIMENTAL RESULTS

In initial experiments a purified calf thymus extract prepared by the method of Hand et al. was used in vivo. For this purpose mice were injected i.v. with 10 to 50 μg of the purified cat thymus factor which had been shown previously to enhance the maturation of immune responsiveness to sheep red cells in newborn mice. Some of the thymus extract-injected mice were infected with varying doses of Friend virus. Other thymus-injected mice were left uninfected. In addition, groups of untreated mice were infected with Friend virus. At various times thereafter, groups of mice were killed and their spleens examined individually for changes in spleen weight as a function of infection. Virus titers were also determined, as was the development of macro foci per spleen. In no case did the calf thymus alone significantly alter the spleen weight of control mice. Furthermore, mice infected with Friend virus invariably developed a large spleen and a high virus titer. The calf thymus extract, injected in various doses and at various time intervals, had no significant effect on the development of such splenomegaly and virus replication.

Additional experimental groups of mice treated with virus and/or calf thymus extract were challenged with 0.5 ml of sheep RBCs at various times. The numbers of antibody-forming cells per spleen were determined 4 days later. The thymus extract appeared to enhance very slightly the antibody response to the SRBCs in normal mice; although such increases were consistent they were not statistically significant. On the other hand, injection of calf thymus extract into leukemic mice resulted in a slight sparing of the immunosuppression induced by the virus. For example, mice given 10 or 50 µg of thymus extract on the day of infection with the virus and at 2- to 3-day intervals thereafter for 1 or 2 weeks showed a two- to fourfold enhancement of PFC responses to sheep red cells during the second or third week of the infection (1,500 to 2,000 PFCs for treated mice vs. 500 to 800 PFCs for untreated, FLV-infected mice). However, control mice given no virus or thymus extract showed a much higher PFC response, i.e., 50,000 or more PFCs. Thus, enhancement of the immune response in the infected mice treated with the calf thymus extract did not increase the PFC response to levels even approaching that of normal mice.

Splenocytes from FLV-infected mice were markedly impaired in immune responsiveness to SRBC in vitro. For example, when spleen cells from infected mice are cultured in vitro in the presence of sheep RBCs, fewer PFCs developed as compared to the response of uninfected control mice (Table 1). The magnitude of this immunodepression was directly related to the length of time the donor mice were infected with virus. When 50 µg of a purified thymus extract prepared by Goldstein et al. (thymosin) was added to varying numbers of splenocytes from either normal or infected mice, there was a significant alteration in the PFC response in vitro by the infected spleen cells. As can be seen in Table 2, splenocytes from FLV-infected mice were markedly depressed in their capability of responding to sheep RBCs in vitro, regardless of the number of cells cultured. For example, even when the number of splenocytes from infected mice was increased 10-fold the number of PFCs induced in vitro was still about half the number induced in cultures containing many fewer normal spleen cells. Addition of thymosin at the time of culture initiation increased the PFC responsiveness of the splenocytes from infected mice. This was most evident when the smallest number of spleen cells was used. For example, cultures containing 1 million spleen cells from infected mice treated with calf thymosin at the time of culture initiation developed about three to five times more PFCs than cultures without thymosin. However, the

TABLE 1. The effect of FLV infection on PFC responses of splenocytes
to SRBC

| Spleen cell source [a] | Antibody response in vitro [b] | |
	PFC/10^6 WBC	Percent of control
Normal mice	986 $\pm$ 128	—
FLV-infected [c]		
-1 day	832 $\pm$ 69	84
-3 days	649 $\pm$ 72	65
-7 days	310 $\pm$ 59	32
-15 days	260 $\pm$ 47	26
-20 days	79 $\pm$ 32	8

[a] Three to five Balb/c mice used for each spleen cell source; 5 X 10^6 viable cells cultured in 1 to 2 ml of medium in triplicate at 37°C. Each culture was immunized with 2 X 10^6 SRBC.

[b] Average response for 5 to 6 cultures per group 4 days after in vitro immunization.

[c] Mice infected by i.p. injection of 10^2 ID $_{50}$ FLV on day indicated before spleen cells obtained.

number of PFCs developing in these cultures was still lower than that occurring in cultures with normal spleen cells. Thymosin, when added in the same concentration to similar numbers of splenocytes from normal mice, had only a slight effect, except in those cultures which had the lowest numbers of cells.

The enhancing effect of thymosin on the PFC response of splenocytes from FLV-infected mice did not appear to be due to a shift in the peak day of the PFC response in vitro. As can be seen in Table 3, the largest number of PFCs appeared in cultures of both control and FLV-infected splenocytes 4 to 5 days after in vitro immunization. Addition of thymosin to cultures of normal cells had very little effect on the PFC responsiveness, except on the peak day when about 20% more hemolysin-forming cells were evident. Very little difference occurred on the other days. Similarly, when thymosin was added to spleen cell cultures from FLV-infected mice, the peak PFC response also occurred on days 4 to 5. However, on each day of culture assay there were more PFCs for splenocytes treated with thymosin in vitro as compared to untreated splenocytes.

The dose of thymosin added to the splenocytes at the time of culture initiation markedly affected the PFC response. As can be seen in Table 4, the largest response occurred with 50 or 100 μg of thymosin per culture. Lesser amounts had little effect. A larger concentration of thymosin was toxic for

TABLE 2. Effect of thymus extract (thymosin) on PFC response of
FLV-infected vs. normal splenocytes in vitro

Spleen cell source	Spleen cell number per culture [a]	Thymus extract [b]	PFC/culture
FLV-infected [c]	10^6	−	325 ± 40
		+	$1,653 \pm 130$
	5×10^6	−	$1,138 \pm 165$
		+	$2,260 \pm 430$
	10^7	−	$1,850 \pm 250$
		+	$3,100 \pm 650$
Normal	10^6	−	$1,931 \pm 398$
		+	$2,586 \pm 682$
	5×10^6	−	$3,050 \pm 675$
		+	$3,878 \pm 976$
	10^7	−	$3,640 \pm 450$
		+	$3,580 \pm 528$

[a] Indicated number of viable spleen cells cultured initially with 2×10^6
SRBC.

[b] Thymosin (50 μg) added per culture on day of culture initiation.

[c] Mice infected 10 to 12 days earlier with 10^2 ID_{50} FLV.

the cells, since depressed PFC responses and lower cell viability occurred
in cultures from both normal and FLV-infected cells.

The time of addition of thymus extract to the cultures of infected spleen
cells markedly influenced the magnitude of the PFC response (Table 5).
Addition of thymosin on the first day after culture initiation resulted in greater
stimulation than addition on the day of culture initiation. When the thymus
extract was added 2 or 3 days after culture initiation, and the number of
PFCs determined on day 4, very little effect was noted. Addition of thymosin
to cultures of normal splenocytes on different days after culture initiation had

TABLE 3. Effect of thymosin on cytokinetics of PFC response of normal
and FLV-infected mouse spleen cells to SRBC

Spleen cell [a]	Thymus extract [b]	Time in days in vitro [c]					
		0	+1	+2	+3	+4	+5
Normal	−	11	73	120	398	645	310
	+	13	48	96	488	964	452
FLV-infected [d]	−	4	18	29	110	125	97
	+	2	28	110	240	378	310

[a] Spleen cells (5×10^6) cultured in vitro with 2×10^6 SRBC.

[b] Thymocin (50 µg) added on day of culture initiation.

[c] Average PFC responses per 10^6 viable spleen cells for 5 to 6 cultures
each day after in vitro immunization.

[d] Mice infected by i.p. injection of 10^2 ID_{50} FLV 12 to 14 days earlier.

TABLE 4. Effect of different doses of thymosin on PFC responses of
splenocytes from FLV and normal mice

Spleen cells [a]	Thymus extract concentration (µg) [b]	PFC/10^6 spleen cells [c]
Normal	0	738 + 64
	10.0	780 + 96
	50.0	698 + 152
	100.0	832 + 180
FLV-infected [d]	0	97 + 18
	10.0	114 + 25
	50.0	238 + 356
	100.0	298 + 78

[a] Spleen cells (5×10^6) immunized in vitro with 2×10^6 SRBC.

[b] Indicated concentration of thymosin added on day of culture initiation.

[c] Average response of 3 to 4 cultures 4 days after in vitro immunization.

[d] Mice infected 10 to 12 days earlier with 10^2 ID_{50} FLV.

TABLE 5. Effect of time of addition of thymus extract to spleen cell cultures from normal or FLV-infected mice on PFC response to SRBC

Time of thymosin addition[a]	PFC/10^6 cells[b]	
	Normal	FLV-infected
None (control)	765 $\pm$ 82	97 $\pm$ 18
Day 0	831 $\pm$ 65	231 $\pm$ 128
+1	971 $\pm$ 138	341 $\pm$ 192
+2	782 $\pm$ 75	129 $\pm$ 32
+3	790 $\pm$ 86	102 $\pm$ 24

[a] Thymosin (50 μg) added to cultures of 5 X 10^6 normal or FLV-infected splenocytes on day indicated after culture initiation.

[b] Average PFC response for 3 to 4 cultures per group 4 days after in vitro immunization with 2 X 10^6 SRBC.

relatively little effect, except for a light to moderate PFC stimulation on cultures treated on day 0 or +1.

DISCUSSION AND CONCLUSIONS

It is quite evident that a variety of "nonspecific" immunologic stimulators may affect immune responsiveness. As a matter of fact, it is now widely accepted that more than one "signal" is necessary for activation of B-lymphoid cells (9). Antigen alone is not considered sufficient by some authors for stimulating an optimum PFC response, at least in vitro. Nonspecific B-cell activators, such as polynucleotides, bacterial lipopolysaccharides, etc., are thought important for the activation of B-cells immunized in vitro with a variety of T-cell-dependent or -independent antigens. The mechanism(s) responsible for such augmented responses are not fully understood. However, it seems likely that some immunostimulatory substances may interact not only with B-cells, but also with other cells such as helper T-cells or antigen "processing" macrophages. Furthermore, it is now also widely accepted that many nonspecific immunologic stimulators have marked effects on biochemical events occurring at the surface membranes of lymphoid cells, including activation of the cyclic AMP system.

Thymus extracts, including purified protein-rich factors derived from the calf thymus, are now known to enhance antibody formation both in vivo and in vitro and also affect the cyclic AMP system by stimulating adenylate cyclase activity (1-3). In this regard, most studies concerning the effects of calf

thymus extract on cellular and biochemical changes of lymphoid cells have
dealt with the responses of normal individuals and cells or cells derived from
immunologically deficient individuals. In the present study splenocytes from
mice infected with a leukemia virus were utilized in a model system to determine if calf thymus extracts affect the immunologic impairment which accompany virus leukemogenesis. Extensive earlier studies had shown that
mice infected with FLV, as well as other murine leukemia viruses, show a
marked impairment of immune competence both in vivo and in vitro (4-6).
Suppressed antibody formation to an antigen such as sheep erythrocytes was
attributed to the effects of the virus on antibody precursor cells, presumably
B-lymphocytes, rather than antibody-forming cells per se. Cultures of
splenocytes from virus-infected mice were markedly impaired in their responsiveness to sheep erythrocytes. Addition of relatively small numbers of
macrophages resulted in enhanced immune responsiveness (10). The mechanism of such reversal of immune suppression in vitro was not entirely clear,
since macrophages may function in a number of several ways. Bacterial
LPS, when added to similar spleen cell cultures from FLV-infected mice,
also partially restored antibody responsiveness. However, LPS also has a
variety of activities, both in vivo and in vitro (11).

The use of calf thymus extracts in similar studies appeared to offer an
alternative approach to an analysis of not only the nature of immunosuppression in leukemic mice but also the ability of nonspecific immunologic stimulators to restore immune responsiveness. In initial experiments calf thymus
extracts injected into FLV-infected animals failed to alter significantly either
the course of the disease or the immunologic impairment induced by the virus.
However, earlier experiments had also shown that macrophages which reverse immunosuppression in vitro have little effect in vivo (10). This was
attributed to the failure of the macrophages to "home" normally into lymphoid
organisms such as the spleen in the infected animals. Thus, it seemed possible that calf thymus extracts, when administered in vivo, did not reach the
appropriate cells in the spleen or lymph nodes of infected animals. Similarly,
the dose or timing of administration of the thymus extracts may not have been
optimal.

In the present study it was found that addition of calf thymus extracts to
splenocyte cultures from FLV-infected mice significantly increased antibody
responsiveness to sheep RBCs. Restoration of immune responsiveness was,
however, only partial. Such failure of complete restoration could be interpreted as due to a defect of immune competence of FLV-infected animals not
only in terms of depressed numbers of antibody precursor cells, but also a
defect in the proliferative response of stimulated cells even after antigen
activation. Addition of calf thymosin on the day of culture initiation resulted
in a three- to fivefold or greater increase in the number of PFCs in most
cultures assayed on the day of peak response. However, even early after
culture initiation there were significantly more PFCs in the cultures of
splenocytes from infected animals treated with thymosin as compared to untreated cultures.

Calf thymosin appeared to have little effect on the PFC responsiveness of
normal spleen cell cultures. Only relatively large amounts of thymosin

(50 to 100 μg) affected PFC responsiveness of normal spleen cells, and this occurred only when thymosin was added on the day of culture initiation or 1 day later.

Both the dose of thymosin and the time of addition relative to the day of culture initiation markedly affected the immune response of spleen cells from infected mice. These and other considerations suggest that the calf thymosin amplified the responsiveness of uninfected B-lymphocytes and also possibly affected helper T-lymphocytes necessary for antibody formation to SRBC. The influence of calf thymosin extracts on the activation of cyclic AMP in B- and T-lymphocytes from leukemia virus-infected mice should be examined. Such studies, when performed, might provide additional information as to the biochemical events involved in the restoration of antibody formation observed in the present study. Furthermore, by means of cell fractionation procedures it should also be possible to determine the cell type influenced by the thymus extracts. Preliminary experiments suggest that although T-cells are stimulated by thymus extract, an increase in B-cell functional activity also occurs. It appears likely that thymosin, representative of thymus extracts which may function as a "hormone" in the immune response mechanism, does have the ability of significantly increasing antibody responsiveness of leukemia virus-impaired splenocytes, at least in terms of antibody formation to sheep erythrocytes in vitro.

SUMMARY

The antibody responsiveness of spleen cells from leukemia virus-infected mice is markedly depressed, both in vivo and in vitro. Culture experiments were performed to determine whether purified calf thymus extract (thymosin) had an effect on the immune responsiveness of immunosuppressed splenocytes in vitro. Cultures of spleen cells from leukemia virus-infected mice developed many more hemolytic plaque-forming cells to sheep cells in vitro when treated at time of culturing initiation or one day thereafter with 50 to 100 μg of thymosin as compared to untreated cultures. Similar or even higher doses of thymosin had no effect on the PFC responses of normal splenocytes in vitro. Both the dose of thymosin and the day of addition to cultures of infected splenocytes affected the restoration of antibody formation. It seemed likely that thymosin, similar to other "nonspecific" immunologic stimulators, affected mainly antibody precursor B-cells, which are depressed or deficient in leukemia virus-infected mice.

ACKNOWLEDGMENTS

The capable technical assistance of Mrs. Leony Mills, Mrs. Susan Spears, and Mr. Chandu Patel during various portions of the study are acknowledged. The immunostimulatory calf thymus factor used for in vivo treatment was prepared by Dr. Terry Hand; thymosin (fraction 5) was kindly supplied by Dr. Allan Goldstein.

REFERENCES

1. Friedman, H. (Ed.) (1975): Thymus factors in immunity. Ann. N.Y. Acad. Sci., 249:1-547.
2. Luckey, T. D. (Ed.) (1973): Thymic Hormones. University Park Press, Baltimore, Md.
3. Trainin, N., and Small, M. (1973): Thymic humoral factors. Contemp. Top. Immunobiol., 2:321-338.
4. Friedman, H., and Ceglowski, W. S. (1971): Immunosuppression by tumor viruses: Effects of leukemia virus infection on the immune response. Prog. Immunol., 1:815-829.
5. Friedman, H., and Ceglowski, W. S. (1975): Immunosuppression in the etiology of cancer. M. D. Anderson Symposium on Fundamentals of Cancer Research (in press).
6. Friedman, H. (1975): Immunosuppression by murine leukemia viruses. In: Viruses and Immunity, edited by C. Koprowski and H. Koprowski, pp. 17-58. Academic Press, New York.
7. Friedman, H., and Ceglowski, W. S. (1974): Virus tumorigenesis and immunity: Influence of immunostimulation and immunosuppression. In: The Role of Immunological Factors in Viral and Oncogenic Processes, edited by R. F. Beers, R. C. Tilghman, and E. G. Bisett, pp. 187-209. Johns Hopkins Press, Baltimore, Md.
8. Hand, T., Ceglowski, W. S., Damrongsak, D., and Friedman, H. (1970): Development of antibody forming cells in neonatal mice; stimulation and inhibition by calf thymus fraction. J. Immunol., 15:446-450.
9. Greaves, M., Janossy, G., Feldmann, M., and Doenhoff, M. (1974): Polyclonal mitogens and the nature of B-lymphocyte activation mechanisms. In: The Immune System, Genes, Receptors and Signals, edited by E. E. Sercarz, A. R. Williamson, and C. Fried Cox, pp. 271-297. Academic Press, New York.
10. Ceglowski, W. S., and Friedman, H. (1975): Failure of peritoneal exudate macrophages to reverse immunologic impairment induced by Friend leukemia virus. Proc. Soc. Exp. Biol. Med., 148:808-811.
11. Bendinelli, M., Kaplan, G. H., and Friedman, H. (1975): Reversal of leukemia virus-induced immunosuppression in vitro by peritoneal exudate macrophages. J. Natl. Cancer Inst., 55:1425-1432.

Control of Neoplasia by Modulation of the Immune System, edited by M. A. Chirigos. Raven Press, New York 1977.

THYMIC TRANSFER FACTOR

E. George Elias

University of Maryland, School of Medicine, Department of Surgery, Baltimore, Maryland 21201

INTRODUCTION

It had been shown that it was possible to transfer immunologically specific generalized delayed hypersensitivity skin reactions (D. H. S.) in animal and in man by means of viable leukocyte transfusion from sensitized donors (1-3). Successful transfer of D. H. S. to 2, 4-dinitrochlorobenzene (DNCB) in guinea pigs using sonicated extract of peritoneal exudate cells was also reported, but large numbers of animals were utilized as donors to accomplish the transfer (4), and these experiments could not be reproduced (5). In the meantime, Lawrence (6,7) reported that extracts of human peripheral blood leukocytes were effective in transferring D. H. S. in man.

The experimental demonstration that thymic hormones affect T-cell differentiation presents some interesting phenomena not encountered with other endocrine glands. It had been reported that the administration of thymic extract to animals with an intact thymus resulted in lymphocytosis (8,9) and lymphopoiesis (10,11). Furthermore, the administration of thymic extracts to neonatally thymectomized mice resulted in a rise in the number of the lymphocytes, prevention of the wasting disease (12), an improvement of the ability of these animals to develop cutaneous hypersensitivity responses (13), and the capability of the spleen cells to mount a graft-versus-host reaction or skin allograft rejection when injected to the appropriate recipient (14,15). All these responses measured T-cell function, and these experiments suggested that T-cell differentiation was stimulated in the thymoprival animal by some component of the injected thymic extract.

The principles underlying the use of the thymus gland for the transfer of D. H. S. were twofold. First, it was assumed that the transfer factor of Lawrence could be an extract of T-cell population, and second, it had been shown that the thymus gland possessed immunological as well as endocrinological functions. The guinea pig system was used in these experiments because these animals had been known to be ideal for the study of D.H.S. in the laboratory, and it seemed to be the most resistent system for all methods of transfer other than with the living cells (1,2).

The principle of transferring D.H.S. to bacterial antigens and chemical allergens could be utilized in the future to transfer specific cell-mediated immunity against neoplasia.

MATERIALS AND METHODS

The animals used in these experiments were female guinea pigs of the Camm/ Hartley strain.[1] Young guinea pigs (GP) that weighed between 150 and 250 g were the donors of thymic extracts, while adult GP weighing between 520 to 900 g were the recipients. The donor guinea pigs were sensitized to DNCB[2] by applying 0.005 ml of 50% DNCB solution in acetone once to the dorsal surface of one ear. The same technique was used for sensitization to OCBC.[2] The donor animals that were sensitized to PPD were each injected with 1 mg of BCG[3] intradermally in the back of the neck.

To test hypersensitivity in the animals (donors or recipients), the following methods were used: For DNCB, 0.1% DNCB cream (in acid mantle vehicle) was applied to an area of skin that had been clipped. For OCBC hypersensitivity, the animals were tested with 12% OCBC dissolved in acetone and olive oil. To test for PPD, $5 \mu g$ of preservative-free PPD[3] in 0.1 ml of buffered saline solution was injected intradermally per animal.

All skin tests, for donors or recipients, were read at 24 and 48 hr after DNCB or OCBC were applied to skin or PPD was injected intradermally. No depilatory material was used in any of the animals before or after applying the allergens or skin testing except in few occasions just prior to obtaining photographs. The intensity of the skin reactions was recorded according to Table 1 and were considered negative if there was 0 or $\pm$ response. On the other hand, reactions of 1+ or more were reported as positive.

The thymic glands were harvested in Hank's buffer saline solution, homogenized, and centrifuged at 250 X g for half an hour. The supernatants were ultracentrifuged at 105,000 X g and then passed through 0.20-μm plain membrane filters.[4] Samples were then taken for quantitative protein determinations (17). The control animals donated TE^0, the DNCB-sensitized animals donated TE^{DNCB}, the OCBC-sensitized animals donated TE^{OCBC}, and those sensitized by BCG donated TE^{PPD}.

It had been reported (16) that the extract of one-fourth of a thymus or less from a sensitized donor, injected into a naive recipient intradermally (i.d.), subcutaneously (s.c.), or intramuscularly (i.m.), was sufficient to establish

---

[1] Obtained from Camm Research Institute, Wayne, New Jersey.

[2] Obtained from Eastman Organic Chemical, Rochester, New York.

[3] Obtained from Connaught Research Laboratories, Willowdale, Ontario, Canada.

[4] Obtained from Nalge Sybron Corp., Rochester, New York.

TABLE 1. Grading the response of delayed cutaneous hypersensitivity in donors or recipients

Response	Symptoms or reactions
To PPD injected intradermally:	
0	None
±	Erythema less than 10 mm, no induration
1+	Erythema more than 10 mm, no induration
2+	Erythema more than 10 mm, mild induration
3+	Erythema more than 10 mm, moderate induration
4+	Necrosis or blebs
To DNCB or OCBC applied to the skin:	
0	None
1+	Patchy erythema
2+	Homogenous erythema
3+	Edema and induration
4+	Necrosis or blisters

transfer of D.H.S. for approximately 4 weeks. The following experiments were designed to elucidate the characteristics of the recipients and those of the donors, to find out the best time for the donor to give the most effective thymic transfer, to document the transfer effect and its specificity, and to establish its ability to cross species.

Characteristics of Recipients

During previous experiments, it was noted that some of the recipients of TE PPD became positive 24 hr after receiving the thymic extract, whereas others remained negative during the first 24 hr but became positive on the 4th to 6th day. In each of these experiments the same preparation of TE PPD was utilized, and the possibility existed that the variant was in the recipient rather than the donors or the extract. To investigate this matter, 11 animals with various weights were utilized as recipients for a single TE PPD preparation. Seven of these recipients weighed between 520 and 660 g, and the other

TABLE 2. Weight of the recipients and its role in expressing D. H. S. after receiving TE PPD

Weight of recipients in grams at time of receiving TE PPD	Days tested for D. H. S. to PPD after TE PPD					
	1	6	13	17	26	38
520	0	++	0	+	+	±
530	0	++	0	0	±	0
540	0	++	0	+	±	0
570	0	±	++	+	±	±
590	0	++	0	±	0	0
630	++	±	+	+	±	0
660	0	±	0	±	0	0
800	++	++	++	++	0	+
800	++	++	0	++	0	0
860	±	+++	++	±	+	+
900	++	++	++	++	0	0

All guinea pigs received 0.25 TE PPD i.d. on day 0. Four control animals (which weighed 550, 565, 810, and 865 g), each received 0.25 TE⁰ and were tested with this group and remained negative.

4 weighed between 800 and 900 g. Each received a standard dose of 0.25[5] TE PPD i.d. All the animals were then subjected to PPD skin testing at variable intervals. Only 1 animal, weighing 630 g, was positive, i.e., expressed D.H.S. to PPD 24 hr after receiving TE PPD. On the other hand, 3 of 4 animals weighing between 800 and 900 g became positive in 24 hr after receiving TE PPD. However, on the 6th day, 8 of 11 recipients expressed D.H.S. to PPD (Table 2). Four control animals each of which received 0.25 TE⁰ i.d. remained negative throughout the 38th day.

[5] Thymic extract of one-fourth of thymus gland.

TABLE 3. Old donors of TE ^{PPD}

Weight of recipient in grams	Days treated for D.H.S. to PPD after TE ^{PPD}			
	1	4	8	12
800	±	±	0	0
860	±	±	±	0
385	±	0	0	0
410	±	0	0	0

Each recipient received 0.25 TE ^{PPD} i.d. obtained from old donors (900 to 1,000 g).

Characteristics of Donors

Because thymic gland degenerates with age and becomes atrophic and in-filtrated with fat, its role in the transfer was investigated. In the following experiment, adult guinea pig donors weighing 900 to 1,000 g each were sensitized in the routine fashion by receiving 1 mg of BCG intradermally in the nape of the neck. Twelve days later, the dorsal hair was clipped and they were skin tested by injecting 0.1 Connaught PPD (5 mg of PPD) intradermally. Twenty-four hours later, the tests showed a 2 to 3+ delayed hypersensitivity reaction. These animals were sacrificed on the 14th day and their thymuses were collected, histological samples were taken, and the rest were minced in Hank's buffered saline solution, homogenated, and extracted in a routine fashion. The resultant TE ^{PPD} from these old animals were then injected into 4 recipients on the same day of preparation. The recipient animals included two adult (800 and 860 g) and two young (385 and 410 g) animals. Each of the recipients received a 0.25 of a TE ^{PPD} i.d. in a standard fashion, then was skin tested as seen in Table 3. All skin tests gave 0 to ± D.H.S. reactions between 1 and 12 days post-TE ^{PPD} injection.

Timing of the Donor

The purpose of the following experiments were to find out when the thymus of sensitized donor animals would be capable of transferring delayed hyper-sensitivity. Young donors each received 1 mg of BCG intradermally in the nape of the neck and were monitored by skin testing for the development of delayed hypersensitivity. A 1+ to 2+ delayed hypersensitivity reaction to 5 mg of PPD was observed between day 7 and day 9, and by day 21 to day 28 a 3+ to 4+ delayed hypersensitivity reaction developed to 5 mg of PPD in this group.

TABLE 4.   Timing of the thymus for transfer of delayed hypersensitivity
to PPD

Donors	Recipients		
No. of days after BCG	Positive skin tests for PPD D.H.S.		
injection to donate TE	Day 1	Day 4	Day 7
1	0/2	0/2	0/2
2	0/2	0/2	0/2
3 [a]	2/6	6/6	6/6
4	0/2	2/2	1/2
7	0/2	1/2	2/2
9 [a]	4/6	6/6	6/6
10	0/2	2/2	2/2
12 [a]	6/8	5/8	3/8
14	0/2	0/2	2/2
17 [a]	4/7	6/7	6/7
21 [a]	1/4	2/4	2/4
24	0/2	0/2	0/2
28 [a]	1/6	1/6	0/6

Each recipient received 0.25 of TE.

All control animals remained negative to skin tests.

[a] Indicates several experiments; the results were summed together.

A similar group of young animals, each of which received 1 mg of BCG
i.d. in the nape of the neck, donated their thymuses on different days after
sensitization. TE PPD were prepared in the routine fashion on days 1, 2, 3,
4, 7, 9, 10, 12, 14, 21, 24, and 28 post-BCG injection. Adult recipients,
each of which received 0.25 TE PPD of each of these preparations, were
tested with PPD as seen in Table 4. Thymic extracts of day 1 and day 2
post-BCG were not capable of transferring D.H.S. From day 3 on, however,
thymic extracts obtained from BCG-injected animals were capable of transferring delayed hypersensitivity.

TABLE 5. Specificity of the transfer by thymic extracts

| Material received | Positive skin testing for D.H.S. 4 days later | |
	OCBC	DNCB
TE DNCB	0/4	4/4
TE OCBC	4/4	0/4

Each recipient received 0.25 of thymic extract i.d. from sensitized animal to DNCB or OCBC. These animals were tested 4 days after receiving the thymic extracts.

Specificity

Two chemical allergens were utilized here: DNCB and OCBC. Of two groups of young donors, one was sensitized to DNCB and donated TE DNCB, whereas the other was sensitized to OCBC and donated TE OCBC. Thymic extracts were prepared in routine fashion. Eight naive recipients were used and each received thymic extract equivalent to one-fourth of a gland. Four received TE DNCB and the other four received TE OCBC. All the animals were then tested 4 days later to both allergens, by the DNCB cream (0.1%) and the OCBC in oil (12%), by applying these separately to their clipped skin. As can be seen in Table 5, animals that received TE DNCB expressed D.H.S. only to DNCB and not to OCBC. On the other hand, animals that received TE OCBC showed D.H.S. to OCBC and not to DNCB.

Cross-Species Transfer (18, 19)

Hartley guinea pigs are not an inbred strain of animals, but we investigated if thymic extract would be capable of transferring delayed hypersensitivity across species at the clinical level. Human volunteers became available for this study under a special protocol study. Most of the volunteers were patients with metastatic cancers that had been repeatedly skin tested and were found to be negative to DNCB and/or PPD. The PPD skin test in man was 5 mg of PPD (250 T.U.) injected i.d. and read at 24 and 48 hr. On the other hand, DNCB-tested patients were skin tested by applying 100 µg of DNCB in acetone to their skin and were examined for D.H.S. 24 and 48 hr later. Those who were found to be negative were retested 2 weeks later with 150 µg of DNCB in acetone. Those who were still negative were admitted to the study of the transfer.

The patients that were admitted to the study each received a single dose of thymic extract (TE PPD or TE DNCB) equivalent to 0.25 of a gland of an animal. They received this injection intradermally. The injection site was observed for any reaction. Prior to the TE injection an intravenous line (i.v.) was started with 5% dextrose in 0.33% normal saline and the vein kept open with slow i.v. drip. Epinephrine and corticosteroids were available at bedside in case of anaphylactoid reaction. The i.v. was maintained for 2 days. The vital signs of the patients were obtained at 4-hr intervals. Besides slight erythema, which lasted for approximately 1 day at the site of injection of the thymic extract, no other reactions were noted. None of the patients had any anaphylactoid reactions, or any significant change in the vital signs. No other medications were given in this period of time.

The same animals that donated TE ^{PPD} or TE ^{DNCB} also donated some of their lymph nodes, which were extracted in the same fashion as the thymuses. To equilibrate the dose level between thymus extracts and lymph node extracts, the proteins were measured. Each thymus gland donated between 14 and 16 mg of protein after ultracentrifugation and millipore filtration. In other words, each patient received approximately 4 mg of protein of thymic extract for the transfer. Control patients received equivalent doses of 4 mg of protein of lymph node extract i.d. All the patients were then tested 4 to 7 days later to DNCB (100 μg/ml in acetone percutaneously) and to PPD (5 mg of PPD intradermally). Four patients that received lymph node extract and were negative to DNCB and PPD remained negative. On the other hand, 7 of 9 patients that received TE ^{DNCB} turned systemically positive, as all were tested on the other forearm. Those who received TE ^{PPD}, 9 of 11 became positive to the PPD skin tests after a standard single injection of thymic extract. Therefore, it seemed that guinea pig thymic extract was capable of transferring D.H.S. to bacterial and chemical allergens cross species to man. Although these patients were supposedly immune-suppressed by their diseases, the transfer of D.H.S. could be established in them.

Two patients showed great clinical significance and should be discussed in some detail: Patient 1 was a male that had massive metastatic colon carcinoma with intestinal obstruction. He was admitted for terminal care. He volunteered to enter the study as all medications had failed to control his disease. He was skin tested with PPD, monilia, mumps, varidase, DNCB, DNFB, and croton oil, and was found negative to all seven. He had been previously sensitized to DNCB and over the last 2 months before his admission he maintained negative DNCB skin reactions to 150 μg in acetone. He was given TE ^{DNCB} i.d. Four days later he was skin tested in the contralateral forearm and he expressed a D.H.S. to DNCB (100 μg) of at least 2+ reaction. Three weeks later, he was retested to the same seven antigens and allergens and was found to be positive only to DNCB.

Patient 2 was a female with massive metastasis from rectal carcinoma. She was admitted to the hospital because of severe leukopenia (white cell count of 800/mm^3) secondary to chemotherapy. She volunteered to enter the study and she received TE ^{DNCB}. Four days later her white cell count was 1,000/mm^3, and she failed to show delayed hypersensitivity to 100 μg of DNCB in acetone. She received 0.25 TE ^{DNCB} and 7 days later she was retested with 150 μg of DNCB and remained negative. At that time, her white cell count was still 1,000/mm^3, and repeated bone marrow aspiration showed hypocellularity of the bone marrow. Unfortunately, she decided to go home and the study was discontinued before her bone marrow recovery. This case seemed to indicate that an intact bone marrow might be necessary for in vivo transfer of D.H.S. with thymic extract.

Proof of Transfer

Most of the results were obtained by observing delayed hypersensitivity reaction of the skin after PPD injection or after applying DNCB to the skin. To prove the transfer of cellular immunity two other methods were used, namely: (a) skin biopsy of histological examination of the tissue, and (b) the macrophage migration inhibition assay.

Skin Biopsies

Recipient guinea pigs were injected with 0.25 TE ^{PPD} i.d. in the nape of the neck. Four days later, the dorsal hair was clipped at a distant site and the animals were tested with 5 mg of PPD intradermally. After 24 hr D.H.S. was noted at the site of PPD. The clipped area was then treated with Nair, a commercial depilatory agent, for 3 min, then washed off. No reaction to Nair was noted. Immediately following this, skin punch biopsy was obtained from the indurated area that showed D.H.S. to PPD and from the normal skin adjacent to it that was similarly treated with Nair. Histological sections were obtained and compared and showed large numbers of lymphocytes infiltrating the dermis at the site of D.H.S. to PPD.

Macrophage Migration Inhibition Assay

Because the transfer effects by thymic extract could last for weeks, it was possible to confirm in vitro the transfer of cellular immunity that took place in vivo. Two equal groups of adult guinea pigs were utilized. In one group, each animal received 0.25 TE ^{PPD} i.d., and in the other group each received 0.25 TE^0. Four days later each animal was injected intraperitoneally (i.p.) with 30 ml of sterile light mineral oil. Three days after the i.p. injection, the animals were sacrificed and the peritoneal exudates were cultivated from the peritoneal cavity in heparinized Hank's buffered saline solution (1,000 I.U. of preservative-free heparin/1,000 ml of Hank's saline solution). The peritoneal exudate of each animal was collected in a separator funnel and allowed to settle, allowing the oil to float to the surface. The peritoneal exudate cells with Hank's buffered saline were then separated from the oil and collected in centrifugation tubes and washed three times with Hank's buffered saline solution. After the last wash, a cell count and viability count was obtained. The viability was 92 to 95% using the exclusion dye method with trypan blue. These cells consisted of 65 to 75% macrophages and 15 to 25% lymphocytes.

The macrophage migration inhibition assays utilizing the capillary tube technique were then carried out in the routine fashion. Each animal's exudate cells were incubated in enriched media only (RPMI-1640 media + 20% GP serum) as control, or in the same media with 25 mg of preservative-free PPD/ml for the test. The surface areas of migration of test chambers were compared to control chambers and the mean migration inhibition indices

(M.I.I.) were obtained. The mean M.I.I. for animals receiving TE ^{PPD} was 30.85 $\pm$ 4.65, whereas that for animals receiving TE^0 was 0 $\pm$ 1.00. This significant difference in inhibition indicated sensitization of the animals that received TE ^{PPD}.

RESULTS

The results obtained from the first experiment seemed to indicate that the older GP recipients expressed an earlier transfer than the younger ones. Three of 4 of the older animals expressed positive D.H.S. to PPD 24 hr after receiving TE ^{PPD}. On the other hand, only 1 of 7 young recipients had positive D.H.S. to PPD in the same period of time. However, most of the recipients, regardless of their weights — i.e., young or old — became positive to PPD skin testing on the 6th day after receiving TE ^{PPD} injection (Table 2). It should also be noted that the effect of a single injection of 0.25 TE ^{PPD} had lasted over 2 weeks, as 7 of 11 recipients continued to express D.H.S. to PPD. This effect seemed to fade away by the 26th day, as only 2 animals remained positive to PPD skin tests.

In the second experiment, the thymic extract obtained from older sensitized donors failed to establish transfer of D.H.S. to PPD, as the recipients express 0 to + reactions as seen in Table 3. The histological examination of the older donor GP thymuses showed lymphocytic infiltration and fatty degeneration of these glands. The main loss of tissue was in the epithelial stroma of the thymuses which was replaced by fat more than lymphocytes. This would suggest that the thymic transfer factor(s) was dependent mainly on the epithelial stroma more so than on the lymphocytes of the gland.

The results of the third experiment showed that thymic extracts obtained from young sensitized donors, 3 days after receiving BCG, was capable of transferring D.H.S. to PPD (Table 4). However, a similar group of young GP that received the same BCG failed to express D.H.S. to PPD 1 week after the primary sensitization. On the other hand, young GP that received BCG expressed more D.H.S. to PPD between 21 and 28 days after primary sensitization, yet the thymic extracts obtained from thymuses of similar donors showed lesser and weaker transfer during this period (Fig. 1).

Experiment 4 was planned to show the specificity of the transfer. As can be seen in Table 5, the animals that received TE ^{DNCB} expressed D.H.S. 4 days later to DNCB but not to OCBC and vice versa. This proved that thymic extract has a specific transfer effect rather than a nonspecific stimulatory one, under these experimental conditions.

It had been shown that thymic extracts from sensitized GP were capable of transferring D.H.S. in the guinea pig system. Furthermore, the results obtained from Experiment 5 suggest that these extracts are also capable of transferring D.H.S. into man, indicating that it is not species-specific. Two interesting phenomena should be noted in the two clinical case reports. The first patient received TE ^{DNCB} and expressed D.H.S. to DNCB only, again suggesting the specificity of the transfer cross species. The second patient, who had hypocellular bone marrow, failed to show transfer effect, and this could indicate the necessity of intact bone marrow in the in vivo system.

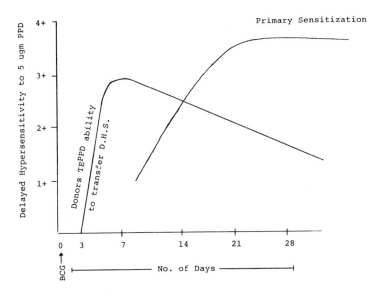

FIG. 1. The relationship in D.H.S. between primary sensitization with BCG and the donor's ability to transfer D.H.S. with thymic extract obtained at different days after BCG sensitization.

The transfer of D.H.S. which was observed by the skin reactions in the recipients was confirmed by skin biopsy and by <u>in vitro</u> assaying the macrophage migration. The skin biopsies obtained from animals that received TE PPD and expressed D.H.S. to PPD skin tests showed massive lymphocytic infiltration at the PPD site. This indicated cell-mediated immunity to PPD in the TE PPD recipients. This was further confirmed by the macrophage migration inhibition assay as the migration of the peritoneal exudate cells from TE PPD recipients were significantly inhibited when incubated in the enriched media with PPD.

DISCUSSION

The results obtained from previous experiments (16, 18, 19) and from the experiments presented above could indicate the following:

1. Thymic extracts obtained from young donor guinea pigs sensitized to bacterial antigens or chemical allergens are capable of transferring D.H.S. to naive animals. The ability of the thymic extract to transfer such D.H.S. is reproducible, as it was successfully seen in several experiments that included different preparations.

2. Such transfer is a passive transfer and not an active immunization, as this effect faded away in approximately 4 weeks; i.e., it was transient, but longer than transfer with other modalities in guinea pigs.

3. It seems that the characteristics of the recipients may influence the onset of the expression of D.H.S. after thymic extract injection. Old recipient animals could express the transfer effect in a shorter period of time than younger ones.

4. Younger donor animals can yield a better transfer factor(s) from the thymus than older ones. This would suggest that this factor could be dependent on the stroma of the gland.

5. This transfer factor(s) could be cultivated from the thymuses of donor animals prior to the expression of D.H.S. by the donor itself to primary sensitization.

6. It seems that the thymic transfer factor is very specific, as no cross-reactivity was noted between DNCB and OCBC.

7. Thymic extract from sensitized animals may be capable of passively transferring cellular immunity to other species; i.e., it is not species-specific.

8. The transfer effect from the thymus was established by cutaneous delayed hypersensitivity skin reactions and was further confirmed by histological examination of the skin and by the macrophage migration inhibition assays.

Finally, thymic extracts could play two roles in modulating the host resistance in human neoplasia: (a) as nonspecific stimulators of cellular response as discussed under thymosin, and (b) by specific transfer of D.H.S. as was shown in this presentation.

SUMMARY

Acellular saline extracts of thymus glands, obtained from young guinea pigs sensitized to bacterial antigens and chemical allergens, could transfer cutaneous D.H.S. to naive guinea pigs. The transfer effect could be obtained from the thymus of the sensitized donor animals even before these could express D.H.S. to the antigen or allergen. Furthermore, the stronger the D.H.S. became in the donors, the weaker was the transfer by their thymic extracts. This thymic factor(s) appeared to be specific in transferring D.H.S., as no cross-reactivity was noted in the recipients between the two chemical allergens used: DNCB and orthochlorobenzenoylchloride (OCBC).

Thymic transfer factor(s) seemed to have a longer transfer effect than transfer with peripheral living cells in the guinea pigs. They also had the ability to establish the transfer earlier in older than in younger recipient animals, and seemed to be capable of establishing the transfer cross species. The transfer of D.H.S. was confirmed histologically and by the macrophage migration inhibition assay.

ACKNOWLEDGMENTS

This work was partially supported by a private donation from Mr. Thomas McMaster, Detroit, Michigan.

REFERENCES

1. Landsteiner, K., and Chase, M. W. (1942): Experiments on transfer of cutaneous sensitivity to simple compounds. Proc. Soc. Exp. Biol. Med., 49:688-690.

2. Chase, M. W. (1945): The cellular transfer of cutaneous hypersensitivity to tuberculin. Proc. Soc. Exp. Biol. Med., 59:134-135.

3. Lawrence, H. S. (1949): The cellular transfer of cutaneous hypersensitivity to tuberculin in man. Proc. Soc. Exp. Biol. Med., 71:516-517.

4. Jeter, W. S., Tremaine, M. M., and Seebohm, P. M. (1954): Passive transfer of delayed hypersensitivity to 2,4-dinitrochlorobenzene in guinea pigs with leukocyte extracts. Proc. Soc. Exp. Biol. Med., 86:251-253.

5. Bloom, B. R., and Chase, M. W. (1967): Transfer of delayed hypersensitivity. Prog. Allergy, 10:151-255.

6. Lawrence, H. S. (1954): The transfer of generalized cutaneous hypersensitivity of the delayed tuberculin type in man by means of constituents of disrupted leukocytes. J. Clin. Invest., 33:951-952.

7. Lawrence, H. S. (1955): The transfer in humans of delayed skin sensitivity to streptococcal M substance and to tuberculin with disrupted leukocytes. J. Clin. Invest., 34:219-230.

8. Bomskow, C. H., and Sladovick, L. (1940): Dtsch. Med. Wochenschr., 66:589.

9. Rehn, E. (1940): Dtsch. Med. Wochenschr., 66:594.

10. Klein, J. J., Goldstein, A. L., and White, A. (1965): Enhancement of in vivo incorporation of labeled precursors into DNA and total protein of mouse lymph nodes after administration of thymic extracts. Proc. Natl. Acad. Sci. (U.S.A.), 53:812-817.

11. Trainin, N., Burger, M., and Kaye, A. M. (1967): Some characteristics of a thymic hormone factor determined by assay in vitro of DNA synthesis in lymph nodes of thymectomized mice. Biochem. Pharmacol., 16:711-720.

12. De Somer, P., Denys, P., Jr., and Leytin, R. (1963): Activity of noncellular calf thymus extract in normal and thymectomized mice. Life Sci., 22:810-819.

13. Jankovic, B. D., Isakovic, K., and Horvat, J. (1965): Effect of lipid fraction from rat thymus on delayed hypersensitivity reactions of neonatally thymectomized rats. Nature, 208:356-357.

14. Bach, J., Dardenne, M., Goldstein, A. L., Guha, A., and White, A. (1971): Appearance of T-cell markers in bone marrow rosette-forming cells after incubation with thymosin, a thymic hormone. Proc. Natl. Acad. Sci. (U.S.A.), 68:2734-2738.

15. Goldstein, A. L., Asamuma, Y., Batkisto, J. R., Hardy, M. A., Quint, J., and White, A. (1970): Influence of thymosin on cell-mediated and humoral immune responses in normal and immunologically deficient mice. J. Immunol., 104:359-366.

16. Elias, E. G., and Cohen, R. M. (1975): Transfer of delayed hyper-sensitivity by thymic extract. Ann. N. Y. Acad. Sci., 249:462-467.

17. Henry, R. J., Sobel, C., and Sigalove, M. (1956): Turbidimetric determination of proteins with sulfosalicylic and trichloroacetic acid. Proc. Soc. Exp. Biol. Med., 97:748-751.

18. Elias, E. G., and Cohen, R. M. (1974): The transfer of delayed hyper-sensitivity to man by guinea pig thymus extract (Abstr.). Clin. Res., 22:417A.

19. Cohen, R. M., and Elias, E. G. (1974): Transfer of delayed hyper-sensitivity to dinitrochlorobenzene and PPD by thymic extract in guinea pig and man. Surg. Forum, 25:316-318.

*Control of Neoplasia by Modulation
of the Immune System*, edited by
M. A. Chirigos. Raven Press, New
York 1977.

EXPERIMENTAL STUDIES OF THYMOSIN IN NZB MICE AND IN SYSTEMIC LUPUS ERYTHEMATOSUS

*, ** Norman Talal, * Michael J. Dauphinee, * Kenneth H. Fye, and
* Haralampos Moutsopoulos

* Clinical Immunology and Arthritis Section, Veterans Administration
Hospital, and
** Department of Medicine, University of California, San Francisco,
San Francisco, California 94143

INTRODUCTION

The introduction of the New Zealand Black (NZB) mouse and the related hybrid NZB/NZW F_1 (B/W) mouse into experimental medicine 20 years ago has contributed greatly to our understanding of autoimmunity in general and systemic lupus erythematosus (SLE) in particular. Several reviews of experimental lupus in the NZ mouse model have been published (1-3).

NZB mice spontaneously develop Coomb's positive hemolytic anemia as their predominant clinical expression of disease. B/W mice develop L. E. cells, antinuclear factor, and immune complex glomerulonephritis as their major clinical features. Antibodies to thymocytes are common in NZB mice, whereas antibodies to nucleic acids are more frequent in B/W mice (4). Female B/W mice have a more accelerated disease and die prematurely in renal failure, generally before 1 year of age. They are the closest model for acute lupus nephritis in young women. Male B/W mice survive longer and may develop lymphoma or macroglobulinemia as they age (5).

Genetic, immunologic, and virologic factors are all intimately involved in the pathogenesis of NZ mouse disease, and by analogy, in human SLE as well (6). Several autosomal genes appear to influence the mouse disease, although exact genetic mechanisms are uncertain. Various immunologic abnormalities are seen in NZ mice, suggesting profound disturbances in several different components of the immune system (Table 1). NZ mice harbor C-type leukemia viruses and produce antibodies to viral antigens. Some of these antiviral immune complexes deposit in the kidney and contribute to the glomerulonephritis (7).

TABLE 1. Immunologic abnormalities in NZB and NZB/NZW mice

---

1. Premature development of competence in B- and T-cells

2. B-cells make excessive antibody responses

3. T-cells are unable to develop and maintain tolerance

4. Loss of T-suppressor cell function

5. Decreased serum "thymic hormone" activity

6. Deficient T-cell functions later in life

7. Loss of recirculating T-lymphocytes

8. Loss of theta-positive cells late in life

9. Spontaneous production of thymocytotoxic antibody

MATERIALS AND METHODS

NZB mice were from our colony maintained at the Vivarium of the University of California, San Francisco. $C_{57}B1/6$ and DBA/2 mice were from Jackson Laboratory, Bar Harbor, Maine. Thymosin fraction 5 was kindly supplied by Dr. Allan L. Goldstein.

Methods for studying thymocyte DNA synthesis in allogeneic recipients and for measuring antigen-induced depression of spleen DNA synthesis have been described previously (8,9).

RESULTS

Thymosin Studies in NZB Mice

NZB mice show a progressive loss of T-cell functions during their life-span (6). Even prior to the onset of autoimmunity, their T-cells are resistant to the development of immunologic tolerance (10). Later in life, they have marked deficiencies of various T-cell effector functions such as reactivity to mitogens and ability to induce graft-versus-host (GvH) disease. At this stage, they also have a deficiency of long-lived recirculating T-cells.

We have reported a thymocyte abnormality in NZB mice detected by measuring the DNA synthetic response to foreign transplantation antigens. NZB thymocytes were injected into lethally irradiated $C_{57}B1/6$ mice and DNA synthesis measured as the incorporation of [125]iododeoxyuridine ([125]IUDR) by spleen- and lymph node-seeking cells. Thymocytes from DBA/2 mice (who are the same H_2 type as NZB) were similarly injected into other $C_{57}B1/6$ mice as controls (8).

DBA/2 thymocytes from 2- and 8-week-old donors and NZB thymocytes from 2-week-old donors showed essentially the same proliferative response upon encountering the foreign histocompatibility antigens of the recipient animals. There was a rapid synthetic response that peaked on day 4 and was over by day 6. By contrast, thymocytes from 8-week-old NZB mice showed a very different response. DNA synthesis was markedly delayed and did not begin until day 4.

These results suggested an alteration in the DNA synthetic response to histocompatibility antigens by NZB thymocytes occurring between 2 and 8 weeks of age. This may reflect an intrinsic abnormality of thymocyte differentiation, perhaps genetically determined or induced by a latent viral infection.

Bach et al. have demonstrated the presence of a thymosin-like material in normal mouse serum that is lacking in the serum of congenitally thymus-deficient ("nude") mice (11). Such thymosin-like activity declined with age in normal mice and declined prematurely in the serum of NZB and NZB/NZW F_1 hybrid mice. By 2 months, a time when abnormal thymocyte proliferation and T-cell resistance to tolerance are already present, serum thymic activity was insignificant in NZB mice. These findings raised the possibility that a deficiency of thymosin could contribute to the T-cell abnormalities characteristic of the NZB strain.

We have studied the ability of thymosin to correct the abnormal DNA synthetic response of NZB thymocytes. We can preserve normal DNA synthesis in 8-week-old thymocytes by treating donor NZB mice with various regimens of thymosin (12). Moreover, we find that the abnormal synthesis of DNA reflects a loss of suppressor T-cells in NZB mice, and that thymosin can preserve suppressor T-cell function.

Many different assay systems have been used to measure the activity of suppressor T-cells. Zatz and Goldstein (9) described a system in which immunization with thymic-dependent antigens caused a transient depression in splenic DNA synthesis detected when radioactive 5-iodo-2-deoxyuridine (^{125}IUDR) was injected 6 hr after antigen. This depression in DNA synthesis was not seen in adult thymectomized mice or with thymic-independent antigens. If ^{125}IUDR was injected 24 hr after antigen, splenic DNA synthesis was increased rather than depressed. They interpreted these results as suggesting the presence of an antigen-activated suppressor cell which nonspecifically and transiently depresses DNA synthesis by splenic cells.

Using this system of antigen-induced depression, we have confirmed the loss of suppressor cells in 2-month NZB mice, and again demonstrated their restoration with thymosin (13). The restoration by thymosin declined between 1 and 2 weeks after treatment, but could be induced again after a second exposure to thymosin. These results suggest a potential for reversible but repeatable restoration of suppressor-cell activity in NZB mice.

Thymosin Studies in SLE and Other Autoimmune Diseases

Since NZB mice are a laboratory model for SLE, we have recently turned our attention to the effects of thymosin fraction 5 on lymphocyte function in

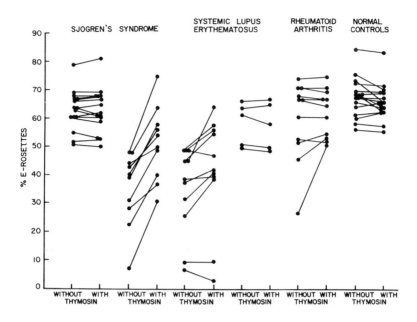

FIG. 1. In vivo effect of thymosin on peripheral T-lymphocytes in patients with collagen vascular disease.

human autoimmune diseases. We have studied the in vitro effect of thymosin on T-cells in patients with SLE, Sjögren's syndrome (SS), and rheumatoid arthritis (RA), using the sheep erythrocyte rosette assay. T-rosette-forming cells were decreased in SLE and SS but not in RA. Incubation with thymosin produced a significant rise in T-rosette-forming cells in most patients with low baseline numbers (Fig. 1). However, whereas all patients with SS showed an increase after thymosin, several patients with SLE showed no response at all. Moreover, serum from 4 active SLE patients blocked T-rosette formation by normal lymphocytes and rendered them unresponsive to stimulation by thymosin. These results suggest the presence of serum-blocking factors in SLE capable of interfering with thymosin binding to cell membrane receptors and thereby interrupting normal mechanisms of T-cell differentiation.

DISCUSSION

Lymphocytes are generally divided into two major classes, bone marrow-derived B-cells and thymic-derived T-cells. B-lymphocytes and their plasma cell progeny mediate humoral immunity through the production of specific antibodies. Autoantibodies are undoubtedly synthesized by B-lymphocytes which, like their more physiological counterparts, contain surface membrane immunoglobulins with antigen-combining sites identical to their secreted antibody product. The proliferation of these autoantibody-producing B-cells is prevented by immunologic control mechanisms which normally act to regulate the immune response and prevent autoimmunity. The major control mechanism involves the action of T-regulatory (helper and suppressor) cells.

T-lymphocytes have two major functions in the immune system. T-effector cells, in analogy with B-lymphocytes, mediate cellular immunity through the production of certain soluble factors (macrophage inhibitory factor, blastogenic factor, etc.). In addition, T-regulatory cells exert a second vital function, i.e., immunologic control. Although various factors (including antigenic load, antibody itself, and accessory cells such as macrophages) exert effects on antibody formation, the major responsibility for regulating this complex phenomenon falls to the T-regulatory cells.

There are two major populations of T-regulatory cells, called helper and suppressor. Helper T-cells promote antibody formation by sending stimulatory signals to the B-cells. Suppressor T-cells diminish antibody responses by sending inhibitory signals to the B-cells. Some antigens require helper cells to produce effective antibody response, whereas others do not. The cellular level at which regulation occurs (B-cell itself, macrophage, or through T-cell interaction), the number of cells involved, and the nature of the regulatory signals are unknown. Whatever the exact mechanisms of regulation, the net effect at the level of the B-cell results either in expansion or repression of the clone and either in increased or decreased antibody concentration.

It follows, therefore, that there are at least two ways to produce autoimmunity (Fig. 2). Either a decrease in the number and/or function of suppressor T-cells, or an increase in the number and/or function of helper T-cells, leads to an unbalanced state of immunologic regulation that could cause the proliferation of B-cell clones capable of producing autoantibodies. A similar mechanism could also lead to the development of malignant lymphomas. A balance of T-cell-derived regulatory signals normally prevents the emergence of autoantibodies and clinical autoimmune disease. Factors associated with autoimmunity (e.g., certain virus infections, a variety of different drugs, the aging process) may act by upsetting this delicate balance and interfering with normal regulatory mechanisms. Indeed, SLE may be primarily a female disease because sex factors interact with T-cell regulation and alter the balance between help and suppression (14).

Abnormalities of both suppressor and helper T-cells are present in NZ mice and influence the time of onset and severity of the autoimmune disease. Suppressor-cell function declines between 1 and 2 months of age, associated with a deficiency of circulating thymic hormone and a resistance to the establishment and maintenance of T-cell tolerance (3). Significant titers of autoantibodies, lymphocytic tissue infiltrates, hemolytic anemia, and glomerulonephritis develop progressively over the next several months. We have previously referred to this overall immunopathologic condition as a phenomenon of B-cell escape from T-cell regulation (6). NZ mice manifest a progressive deficiency of other T-cell functions over time. Antibodies cytotoxic to T-lymphocytes may contribute to their T-cell abnormalities. Ultimately, gross defects of T-effector function, malignant lymphomas, and monoclonal macroglobulinemia may appear (Fig. 3).

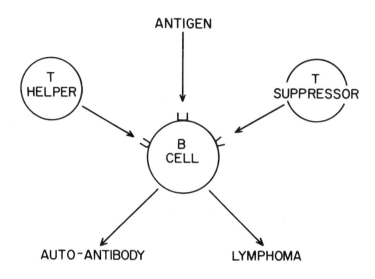

FIG. 2

This pathogenetic concept puts great emphasis on a deficiency of thymic hormone contributing to the progressive T-cell abnormalities of NZ mice. Our experimental results suggest that thymosin can restore suppressor-cell function in NZ mice. Nevertheless, treatment of NZB/NZW mice with thymosin has been disappointing to date. Our best results have been only a modest delay in the onset of autoimmunity. We feel that the simple hypothesis of a deficiency in thymic hormone and suppressor T-cells is inadequate to explain the disease fully, and have begun to think in terms of a balance between suppressor and helper T-cells (Fig. 2).

We are accumulating evidence that helper T-cell activity may be hyperactive at some periods in the life of NZ mice. We have reported on a possible abnormal thymic microenvironment which resulted in increased T-cell differentiation in X-irradiated bone marrow-repopulated NZB mice (15). The deficiency of circulating thymic hormone may be only one component of a thymic hormone abnormality. There may be other thymic epithelial products produced which can act locally in the thymus to cause accelerated T-cell maturation and contribute further to an unbalanced state of T-cell regulation.

Furthermore, we have observed an accelerated switch from IgM to IgG anti-DNA antibodies in female NZB/NZW mice who develop severe SLE glomerulonephritis and die earlier than males (14). Since switching involves T-regulatory cells (16), this result suggests excessive helper activity for the DNA response in female NZB/NZW mice.

Our results with SLE lymphocytes suggest another mechanism for T-cell abnormalities and apparent ineffectiveness of thymic hormones in autoimmune disorders. Lymphocytes contain receptors for many different hormones,

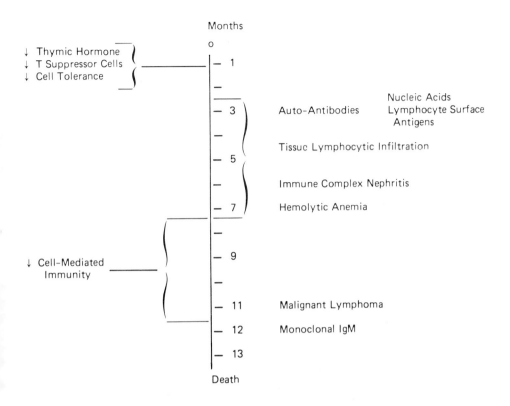

FIG. 3. Immunologic and immunopathologic events throughout the life-span of NZB and NZB/NZW mice.

including insulin and hydrocortisone. Antibodies to lymphocyte surface membranes occur frequently in SLE and may contribute to abnormal T-cell function. Serum "blocking factors" in SLE may consist of such antilymphocyte antibodies as well as circulating immune complexes. Moreover, blocking factors are shed from SLE lymphocytes during overnight culture. Blocking of specific hormone receptor sites on lymphocyte membranes must now be added to the list of abnormalities related to these antibodies. Antibodies to other receptors (for example, to insulin, acetylcholine, and TSH receptors) have been implicated as causative factors in diabetes mellitus, myasthenia gravis, and hyperthyroidism, respectively (17). Antibody blockade of receptor sites on lymphocytes may be another mechanism contributing to altered T-cell regulation and function in SLE.

SUMMARY

NZB mice are genetically predisposed to an autoimmune disease resembling SLE. A deficiency of suppressor T-cells and of thymic hormone characterize these mice. Treatment with thymosin can restore suppressor cell function but does not significantly modify disease. An imbalance of regulatory (helper and suppressor) T-cell function rather than a simple deficiency of suppressor T-cells may best explain disease in these mice.

Many patients with SLE and Sjögren's syndrome have decreased T-rosette-forming cells in peripheral blood. Incubation with thymosin will generally stimulate T-rosette formation when baseline values are low. However, some patients with active SLE have serum inhibitory factors which can decrease rosette-forming cells and block the stimulation by thymosin. Such "blocking factors" (presumably antilymphocyte antibodies) constitute a mechanism whereby thymosin-induced T-cell differentiation and function can be impaired in SLE.

REFERENCES

1. Howie, J. B., and Helyer, B. J. (1968): The immunology and pathology of NZB mice. Adv. Immunol., 9:215-266.
2. Mellors, R. C. (1966): Autoimmune and immunoproliferative diseases of NZB/B1 and hybrids. Int. Rev. Exp. Pathol., 5:217-252.
3. Talal, N. (1974): Autoimmunity and lymphoid malignancy in New Zealand mice. In: Progress in Clinical Immunology, Vol. 2, pp. 101-120. Grune & Stratton, New York.
4. Goldblum, R., Pillarisetty, R., and Talal, N. (1975): Independent appearance of anti-thymic and anti-RNA antibodies in NZB/NZW F_1 mice. Immunology, 28:621-628.
5. Sugai, S., Pillarisetty, R. J., and Talal, N. (1973): Monoclonal macroglobulinemia in NZB/NZW F_1 mice. J. Exp. Med., 138:989-1002.
6. Talal, N. (1970): Immunologic and viral factors in the pathogenesis of systemic lupus erythematosus. Arthritis Rheum., 13:887-894.
7. Yoshiki, T., Mellors, R. C., Strand, M., and August, J. T. (1974): The viral envelope glycoprotein of murine leukemia virus and the pathogenesis of immune complex glomerulonephritis of New Zealand mice. J. Exp. Med., 140:1011-1027.
8. Dauphinee, M. J., and Talal, N. (1973): Alteration in DNA synthetic response of thymocytes from different aged NZB mice. Proc. Natl. Acad. Sci. (U.S.A.), 70:37-39.
9. Dauphinee, M. J., and Talal, N. (1975): Antigen-induced depression of DNA synthesis in NZB mice. J. Immunol., 114:1713-1716.
10. Staples, P. J., Steinberg, A. D., and Talal, N. (1970): Induction of immunologic tolerance in older New Zealand mice repopulated with young spleen, bone marrow, or thymus. J. Exp. Med., 131:1223-1238.

11. Bach, J. F., Dardenne, M., and Salomon, J. C. (1973): Studies of thymus products IV. Absence of serum thymic activity in adult NZB and (NZB X NZW) F1 mice. Clin. Exp. Immunol., 14:247-256.

12. Dauphinee, M. J., Talal, N., Goldstein, A. L., and White, A. (1974): Thymosin corrects abnormal DNA synthetic response of NZB mouse thymocytes. Proc. Natl. Acad. Sci. (U.S.A.), 71:2637-2641.

13. Dauphinee, M. J., and Talal, N. (1975): Reversible restoration by thymosin of antigen-induced depression of spleen DNA synthesis in NZB mice. J. Immunol., 114:1713-1716.

14. Papoian, R., Pillarisetty, R., and Talal, N. (1975): Regulated sequential development of spontaneous nucleic acid antibodies in NZB/NZW F1 mice. (Submitted for publication.)

15. Dauphinee, M. J., Palmer, D. W., and Talal, N. (1975): Evidence for an abnormal microenvironment in the thymus of New Zealand Black mice. J. Immunol., 115:1054-1059.

16. Davie, J. M., and Paul, W. E. (1974): Role of T lymphocytes in the humoral immune response. I. Proliferation of B lymphocytes in thymus-deprived mice. J. Immunol., 113:1438-1445.

17. Carnegie, P. R., and Mackey, I. R. (1975): Vulnerability of cell-surface receptors to autoimmune reactions. Lancet, 21:684-687.

Control of Neoplasia by Modulation of the Immune System, edited by M. A. Chirigos. Raven Press, New York 1977.

IMMUNOLOGIC EFFECTS OF THYMOSIN IN YOUNG AND AGED AKR MICE

Anna D. Barker and Victor S. Moore

Biomedical Sciences Research Section, BATTELLE, Columbus Laboratories, Columbus, Ohio 43201

INTRODUCTION

Recent evidence indicates that the endocrine activity of the reticular-epithelial thymus plays a central role in the maturation of immature (presumably bone marrow-derived) prethymic cells (1, 2), intrathymic differentiation of thymocytes (3), and may effect subsequent differentiation of thymus-derived lymphocytes (T-cells). Thymosin, a thymic hormone (4, 5), has been shown to: induce precursor cells to express T-cell surface markers and perform T-cell functions (6, 7), restore and/or enhance a variety of cell-mediated immune responses in vivo (8-12); restore normal DNA synthetic patterns in New Zealand black (NZB) mice (13); increase the numbers of T-cell rosettes in patients with primary immunodeficiency diseases and neoplastic diseases (14, 15); and induce immunotherapeutic effects in animal leukemia models (16, 17).

Mice of the AKR strain uniformly develop a vertically transmitted viral-induced spontaneous lymphoid leukemia of thymus origin (18). Although the thymus has been established as the target organ in this disease (19), the mechanism of this thymus-dependent leukemogenesis is not presently understood. The present study was designed to determine the effects of thymosin on selected immunologic responses in young and aged AKR mice.

Although certain cell-mediated and humoral immune responses are reported to be near normal in young (preleukemic) AKR mice (20-23), increased immunologic dysfunction is associated with aging and subsequent disease onset (24, 25) in these animals. The role of thymic hormones in the immunologic changes and associated leukemogenesis observed in AKR mice has not been investigated.

The present study reports the effects of chronic in vivo thymosin fraction 5 or control spleen extract fraction 5 treatment of 6- to 8-week old (preleukemic) and 7- to 8-month-old (without overt disease) mice on: (a) mitogen responsiveness; (b) splenic IgM and IgG plaque formation following sheep erythrocyte immunization; and (c) the migration patterns in syngeneic recipients of lymphocytes from treated mice. The data from these experiments demonstrate that the in vivo effects of thymosin fraction 5 are dependent both on the age of these mice and the T-cell subpopulation tested.

MATERIALS AND METHODS

Mice

Six-week-old and 7- to 8-month-old (retired breeders) female AKR mice were purchased from Jackson Laboratories, Bar Harbor, Maine. All mice were housed in plastic cages and allowed Purine Laboratory Chow and water ad libitum. The aged mice were palpated at regular intervals for the presence of splenomegaly, lymphadenopathy, and/or thymic enlargement.

Thymosin

Bovine thymosin (fraction 5) and a control bovine spleen extract (fraction 5) were provided by Dr. Allan Goldstein. Thymosin, fraction 5, and the control spleen extract, fraction 5, will subsequently be referred to as thymosin or control extract. As recommended by Dr. Goldstein, the lypholized thymosin and control spleen extracts were reconstituted with pyrogen-free normal saline, passed through a 0.22-μm millipore filter and stored in 1,000-μg aliquots at -70°C. Thymosin and the control extract were thawed and diluted to the desired concentration in Hank's balanced salts solution (HBSS) (pH 7.2) just prior to administration. In the experiments reported here, the standard dose per animal of thymosin or the control spleen extract was 50 μg/injection.

Mitogen Studies

Lymphoid organs (thymuses, spleens, nodes) were removed (5 mice/group), separately pooled, lymphocyte suspensions prepared, and contaminating erythrocytes removed by centrifugation through a ficoll-hypaque gradient. The lymphocytes were resuspended in Dulbecco's media supplemented with 10% calf serum and 100 units of penicillin and 100 μg of streptomycin/ml. Lymphocytes (5 X 10^5 cells/0.1 ml), test mitogens, concanavalin A (Con A) at a concentration of 1 μg/0.1 ml or phytohemagglutinin (PHA) at a concentration of 0.5 μg/0.1 ml, or complete media (0.1 ml) were placed in microtest II plates (Falcon Plastics, Oxnard, California). All mitogen-containing and control cultures were prepared in quadruplicate and incubated at 37°C in a humidified CO_2 (5%) incubator for 72 hr. The cultures were pulsed with 1 μCi of ^{3}H-thymidine (New England Nuclear, Boston, Massachusetts) during the final 24 hr of incubation. The samples were harvested on a Multiple Automatic Sample Handler (Otto Hiller Company, Madison, Wisconsin), the filter strips dried, and subsequently placed in scintillation fluid for counting on a liquid scintillation spectrometer. The stimulation index was obtained by dividing the mean counts per minute (cpm) in the mitogen-containing cultures by the mean cpms in the unstimulated control cultures.

Assay for Numbers of IgM and IgG Plaque-Forming Cells (PFC)

The details of the hemolytic plaque technique, modified from that of Jerne et al. (26), has been reported (27). Plaques were visualized using a high-quality light source and the mean number of plaques/10^6 nucleated spleen cells for four plates was determined.

Lymphocyte Migration Studies

The thymuses, spleens, and lymph nodes were removed from thymosin or spleen control extract-treated mice, separately pooled (Dulbecco's media plus 10% calf serum) at 4° C, and the lymphocyte suspensions were prepared by gently homogenizing the tissue in Dulbecco's media supplemented with 10% calf serum. Contaminating erythrocytes were removed by centrifugation through a ficoll-hypaque gradient, followed by three washes in HBSS. The lymphocyte subpopulations were resuspended in Dulbecco's media supplemented with 20% calf serum and labeled with sodium chromate ^{51}Cr (New England Nuclear, Boston, Massachusetts) for 1 hr at 37°C (100 μCi/10^8 cells). The labeled lymphocytes were washed three times in HBSS, resuspended in HBSS, and injected intravenously into 6- to 8-week-old AKR mice (4 to 5 mice/lymphocyte subpopulation) at a concentration of 10^7 labeled lymphocytes/mouse. The mice were sacrificed 24 hr later and the percentage of cell-associated radioactivity localizing in the thymus, spleen, lymph nodes, and liver of syngeneic recipients was determined by counting individual lymphoid organs in a gamma counter. The method of Zatz and Lance (28) was employed to estimate the total lymph node compartment.

RESULTS

Groups (25 to 30 mice/group) of 7- to 8-month-old AKR mice, without any overt signs of lymphoma (splenomegaly, lymphadenopathy, thymic enlargement), and 6- to 8-week-old preleukemic AKR mice were administered 7 intraperitoneal injections of thymosin or control spleen extract (50 μg/injection) at 48-hr intervals. The treatment regimen and assay sequence are shown in Table 1. In addition to the 7 injections, mice employed in the splenic IgG PFC assay and the lymphocyte migration studies received additional injections on day 18 and on days 18 and 21, respectively. These data represent four replicate experiments using this regimen.

TABLE 1. Treatment regimen and assay sequence

Dose and route	Treatment (day)	Assay sequence (days)
Dose: 50 μg	0	
Thymosin fraction	2	
5 or control	4	
Spleen extract	6	
Fraction 5	8	
	10	
Route: intraperitoneal	12	13 mitogen studies
		14 SRBC immunization
		16 mitogens harvested
	18[a]	18 splenic IgM PFC response
	21	21 splenic IgG PFC response
		22 lymphocyte migration studies
		23 percent localization — lymphocyte migration studies

[a] Young and aged AKR mice employed in the IgG PFC determinations received one additional injection on day 18, and those used in the lymphocyte migration studies received two on days 18 and 21.

Mitogen Studies

Thymus and spleen cells from 6- to 8-week-old preleukemic AKR mice chronically treated with thymosin exhibited approximately a twofold decrease in responsiveness to Con A (Table 2). As shown in Table 2, the opposite effect was noted in lymph node cells from the thymosin-treated mice, with a stimulation index in response to Con A approximately seven times that observed in the control extract-treated group. The only notable changes in the PHA stimulation index was also seen in lymph node lymphocytes from thymosin-treated young AKR mice. It should be noted that an increase in the spontaneous incorporation of ^{3}H-thymidine was consistently observed in spleen cells from both the thymosin-treated young and aged animals. The data in Table 3 show that the pattern of Con A responsiveness of lymphocytes from the thymuses, spleens, and lymph nodes of thymosin-treated aged AKR

TABLE 2. Mitogen responsiveness in young AKR mice following chronic thymosin treatment

Treatment[a]	Organ tested	Cell controls (cpm)	Stimulation index[b]	
			Con A	PHA
Thymosin	Thymus	336 ± 83[c]	2.79 ± 0.77	0.57 ± 0.09
Control extract	Thymus	223 ± 51	8.87 ± 1.00	1.82 ± 0.23
Thymosin	Spleen	1,338 ± 78	7.98 ± 0.48	1.50 ± 0.18
Control extract	Spleen	302 ± 48.5	18.07 ± 1.04	1.52 ± 0.11
Thymosin	Nodes	121 ± 9	116.00 ± 5.28	5.29 ± 0.49
Control extract	Nodes	178 ± 44	15.61 ± 4.36	3.48 ± 0.62

[a] Six- to eight-week-old AKR mice received thymosin or control spleen extract (50 μg/injection).

[b] Ratio of mitogen-stimulated cells/unstimulated control cells.

[c] Standard error of the mean.

mice was essentially the same as that seen in young AKR mice. Thymosin treatment had no appreciable effect (slight decrease in thymus cells) on the Con A stimulation index of splenic lymphocytes from aged mice, but as noted in the young mice a significant increase in Con A reactivity occurred in the lymph node lymphocytes (approximately a fourfold increase). The PHA reactivity of splenic, thymic, or lymph node lymphocytes from thymosin- or control extract-treated aged AKR mice did not differ significantly. Although Con A responses were generally quantitatively higher in young mice, with the exception of thymus cells from thymosin-treated aged animals, the PHA stimulation index was greater in the aged mice in all test groups.

IgM and IgG PFC Responses

As shown in Table 4, aged thymosin-treated AKR mice exhibited a marked increase in the total number of splenic IgM and IgG plaque-forming cells/10^6 nucleated spleen cells. The most significant increase was noted in the

TABLE 3. Mitogen responsiveness in aged AKR mice following chronic thymosin treatment

Treatment[a]	Organ tested	Cell controls (cpm)	Stimulation index[b]	
			Con A	PHA
Thymosin	Thymus	441 + 79[c]	5.64 + 0.78	1.47 + 0.16
Control extract	Thymus	157 + 34	7.69 + 0.06	3.43 + 0.37
Thymosin	Spleen	759 + 50	6.66 + 0.35	1.67 + 0.19
Control extract	Spleen	876 + 126	5.65 + 0.35	1.85 + 0.26
Thymosin	Nodes	144 + 33	98.62 + 5.06	6.64 + 0.67
Control extract	Nodes	257 + 22	23.94 + 1.38	6.72 + 0.28

[a] Seven- to eight-month-old AKR mice without detectable lymphoma received thymosin or control spleen extract (50 µg/injection).

[b] Ratio of mitogen-stimulated cells/unstimulated control cells.

[c] Standard error of the mean.

number of IgM PFC present in the spleens of aged AKR mice following chronic thymosin treatment (3.3 times control extract-treated group). The opposite effect was seen in the young animals in which chronic thymosin treatment resulted in a moderate decrease in both the splenic IgM and IgG response. This was most notable in the decreased number of IgM splenic plaques.

Lymphocyte Migration Studies

The migration patterns of thymus, spleen, and lymph node lymphocytes from both thymosin- and control extract-treated aged and young AKR mice were determined. The "homing" patterns of these lymphoid subpopulations did not change in young AKR mice following thymosin administration (Table 5). A slight decrease in the localization of labeled lymphoid cell subpopulations from thymosin-treated young mice was observed in the spleens and lymph nodes of syngeneic recipients. The percent localization of labeled lymph node cells from young thymosin- and control extract-treated animals in recipient lymph nodes was generally greater than previously reported

TABLE 4. IgM and IgG response of spleen cells from young and aged
AKR mice following chronic thymosin treatment

Treatment [a]	PFC/10^6 nucleated spleen cells [b]	
	IgM	IgG
6 to 8-week-old Mice		
Thymosin	93.6 $\pm$ 7.2[c]	62.9 $\pm$ 6.3
Control extract	154.3 $\pm$ 12.2	76.0 $\pm$ 7.0
7 to 8-month-old Mice		
Thymosin	309.6 $\pm$ 6.1	133.3 $\pm$ 15.0
Control extract	92.6 $\pm$ 2.8	108 $\pm$ 2.89

[a] Following thymosin or control extract treatment mice were challenged with 0.5 ml of a 25% suspension of SRBC.

[b] Standard plaque assays were performed 4 days postinjection of SRBC for IgM plaques, 7 days for IgG plaques.

[c] Standard error of the mean.

values. This may be a function of the number and types of nodes removed in estimating the total lymph node compartment. As shown in Table 6, chronic thymosin treatment resulted in an increase in the percent of thymus cells from thymosin-treated aged AKR mice localizing in recipient spleen and node tissues. However, the most notable increase was seen in the spleen and lymph node localization of ^{51}Cr-labeled lymph node cells derived from thymosin-treated aged AKR mice. The percent localization in the spleen of lymph node cells from the thymosin-treated aged animals increased from 9.1% to 13.3%, while the percent of lymph node-seeking cells was 25.42% as compared with 14.2% localization of lymph node cells from the control extract-treated group (Table 6).

TABLE 5. Migration patterns of ^{51}Cr-labeled lymphocytes from young AKR mice following chronic thymosin treatment

Cell source	Treatment	Percent organ localization [a]				
		Thymus	Spleen	Lymph nodes	Liver
Thymus	Thymosin	0.06 ± 0.03 [b]	17.74 ± 0.82	7.32 ± 0.18	25.6 ± 1.4
Thymus	Control extract	0.06 ± 0.02	17.86 ± 0.09	8.93 ± 0.26	24.0 ± 1.4
Spleen	Thymosin	0.01 ± 0	5.00 ± 0	3.00 ± 0.80	21.9 ± 1.2
Spleen	Control extract	0.07 ± 0.02	7.36 ± 0.66	4.46 ± 0.55	28.6 ± 4.2
Lymph nodes	Thymosin	0.06 ± 0.01	10.90 ± 0	25.40 ± 1.90	16.7 ± 0.3
Lymph nodes	Control extract	0.13 ± 0.05	14.7 ± 1.04	28.80 ± 1.80	20.2 ± 4.4

[a] 10^7 ^{51}Cr-labeled lymphocyte subpopulations were injected intravenously into syngeneic recipients and the percent localization determined 24 hr later.

[b] Standard error of the mean.

TABLE 6. Migration patterns of ^{51}Cr-labeled lymphocytes from aged AKR mice following chronic thymosin treatment

Cell source	Treatment	Percent organ localization [a]			
		Thymus	Spleen	Lymph nodes	Liver
Thymus	Thymosin	0.06 ± 0.03 [b]	16.16 ± 0.90	9.32 ± 0.59	22.6 ± 1.3
Thymus	Control extract	0.09 ± 0.001	14.00 ± 1.20	7.40 ± 0.36	16.8 ± 3.5
Spleen	Thymosin	0.04 ± 0.005	6.00 ± 1.00	3.00 ± 0.35	24.3 ± 1.6
Spleen	Control extract	0.08 ± 0.02	7.70 ± 0.80	4.40 ± 0.20	33.1 ± 4.5
Lymph nodes	Thymosin	0.10 ± 0.03	13.30 ± 0.70	25.42 ± 1.60	19.6 ± 0.7
Lymph nodes	Control extract	0.04 ± 0.01	9.10 ± 0.30	14.20 ± 1.20	13.9 ± 0.02

[a] 10^7 ^{51}Cr-labeled lymphocyte subpopulations were injected intravenously into syngeneic recipients and the percent localization determined 24 hr later.

[b] Standard error of the mean.

DISCUSSION

The development of spontaneous lymphoid leukemia in AKR mice is preceded by a latent period of 6 to 12 months, with most mice dying between 8 and 9 months of age. It is well documented that leukemogenesis in these animals is vertically transmitted and related to chronic infection with Gross leukemia virus. Although the thymus is apparently the site of lymphocyte neoplastic transformation (19), neither the possible microenvironmental effects of the endocrine thymus nor the progressive immunologic dysfunction associated with aging in these animals is understood in relation to spontaneous leukemogenesis.

Metcalf (19) demonstrated that the development of neoplastic lymphoma cells in the AKR thymus is preceded (4 months) by depletion of small cortical lymphocytes and the development of lymphoid follicles in the medulla. It was suggested that one possible explanation for these pathologic changes in preleukemic mice was a result of derangement in the function of the thymic reticular epithelial cells. The epithelial stroma of the thymus has been suggested as the source of thymic hormones, and recent evidence indicates that the human thymic epithelial cells cultured in vitro may be the source of biologically active thymic hormones (29).

The apparent shift in immunologic homeostasis due to thymic changes in preleukemic AKR mice is reflected in progressive alterations in both humoral and cell-mediated responses. The response of spleen cells from AKR mice to sheep red blood cells declines with age, and minimal responsiveness is seen in leukemic animals (20, 21). A decrease in the reactivity of spleen cells to PHA with age and disease onset has been reported (23, 24), whereas thymus cells tend to acquire increased PHA responsiveness (23, 24). A progressive reduction in the number of Con A-responsive cells has been noted in both thymus and spleen with increasing age (23, 30). These changes in PHA and Con A reactivity were associated with a concomitant decline in the numbers of lymph node-seeking cells (24).

In the present studies, aged AKR mice demonstrated significant increases in all of the immunologic parameters measured, following chronic thymosin treatment. In contrast, only mitogen responsiveness was differentially enhanced in thymosin-treated young animals. As noted by other investigators (23, 24, 30), Con A reactivity of thymus and spleen cells from control mice was slightly higher in young animals, and the PHA response of thymus cells from aged control animals was increased over that noted in young mice.

The decrease in Con A reactivity observed in thymus and spleen cells from thymosin-treated young mice may be a result of differentiation of Con A reactive cells which localize in lymph nodes, or simply a result of a thymosin-mediated shutdown of the normal immunoregulatory processes which induce prethymic cells (presumably bone marrow-derived) to differentiate and enter the thymus. Although the former seems likely in view of the significant increase in the Con A stimulation index of lymph node cells from thymosin-treated young mice, no significant increases in the numbers of T-cell subpopulations localizing in nodes were observed in the young thymosin-treated animals. These results suggest a qualitative as opposed to a quantitative change in the T-cell subpopulations in the nodes of these young animals. This explanation (i.e., differentiation of thymic and/or splenic T-cells) seems more applicable to the increased Con A reactivity noted in lymph node cells from aged thymosin-treated animals, in view of the increased localization of lymph node-derived cells in recipient nodes and the associated decrease in the Con A responsiveness of spleen cells from this group. The quantitative dimunition of this response may reflect a decrease in the numbers of thymosin-reactive thymus and/or prethymic cells with increasing age.

Although other investigators have observed increases in numbers of IgM and IgG splenic PFC following thymosin treatment, the marked increase seen in aged thymosin-treated AKR mice has not been previously reported. The opposite effect recorded in the thymosin-treated young mice would seem to rule out B-cell stimulation as an appropriate explanation, and points to proliferation and/or differentiation of a helper T-cell subpopulation in the aged animals.

The major difference in the lymphocyte migration studies (i.e., increased "homing" of lymph node cells from aged thymosin-treated AKR mice to recipient nodes) between the thymosin-treated young and aged animals may simply reflect reduced thymosin levels in the latter group. Assuming "physiologic thymosin levels" in young mice, no significant effects, or possibly a decrease, in numbers of lymph node-seeking cells might be expected in the presence of increased thymosin concentrations. It cannot be precluded at this time that a thymosin-reactive lymph node population of cells exist in aged and/or young animals or that thymosin induces the differentiation of lymphoid cells from the bone marrow, spleen, and/or thymus in both groups of animals. However, the data show that aged AKR mice are more thymosin-reactive than the preleukemic animals.

It is not possible at this time to offer a comprehensive explanation for the differential effects of thymosin observed in young and aged AKR mice. However, Proffitt et al. (31) have recently shown that thymocytes which carry murine leukemia viruses are reactive against normal syngeneic cells. This pattern of "autoreactivity" is postulated to exist in both NZB and AKR mice, and the continued proliferation of these cells is thought to result in lymphoproliferative disease. These observations are of interest in that "suppression" in aged AKR mice may be directed toward normal cells. These cells may be triggered to proliferate and/or differentiate in the presence of elevated thymosin levels.

Also to be considered is the recent report by Cantor and Boyse (32) that the Ly alloantigens are differentially expressed on cells undergoing thymus-dependent differentiation. Enrichment of a T-cell population for Ly.1+ cells results in a subpopulation capable of helper but not killer function. T-cell mediated killing appears to involve two different T-cell subpopulations and is maximum when the preparations are enriched for Ly2.3+ cells. Thus, these authors conclude that T-cell commitment is a differentiative process which takes place before antigen encounter.

These data reflect the complex nature of the T-cell differentiation process. Thymosin may act on prethymic, thymic, and peripheral thymus-derived lymphocytes. The mechanism of thymosin-lymphoid cell interactions must be elucidated if we are to understand the role of thymic hormones on T-cell subpopulations and ultimately on T-cell differentiation.

The experiments presented and additional unpublished data indicate that thymosin differentially modulates the immune response in preleukemic and more markedly in aged (without overt disease) AKR mice. It is anticipated that the experiments reported here will provide data which will allow for a better understanding of normal immunoregulatory processes and how they are altered in the neoplastic state. These types of studies may ultimately provide a sound basis for thymosin therapy of neoplastic disease via manipulation of the host's immune mechanism.

SUMMARY

Bovine thymosin fraction 5 or a control spleen extract fraction 5 were administered to 6- to 8-week-old and 7- to 8-month-old AKR mice. Mice received 7 to 9 injections of thymosin or control extract and were subsequently assayed for responsiveness to Con A and PHA, numbers of splenic IgM and IgG PFC, and lymphocyte migration patterns. Preleukemic thymosin-treated AKR mice demonstrated a moderate increase in Con A reactivity in thymic- and splenic-derived lymphocytes, and a sevenfold increase in lymph nodes lymphocytes. PHA responsiveness was also increased in lymph node cells from this group. A fourfold increase in Con A reactivity of lymph node cells from thymosin-treated aged mice was noted. The numbers of splenic IgM and IgG PFC were significantly increased in thymosin-treated aged AKR mice, whereas a decrease was seen in young mice. The percent of ^{51}Cr-labeled lymph node cells from thymosin-treated aged mice localizing in the spleens and nodes of recipients was significantly increased over that in spleen extract-treated animals. Thymosin produced no marked changes in the "homing" patterns of lymphocytes from young thymosin-treated animals. The increase in Con A reactive cells in both young and aged AKR mice probably represents a thymosin-reactive subpopulation of thymocytes. Reduced thymosin levels and/or thymosin-mediated differentiation of suppressor cells in aged animals are postulated as the mechanism(s) responsible for the significant increase in immune competence observed in this group.

ACKNOWLEDGMENTS

This research was supported in part by grant 4 S01 RR05723-04 from the National Institutes of Health.

The authors wish to express their gratitude to Karen Huston for her expert assistance in the preparation of this manuscript, and to Gregory Stelzer for his excellent technical assistance.

REFERENCES

1. Komuro, K., and Boyse, E. A. (1973): Induction of T-lymphocytes from precursor cells in vitro by a product of the thymus. J. Exp. Med., 138:479-482.

2. Goldstein, A. L., Guha, A., Howe, M. L., and White, A. (1971): Ontogenesis of cell-mediated immunity in murine thymocytes and spleen cells and its acceleration by thymosin, a thymic hormone. J. Immunol., 106:773-780.

3. Raff, M. C., and Cantor, H. (1971): Subpopulations of thymus cells and thymus-derived lymphocytes. In: Progress in Immunology, edited by B. Amos, p. 83. Academic Press, New York.

4. Goldstein, A. L., Slater, F. D., and White, A. (1966): A preparation, assay, and partial purification of a thymic lymphocytopoietic factor (thymosin). Proc. Natl. Acad. Sci. (U.S.A.), 56:1010-1017.

5. Goldstein, A. L., Guha, A., Zatz, M. M., Hardy, M. A., and White, A. (1972): Purification and biologic activity of thymosin, a hormone of the thymosin gland. Proc. Natl. Acad. Sci. (U.S.A.), 69:1800-1803.

6. Komuro, K., and Boyse, E. A. (1973): In vitro demonstration of thymic hormone in the mouse by conversion of precursor cells into lymphocytes. Lancet, 1:740-743.

7. Miller, H. C., Schmiege, S. K., and Rule, A. (1973): Production of functional T-cells after treatment of bone marrow with thymic factor. J. Immunol., 111:1005-1009.

8. Tehila, U., and Tranin, N. (1975): Increased reactivity of responding cells in the mixed lymphocyte reaction by a thymic humoral factor. Eur. J. Immunol., 5:85-88.

9. Goldstein, A. L., Asanuma, Y., Battisto, J. R., Hardy, M., Quint, J., and White, A. (1970): Influence of thymosin on cell-mediated and humoral immune response in normal and immunologically deficient mice. J. Immunol., 104:359-366.

10. Kook, A. I., and Tranin, N. (1975): Intracellular events involved in the induction of immune competence in lymphoid cells by a thymus humoral factor. J. Immunol., 114:151-157.

11. Tranin, N., Carnaud, C., and Ilfeld, D. (1973): Inhibition of in vitro autosensitization by a thymic humoral factor. Nature (New Biol.), 245:253-255.

12. Dardenne, M., and Bach, J. F. (1973): Studies on thymus products. I. Modification of rosette-forming cells by thymic extracts. Determination of the target RFC subpopulation. Immunology, 25:343-352.

13. Dauphinee, M. J., Talal, N., Goldstein, A. L., and White, A. (1974): Thymosin corrects abnormal DNA synthetic response of NZB mouse thymocytes. Proc. Natl. Acad. Sci. (U.S.A.), 71:2637-2641.

14. Wara, D. W., Goldstein, A. L., Doyle, N. E., and Ammann, A. J. (1975): Thymosin activity in patients with cellular immunodeficiency. N. Engl. J. Med., 292:70-74.

15. Goldstein, A. L., Thurman, G. B., Cohen, G. H., and Hooper, J. A. (1975): Thymosin: Chemistry, biology, and clinical applications. In: Biological Activity of Thymic Hormones, pp. 19-21. Kouyker Scientific Publications, Rotterdam.

16. Khaw, B., and Rule, A. H. (1973): Immunotherapy of the Dunning leukemia with thymic extracts. Br. J. Cancer, 28:288-292.

17. Barker, A. D., and Moore, V. S. (1975): Immunotherapeutic effects of thymosin in first-transplant AKR leukemias. (In Preparation.)

18. Gross, L. (1951): Spontaneous leukemia developing in C3H mice following inoculation in infancy with AK leukemic extracts or AK embryos. Proc. Soc. Exp. Biol. Med., 76:27-32.

19. Metcalf, D. (1966): Histologic and transplantation studies on preleukemic thymus of the AKR mouse. J. Natl. Cancer Inst., 37:425-442.

20. Barker, A. D., Rheins, M. S., and St. Pierre, R. L. (1973): The effect of rabbit anti-mouse brain associated serum on the immunologic responsiveness of AKR mice. Cell Immunol., 7:85-91.

21. Hargis, B. J., and Malkiel, S. (1972): The immunocapacity of the AKR mouse. Cancer Res., 32:291-297.

22. Metcalf, D., and Moulds, R. (1967): Immune responses in preleukemic and leukemic AKR mice. Int. J. Cancer, 2:53-58.

23. Nagaya, H. (1973): Thymus function in spontaneous lymphoid leukemia. II. In vitro response of preleukemic and leukemic cells to mitogens. J. Immunol., 111:1052-1060.

24. Zatz, M. M., Goldstein, A. L., and White, A. (1973): Lymphocyte populations of AKR/J mice. I. Effect of aging on migration patterns, responses to PHA, and expression of theta antigen. J. Immunol., 111:1514-1525.

25. Oldstone, M. B., Aoki, T., and Dixon, F. J. (1972): The antibody response of mice to murine leukemia virus in spontaneous infection: Absence of classical immunological tolerance. Proc. Natl. Acad. Sci. (U.S.A.), 69:134-138.

26. Jerne, K., Nordin, A. A., and Henry, C. (1963): The agar plate technique for recognizing antibody producing cells. In: Cell-Bound Antibodies, edited by B. Amos and H. Koprowski, p. 109. Wistar Institute Press, Philadelphia.

27. Barker, A. D., Rheins, M. S., David, G. W., and Wilson, H. E. (1973): Immunologic responsiveness of young AKR mice to iodoacetate and iodoacetate-treated tumor cells. Immunol. Commun., 2:343-352.

28. Zatz, M. M., and Lance, E. M. (1970): The distribution of chromium 51-labeled lymphoid cells in the mouse. Cell. Immunol., 1:3-18.

29. Pyke, K. W., and Gelfand, E. W. (1974): Morphological and functional maturation of human thymic epithelium in culture. Nature, 251:421-423.

30. Zatz, M. M. (1975): Lymphocyte populations of AKR/J mice. III. Changes in the preleukemic state. J. Immunol., 115:1168-1170.

31. Proffitt, M. R., Hirsch, M. S., Gheridian, B., McKenzie, I. F., and Black, P. H. (1975): Immunological mechanisms in the pathogenesis of virus-induced murine leukemia. I. Autoreactivity. Int. J. Cancer, 15:221-229.

32. Cantor, H., and Boyse, E. A. (1975): Functional subclasses of T-lymphocytes bearing different Ly antigens. I. The generation of functionally distinct T-cell subclasses is a differentiative process independent of antigen. J. Exp. Med., 141:1376-1389.

Control of Neoplasia by Modulation of the Immune System, edited by M. A. Chirigos. Raven Press, New York   1977.

IN VITRO EFFECT OF THYMOSIN ON T-CELL LEVELS IN CANCER PATIENTS RECEIVING RADIATION THERAPY

*Daniel E. Kenady, *Claude Potvin, **Richard M. Simon, and *Paul B. Chretien

*Surgery Branch and **Biostatistics and Data Management Section, Division of Cancer Treatment, National Cancer Institute, National Institutes of Health, Bethesda, Maryland 20014

INTRODUCTION

Recently, thymosin, an extract of fetal calf thymus (10), improved cellular immune responses in children with thymic deficiencies (20).   The patients had low thymus-derived lymphocyte (T-cell) levels which increased after incubation in vitro with thymosin.   After treatment with thymosin, their circulating blood T-cell levels increased and did not increase further after incubation with thymosin.   These correlations suggest that if cancer patients have impaired cellular immunity that is secondary to deficiency of factors vital for maturation of T-cell precursors, thymosin may be similarly effective in increasing T-cell levels and other parameters of cellular immunity.

If the thymus gland is the principal source of factors that lead to maturation of T-cell precursors (1, 4, 12, 19), irradiation of the mediastinal region may cause a decline in cellular immune responses due to deleterious effects of irradiation on this function of the gland.   If this mechanism is a major contributor to the decline in cellular immunity during mediastinal irradiation (5, 6, 9, 17, 18), then T-cell levels in blood specimens from patients during mediastinal irradiation may increase after incubation with thymosin as occurred in children with thymic deficiencies.

This study was designed to explore these hypotheses by determining the comparative effects of thymosin in vitro on T-cell levels in cancer patients receiving radiotherapy via mediastinal, head and neck, and pelvic portals.

MATERIALS AND METHODS

Patients

Three hundred eighty-eight determinations were made in cancer patients receiving radiation therapy via head and neck, mediastinal, and pelvic portals (Table 1). All patients had clinically localized tumors that were encompassed by the radiation portal. The head and neck cancers were squamous carcinomas. The mediastinal cancers were localized, inoperable bronchogenic and esophageal carcinomas. The bronchogenic cancers were squamous, adeno-, oat cell, and undifferentiated carcinomas. Esophageal cancers were all squamous carcinomas. The pelvic cancers consisted of squamous carcinomas of the cervix; adenocarcinomas of the colon, rectum, uterus, prostate, and ovary; transitional cell carcinomas of the bladder; and testicular carcinomas. The mean age of all irradiated patients was 55, with a range of 18 to 85 years.

Concurrently, 74 patients with head and neck, mediastinal, or pelvic malignancies were studied prior to therapy. These control groups were similar to irradiated patients in tumor histology, clinical stage, sex, and race. Their mean age was 58, with a range of 30 to 75.

Normals

Two hundred seventy-seven healthy volunteers were also studied concurrently. Sixty percent were male and 85% were Caucasian. Their mean age was 42, with a range of 18 to 85. Volunteers with a history of malignancy, systemic disease, or recent viral infections were excluded.

Spontaneous Lymphocyte Rosette Assay (T-Cell Assay)

Peripheral blood thymus-derived lymphocytes (T-cells) were quantitated by the formation of spontaneous rosettes when mixed with sheep erythrocytes by a technique previously described (15). Triplicate samples were prepared for T-cell determination and three additional samples were prepared in an identical fashion with the addition to each tube of 0.1 ml of phosphate-buffered saline containing 100 μg of thymosin fraction 5 (11) (provided by Dr. Allan Goldstein and Hoffmann-LaRoche Laboratories) prior to incubation. The tubes were coded similarly, so as to prevent identification of the blood donor or of the tubes containing thymosin by the person performing the T-cell determinations.

The effect of thymosin was determined by subtracting the mean of the triplicate samples without thymosin from the mean of the triplicate samples with thymosin.

TABLE 1. Distribution of determinations in the study for each radiation portal and cumulative radiation dose

Cumulative radiation dose (rads)	Portal		
	Head and neck	Mediastinal	Pelvic
0	[22]	[22]	[30]
< 1,000	21[a] (17%)	23 (15%)	20 (17%)
1,000-2,000	20 (17%)	23 (15%)	18 (16%)
2,000-3,000	23 (19%)	32 (21%)	20 (17%)
3,000-4,000	21 (17%)	30 (20%)	19 (17%)
4,000-5,000	20 (17%)	28 (18%)	24 (31%)
5,000-6,000	15 (13%)	17 (11%)	14 (12%)
Totals[b]	120	153	115

[☑] = untreated patients.

(☑) = percent of the total number of determinations for each portal during radiation therapy.

[a] = number of patients studied who had received the cumulative radiation dose given.

[b] = total numbers of determinations during radiation therapy. Some patients were studied at more than one treatment interval during therapy.

Statistical Methods

Comparisons of parameters among groups of individuals were performed using Student's t-test. All p values correspond to two-tailed statistical tests.

RESULTS

Total Leukocyte Counts

The mean total leukocyte count in normals was 5,300. The mean leukocyte count in each group of untreated patients was significantly higher than in normals ($p < 0.005$), and also higher than the mean count in each respective patient group during radiotherapy (head and neck, $p < 0.025$; mediastinal and pelvic, $p < 0.001$) (Table 2).

TABLE 2. Peripheral blood leukocyte and lymphocyte determinations in the populations studied

	N	Leukocytes/mm³ Mean	SEM[a]	Percent lymphocytes Mean	SEM	Total lymphocytes/mm³ Mean	SEM	Percent T-cells Mean	SEM	Total T-cells/mm³ Mean	SEM	ΔT[b] Mean	SEM
Normals	277	5,300	81	36.7	0.5	1,912	35	68.4	0.5	1,301	26	1.3	0.5
Untreated cancer patients													
Head and neck	22	6,610	398	30.1	1.8	1,956	155	60.6	3.0	1,222	129	4.4	1.7
Mediastinal	22	7,110	394	26.2	1.6	1,780	116	62.0	2.0	1,115	86	1.9	1.7
Pelvic	30	6,440	280	31.6	2.1	1,945	124	62.9	1.7	1,243	95	4.2	1.4
Cancer patients during radiation therapy													
Head and neck	120	5,610	155	25.6	0.9	1,374	55	59.2	1.0	821	37	0.7	0.8
Mediastinal	153	5,580	148	16.6	0.7	886	41	55.2	1.2	499	26	3.1	0.8
Pelvic	115	4,910	153	19.3	0.8	957	56	55.7	1.3	551	36	-0.1	1.0

[a] Standard error of the mean.

[b] ΔT = Percent T-cell level after incubation with thymosin minus initial percent T-cell level.

Lymphocyte Levels

The mean percent lymphocyte level in normals (36.7) was higher than in each untreated patient group ($p < 0.005$ to 0.001) and each group during radiotherapy ($p < 0.001$). The mean level in each group during radiotherapy was also lower than in each respective untreated patient group (head and neck, $p < 0.05$; mediastinal and pelvic, $p < 0.001$). The mean total lymphocytes/ per cubic millimeter in normals and untreated patients did not differ. However, the mean levels in patients during radiotherapy were lower than in both normals and untreated patients ($p < 0.001$). The levels in patients during mediastinal and pelvic irradiation were also lower than in patients with head and neck irradiation ($p < 0.001$) and were similar to each other (Table 2).

T-Cell Levels

The mean percent T-cell level in normals (68.4) was higher than in each untreated group ($p < 0.025$ to 0.005) and in each group during radiotherapy ($p < 0.001$). The mean percent T-cell level in patients with head and neck irradiation did not differ from that in their untreated counterparts. However, the levels in patients with mediastinal and pelvic carcinomas during irradiation were lower than in their respective untreated counterparts ($p < 0.01$ and $p < 0.005$, respectively) and did not differ from each other. Among untreated patients, only in those with mediastinal malignancies was the mean total T-cells per cubic millimeter lower than in normals ($p < 0.05$). During radiation therapy, the mean total T-cell level in each group was lower than in normals ($p < 0.001$) and also lower than in each corresponding untreated group ($p < 0.001$). Total T-cell levels in patients during mediastinal and pelvic irradiation were also significantly lower than in patients with head and neck irradiation ($p < 0.001$) and were similar to each other (Table 2).

Effect of Thymosin on T-Cell Levels

After incubation with thymosin, the mean T-cell level in normals increased significantly ($p < 0.005$). In untreated patients with head and neck and pelvic malignancies the levels also increased significantly ($p < 0.01$ and < 0.005, respectively). These increases did not differ from the increase in normals. In untreated patients with mediastinal malignancies, however, the increase was not significant. Mean T-cell levels in patients with head and neck and pelvic malignancies during irradiation did not change significantly after incubation with thymosin, and in patients with pelvic malignancies the change was less than in untreated patients ($p < 0.05$). However, in patients with mediastinal malignancies during irradiation the mean level increased ($p < 0.001$), and the increase was greater than in normals ($p < 0.05$) (Table 2).

These results show that T-cell levels of patients with head and neck malignancies during irradiation did not differ significantly from untreated patients, and after incubation with thymosin, the mean levels did not change significantly; but T-cell levels in patients with mediastinal and pelvic malignancies during radiation therapy were significantly lower than in their untreated counterparts and patients with head and neck malignancies during radiation therapy, and did not differ from each other. However, after incubation with thymosin, the levels in patients with mediastinal malignancies increased by a greater increment than in normals, whereas the levels in patients with pelvic malignancies did not change significantly. The change in patients with pelvic malignancies during radiation therapy was significantly less than in comparable untreated patients.

DISCUSSION

The demonstrations that transplants of thymus gland (2) and thymosin (20), an extract of the thymus gland, restore cellular immunity in children with thymic deficiencies support previous experimental studies which demonstrate that the factors elaborated by the thymus are essential for development and maintenance of normal cellular immune competence (3, 13, 14). Evidence that thymus extracts restore cellular immunity after lethal irradiation in experimental animals (7, 8) may have clinical relevance to the decreases in cellular immunity in patients during radiation therapy. If so, the observation in patients with thymic deficiency who were treated with thymosin that the T-cell levels increased spontaneously after incubation with thymosin before treatment, and after treatment no longer increased after incubation with thymosin, appears to provide a method for determining if the decrease in cellular immunity in patients receiving mediastinal irradiation may be due to a deleterious effect of irradiation on functions of the thymus gland that maintain cellular immune competence.

The correlations between the in vitro and in vivo effect of thymosin in the patients with thymic deficiency treated with thymosin suggest that in patients with head and neck and pelvic malignancies, the significantly lower mean responses to thymosin of patients during radiation therapy may be due to a diminution in the blood levels of T-cell precursors. Evidence has been presented which suggests that the increase in T-cell levels after in vitro incubation with thymosin is due to a conversion of a subpopulation of lymphocytes which do not exhibit rosette-forming capabilities to one that forms spontaneous rosettes with sheep erythrocytes (T-cells) (16). A decrease in thymosin-responsive cells in these two patient groups could be explained by a deleterious effect of radiation therapy on these cells. Sites of this effect that can be postulated are the circulating blood and bone marrow. In view of the limited area of bone marrow included in head and neck radiation portals, irradiation of the cells in the circulating blood is more plausible as the cause of the diminution of these cells in patients with head and neck carcinomas. That the principal site of the effect on precursors is not the circulating blood in patients during pelvic irradiation is evidenced by the greater responses to thymosin in patients during irradiation for mediastinal malignancies, in whom the most extensive irradiation of the circulating blood occurs.

In patients with mediastinal malignancies, the unique finding of an increase in T-cells after incubation with thymosin in patients during radiation therapy that exceeded the increase in normals suggests a marked increase in T-cell precursors in the circulating blood. This can best be explained by a suppression of functions of the thymus gland essential for the maturation of T-cell precursors by a direct effect of irradiation on the gland. Also, irradiation of T-cells in the circulating blood and thoracic duct would account for the decrease in the circulating levels of T-cells that was similar to the decrease in patients during pelvic irradiation. However, a major conclusion that derives from these data is that although the T-cell levels in patients during mediastinal irradiation and patients during pelvic irradiation are decreased similarly, the greater increase in T-cell levels after thymosin in patients during mediastinal irradiation delineates a qualitative difference in the nonrosetting lymphocytes in these two patient groups. Thus, in patients during irradiation for pelvic malignancies, T-cell levels do not increase after thymosin because of low levels of circulating T-cell precursors, best explained by irradiation of the pelvic bone marrow, but in patients during mediastinal irradiation the increase in T-cell levels after thymosin suggests a higher blood level of T-cell precursors, best explained by a radiation-induced diminution of a function of the thymus gland.

SUMMARY

Comparisons were made among the effects of thymosin in vitro on percent T-cells in blood specimens from patients receiving radiation therapy for head and neck, mediastinal, and pelvic malignancies. Untreated patients with these malignancies and normal adults were studied concurrently. In untreated patients, mean percent T-cells were less than in normals. During irradiation, levels in patients with head and neck malignancies did not differ from untreated patients; but in patients with mediastinal and pelvic malignancies, the levels were less than in their untreated counterparts and were similar to each other. T-cell levels after incubation of lymphocytes with thymosin increased by a similar increment in normals and in the untreated patients. During irradiation, the mean levels did not change significantly in patients with head and neck and pelvic malignancies, but in patients with mediastinal malignancies the levels increased more than in normals. The results can be explained by an increase in circulating thymosin-responsive lymphocytes during mediastinal irradiation due to suppression of thymic function, and a decrease in these cells during pelvic irradiation due to a deleterious effect on precursors in pelvic bone marrow.

REFERENCES

1. Aiuti, F., Schirrmacher, V., Ammirati, P., and Fiorilli, M. (1975): Effect of thymus factor on human precursor T lymphocytes. Clin. Exp. Immunol., 20:499-503.

2. Ammann, A. J., Wara, D. W., Salmon, S., and Perkins, H. (1973): Thymus transplantation: Permanent reconstitution of cellular immunity in a patient with sex-linked combined immunodeficiency. N. Engl. J. Med., 289:5-9.

3. Bach, J-F., Dardenne, M., and Davies, A. J. S. (1971): Early effect of adult thymectomy. Nature (New Biol.), 231:110-111.

4. Bach, J-F., Dardenne, M., Goldstein, A. L., Guha, A., and White, A. (1971): Appearance of T-cell markers in bone marrow rosette-forming cells after incubation with thymosin, a thymic hormone. Proc. Natl. Acad. Sci. (U.S.A.), 68:2734-2738.

5. Braeman, J., and Deeley, T. J. (1972): Immunological studies in irradiation of lung cancer. Ann. Clin. Res., 4:355-360.

6. Check, J. H., Damsker, J. I., Brady, L. W., and O'Neill, E. A. (1973): Effect of radiation therapy on mumps-delayed type hypersensitivity reaction in lymphoma and carcinoma patients. Cancer, 32:580-584.

7. Cross, A. M., Leuchar, S. E., and Miller, J. F. A. P. (1964): Studies on the recovery of the immune response in irradiated mice thymectomized in adult life. J. Exp. Med., 119:837-850.

8. Dauphinee, M. J., Talal, N., Goldstein, A. L., and White, A. (1974): Thymosin corrects the abnormal DNA synthetic response of NZB mouse thymocytes. Proc. Natl. Acad. Sci. U.S.A., 71:2637-2641.

9. Dellon, A. L., Potvin, C., and Chretien, P. B. (1975): Thymus-dependent lymphocyte levels during radiation therapy for bronchogenic and esophageal carcinoma: Correlations with clinical course in responders and nonresponders. Am. J. Roentgenol. Radium Ther. Nucl. Med., 123:500-511.

10. Goldstein, A. L., Slater, F. D., and White, A. (1966): Preparation, assay, and partial purification of a thymic lymphocytopoietic factor (thymosin). Proc. Natl. Acad. Sci. (U.S.A.), 56:1010-1017.

11. Hooper, J. A., McDaniel, M. C., Thurman, G. B., Cohen, G. H., Schulof, R. S., and Goldstein, A. L. (1975): Purification and properties of bovine thymosin. Ann. N.Y. Acad. Sci., 249:125-144.

12. Komuro, K., and Boyse, E. A. (1973): In-vitro demonstration of thymic hormone in the mouse by conversion of precursor cells into lymphocytes. Lancet, I:740-743.

13. Miller, J. F. A. P. (1961): Immunologic function of the thymus. Lancet, II:748-749.

14. Miller, J. F. A. P. (1965): Effect of thymectomy in adult mice in immunological responsiveness. Nature, 208:1337-1338.

15. Potvin, C., Tarpley, J. L., and Chretien, P. B. (1975): Thymus-derived lymphocytes in patients with solid malignancies. Clin. Immunol. Immunopathol., 3:476-481.

16. Scheinberg, M. A., Cathcart, E. S., and Goldstein, A. L. (1975): Thymosin-induced reduction of "null cells" in peripheral-blood lymphocytes of patients with systemic lupus erythematosus. Lancet, I:424-426.

17. Stratton, J. A., Byfield, P. E., Byfield, J. E., Small, R. C., Benfield, J., and Pilch, Y. (1975): A comparison of the acute effects of radiation therapy, including or excluding the thymus, on the lymphocyte subpopulations of cancer patients. J. Clin. Invest., 56:88-97.

18. Thomas, J. W., Coy, P., Lewis, H. S., and Yuen, A. (1971): Effect
     of therapeutic irradiation on lymphocyte transformation in lung cancer.
     Cancer, 27:1046-1050.
19. Vogel, J. E., Incefy, G. S., and Good, R. A. (1975): Differentiation
     of population of peripheral blood lymphocytes into cells bearing sheep
     erythrocyte receptors in vitro by human thymic extract. Proc. Natl.
     Acad. Sci. (U.S.A.), 72:1175-1178.
20. Wara, D. W., Goldstein, A. L., Doyle, N. E., and Ammann, A. J.
     (1975): Thymosin activity in patients with cellular immunodeficiency.
     N. Engl. J. Med., 292:70-74.

Control of Neoplasia by Modulation of the Immune System, edited by M. A. Chirigos. Raven Press, New York 1977.

IN VITRO AND IN VIVO EFFECT OF THYMOSIN VERSUS FETAL THYMUS TRANSPLANTATION ON CELLULAR FUNCTION IN PRIMARY IMMUNODEFICIENCY DISEASE

Arthur Ammann and Diane W. Wara

Department of Pediatrics, Immunology Section, and Pediatric Clinical
Research Center, University of California,
San Francisco, California 94117

INTRODUCTION

The importance of thymic humoral factors in the regulation of cell-mediated immunity first became apparent with the demonstration that a thymus transplanted in a cell-impermeable millipore chamber was capable of providing reconstitution of cellular immunity in neonatally thymectomized mice. Since these initial observations, numerous thymic hormones have been described and evaluated for their ability to reconstitute cell-mediated immunity or to interact with B-cells in providing a normal antibody response (1). Thymic factor is a substance first described by Bach and Dardenne (2), in the serum of adult mice, which is capable of producing enhanced antigen binding by mouse lymphocytes. This factor was shown to disappear from the serum following thymectomy. A similar factor was described in the serum of human patients (3). Thymopoietin (initially called thymin) was originally described in patients with myasthenia gravis (4). Subsequently, it was shown that thymopoietin had the capacity to differentiate bone marrow or spleen precursor cells into thymocytes with characteristic T-cell markers. A thymic humoral factor isolated from the thymus of mice or calves has been shown by Trainin et al. to restore the ability of mouse spleen cells obtained from neonatally thymectomized mice to react in a graft-versus-host assay (5).

A variety of other factors have been described. Hand et al. (6) described a lymphocyte-stimulating hormone (LSH) which could increase the lympho-cyte-polymorphonuclear leukocyte ratio in mice (7). Stimulation of IgG antibody response in vitro by a T-cell replacing factor (TRF) has been demonstrated by Schimpl and Wecker (8). This factor was produced by a mixture

315

of allogeneic mouse spleen, lymph node, and thymus cells and could functionally replace T-cells in a primary IgM antibody response to sheep red
blood cells in vitro. Other antibody-enhancing factors produced by thymus
cells have been studied by Okumura et al. (9), Ruben and Coons (10),
Sjöberg et al. (11), and Gorczynski et al. (12). These factors are all produced by T-cells and have in common the ability to enhance antibody formation.

The first convincing evidence of a thymic humoral substance in humans
was provided by Steele et al. (13). A 10-week-old female infant with cellular
immunodeficiency and hypoparathyroidism (DiGeorge syndrome) was transplanted with a fetal thymus in a millipore diffusion chamber. Six hours following transplantation an increase in the peripheral blood lymphocyte response to phytohemagglutinin was demonstrated. Although patients with this
disorder previously had been successfully transplanted with a fetal thymus,
it was not certain whether the effect was a result of cellular repopulation or
of a thymic factor.

Because of increasing evidence that the thymus elaborated potent humoral
factors which could affect cell-mediated immunity, we chose to evaluate a
variety of immunodeficient patients for potential treatment with a thymic
hormone and to compare the effect with fetal thymus transplantation. Our
studies utilized thymosin fraction 5, obtained from A. Goldstein, in an
in vitro T-cell rosette assay system. Thymosin was chosen because it had
been well studied and characterized. It had been shown in neonatally
thymectomized mice to decrease the incidence of wasting disease, to increase the development of the cell-mediated immune response, to increase
the ability to develop a normal graft-versus-host reaction, to increase the
ability to reject histoincompatible skin grafts, and to increase the number of
T-cells with T-cell-specific markers following in vitro incubation with mouse
spleen or bone marrow cells (14).

Thymus transplantation was accomplished utilizing 16 to 18-week gestational age thymus obtained from prostaglandin-induced abortuses. The
thymus was transplanted intraperitoneally.

IN VITRO LYMPHOCYTE STIMULATION WITH PHYTOHEMAGGLUTININ IN MICROCULTURE

Peripheral blood lymphocytes are isolated by Hypaque-Ficoll gradient for
stimulation in vitro by phytohemagglutin (PHA) (Burroughs-Wellcome). The
cell suspension is adjusted to 2×10^6 lymphocytes/ml using RPMI-1640
(15 mM HEPES buffer) with 15% human plasma. PHA is added in concentrations varying from 0.5 to 10.0 μg/ml of cell suspension. These cell suspensions, each containing 2×10^6 lymphocytes/ml, are immediately aliquoted
into microtiter plates: 0.2 ml of cell suspension per well. The microtiter
plates are incubated at 36°C for 96 hr in a 5% CO_2 incubator. ^{14}C-thymidine,
0.1 μCi, is added to each well and incubated for an additional 14 hr. DNA
is then precipitated, solubilized, and counted in a scintillation counter.
Normal in vitro lymphocyte stimulation with PHA in microculture is: resting
$\pm$ 1 SD equals 52 $\pm$ 15; maximum stimulated counts achieved at any of five

PHA concentrations utilized equals $5,600 \pm 1,640$. In our laboratory, any stimulated count greater than 2,020 is considered normal by this technique.

MIXED LYMPHOCYTE CULTURE

Peripheral blood lymphocytes are isolated by Hypaque-Ficoll gradient for stimulation in mixed lymphocyte culture (MLC). Lymphocytes are adjusted to a concentration of 1×10^6 cells/ml using RPMI-1640 (15 mM HEPES buffer) with 15% human plasma. Each patient's cells are stimulated by lymphocytes from a nonrelated adult control. Stimulating cells from both the patient and the control are treated with 3,000 rads. One million responding cells from the patient are incubated with 1×10^6 lymphocytes from the control in 2 ml of media at $37^\circ C$ in 5% CO_2 for 96 hr. One microcurie of ^{14}C-thymidine is then added to each cell suspension and the incubation is continued for an additional 18 hr. DNA is then precipitated, solubilized, and counted in a scintillation counter. The patient's lymphocyte resting state is determined by incubating the patient's untreated lymphocytes with his own lymphocytes following 3,000 rads of irradiation. Normal stimulated in vitro lymphocyte response in MLC $\pm$ 1 SD equals $5,000 + 1,500$ counts per minute.

PERCENT T-CELL ROSETTE FORMATION

Peripheral blood lymphocytes are isolated by Hypaque-Ficoll gradient and adjusted to 4×10^6 cells/ml Hanks Balanced Salt Solution (HBSS) supplemented with 10% sheep red blood cell absorbed fetal calf serum. Sheep red blood cells (GIBCO) are washed twice and adjusted to a 1% suspension in fetal calf serum supplemented HBSS. 0.25 ml of the lymphocyte suspension is incubated with 0.25 ml of the sheep red blood cell suspension at $37^\circ C$ for 5 min, centrifuged at 200 X 2 for 5 min, and then incubated at $4^\circ C$ for 18 hr. Cell suspensions are observed under phase microscopy and percentage of spontaneous rosette forming cells determined. A rosette-forming cell is defined as a lymphocyte with three or more adherent sheep red blood cells. Normal mean spontaneous rosette-forming cells $\pm$ 1 SD equals $73 \pm 7\%$. Greater than 59% spontaneous rosette-forming cells is considered normal by current methodology.

THYMUS TRANSPLANTATION

Thymus transplantation is performed as follows: Fetal thymus glands are obtained either from prostaglandin-induced abortions or by hysterotomy. Gestational age of the fetus is obtained by history and by using measurements of crown-rump and crown-heel lengths. The fetus is dissected under sterile conditions in a laminar flow hood. Incisions are made horizontally along the diaphragm and laterally along the thorax to form a triangle with the apex at the sternal notch. The flap is lifted and the entire thymus dissected and placed in RPMI 1640 (15 mM HEPES) culture media at ambient temperatures.

At no time does more than 6 hr elapse from the time of dissection to the time of implantation. The patients are premedicated with Demerol and Thorazine. Routine sterile procedures are used to prepare the site of implantation, which is in the midline of the abdomen half way between the symphysis and umbilicus. A number-14 "intracath" is utilized (Becton Dickinson, Rutherford, New Jersey, "Longdwell #14"). Prior to implantation the culture media is removed and the thymus placed in a small sterile Petri dish. Scissors are used to mince the tissue. The minced thymus is drawn into a 10-ml syringe with normal saline and attached to a three-way stopcock in the vertical position. This allows the minced pieces of thymus to settle to the bottom of the syringe. The entire amount is injected intraperitoneally with the exception of a small piece of tissue for HL-A typing and/or histology. A second syringe filled with normal saline is placed in the horizontal position on the three-way stopcock. This is used to flush into the empty syringe which contained the thymus. The normal saline in the vertical syringe is then flushed into the peritoneum. The flush is repeated three times and the "intracath" is then withdrawn. The site is covered with a sterile 4 X 4 gauze for 24 hr. Normal saline is used for injection of the thymus because one patient experienced signs of sterile peritonitis for 24 hr following a transplant when culture media was used.

THYMOSIN INCUBATION STUDIES

Bovine thymosin fraction 5, prepared by Dr. Allan Goldstein, is added to cell suspensions in concentrations varying from 50 to 500 µg/ml. After the addition of thymosin, the suspensions were incubated for 5 min at 37°C, centrifuged for 5 min at 200 X g, and then incubated for 18 hr at 4°C. Triplicate wet cell preparations are examined under phase microscopy. For each preparation, 200 lymphocytes are counted and the proportion binding three or more sheep erythrocytes determined (normal 56 $\pm$ 5%). Monocytes or polymorphonuclear cells forming rosettes are excluded.

THYMOSIN ADMINISTRATION

Following an initial test dose of thymosin (1 mg) given intradermally, thymosin (1 mg/kg given subcutaneously) is administered each day for 2 to 4 weeks. Subsequently, thymosin is given once each week. The following studies are performed at 3-month intervals: quantitative immunoglobulins, T-cell rosettes, lymphocytes response to mitogens and allogeneic cells, autoantibodies, BUN, creatinine, Na^+, K^+, SGOT, SGPT, alkaline phosphatase, Ca^+, total white blood cell count, and differential and hematocrit.

RESULTS

In vitro incubation of thymosin, in a concentration varying from 50 µg/ml to 500 µg/ml of cell suspension, dramatically increased the percent T-cell

TABLE 1. In vitro response of T-cell rosettes to thymosin

Immunodeficiency disorder	Initial % TCR	Final % TCR	% Increase[a]
Cellular I.D. with Abnormal I.G. synthesis	42	78	86
Cellular I.D. with Abnormal I.G. synthesis	32	79	147
Cellular I.D. with Abnormal I.G. synthesis	23	47	101
Cellular I.D. with Abnormal I.G. synthesis	10	53	430
Wiskott-Aldrich syndrome	38	49	29
Wiskott-Aldrich syndrome	52	78	50
Wiskott-Aldrich syndrome	51	66	29
Wiskott-Aldrich syndrome	38	38	0
Wiskott-Aldrich syndrome	21	34	62
Ataxia-telangiectasia	29	44	52
Di George syndrome	26	49	88
Di George syndrome[b]	41	45	10
SCID	6	9	50
SCID	4	8	50
SCID	7	8	14
SCID	2	4	50

[a] Percent increase felt not be significant unless greater than 50% in patients whose initial percent is greater than 20%.

[b] Patient had a graft-versus-host reaction at time of studies.

I.G. = immunoglobulin; I.D. = immunodeficiency; SCID = severe combined immunodeficiency disease; TCR = T-cell rosettes.

rosettes in vitro in certain patients with cellular immunodeficiency disorders (Table 1). The increase in percent T-cell rosettes had a dose-response relationship with the thymosin concentration in vitro (15, 16).

In those individuals who had depressed T-cell rosettes, the percent increase (percent increase = final percent minus initial percent divided by initial percent) ranged from 0 to 430%. Four patients with severe combined immunodeficiency disease who presumably lack a stem cell population had severely depressed T-cell rosettes which failed to respond significantly following in vitro thymosin incubation. These studies suggest that stem cells, which have not yet come under thymic influence, are necessary for thymosin affect. An alternative explanation is that cells which have come under minimal thymic influence can be expanded under the influence of a thymic hormone such as thymosin.

The most dramatic increase in T-cell rosette formation following thymosin incubation occurred in 4 patients with cellular immunodeficiency and immunoglobulin synthesis (Nezelof's syndrome). These patients, although severely immunodeficient, are felt to have stem cells but deficient thymic function and thus abnormal stem cell maturation in vivo. Percent increase of T-cell rosettes following thymosin incubation in this group of patients ranged from 86 to 430%.

Similar, but less dramatic results were obtained in patients with the Wiskott-Aldrich syndrome and ataxia-telangiectasia. Although the percent increase of T-cell rosettes was in a lower range than that observed in patients with cellular immunodeficiency with abnormal immunoglobulin synthesis, the baseline rosettes were in a more normal range. Incubation of depressed T-cell rosettes with thymosin did not increase T-cell rosettes to values above normal.

An interesting observation was made following the testing of 2 patients with DiGeorge syndrome. In one patient depressed T-cell rosettes responded to thymosin incubation with an 88% increase over baseline values. This patient did not receive any immunotherapy and, when followed over a 1-year period, spontaneously developed normal cell-mediated immunity. The patient had also received several blood transfusions prior to the time a diagnosis was made and did not experience a graft-versus-host reaction. The second patient did not have a significant increase in T-cell rosettes following thymosin incubation. The initial percent total rosettes were somewhat higher in this patient (41%), and the incubation was performed at a time when a graft-versus-host reaction was in progress. The patient had received whole blood transfusions for anemia before a diagnosis of DiGeorge syndrome was made. The failure of the T-cell rosettes in the patient to respond to thymosin incubation suggests that there may be two forms of DiGeorge syndrome. In one, a thymic remnant and a stem cell population are present, providing a population of lymphocytes capable of responding to thymosin. In the other, the defect is probably at a stem cell level, as indicated by lymphocyte unresponsiveness to in vitro thymosin incubation and by the presence of a graft-versus-host reaction following a blood transfusion.

Four patients were selected for treatment with thymosin therapy in vivo (Table 2). The selection was based on (a) the lack of a suitable histocompatible and/or mixed lymphocyte culture-identical donor for bone marrow transplantation, (b) the failure to respond to other therapeutic measures such as antibiotic treatment and transfer factor, and (c) the in vitro responsiveness of lymphocytes to incubation with thymosin. Three of the patients selected had cellular immunodeficiency with abnormal immunoglobulin synthesis and one patient had the Wiskott-Aldrich syndrome. The duration of therapy ranged from 18 months (case 1) to 1.5 months (case 4).

Table 3 summarizes pertinent immunologic data on the 4 patients treated prior to and following thymosin therapy. An effect on B-cell immunity was observed in case 1 (thymic hypoplasia with immunoglobulin synthesis) with a normalization of IgG values. IgM and IgA remained relatively unchanged. Despite the increased concentration of serum IgG, no active antibody synthesis following immunization could be demonstrated. T-cell rosettes

TABLE 2. Immunologic evaluation pre- and postthymosin therapy

	Prethymosin	Postthymosin
Case 1 (treatment 18 months)		
Immunoglobulins G	220	1,500
M	50	65
A	840	1,220
TCR %/absolute #	10/338	55/660
PHA (R/S) in cpm	222/2,443	493/12,400
MLC (R/S)	85/631	103/232
Case 2 (treatment 10 months)		
Immunoglobulins G	940	940
M	380	380
A	80	80
TCR	10/20	63/334
PHA	93/158	50/2,868
MLC	69/134	1,212/5,862
Case 3 (treatment 10 months)		
Immunoglobulins G	975	690
M	27	30
A	480	410
TCR	21/231	59/598
PHA	116/499	602/62,367
MLC	54/726	52/170
Case 4 (treatment 1.5 months)		
Immunoglobulins G	600	N.D.
M	250	
A	4	
TCR	52/1,040	71/1,420
PHA	473/8,116	351/6,178
MLC	384/3,729	410/1,547

Abbreviations: TCR = T-cell rosettes; PHA = phytohemagglutinin;
MLC = mixed lymphocyte culture; N.D. = not done; R/S = resting/stimulated;
cpm = counts per minute.

increased both in percent and absolute numbers. Delayed hypersensitivity
skin tests to mumps and candida antigens became positive. Although a
definite increase in in vitro lymphocyte response to PHA was observed, there
was no change in lymphocyte response to allogeneic cells.

TABLE 3. Comparison of thymosin and fetal thymus in various immunodeficiency disorders in vivo

Disorder	Thymosin	Fetal thymus
SCID	No effect on AMI or CMI	No effect on AMI Normal CMI
Di George syndrome	Normalization of CMI (1 case treated)	Normalization of AMI and CMI
Cellular immuno-deficiency with abnormal immunoglobulin synthesis	No effect on AMI (2/4 cases), increase in IgG (1 case) Partial reconstitution of CMI, TCR, PHA, or MLC	Variable effect on immuno-globulins, partial reconstitution of antibody response, complete response, complete reconstitituon of CMI (3/5)

Abbreviations: SCID = severe combined immunodeficiency disease; AMI = antibody-mediated immunity; CMI = cell-mediated immunity; TCR = T-cell rosettes; PHA = phytohemagglutinin; MLC = mixed lymphocyte culture.

No change in immunoglobulin values occurred in the second case (thymic hypoplasia with immunoglobulin synthesis). T-cell rosettes increased in percentage and absolute numbers. Delayed hypersensitivity skin test to mumps antigen became positive. A gradual increase in in vitro lymphocyte response to PHA occurred but remained subnormal. A normalization of lymphocyte response to allogeneic cells occurred. In this patient in vitro incubation of lymphocytes with thymosin prior to in vivo therapy had resulted in a normalization of responsiveness of both T-cell rosettes and lymphocyte response to allogeneic cells.

The third case, a patient with Wiskott-Aldrich syndrome, had no alteration in immunoglobulin values following thymosin therapy. The percent T-cell rosettes and the absolute numbers increased gradually. The response of peripheral blood lymphocytes to PHA became normal but the lymphocyte response to allogeneic cells remained unchanged.

The fourth patient was treated for a short duration (1.5 months). The patient had previously received four fetal thymus transplants in conjunction with transfer factor. This had resulted in normalization of cell-mediated immunity but was followed by gradual deterioration in function. The patient was therefore given a trial of thymosin therapy. No alteration in immunoglobulin levels or response of lymphocytes in vitro to PHA or allogeneic cells was observed during the treatment period. T-cell rosettes, which were moderately depressed prior to treatment, increased to normal.

The studies of antibody- and cell-mediated immunity in patients receiving thymosin therapy indicate that the effect on immunologic function is variable. Immunoglobulin values increased in only one patient and were not associated with active antibody synthesis. The in vitro lymphocyte response to PHA following treatment varied. Two of the 4 patients showed improvement, but normal responsiveness was obtained in only one. Only one patient showed an increased responsiveness to allogeneic cells with a normal value achieved.

Both percent and absolute T-cell rosettes increased following in vivo thymosin therapy in all 4 patients. Delayed hypersensitivity skin tests to recall antigens became positive in 2 patients.

The clinical response of the 4 patients varied following treatment. Case 1 improved clinically, with a diminution in the number of infections and improved growth and development. During the entire treatment course she has been admitted to the hospital only for routine evaluation and for a single episode of draining otitis media. Case 2 improved significantly, with a reduction in the number of respiratory infections. However, during the spring season she appeared to have an increase in allergic symptomatology. At this time it was not known whether thymosin therapy was related to the exacerbation of her allergies. Thymosin therapy was continued. During the fall, her allergic symptomatology again increased. Thymosin administration subcutaneously was associated with local swelling and urticaria. On two occasions it appeared that respiratory wheezing occurred transiently following the injections. It was felt that the patient might have developed an allergic response to thymosin, IgE activity against thymosin was demonstrated in vitro, and therapy was discontinued. Subsequently, the T-cell rosettes decreased to the previously observed abnormal values and the response of lymphocytes to PHA and allogeneic cells became markedly depressed. The third case (Wiskott-Aldrich) had significant clinical improvement following the initiation of thymosin therapy. Eczema which had been present in varying degrees improved. The patient had fewer episodes of recurrent herpes stomatitis, and when these occurred they were less severe than previously observed. The patient did not have any alteration in the number or severity of bleeding episodes related to thrombocytopenia. The fourth patient was not felt to have received treatment for a sufficient time period to evaluate any alteration in clinical status.

Figures 1 to 3 summarize the immunologic alterations which occurred following fetal thymus transplantation in 3 of 5 patients with a variety of cellular immunodeficiency disorders (17). Three of the patients had cellular immunodeficiency with abnormal immunoglobulin synthesis, one patient had ataxia telangiectasia, and one patient had the Wiskott-Aldrich syndrome.

Two of the 3 patients with cellular immunodeficiency and abnormal immunoglobulin synthesis responded to fetal thymus transplantation with normalization of all aspects of cell-mediated immunity (Figs. 1 and 2). Two of the patients demonstrated evidence of active antibody formation following immunization. One patient developed normal levels of immunoglobulin G and M but maintained absent serum IgA. One patient with ataxia-telangiectasia developed normal cell-mediated immunity following fetal thymus transplant (Fig. 3). Two of the patients, one with cellular immunodeficiency and abnormal

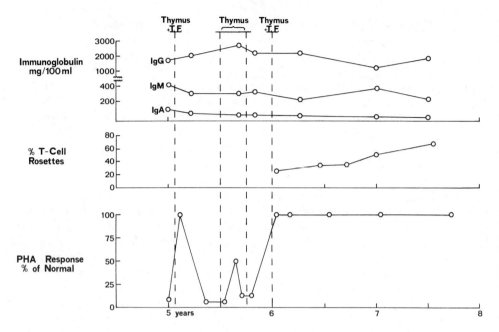

FIG. 1. Studies of antibody- and cell-mediated immunity in a patient with cellular immunodeficiency and abnormal immunoglobulin synthesis following transfer factor (T. F.) and fetal thymus transplantation.

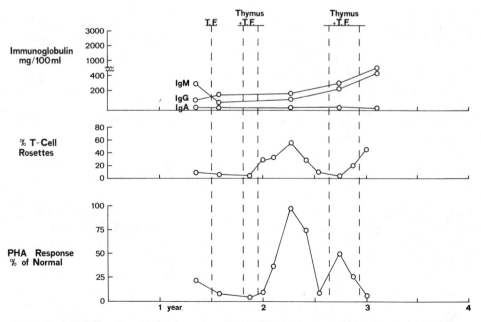

FIG. 2. Studies of antibody- and cell-mediated immunity in a patient with cellular immunodeficiency and abnormal immunoglobulin synthesis following transfer factor (T. F.) and fetal thymus transplantation.

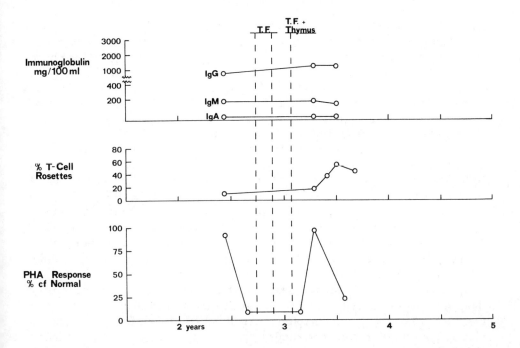

FIG. 3. Studies of antibody- and cell-mediated immunity in a patient with cellular ataxia-telangiectasia following transfer factor (T. F.) and fetal thymus transplantation.

immunoglobulin synthesis and the other with Wiskott-Aldrich syndrome, failed to demonstrate a significant increase in cell-mediated immunity following fetal thymus transplant.   The patient with the Wiskott-Aldrich syndrome expired prior to a time when the full effect of a fetal thymus transplant might have been observed.

The duration of reconstitution following fetal thymus transplantation varied from several months to as long as 2-1/2 years.   The explanation for the variable duration is not apparent and does not appear to be related to the age of the fetal thymus nor to the presence or absence of a strong response of the patient's lymphocytes to allogeneic cells.

In this group of patients there was no evidence of graft-versus-host reaction or subsequent chimerism following fetal thymus transplantation.   This is in contrast to patients with severe combined immunodeficiency disease who develop graft-versus-host reaction and cellular chimerism following the transplantation of fetal thymus glands (18).

DISCUSSION

Of the many thymic factors and thymic hormones described, thymosin appeared to us to be the most likely candidate for a study on the in vitro effect of a thymic hormone on cell-mediated immunity in immunodeficient patients. Thymosin has been shown to be effective in reconstituting deficient cell-mediated immunity secondary to thymectomy in the mouse. Reconstitution of lymphocyte responsiveness to mitogens and allogeneic cells had been demonstrated and restoration of graft-versus-host potential had been observed. Additional evidence for a direct effect of thymosin on immunocompetent cells was the demonstration of the appearance of thymic-specific antigens on precursor spleen and bone marrow cells in the mouse. The in vitro testing of thymosin in humans was limited by the lack of a suitable assay procedure. After considerable testing we observed that the T-cell rosette assay appeared to be a sensitive indicator of thymosin activity in vitro. This effect was felt to be specific because (a) material prepared in an identical manner to thymosin but obtained from liver and spleen did not have comparable effects, (b) other immunotherapeutic agents derived from lymphocytes such as transfer factor did not have comparable effects, (c) thymosin incubation with lymphocytes in vitro resulted in an increase in T-cell rosettes only in those disorders with evidence of defective precursor cells and not in immunodeficiency disorders associated with stem cell defects.

Utilizing the T-cell rosette assay system, a number of immunodeficiency disorders were evaluated. Thymosin had the most marked effect in those disorders associated with partial defects of cell-mediated immunity. No effect was observed in stem cell disorders such as severe combined immunodeficiency disease.

Utilizing the in vitro responsiveness of T-cell rosettes to thymosin, 4 patients were chosen for therapy. The most consistent alterations observed in the patients following therapy paralleled the observations made in in vitro studies. That is, patients who had the greatest response of T-cell rosettes in vitro also had the most significant response following treatment in vivo. Two of the 4 patients had some evidence of increased responsiveness of lymphocytes to phytohemagglutinin. One patient developed a normal mixed lymphocyte culture response.

One patient, who had been followed for 5 years with an abnormal immunoglobulin pattern, developed normalization of IgG after prolonged thymosin therapy. Although the IgG increased significantly in quantity, no evidence of active antibody synthesis was obtained following immunization.

The results of in vivo treatment of patients with immunodeficiency suggest that thymosin has a partial effect on reconstituting cell-mediated immunity. There is very little effect on antibody-mediated immunity. When these results are compared to those obtained following the use of fetal thymus transplantation in patients with similar immunodeficiency disorders, it is apparent that a more complete reconstitution of immunity is achieved by means of fetal thymus transplantation. This strongly suggests that thymosin may be one of several hormones elaborated by the thymus.

Thymosin may be useful in several areas in the field of immunodeficiency. First, the in vitro testing of cells from immunodeficient patients may result in a more accurate diagnosis. This is illustrated by the variable effect of thymosin in vitro in the 2 patients with DiGeorge syndrome. The patient who failed to show any response to in vitro thymosin expired with a severe graft-versus-host reaction following a blood transfusion. It is possible that a fetal thymus transplant might also have caused a fatal graft-versus-host reaction in this patient if this treatment had been given. Second, thymosin may provide a safe immunotherapeutic agent for the treatment of selected immunodeficiency disorders in vivo. If certain disorders, such as the DiGeorge syndrome, can be shown to respond to thymosin in vivo, then the risk of a fetal thymus transplant may be unnecessary. Third, thymosin may be useful in the selective reconstitution of depressed immunity in secondary immunodeficiency disorders. If thymosin has an effect on expanding depressed T-cell populations, then the use of thymosin in conjunction with a specific immunotherapeutic agent such as transfer factor might provide a rational approach in the treatment of both primary and secondary immunodeficiency disorders.

SUMMARY

Thymosin incubation in vitro increases T-cell rosettes in a dose-response relationship in primary immunodeficiency disorders. Thymic precursor cells appear to be necessary for this effect. No effect on T-cell rosettes was observed in patients with stem cell defects.

Treatment of immunodeficient patients with thymosin resulted in an increase in the percent of T-cell rosettes as well as the absolute numbers. The degree of increase closely paralleled that observed following in vitro testing. Thymosin does not appear to have as complete an effect on reconstitution of cell-mediated and antibody-mediated immunity as does fetal thymus transplantation in similar immunodeficiency disorders. It is postulated that thymosin is one of several thymic hormones elaborated by the thymus gland. The role of thymosin in the treatment of primary and secondary immunodeficiency disorders must await larger clinical trials.

REFERENCES

1. Trainin, N. (1974): Thymic hormones and the immune response. Physiol. Rev., 54:272.

2. Bach, J. F., and Dardenne, M. (1972): Thymus dependency of rosette-forming cells: Evidence for a circulating thymic hormone. Transplant. Proc., 4:345.

3. Bach, J. F., Papiernik, M., Levasseur, P., Dardenne, M., Barois, A., and Brigand, H. L. (1972): Evidence for a serum factor secreted by the human thymus. Lancet, 2:1056.

4. Basch, R. S., and Goldstein, G. (1975): Antigenic and functional evidence for the in vitro inductive activity of thymopoietin (thymin) thymocyte precursors. Ann. N.Y. Acad. Sci., 249:290.

5. Trainin, N., Small, M., and Globerson, A. J. (1969): Immunocompetence of spleen cells from neonatally thymectomized mice conferred in vitro by a syngeneic thymus extract. J. Exp. Med., 130:765.

6. Hand, T. P., Ceglowski, S., Damorongsak, D., and Friedman, H. J. (1970): Development of antibody-forming cells in neonatal mice: Stimulation and inhibition by calf thymus fractions. J. Immunol., 105:442.

7. Robey, G., Campbell, B. J., and Luckey, T. D. (1972): Isolation and characterization of a thymic factor. Infect. Immun., 6:682.

8. Schimpl, A., and Wecker, E. (1973): Stimulation of IgG antibody response in vitro by T cell replacing factor. J. Exp. Med., 137:547.

9. Okumura, K., Shinohara, N., and Kern, M. (1974): Differentiation of lymphoid cells: Enhancement of the induction of immunoglobulin reduction by thymus cells and a product secreted by thymus cells. J. Immunol., 113:2027.

10. Ruben, A. S., and Coons, A. H. (1972): Specific heterologous enhancement of immune responses. J. Exp. Med., 136:1501.

11. Sjöberg, O., Andersson, J., and Moller, G. (1972): Reconstitution of the antibody response in vitro of T cell deprived spleen cells by supernatants from spleen cell cultures. J. Immunol., 109:1379.

12. Gorczynski, R. M., Miller, R. G., and Phillips, R. A. (1973): Reconstitution of T cell depleted spleen cell populations by factors derived from T cells. III. Mechanism of action of T cell derived factors. J. Immunol., 111:900.

13. Steele, R. W., Limas, C., Thurman, G. B., Schuelein, M., Baur, H., and Bellanti, J. A. (1972): Familial thymic aplasia: Attempted reconstitution with fetal thymus in a millipore diffusion chamber. N. Engl. J. Med., 287:787.

14. Hooper, J. A., McDaniel, M. C., Thurman, G. B., Cohen, G. H., Schulof, R. S., and Goldstein, A. L. (1975): Purification and properties of bovine thymosin. Ann. N.Y. Acad. Sci., 249:125.

15. Wara, D., and Ammann, A. J. (1975): Activation of T cell rosettes in immunodeficient patients by thymosin. Ann. N.Y. Acad. Sci., 249:308.

16. Wara, D. W., Goldstein, A. L., Doyle, N. E., and Ammann, A. J. (1975): Thymosin activity in patients with cellular immunodeficiency. N. Engl. J. Med., 292:70.

17. Ammann, A. J., Wara, D., Salmon, S., and Perkins, H. (1973): Thymus transplantation. Permanent reconstitution of cellular immunity in a patient with sex-linked combined immunodeficiency. N. Engl. J. Med., 289:5.

18. Ammann, A. J., Wara, D. W., Salmon, S., Perkins, H. (1973): The in vitro and in vivo effect of thymosin versus fetal thymus transplantation on cellular function in primary immunodeficiency disease. N. Engl. Med. J., 289:5.

Control of Neoplasia by Modulation of the Immune System, edited by M. A. Chirigos. Raven Press, New York 1977.

IN VITRO AND IN VIVO STUDIES OF THYMOSIN ACTIVITY IN CANCER PATIENTS

Larry A. Schafer, Jordan U. Gutterman, Evan M. Hersh, Giora M. Mavligit, and *Allan L. Goldstein

Section of Immunology, Department of Developmental Therapeutics, M. D. Anderson Hospital and Tumor Institute, 6723 Bertner Avenue, Houston, Texas 77025, and
*Division of Biochemistry, University of Texas Medical Branch, Galveston, Texas 77550

INTRODUCTION

At some developmental stages in mammals, the thymus gland comprises up to 25% of the total lymphoid mass. It is interesting, therefore, that the importance of the thymus gland in the lymphoid system has been appreciated only in recent years. Investigators, pursuing findings associated with neonatal thymectomy and studies in children with congenital immunodeficiency syndromes (2-4), have established in the last 15 years that a normal functioning thymus gland is needed for the appearance and proper function of cell-mediated immunity (1,5,6). It has been determined that at least part of the activity of the normal thymus is endocrine, a conclusion supported by investigations of thymus tissue implanted in cell-impermeable chambers (7-9) and by studies of cell-free thymic extracts (1,10-13). Although the mass of the thymus gland "atrophies" with age due to disappearance of its lymphoid elements, the reticulo-endothelial components remain much longer. It is these cells which probably secrete thymic hormone(s) (14-15).

The hormone(s) has antitumor action in several animal models. Thymosin, the thymic extract used in our studies, partially restores cell-mediated immunity (CMI) in neonatally thymectomized animals and in congenitally athymic (nude) mice (16-17). It prolongs survival in neonatal CBA/Wh mice inoculated with Moloney sarcoma virus (MSV) (18). In inbred rats with Dunning leukemia (a disease of monocytes), thymosin protects 60% of affected animals (disease-free 1 year after onset of leukemia) as compared to 0% protection (mean survival 16 days) in rats not receiving thymosin (19).

Barker (20) has shown that thymosin may not only reduce Rauscher leukemia virus titer, but, based on the timing of giving thymosin, may enhance Rauscher leukemia cell proliferation.

A rationale exists for trials of thymosin in humans with malignancy, which can be summarized as follows:

1. Thymosin is active in several animal tumor models (18-21).

2. It has been effective on a long-term basis in some childhood immunodeficiency syndromes (21-24).

3. It is not toxic in animals (25), in spite of the administration of massive doses for prolonged periods, nor is it damaging to humans receiving protracted courses of thymosin (21, 22, 24-26).

4. Cancer prognosis often correlates directly with patients' immune status (27-29).

5. Additionally, improved survival and prolonged disease-free intervals occur when patients' immune status is augmented by immune manipulation with other agents (30-33).

Because the deficient tests of immunity associated with certain types of congenital immunoincompetence and with cancer parallel the immunodeficiency associated with thymic insufficiency, and because several congenital immunodeficiency syndromes and animal tumor models respond to thymosin, an in vitro and in vivo trial of thymosin administration was conducted, the results of which comprise this report. Thymosin, fraction 5, was studied in vitro in lymphocyte cultures, using cells from both normal subjects and cancer patients. Thymosin, fraction 5, was also given to patients with far advanced malignancy.

MATERIALS AND METHODS

The in vitro studies were performed using cells from 24 normal subjects and 47 cancer patients. Lymphocytes from these individuals were isolated from whole blood, and blastogenesis microcultures were set up according to standard methods (34-36). Particular attention was directed to results obtained with cultures of lymphocytes and thymosin alone, lymphocytes and allogeneic irradiated lymphocytes (mixed lymphocyte culture, or MLC) and lymphocytes and mitogens, especially phytohemagglutinin (PHA).

In Vitro Studies

First, in vitro studies were conducted to determine whether thymosin, in and of itself, affected ^{3}H-thymidine incorporation by normal human lymphocytes. To do this, thymosin was added alone, as the only foreign substance, to normal lymphocytes and their blastogenic response was assessed. The effects of thymosin on MLCs between normal donor lymphocytes were examined next. In each case, MLC response without thymosin was compared to MLC with thymosin.

Identical experimental conditions, using unstimulated lymphocytes from 47 patients with disseminated cancer, were examined next. As with normal donors, changes in ^{3}H-thymidine incorporation in the presence of thymosin alone and changes in MLC response with and without thymosin were emphasized.

In Vivo Investigations

Patients with histologically proven, disseminated malignancy and a known limited life expectancy were selected. They were immunodeficient[1] and were not candidates for, or recipients of, other immunotherapy. They received only thymosin, or, if other drugs were used, thymosin was given between cycles of chemotherapy. Patients selected had no history of beef product allergy. They did not react to an intradermal test dose of 0.01 mg of thymosin. Participating patients comprehended the experimental nature of the phase I trial and granted informed consent.

Daily doses of subcutaneous or intramuscular thymosin ranged from 1 mg/m^2 of body surface area to 60 mg/m^2. Although several patients received repeated courses of thymosin, only the first courses of each of the 32 treated patients are analyzed in this chapter. Of these 32 first courses, 94% were for 7 days and 6% were for more than 7 days. Each patient was skin-tested with dermatophytin (Derm), Candida, mumps, and streptokinase-streptodornase (SK-SD, or varidase); these four recall antigens are grouped together for subsequent discussion. Intermediate strength PPD (I-PPD), and keyhole limpet hemocyanin (KLH) were also followed. KLH was interpreted as a recall antigen in 28 of the initial 32 courses, because all 28 patients had been sensitized to and challenged one or more times with KLH before and after thymosin administration. Skin tests were repeated immediately after completing thymosin and again 1 or 2 weeks later.

The percent E-rosetting lymphocytes were followed serially, according to the skin test (ST) schedule. The rosettes were prepared using a modification (37) of the methods of Jondal et al. and Bentwich et al. (38, 39). E-rosette testing was performed before and after in vivo thymosin.

In addition to the immunological parameters monitored, the following clinical and laboratory parameters were also evaluated frequently: physical condition; immediate and delayed (24 and 48 hr) reaction at the injection site; blood count with platelets and differential; SMA survey; quantitative immunoglobulins; protein electrophoresis; prothrombin time; partial thromboplastin time; chest film; electrocardiogram; electrolytes; and tumor(s) size(s). The patient's thymosin courses were chronologically related to previous and concomitant medications, surgery, and radiotherapy.

---

[1] Immunodeficiency: two or fewer positive skin tests to a battery of five recall antigens and/or less than 50% E-rosetting lymphocytes.

TABLE 1. Normal donor lymphocytes (L) with no baseline response to thymosin (T)

Donor	Baseline cpm/10^6 L without T	Baseline cpm with T	Ratio
1	411	695	(1.69)
2	574	572	(1.00)
3	651	958	(1.47)
4	671	749	(1.12)
5	968	1,447	(1.49)
6	984	1,584	(1.61)
7	1,030	910	(0.88)
8	1,104	1,123	(1.02)
9	1,184	1,946	(1.64)
10	1,566	952	(0.61)
11	3,149	2,061	(0.65)
12	3,353	2,873	(0.86)
13	4,352	5,230	(1.20)
14	5,850	4,667	(0.80)
Mean	1,846	1,840	(1.15)
Median	1,140	1,162	(1.07)
Standard error	445	1,465	(0.10)
		$p = 0.78$	

RESULTS

Studies are discussed in three separate sections: In vitro results using normal subjects' lymphocytes, in vitro results with cancer patients' cells, and in vivo results after the first course of thymosin in 32 cancer patients.

TABLE 2. Normal donor lymphocytes (L) with $\geq 100\%$ increase in baseline cpm with thymosin (T)

Donor	Baseline cpm/10^6 L without T	cpm with T	Ratio
1	92	532	(5.78)
2	157	376	(2.39)
3	268	1,267	(4.73)
4	326	928	(2.85)
5	393	1,240	(3.16)
6	397	1,030	(2.59)
7	533	2,527	(4.74)
8	546	4,848	(8.88)
9	1,080	4,751	(4.40)
10	1,380	4,687	(3.40)
Mean	517	2,219	(4.29)
Median	395	1,135	(3.90)
Standard error	129	584	(0.62)

Normal Subjects' Lymphocytes In Vitro

Twenty-four normal subjects were studied by adding only thymosin to their otherwise unstimulated lymphocytes in routine microculture systems (36). The subjects were then grouped according to their response to thymosin and the response groups were compared to one another statistically.

The normal subjects could be separated into two groups. Group 1 (Table 1) included 14 donors with no thymosin effect.[2] Although each value in Table 1 is the mean of three or more replicates, there was, nevertheless, a wide range of baseline cpm of the unstimulated lymphocytes, presumably reflecting a spectrum of in vivo lymphocyte stimulation at the time blood was obtained. Group 2 (Table 2) consisted of 10 normal donors whose baseline thymidine incorporation was increased with thymosin. These 10 individuals

---

[2] No thymosin effect: no change in counts per minute (cpm) per 10^6 lymphocytes >100% more than, or >50% less than, baseline cpm.

TABLE 3. Changes in baseline thymidine incorporation by lymphocytes from normal human donors associated with the in vitro addition of thymosin (T)

	Group 1 Subjects with no change in cpm[a] with T	Group 2 Subjects with ≥ 100% Increased cpm[a] with T	p[b]
n	14	10	
cpm[a] without T (mean ± SEM)	1,846 ± 445	517 ± 395	0.017
cpm[a] with T (mean ± SEM)	1,840 ± 391	2,219 ± 1,135	not significant

[a] cpm = counts per minute per 10^6 lymphocytes.

[b] p = Student's t-test.

composing group 2 also showed a broad spread of unstimulated, baseline cpm, which, although individual counts overlapped between groups 1 and 2, was nevertheless a statistically different set of values from those occurring in response group 1 (p = 0.017, Student's t-test).

Groups 1 and 2, defined and originally established according to the individual donor's response to thymosin, are summarized and compared in Table 3. Mean cpm in group 1 were 1,846 without thymosin and 1,840 with it. Mean cpm in group 2 were 517 without thymosin and 2,219 with thymosin. Thus, Table 3 suggests that normal subjects whose baseline blastogenesis was increased with thymosin had, as a group, significantly lower baseline counts than subjects showing no change with thymosin. Table 3 additionally demonstrates that adding thymosin to otherwise unstimulated lymphocytes normalized differences between the cpm of the two response groups; thymosin did not produce supranormal "baseline" lymphocyte activity. Finally, thymosin was not mitogenic.

Table 4 (similar to Table 3) displays summary counts for normal donors concerning MLC responses with and without thymosin. Three groups could be defined depending on whether MLC was increased, unaffected, or decreased in the presence of thymosin. Group 1, with 9 donors, had cpm decreased by thymosin. Without thymosin, cpm were 75,500; with it, cpm were approximately 20,000. Group 2 showed counts without thymosin of 76,500, and with thymosin 74,000. These 7 subjects obviously showed no change in the presence of thymosin. Group 3, also with 7 volunteers, had nonthymosin counts of 12,650 and thymosin-related counts of 50,300. By statistical evaluation, as condensed in Table 4, the counts without thymosin

TABLE 4.   Changes in mixed lymphocyte culture (MLC) response of normal
human lymphocytes after the in vitro addition of thymosin (T)

	Group 1 ≥50% Decrease in cpm [a] with T	Group 2 No change in cpm [a] with T	Group 3 ≥100% Increase in cpm [a] with T	p [b] Value
n	9	7	7	
cpm [a] without T (mean ± SEM)	75,481 ± 20,277	76,517 ± 30,681	12,648 ± 3,722	0.018 (3 vs. 1) 0.016 (3 vs. 2)
cpm [a] with T (mean ± SEM)	19,972 ± 6,467	74,043 ± 28,344	50,337 ± 12,179	0.034 (3 vs. 1) N.S. [c] (3 vs. 2)

[a] cpm = counts per minute per 10^6 lymphocytes.

[b] p = Student's t-test.

[c] N.S. = not significant.

for group 3 were significantly different from the baseline counts in response groups 1 and 2.

The similarities between thymosin-responsive groups, as compared to thymosin-suppressed or thymosin-unchanged groups, are striking. Whether evaluating unstimulated lymphocytes or lymphocytes in MLC, thymosin augmented T-lymphocyte activity toward (but not beyond) the normal range in those subjects who, as a group, had statistically significantly depressed nonthymosin counts to begin with. In these 24 normal subjects, therefore, thymosin seemed to modulate lymphocyte ^{3}H-thymidine incorporation, especially showing activity in correcting initially depressed lymphocyte blastogenesis. These findings persist when standard mitogens, such as PHA, are similarly examined.

Cancer Patients Lymphocytes In Vitro

Identical experimental conditions to those used with normal subjects were employed in the study of the lymphocytes from 47 cancer patients with disseminated disease. The effects of in vitro thymosin on the unstimulated lymphocytes from these patients (Table 5) can be separated into the same three response groups shown in Table 4. Table 5 shows that the "resting" lymphocytes from cancer patients responded to thymosin alone much as the lymphocytes from normal subjects, as already detailed in Tables 1, 2, and 3.

TABLE 5. Response of cancer patients' lymphocytes in vitro to the addition of thymosin: changes in baseline blastogenesis in the presence of thymosin (T)

	Group 1 Patients whose cpm [a] decreased by $\geq 50\%$ with T	Group 2 Patients whose cpm [a] showed no change with T	Group 3 Patients whose cpm [a] in- creased $\geq 100\%$ with T
n	11	23	12
cpm [a] without T [b]	$2,135 \pm 545$	$1,389 \pm 229$	962 ± 294
cpm [a] with T [b]	530 ± 67	$1,306 \pm 275$	$3,993 \pm 940$

[a] cpm = counts per minute.

[b] Results are expressed as the mean $\pm$ SEM.

TABLE 6. Response of cancer patients' lymphocytes in vitro to the addition of thymosin: changes in mixed lymphocyte culture responses in the presence of thymosin (T)

	Group 1 Patients whose cpm [a] decreased by $> 50\%$ with T	Group 2 Patients whose cpm [a] showed no change with T	Group 3 Patients whose cpm [a] in- creased $>100\%$ with T
n	15	20	9
cpm [a] without T [b]	$6,730 \pm 3,274$	$7,382 \pm 3,027$	$5,783 \pm 1,996$
cpm [a] with T [b]	$2,243 \pm 998$	$6,550 \pm 2,650$	$25,467 \pm 6,467$

[a] cpm = counts per minute.

[b] Results are expressed as the mean $\pm$ SEM.

TABLE 7. Thymosin dosage schedules

Dosage (mg/m²)	Number of first therapy courses at that dosage	Duration of first T course		
		7 days	10 days	14 days
1-3	10	10	0	0
10-20	12	11	0	1
30-60	10	9	1	0

The MLC responses of cancer patients' lymphocytes to the addition of thymosin, still using the same experimental techniques, are summarized in Table 6. The same three response groups as depicted in Tables 4 and 5 are apparent and strikingly approximate the changes in the MLCs of normal donors' lymphocytes.

In Vivo Effects of the First Course of Thymosin in 32 Patients with Disseminated Malignancy

Clinical Parameters

Patients received 1 to 3, 10 to 20, or 30 to 60 mg of thymosin subcutaneously or intramuscularly daily, as shown in Table 7. The 32 initial courses of thymosin fell roughly into three equal groups according to the dosage categories defined. Twenty-six of the 32 thymosin courses were given without any detectable toxicity. One patient experienced an unexplained, febrile, "flu-like" illness for one day midway through this 7 days of treatment. Another patient with multiple myeloma developed his fifth lobar bacterial pneumonia during thymosin therapy. Finally, 4 of the 32 patients experienced inconstant local reactions to thymosin. These would appear one day but not the next. Their intensity never progressed; they did not necessitate discontinuation of thymosin or reduction in dosage.

Patients' diagnoses are shown in Table 8, along with the number of patients with each diagnosis and the number of thymosin courses each group of patients received. There was no attempt to select patients with specific malignancies initially, but after it seemed that thymosin was well tolerated, patients with leukemia and lymphoma were sought for thymosin treatment.

In 5 patients, possible clinical benefit from thymosin was suspected. Their diagnoses were "smoldering" acute myelogenous leukemia, acute lymphocytic leukemia, multiple myeloma, disseminated melanoma, and chronic lymphocytic leukemia. Accelerated disease possibly related to thymosin was detected in a young man with choriocarcinoma. In the other 26 patients, no clinical effects were apparent. Considering the spectrum of

TABLE 8. Diagnosis of patients receiving thymosin

Diagnosis	Number of patients	Total number of courses
Acute leukemia	6	19
Chronic lymphocytic leukemia	5	17
Disseminated melanoma	4	14
Multiple myeloma	4	9
Chronic myelocytic leukemia	2	5
Hairy cell leukemia	2	3
Hodgkin's disease	1	5
Head and neck squamous	1	2
Mycosis fungoides	1	2
Breast carcinoma	1	1
Choriocarcinoma (male)	1	1
Gall-bladder carcinoma	1	1
Gastroesophageal carcinoma	1	1
Leiomyosarcoma	1	1
Pancreatic carcinoma	1	1
	32	82

tumors treated, the generally far-advanced stages of patients' diseases, and the short periods of thymosin administration, no attempts to draw conclusions concerning thymosin's clinical activity were considered appropriate.

Immunological Evaluation

In Table 9, skin test changes after in vivo thymosin are summarized. In the first row changes in the number of positive skin tests to four standard recall antigens are displayed. The inevaluable patients include subjects who were anergic because of immediate resumption of combination chemotherapy, one patient whose forearm had to remain covered by a surgical dressing applied a few hours after the skin tests, and one patient whose skin test record was lost. Changes in KLH and PPD skin tests are shown in the second and third horizontal rows, respectively. The criteria employed to

TABLE 9. Skin test changes after in vivo thymosin

Test	Increase	No change	Decrease	Inevaluable
4 recall antigens[a] (change in number positive)	11	9	9	3
KLH response (neg → pos, or pos → neg, or 100% increase or 50% decrease)	10	15	3	4
PPD response (same criteria as used in KLH)	11	17	0	4

[a] Derm, Candida, SK-SD, and mumps.

define changes in KLH and PPD reactivity are elaborated in Table 9. In matched patients with similarly severe disseminated malignancy, it is unusual to find the degree of increased skin test positivity observed in these 32 patients (40).

The patients themselves made two observations about which we would not have inquired. Six noted that pretreatment skin tests enlarged when thymosin was started, even if the original reactions had begun to fade. Second, 5 patients reported that skin tests remained positive for 4 or 5 days during thymosin administration, an occurrence they had not experienced before receiving thymosin.

In Table 10, results of E-rosette determinations are summarized. Patients are separated into two groups depending on whether initial E-rosette percentages were less than 50% or equal to or greater than 50%. Rosette percentages significantly increased after in vivo thymosin in those subjects (approximately two-thirds of the total) whose initial percent T-lymphocytes was less than 50%. Conversely, E-rosette percentages were not statistically changed by in vivo thymosin administration when rosette values were originally equal to or greater than 50%. The rosette changes following in vivo thymosin parallel Kenady et al. 's detailed in vitro studies (41) as well as studies with levamisole and lymphocytes from patients with Hodgkin's disease (42).

Changes in lymphocyte incorporation of ^{3}H-thymidine after in vivo thymosin treatment are displayed in Table 11. These blastogenesis changes are quite similar to alterations in cancer patients' thymidine incorporation following in vitro thymosin (which were summarized in Table 5). This

TABLE 10. "Total" E-rosette percentages before and after in vivo thymosin (T)

Percentage of initial rosette-positive lymphocytes	Number of patients	E-rosette percentages before T (mean ± SEM)	E-rosettes after in vivo T (mean ± SEM)	p value (Student's t-test)
Less than 50%	20	34 ± 4	46 ± 3	p < 0.001
Greater than 50%	11	63 ± 3	57 ± 4	p = N.S.

TABLE 11. Changes in cancer patients' baseline blastogenesis after in vivo thymosin (T)

	Group 1 ≥ 50% Decrease in cpm after in vivo thymosin	Group 2 No change in cpm after in vivo thymosin	Group 3 100% Increase in cpm after in vivo thymosin	p Value (Student's t-test)
n	4	17	7	
cpm before T (mean ± SEM)	1,692 ± 149	1,157 ± 143	645 ± 107	p = 0.003 (3 vs. 1) p = 0.04 (3 vs. 2)
cpm after T (mean ± SEM)	560 ± 39	1,041 ± 115	2,825 ± 575	p = 0.002 (3 vs. 1) p = 0.07 (3 vs. 2)

agreement between changes in vitro and subsequently in vivo suggest that thymosin's activity on cultured but unstimulated lymphocytes in vitro may help predict thymosin's effect in vivo on cancer patients' T-lymphocytes.

Table 12 presents the effects of in vivo thymosin on MLC responsiveness. The distribution of patients among the three response groups and the nature of the changes induced are compatible with and complementary to similar changes in vitro in both normals (Table 4) and cancer patients (Table 6) when thymosin is added. Thus the in vitro MLC response to exogenous

TABLE 12. Cancer patients' MLC blastogenesis responses before and after in vivo thymosin (T)

	Patients with 50% decrease in cpm after T	Patients with no change after T	Patients with ≥ 100% increase after T	p Value
n	9	14	5	
cpm before T (mean ± SEM)	11,117 ± 5,133	4,772 ± 1,859 (1 vs. 2: N.S.)	985 ± 149	1 vs. 3: N.S. 2 vs. 3: N.S.
cpm after T (mean ± SEM)	1,606 ± 930	4,245 ± 1,339 (1 vs. 2: N.S.)	13,756 ± 10,952	1 vs. 3: N.S. 2 vs. 3: N.S.

thymosin may assist physicians in anticipating in vivo responses, exactly as in vitro changes of unstimulated, cultured lymphocytes to added thymosin may help predict in vivo responses to thymosin.

DISCUSSION

The in vitro and in vivo investigation described in this chapter consistently suggest that thymosin partially corrects deficient numbers and function of normal donors' and cancer patients' T-lymphocytes. These results extend Kenady et al.'s in vitro studies of E-rosettes (41) and are compatible with investigations in other laboratories (22,43,44).

Specifically, the in vitro results show an increase to or toward normal of initially depressed baseline and MLC blastogenic responses in the presence of thymosin, whether normal or cancer patients' lymphocytes are studied. Investigations from other laboratories may offer an explanation for these observations, as well as the occasionally decreased activity produced by thymosin in lymphocytes originally functioning normally. Thymosin appears to increase T-lymphocyte intracellular cyclic AMP (44). For example, when prethymus, immature (T_0) T-cells predominate in a population of lymphocytes, thymosin helps shift the T-lymphocyte characteristics toward those of mature (T_2) lymphocytes (43), a finding directly related to increased intracellular cyclic AMP. On the other hand, too much cyclic AMP within mature lymphocytes may suppress the activity of those cells (43).

The in vivo results reported here serve to spur further investigations of thymosin in human malignancy, but the potential thymosin demonstrates for possible beneficial and detrimental in vivo activity must lead to careful selection of patients for thymosin administration. With this cautious note in mind, continued phase I and beginning phase II studies are in progress at M. D. Anderson Hospital and at other institutions, in collaboration with Hoffmann-LaRoche. Our group is concentrating on malignant melanoma (regionally recurrent with metastases in regional lymph nodes, but disease-free after recent surgery and staging for disseminated disease); our attention and therapy are also being directed at chronic lymphocytic leukemia, multiple myeloma, remission maintenance of adult acute leukemia, "hairy cell" leukemia, and Mycosis fungoides.

Accumulating evidence suggests that thymosin therapy may be helpful in B-lymphocyte malignancies (45-49). The postulated mechanism of activity against these tumors is a reactivation by thymosin of suppressor T-lympho-cytes, which in turn should block B-cells from behaving abnormally (49-51). Whether B-cell malignancies will be responsive as postulated remains to be determined.

SUMMARY

The lymphocytes of 24 normal donors and 47 cancer patients were studied in vitro with and without thymosin, using standard lymphocyte culture tech-niques. Subjects were grouped according to the response of their lympho-cytes to thymosin. The groups of subjects whose lymphocyte ^{3}H-thymidine incorporation was augmented in the presence of thymosin showed statistically significant depression of prethymosin (baseline) counts per minute per 10^6 lymphocytes (cpm) as compared to all other subjects' baseline counts. Thus, thymosin seemed to augment initially subnormal blastogenic activity, tending to raise it into the normal range. Thymosin did not itself act as a mitogen or antigen and did not produce supranormal blastogenesis.

Eighty-two in vivo thymosin courses were given to 32 patients. In this chapter, the first thymosin course received by each of the 32 patients is analyzed. Immunological restoration of the parameters surveyed — skin tests, E-rosettes, blastogenic responses — tended to occur in patients with originally depressed T-cell function and numbers. No change, or even some depression in immunological parameters, developed in patients with initially intact T-cell responses. Four of 32 patients experienced toxicity, in each case transient local inflammation. Clinical effects of thymosin on patients' malignancies were equivocal, a finding which is not unexpected in a clinical trial where no systematic look at a specific disease was attempted. The in vitro and in vivo findings in this study indicate that thymosin may modulate and partially normalize human T-cell numbers and function.

ACKNOWLEDGMENTS

This work was supported in part by contract N01-CB-33888 and grants CA-05831, CA-14108, CA-15419, and CA-16964 from the National Cancer Institute, National Institutes of Health, Bethesda, Maryland 20014. Jordan U. Gutterman and Giora M. Mavligit are the recipients, respectively, of career development awards CA-71007-01 and CA 1 K0 4 CA 00130-01 from the National Institutes of Health.

REFERENCES

1. Trainin, N. (1974): Thymic hormones and the immune response. Physiol. Rev., 54:272-315.
2. Miller, J. F. A. P. (1961): Immunological function of the thymus. Lancet, 2:748-749.
3. Good, R. A., Gabrielson, A. E., Peterson, R. D. A., Finstad, J., and Cooper, M. D. (1966): The development of the central and peripheral lymphoid tissue: Ontogenic and phylogenetic considerations. In: Thymus: Experimental and Clinical Studies, edited by G. E. W. Wolstenholme and R. Porter, pp. 181-213. A Ciba Foundation Symposium, London.
4. Lischner, H. W., Punnet, H. H., and Di George, A. M. (1967): Lymphocytes in congenital absence of the thymus. Nature, 214:580-582.
5. Good, R. A., and Gabrielson, A. E. (Eds.) (1964): The Thymus in Immunobiology: Structure, Function, and Role in Disease. Hoeber (Harper & Row), New York.
6. White, A., and Goldstein, A. L. (1975): The endocrine role of the thymus, and its hormone thymosin in the regulation of the growth and maturation of host immunological competence. Adv. Metab. Dis., 8:361-376.
7. Wong, F. M., Taub, R. N., Sherman, J. D., and Dameshek, W. (1966): Effect of thymus enclosed in millipore diffusion envelopes on thymectomized hamsters. Blood, 28:40-53.
8. Stutman, O., Yunis, E. J., and Good, R. A. (1969): Carcinogen-induced tumors of the thymus. III. Restoration of neonatally thymectomized mice with thymomas in cell-impermeable chambers. J. Natl. Cancer Inst., 43:499-508.
9. Stutman, O., Yunis, E. J., and Good, R. A. (1969): Carcinogen-induced tumors of the thymus. IV. Humoral influences of normal thymus and functional thymomas and influence of postthymectomy period on restoration. J. Exp. Med., 130:809-820.
10. Bomskov, C., and Sladovic, L. (1940): Der Thymus als Innersekretorisches. Org. Dtsch. Med. Wochenschr., 66:589-594.
11. Goldstein, A. L., Thurman, G. B., Cohen, G. H., and Hooper, J. A. (1974): Thymosin: Chemistry, biology, and clinical applications. In: Biological Activity of Thymic Hormones, edited by R. W. Van Bekkum, pp. 173-197. Kooyker Scientific Publications, Rotterdam.
12. Goldstein, G. (1975): The isolation of thymopoietin (thymin). Ann. N.Y. Acad. Sci., 249:177-185.
13. Bach, J. F., Dardenne, M., Pleau, J. M., and Block, M. A. (1975): Isolation, biochemical characteristics, and biological activity of a circulating thymic hormone in the mouse and in the human. Ann. N.Y. Acad. Sci., 249:186-210.

14. Shelton, E. (1966): Differentiation of mouse thymus cultured in diffusion chambers. Am. J. Anat., 119:341-358.

15. Clark, S. L., Jr. (1966): Cytological evidence of secretion in the thymus. In: Thymus: Experimental and Clinical Studies, edited by G. E. W. Wohlstenholme, and R. Porter, pp. 3-30, A Ciba Foundation Symposium, London.

16. Asanuma, Y., Goldstein, A. L., and White, A. (1970): Reduction in the incidence of wasting disease in neonatally thymectomized CBA/Wh mice by the injection of thymosin. Endocrinology, 86:600-610.

17. Goldstein, A. L., Asanuma, Y., Battisto, J. R., Hardy, M. A., Quint, J. and White, A. (1970): Influence of thymosin on cell-mediated and humoral immune responses in normal and in immunologically deficient mice. J. Immunol., 104:359-364.

18. Zisblatt, M., Goldstein, A. L., Lilly, F., and White, A. (1970): Acceleration by thymosin of the development of resistance to murine sarcoma virus-induced mice. Proc. Natl. Acad. Sci. (U.S.A.), 66:1170-1174.

19. Khaw, B. A., and Rule, A. H. (1973): Immunotherapy of the Dunning leukemia with thymus extracts. Br. J. Cancer, 28:288-292.

20. Barker, A. (1975): Personal communication.

21. Goldstein, A. L., Cohen, G. H., Rossio, J. L., Thurman, G. B., and Ulrich, J. T. (1976): Use of thymosin in the treatment of primary immunodeficiency diseases and cancer. Med. Clin. North Am. (in press).

22. Wara, D. W., Goldstein, A. L., Doyle, N. E., and Ammann, A. J. (1975): Thymosin activity in patients with cellular immunodeficiency. N. Engl. J. Med., 292:70-74.

23. Wara, D. W., and Ammann, A. J. (1975): Effect of thymosin on B-lymphocyte function. N. Engl. J. Med., 293:507.

24. Goldstein, A. L., Griscelli, C., August, C. S., Hill, H. R., Reid, R., Waldmann, T., and Ammann, A. J. (1975): Unpublished observations.

25. Goldstein, A. L. (1975): Unpublished observations.

26. Schafer, L. A., Goldstein, A. L., Gutterman, J. U., and Hersh, E. M. (1976): In vitro and in vivo studies with thymosin in cancer patients. Ann. N.Y. Acad. Sci. (in press).

27. Hersh, E. M., Gutterman, J. U., and Mavligit, G. M. (1976): Immunocompetence, immunodeficiency, and prognosis in cancer. Ann. N.Y. Acad. Sci. (in press).

28. Eilber, F. R., and Morton, D. L. (1970): Impaired immunological reactivity and recurrence following cancer surgery. Cancer, 25:362-367.

29. Chretien, P. B., Crowder, W. L., Gertner, H. R., Sample, W. F., and Catalona, W. J. (1973): Correlation of pre-operative lymphocyte reactivity with the clinical course of cancer patients. Surg. Gynecol. Obstet., 136:380-384.

30. Gutterman, J. U., Mavligit, G. M., Gottlieb, J. A., Burgess, M. A., McBride, C. E., Einhorn, L., Freireich, E. J., and Hersh, E. M. (1974): Chemoimmunotherapy of disseminated malignant melanoma with DTIC and BCG. N. Engl. J. Med., 291:592-597.

31. Gutterman, J. U., Hersh, E. M., Rodriguez, V., McCredie, K. B., Mavligit, G. M., Reed, R. C., Burgess, M. A., Smith, T., Gehan, E., Bodey, G. P., Sr., and Freireich, E. J. (1974): Chemoimmunotherapy of adult acute leukemia: Prolongation of remission in myeloblastic leukaemia with BCG. Lancet, 2:1405-1409.

32. Torisu, M. (1976): Immunotherapy of cancer patients with BCG: Summary of four years experience in Japan. Ann. N.Y. Acad. Sci. (in press).

33. Israel, L. (1976): Regressions of disseminated cancer following intravenous administration of Corynebacterium parvum. Ann. N.Y. Acad. Sci. (in press).

34. Boyum, A. (1968): Separation of lymphocytes from blood and bone marrow. Scand. J. Clin. Lab. Invest., 21 (Suppl. 97):77-89.

35. Hartzman, R. J., Segall, M., Bach, M. L., and Bach, F. H. (1971): Histocompatibility matching. VI. Miniaturization of the mixed leukocyte culture test: A preliminary report. Transplantation, 11:268-273.

36. Thurman, G. B., Strong, D. M., Ahmed, A., Green, S. S., Sell, K. W., Hartzman, R. J., and Bach, F. H. (1973): Human mixed lymphocyte cultures: Evaluation of a microculture technique utilizing the multiple automated sample harvester (MASH). Clin. Exp. Immunol., 15:289-302.

37. Schafer, L. A., Gutterman, J. U., Mavligit, G. M., Reed, R. C., and Hersh, E. M. (1975): Permanent slide preparations of T-lymphocyte-sheep red blood cell rosettes. J. Immunol. Methods, 8:241-250.

38. Jondal, M., Holm, G., and Wigzell, H. (1972): Surface markers on human T and B lymphocytes. I. A large population of lymphocytes forming non-immune rosettes with sheep red blood cells. J. Exp. Med., 136:207-215.

39. Bentwich, Z., Douglas, S. D., Siegal, F. P., and Kunkel, H. G. (1973): Human lymphocyte-sheep erythrocyte rosette formation: Some characteristics of the interaction. Clin. Immunol. Immunopath., 1:511-522.

40. Gutterman, J. U. (1975): Unpublished observations.

41. Kenady, D. E., Potvin, C., Simon, R. M., and Chretien, P. (1976): In vitro effect of thymosin on T-cell levels in cancer patients receiving radiation therapy. This Volume.

42. Ramot, B., and Biniaminov, M. (1976): The effect of levamisole on lymphocytes of Hodgkin's disease patients in vivo and in vitro. This Volume.

43. Aiuti, F., Schirrmacher, V., Ammirati, P., and Fivrilli, M. (1975): Effect of thymus factor on human precursor T-lymphocytes. Clin. Exp. Immunol., 20:499-503.

44. Rotter, V., and Trainin, N. (1975): Increased mitogenic reactivity of normal spleen cells to T lectins induced by thymus humoral factor (THF). Cell. Immunol., 16:413-421.

45. Dauphines, M. J., Talal, N., Goldstein, A. L., and White, A. (1974): Thymosin corrects the abnormal DNA synthetic response of NZB mouse thymocytes. Proc. Natl. Acad. Sci. (U.S.A.), 71:2637-2641.

46. Gershwin, M. E., Ahmed, A., Steinberg, A. D., Thurman, G. B., and Goldstein, A. L. (1974): Correction of T-cell function by thymosin in New Zealand mice. J. Immunol., 113:1068-1071.
47. Scheinberg, M. A., Goldstein, A. L., and Cathcart, E. S. (1976): Thymosin restores T-cell function and reduces the incidence of amyloid disease in casein-treated mice. J. Immunol., 116:156-158.
48. Gershwin, M. E., and Steinberg, A. D. (1975): Suppression of auto-immune hemolytic anemia in New Zealand (NZB) mice by syngeneic young thymocytes. Clin. Immunol. Immunopathol., 4:38-45.
49. Talal, N., Dauphinee, M. J., Fye, K. H., and Moutsopoulos, H. (1976): Experimental studies of thymosin in NZB mice and in systemic lupus erythematosus. This Volume.
50. Decker, J. L., Steinberg, A. D., Gershwin, M. E., Seaman, W. E., Klippel, J. H., Plotz, P. H., and Paget, S. A. (1975): Systemic lupus erythematosis: Contrasts and comparisons. Ann. Int. Med., 82:391-404.
51. Scheinberg, M. A., and Cathcart, E. S. (1975): Amyloid disease and polyclonal B cell activation. Clin. Res., 23:342A.

Control of Neoplasia by Modulation of the Immune System, edited by M. A. Chirigos. Raven Press, New York 1977.

INTERFERON-DIRECTED INHIBITION OF CHRONIC MURINE LEUKEMIA VIRUS PRODUCTION IN CELL CULTURES

*Robert M. Friedman, *Francis T. Jay, *Esther H. Chang, *Maureen W. Myers, *Janet M. Ramseur, **Sharon J. Mims, **Timothy J. Triche, and †Paul K. Y. Wong

*Laboratory of Experimental Pathology, National Institute for Arthritis, Metabolism and Digestive Diseases, and **Laboratory of Pathology, National Cancer Institute, National Institutes of Health, Bethesda, Maryland 20014 and †Department of Microbiology, University of Illinois, Urbana, Illinois 61801

INTRODUCTION

During the past three years several laboratories have demonstrated an interferon-induced inhibition of murine leukemia virus production in tissue culture (1-4). This inhibition has several unexpected features. These include: (a) the inhibition takes place in chronic murine leukemia virus-infected cell lines, cells producing murine leukemia virus long before interferon treatment; (b) in spite of marked inhibition of extracellular virus concentrations, intracellular markers for virus replication are not inhibited by interferon; and (c) the site of the block appears to be at a late step in the virus replication cycle, probably a step involving virus release from the cell.

The following is a review of recent studies in our laboratory which have been carried out on the inhibition of murine leukemia virus by interferon.

MATERIALS AND METHODS

Cells

AKR, C^- cells were obtained from W. Rowe, National Institute of Allergy and Infectious Diseases. They were negative for RNA tumor virus production and for viral p30 (gs) antigen in an immunofluorescence assay. Their culture fluids contained no viral reverse transcriptase activity. A culture of these cells spontaneously became chronic MLV producing and is termed AKR, C^+.

347

All of the cells in an AKR, C^+ culture produced viral p30 (gs) antigen. Other properties of AKR, C^+ have been described (3). New Zealand black (NZB) cells derived from a NZB mouse embryo were also obtained from Dr. Rowe. An endogenous, xenotropic MLV is present in the cultures. NZB 2C cells were derived by Dr. Rowe from a clone of the NZB cells. SC-1 is a line derived from a wild mouse embryo. The culture of SC-1 used had been infected with a B-tropic MLV taken from a BALB mouse tumor. KBALB-V_1, from S. Aaronson, National Cancer Institute (NCI), is a BALB-3T3 cell line transformed by Kirsten sarcoma virus and infected with the BALB-V_1 virus, an N-tropic virus. KBALB-R, also 3T3 cells from Dr. Aaronson, had been transformed by Kirsten sarcoma virus and infected with the Rauscher leukemia virus (NB tropic). JLS-V9 from N. Wivel (NCI) also carries the Rauscher leukemia virus. All of these cell lines were chronic producers of MLV; none was a transformed cell line. TB cells were obtained from Dr. Wong's laboratory and are derived from CFW/D mouse bone marrow and thymus (5).

Interferon and Interferon Assays

The mouse interferon used was prepared by the method of Ogburn and Paucker in K. Paucker's laboratory (6). The preparation had a specific activity of at least 5×10^7 mouse interferon international reference units per milligram of protein. The antiviral activity of this preparation had the chemical and physical properties usually ascribed to interferon.

Interferon was assayed by either a plaque inhibition or a cytopathic effect inhibition assay in L_y cells. In either assay vesicular stomatitis virus was employed as the test virus (3).

Assay for Viral p30 (gs) Antigens

A radioimmunoprecipitation inhibition assay for viral p30 (gs) antigens was employed (7). Because of the use of a new antiserum provided by J. Gruber of the Program Resources and Logistics Branch, NCI, the average level of p30 (gs) antigen in AKR, C^+ cells in this study (3.4 μg/mg of protein) was higher than the value of about 1 μg/mg of protein previously reported from this laboratory.

Transcriptase Assays

The conditions for assay of viral and cellular polymerases were similar. The 100-μl incubation mixtures contained 50 mM Tris-HCl, pH 8.0, 60 mM KCl, 1 mM $MnCl_2$, 2.5 mM dithiothreitol 0.05% Triton X-100, 0.04 A_{260} units of polyriboadenylic acid·oligodeoxythymidylic acid (rA·dT), polydeoxyadenylic acid·oligodeoxythymidylic acid (dA·dT), or polyribocytidylic acid·oligodeoxyguanylic acid (rC·dG) and 10 μl of cell extract and 10 μl of 0.2 mM TTP or dGTP containing 20 μCi of tritiated TTP or dGTP at a specific activity of 10 Ci/mmole. The incubation was carried out for 30 or 45 min at 37°C. Acid-precipitable radioactivity was collected on membrane filters (Millipore Corp.) and was estimated in a liquid scintillation counter.

Tissue culture fluid containing virus was prepared for assay of reverse transcriptase activity by sedimentation first at 10,000 X g for 20 min to remove cell debris and then sedimentation at 48,000 X g for 2 hr. The level of enzyme activity has previously been shown to parallel closely that of virus infectivity. Cytoplasmic extracts were prepared by scraping AKR monolayers containing about 10^8 cells into buffer (10 mM NaCl, 10 mM Tris-HCl, pH 7.4, and 1.5 mM $MgCl_2$) and homogenizing the cells in a Dounce homogenizer. The extracts were then sedimented at 10,000 X g for 10 min, and the supernatants were sedimented at 40,000 X g for 1 hr. The resulting sediments were prepared for assay by resuspending them in 0.5 ml of 10 mM Tris-HCl, pH 7.4, 1 mM EDTA, 100 mM NaCl, and 2.5 mM dithiothreitol. Results similar to those reported were obtained by us when cytoplasmic extracts prepared with Triton X-100 or with NP-40 were employed. In the latter case, however, background incorporation of radioactivity by extracts was high.

Preparation of Cells for Scanning Electron Microscopy (SEM)

The cells were grown in Falcon plastic flasks, and treated with 30 units/ ml of interferon. They were then trypsinized every 48 hr before reaching confluency and fresh medium containing interferon was added. After a 5- to 6-day interferon treatment the cells were seeded in Petri dishes containing 6-mm glass coverslips (Corning) 48 hr before sample collection. The 80% confluent monolayers were washed five times in phosphate-buffered saline (PBS), pH 7.4, and fixed in 2.5% glutaraldehyde in PBS pH 7.4 for 1 hr at room temperature. After washing three times with PBS, the monolayers were postfixed 30 min in OsO_4, rinsed, and dehydrated through gradients of ethanol and amyl acetate. Immediately after dehydration, the cells were critical-point dried in CO_2 in a Denton Vacuum critical-point drying apparatus, DCP-1 (Cherry Hill, New Jersey) (8). The samples were then rotary coated with a 15- to 20-nm layer of gold-palladium in a vacuum evaporator, High Vacuum Equipment Corp. evaporator (Hingham, Massachusetts) and were viewed in an Etec scanning electron microscope at a nominal resolution of approximately 15 to 20 nm.

Virus

The spontaneously arising temperature-sensitive (ts) mutant of the Moloney strain of murine leukemia virus (MLV) was isolated as described in detail previously (9). It is designated ts-3.

Chromatographic Procedures

(1) Preparation of crude enzyme extract. AKR, C^+ or AKR, C^- cells were cultured in disposable roller bottles (Bellco Biological Glassware) with McCoy's 5a modified medium supplemented with 10% fetal calf serum

at 37° C. Cells were grown to subconfluency and washed twice with phosphate-buffered 0.14 M NaCl (PBS). A cell suspension in PBS was sedimented at 700 rpm for 5 min in an IEC model RP-2 centrifuge and washed twice more with PBS. The cell pellet was suspended in hypotonic buffer (50 mM Tris-HCl, pH 7.5, 1 mM EDTA, 1 mM DTT) and allowed to stand for 5 min before homogenizing with 20 strokes in a Dounce homogenizer using a tight-fit pestle. Tris-HCl, pH 7.5, KCl, glycerol, Triton X-100, and dithiothreitol (DTT) were added to final concentrations similar to those in the extraction buffer (50 mM Tris-HCl, pH 7.5, 1 M KCl, 10% glycerol, 0.3% Triton X-100, 1 mM DTT). The suspension was further homogenized with 5 strokes and allowed to stand for 30 min. The supernatant was removed after centrifugation at 17,300 X g for 15 min and the pellet was reextracted with lysing buffer and 5 strokes in a Dounce homogenizer. The supernatant was obtained as before and the two supernatant fractions were pooled and dialyzed in standard buffer, pH 7.5 (50 mM Tris-HCl, 1 mM DTT, 10% glycerol), for 2 to 3 hr.

The cell extract was allowed to pass through a column of DE-23 cellulose (15 ml; Whatman Biochemicals Ltd.) and the column was washed with 3 column volumes of standard buffer, pH 7.5, containing 0.3 M KCl. The column flow-through and the column wash were pooled and concentrated by dialysis in 30% polyethylene glycol (20,000 M.W.) in standard buffer, pH 7.5. After concentration, the crude enzyme extract was dialysed against standard buffer, pH 7.5, and stored at -70°C after clarification by centrifugation. All procedures were carried out at 0 to 4° C unless otherwise specified.

(2) DE-52 cellulose column chromatography. Urea and Triton X-100 were added to the crude enzyme preparation to final concentrations of 1 M and 0.1%, respectively. The preparation was then dialyzed against standard buffer, pH 7.8, containing 1 M urea and 0.1% Triton for 2 hr before loading on to a DE-52 cellulose column, 1 X 25 cm, previously equilibrated with the same buffer. The column was washed with 10 ml of buffer and developed with 400 ml of 0 to 0.4 M KCl gradient in standard buffer, pH 7.8 (containing no urea or Triton). Fractions of 80 drops (approx. 2 ml) were collected and assayed by the above procedure except that the reaction was incubated at 37°C for 10 min and an aliquot was deposited onto a Whatman 3-mm filter paper disc for precipitation and washing in 5% TCA containing 20 mM sodium pyrophosphate at 0° C. The disc was dehydrated in alcohol and ether and dried for counting by liquid scintillation with a toluene-PPO-POPOP scintillation fluid.

RESULTS AND DISCUSSION

Effect of Interferon on MLV Production in AKR Cells

Table 1 presents a summary of our findings relating to the effects of interferon treatment on several intra- and extracellular markers of murine leukemia virus production in cultures of AKR mouse fibroblasts. All three assays of virus production and release of virus into extracellular fluid (Table 1, columns A, B, and C) indicated that at both concentrations of interferon employed, there is marked inhibition of virus production. It is

TABLE 1. Effects of interferon treatment on intracellular and extracellular viral markers in AKR cell cultures

Interferon concentration[a]	Extracellular			Intracellular	
	A	B	C	B'	C'
	Virus titer [b]	Reverse transcriptase activity [c]	p30 antigen conc. [d]	Reverse transcriptase activity [c]	p30 antigen conc. [e]
0	4.7	19	512	14	0.93
10	3.5	NA[f]	8	NA[f]	3.0
30	3.2	2.0	2	12	4.2

[a] International mouse reference units per milliliter.

[b] 2 $\log_{10}$ of infectious virus per milliliter in an XC plaque assay.

[c] Picomoles of dGMP incorporated per 25 µl of 100X concentrated culture fluid or per 10 µl of cytoplasmic extract.

[d] Terminal dilution of antigen giving significant activity in the radioimmunoprecipitation inhibition assay. Protein content of pelleted virus was too low to determine accurately.

[e] Milligrams of antigen per milligram of cell protein.

[f] Not assayed for enzyme activity at this concentration of interferon.

possible that interferon might cause cells to release an incomplete virus which is lacking in transcriptase and therefore noninfectious; however, such a virus, lacking in p30 group-specific antigen, is unlikely.

On the other hand, production of intracellular markers of virus replication (Table 1, columns B' and C') was not inhibited by interferon treatment. In fact, concentrations of p30 antigen are consistently increased in interferon-treated cells and the increase has been shown to be proportional to the interferon concentration employed.

These results are paradoxical: In the face of marked inhibition of virus production, the production of virus specific proteins was not impaired.

Nature of Intracellular Polymerase

Although the use of rC·dG as a template is reported to be a specific assay for a viral reverse transcriptase, the large number of DNA polymerase activities present in animal cells makes further characterization of such enzyme activities mandatory (10). We have employed a chromatographic

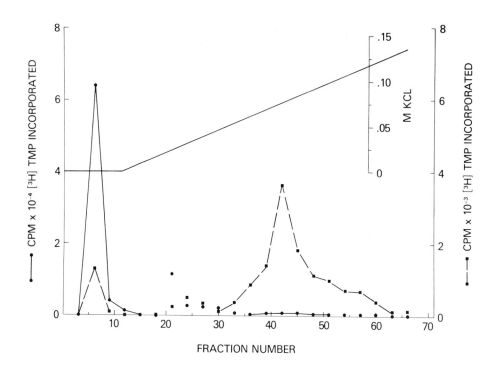

FIG. 1. Fractionation of crude DNA polymerases from AKR, C⁻ cells on
DEAE-cellulose column. The cell extract, equilibrated in standard buffer,
pH 7.8 (20 mM Tris-HCl, pH 7.8, 1 mM DTT, 10% glycerol) containing 1 M
urea and 0.1% Triton X-100, was loaded on to a DE-52 cellulose column,
1 X 25 cm, previously equilibrated in the same buffer. The column was
washed with 10 ml of the same buffer and developed with 400 ml of 0 to 0.4 M
KCl gradient in standard buffer, pH 7.8 (containing no urea or Triton).
Fractions of 80 drops (approx. 2 ml) were collected and aliquots were assayed
for polymerase activities in response to each of the templates, as described
in "Materials and Methods." Incorporation of [³H]TMP (5 Ci/mmole) in
response to dA·dT, ●——●, and rA·dT, ■——■ into acid precipitable counts
(cpm/18 μl eluate/10 min at 37°C) is shown.

procedure on DEAE-cellulose to separate viral from cellular polymerases.
The presence of M urea in the first part of the elution procedure which employed a very low ionic strength greatly reduced nonspecific elution of
enzyme activities from the column.

In AKR cells not producing MLV, two peaks of polymerase activity were
observed, one eluted before addition of KCL, the other, at 0.08 M KCl
(Fig. 1). In the first peak, most of the activity was responsive to the dA·dT
template; the activity eluted at the higher salt concentration responded best
to the rA·dT template. No activity was stimulated by the rC·dG template in
these cell extracts; the two activities found apparently corresponded to
cellular DNA polymerases β and γ.

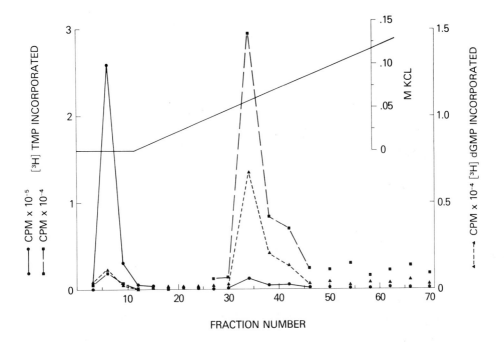

FIG. 2.   Fractionation of crude DNA polymerase from AKR, C$^+$ cells on DEAE-cellulose column.   See Fig. 1 legend for experimental detail.   Incorporation of [^{3}H]TMP (5 Ci/mmole) in response to dA·dT, ●——●, and rA·dT, ■——■; and [^{3}H]dGMP (5 Ci/mmole) in response to dG·rC, ▲——▲, templates into acid precipitable counts (cpm/18 μl eluate/10 min at 37°C) is shown.

In AKR cells producing virus, an additional activity was found eluting at 0.06 M salt (Fig. 2).   This activity was responsive to the rA·dT and the rC·dG templates; it thus appeared to be a viral reverse transcriptase. Therefore, it is possible to isolate and to characterize the activity assayed for by the rC·dG template.   This suggested that we were indeed dealing with a viral activity and that the relevant findings in Table 1 fairly accurately indicated viral enzyme production.

Effect of Interferon in MLV-Producing Mouse Cell Lines

When several MLV producing cell lines were tested, the inhibition of MLV production with interferon treatment was roughly proportional to the sensitivity of a particular cell line to the antiviral activity of interferon when assayed against VSV infections (Table 2).   The cell lines could be classified into one of three groups: A, interferon sensitive; B, moderately sensitive; and C, relatively insensitive.   The tropism of the virus (11) or whether the virus infection was exogenous or endogenous had no effect on the sensitivity

TABLE 2. Inhibition of reverse transcriptase activity in culture fluids of interferon-treated, chronically infected mouse cell lines

Group	Cell line	Relative sensitivity to interferon [a]	Tropism of virus [b]	Percent reduction in extracellular trans-criptase activity [c]
A	AKR	1.0	N, en	94
	NIH	1.0	NB, ex	87
B	KBALB-V$_1$	0.3	N, ex	77
	SC-1	0.3	B, ex	75
	NZB	0.2	X, en	43
C	KBALB-R	< 0.1	NB, ex	0
	JLS-V9	< 0.1	NB, ex	0
	NZB2C	< 0.1	X, en	0

[a] Monolayers of each cell line were assayed in microtiter plates by treatment for 18 hr with a concentration range (1 to 30 U/ml) of interferon. The cells were washed and infected with VSV at a multiplicity of 1. After 48 hr the cytopathic effect of the virus was observed, and the lowest concentration of interferon which completely protected the monolayers was noted. Relative sensitivity was estimated by the ratio of the concentration which protected AKR, C^+ (3 U/ml) to the concentration which protected other cell lines.

[b] Tropism of the endogenous (en) or exogenous (ex) murine leukemia virus infecting the culture. N, N-tropic; B, B-tropic; X, xenotropic; NB, N and B tropic.

[c] Percentage reduction in extracellular reverse transcriptase activity following treatment of cultures with 10 units/ml of interferon.

of a system to interferon. In one case a clone of NZB cells, NZB-2C, was relatively insensitive to interferon whereas the parent NZB cell line was moderately sensitive. Both cell lines produced the same xenotropic virus. In another case, two different KBALB cultures were infected with different viruses, an interferon-insensitive exogenous NB Rauscher-type agent (KBALB-R) or an exogenous N-tropic BALB/C MLV (KBALB-V$_1$). The former cell line was relatively insensitive to interferon, the latter, moderately sensitive. In both systems of NZB or KBALB varients, the cells insensitive to interferon showed no effect on MLV production after interferon treatment, whereas the moderately sensitive cell lines showed a significant response to interferon.

In one case the Rauscher-type MLV from a relatively insensitive cell line, JLS-V9, was employed to infect interferon-sensitive NIH cells. In this case, the replication of the virus was sensitive to interferon.

These results indicated that MLV production in several cell systems is sensitive to interferon treatment. The degree of sensitivity depended on the sensitivity of the cells to the antiviral activity of interferon, and not on an inherent sensitivity or resistance of different MLV strains to interferon. So far, all MLV strains tested have been sensitive to interferon.

Morphological Correlation with Interferon Inhibition of MLV Production

The results discussed so far indicated that interferon inhibits production of extracellular MLV but does not seem to inhibit synthesis of viral proteins. This apparent paradox was partially resolved by morphological studies. During the course of examining by conventional transmission electron microscopy (TEM) interferon-treated and control AKR cells producing MLV, it became obvious that, in the interferon-treated cells, budding virus particles were relatively easy to find although extracellular virus was difficult to locate. Quantitating these findings proved difficult with TEM, so we turned to scanning electron microscopy (SEM). When AKR cells were viewed by SEM, their surfaces were usually smooth; however, even in cells with extensive formation of microvilli, the smooth 100-nm budding virus particles were easy to identify (Fig. 3). In control cells an average of 2.17 virus particles was found per square micron of cell surface (Fig. 3B), whereas in interferon treated cells there were 6.06 (Fig. 3A); the difference was highly significant ($p < 0.001$).

The explanation for our previous findings appears to be that, in interferon-treated cells, virus was prevented from detaching from the cell surface. Therefore, virus production was inhibited but not the production of the viral proteins assayed. The density of budding virus particles on the cell surface was significantly increased in the interferon-treated cells.

Locus of Interferon Action — Studies with the ts-3 Mutation

The striking findings in interferon-treated cells viewed in the SEM are very similar to those recently reported in experiments carried out with an MLV mutant, ts-3, at nonpermissive conditions (9). In both cases, a marked increase in virus particles was seen on the cell surface, the scanning micrographs being indistinguishable.

Since the ts-3 mutation would appear to involve a single genetic locus, we attempted to define the interferon sensitive point in MLV replication in terms of the ts-3 site. Therefore, ts-3-infected TB cells were incubated at nonpermissive conditions (39.5°C) and treated with interferon for 26 hr, sufficient time to establish an antiviral state. The temperature was then

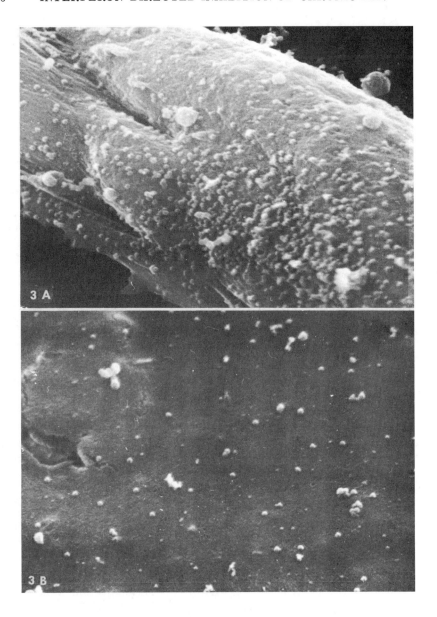

FIG. 3. An interferon-treated AKR, C^+ cell (A). The density of budding virions on the surface of these cells is greatly increased compared to that in the untreated cells (B). (13,440X).

dropped to the permissive level, $34°C$, and virus production monitored by collecting fluids at intervals over the first hour after the temperature downshift and assaying them for viral reverse transcriptase activity.

Almost immediately after the temperature downshift, virus production increased in both the interferon-treated and control cultures (Fig. 4);

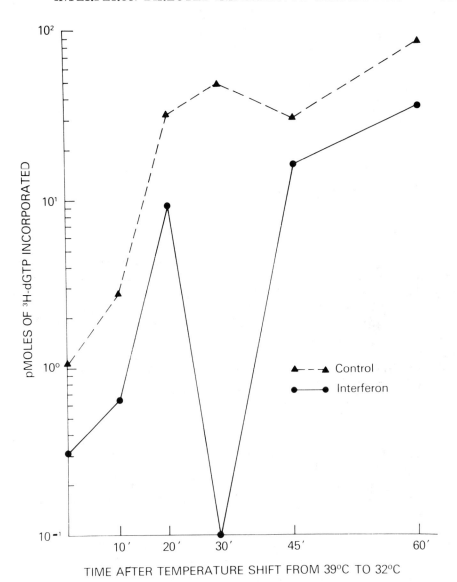

FIG. 4. Ts-3-infected TB cells were incubated at 39.5°C and treated with 100 units/ml of interferon when monolayer reached 70 to 75% confluency. After 26 hr of interferon treatment, the medium was changed and the temperature shifted from 39.5°C to 34°C. At the indicated time intervals culture fluids were collected. Reverse transcriptase assay was performed as described in "Methods and Materials." The values reported for enzyme activity at each time point represent the amount of virus released since the previous collection.

however, instead of following parallel courses throughout the time period, virus production in the interferon-treated cultures regularly dropped off markedly about 30 min after temperature reversal. This finding has consistently been seen in five experiments.

The interpretation of this experiment is difficult but could reasonably be made as follows. The interferon-sensitive locus is unlikely to be after the ts-3 site because, if it were, the virus production in the interferon-treated cultures would not resume following a temperature downshift. On the other hand, the discontinuous production of virus observed in interferon-treated cultures (Fig. 4) suggests that the interferon-sensitive locus is before or, possibly, is the same as the ts-3 site.

SUMMARY

Production of murine leukemia viruses (MLV) is inhibited in interferon-treated mouse fibroblast cultures; however, intracellular concentrations of viral p30 (gs) antigen and viral reverse transcriptase are not decreased, and in the case of the p30 antigen are actually increased. These findings are due to an inhibition of virus release from the cell surface into the extracellular fluid, a phenomenon which was assayed by scanning electron microscopy. Studies with a late temperature-sensitive mutant of murine leukemia virus have been useful in helping to define the genetic locus of the interferon-induced inhibition.

REFERENCES

1. Horvath, A. E., and Friedman, R. M. (1971): Nucleic acid and proteins isolated from a strain of murine sarcoma virus (MSV-O). Proc. Soc. Exp. Biol. Med., 137:1075-1081.
2. Billiau, A., Sobis, H., and De Somer, P. (1973): Influence of interferon in virus particle formation in different oncornavirus carrier cell lines. Int. J. Cancer, 12:646-653.
3. Friedman, R. M., and Ramseur, J. M. (1974): Inhibition of murine leukemia virus production in chronically infected AKR cells: A novel effect of interferon. Proc. Natl. Acad. Sci. (U.S.A.), 71:3542-3544.
4. Pitha, P. M., Rowe, W. P., and Oxman, M. N. (1976): Effect of interferon on exogenous, endogenous, and chronic murine leukemia virus infection. Virology (in press).
5. Ball, J. K., McCarter, J. A., and Sunderland, S. M. (1973): Evidence for helper independent murine sarcoma virus. I. Segregation of replication-defective and transformation-defective viruses. Virology, 56:268-284.
6. Ogburn, C. A., and Paucker, K. (1973): Purification of mouse interferon by affinity chromatography on anti-interferon globin-sepharose. J. Immunol., 11:1206-1218.
7. Scolnick, E. M., Parks, W. P., and Livingston, D. M. (1972): Radioimmunoassay of mammalian type C viral proteins. I. Species specific reactions of murine and feline viruses. J. Immunol., 109:570-577.

8. Anderson, T. F. (1951): Techniques for the preservation of three dimensional structure in preparing specimens for the electron microscope. Trans. N. Y. Acad. Sci., 13:130-134.

9. Wong, P. K. Y., and McCarter, J. A. (1974): Studies of two temperature-sensitive mutants of Moloney murine leukemia virus. Virology, 58:396-408.

10. Green, M., and Gerard, G. F. (1974): RNA-directed DNA polymerase — properties and function in oncogenic RNA viruses and tumors. Prog. Nucleic Acid Res. Mol. Biol., 14:187-334.

11. Levy, J. A. (1973): Xenotropic viruses: Murine leukemia viruses associated with NIH Swiss, NZB, and other mouse strains. Science, 182:1151-1153.

*Control of Neoplasia by Modulation
of the Immune System,* edited by
M. A. Chirigos. Raven Press, New
York 1977.

EFFECT OF INTERFERON ON EXOGENOUS, ENDOGENOUS, AND CHRONIC MURINE LEUKEMIA VIRUS INFECTION

*Paula M. Pitha and **Wallace P. Rowe

*Oncology Center, The Johns Hopkins University School of Medicine,
Baltimore, Maryland 21205, and **Laboratory of Viral Diseases, National
Institute of Allergy and Infectious Diseases, National Institutes of Health,
Bethesda, Maryland 20014

INTRODUCTION

It is generally believed that interferon inhibits the multiplication of oncogenic viruses and blocks virus-induced cell transformation by interfering
with the expression of nonintegrated viral genes.

In the present work, we examined whether the ability of the interferon
system to recognize the exogenous viral genome, but not the integrated one,
which was observed with Simian virus 40 (SV40) (1), applies also to murine
leukemia virus (MLV). It has previously been shown that both replication
and cellular transformation caused by MLV and murine sarcoma virus (MSV)
are inhibited in cells pretreated with interferon (2-5). However, in those
studies, virus replication was not measured under single-cycle conditions, and
the involvement of helper viruses (6) makes the systems examined too complex to permit this question to be answered unambiguously. Furthermore,
these studies were performed with unpurified interferon, and thus the observed effects might have been due to inhibition of cellular metabolism rather
than to the direct antiviral action of interferon, since the efficiency of infection in this system is dependent on the competence of the cell to synthesize
DNA and to undergo mitosis (7).

The availability of highly purified mouse interferon (5×10^7 units/mg of
protein) (8), and the existence of virus-free AKR mouse embryo cell lines in
which the MLV genome is part of the cell genome and can be induced by
IdUrd treatment (9), enabled us to study the effect of interferon on acute
exogenous virus infection, on the induction of the integrated viral genome,
and on persistent infection in a single virus cell system. The results reported
here indicate that interferon produces a temporary inhibition of the replication of both exogenous and endogenous MLV. However, in contrast to the

361

effect of interferon observed in other virus-cell systems, the inhibition of MLV replication is not due to a general inhibition of viral protein synthesis, but rather to interference with some later step(s) in the virus growth cycle. The results of these studies have been presented in detail elsewhere (14).

MATERIALS AND METHODS

Cells and viruses. The virus-negative AKR mouse embryo cell line, AKR-2B (9), the SC-1 mouse cell line (10), primary NIH Swiss mouse embryo cells, and XC cells (11, 16) were grown in Eagle's minimal essential medium with 10% heated fetal bovine serum (FBS). Chronically infected AKR cells were obtained by infecting virus-negative AKR-2B cells with AKR-L1 virus; at the time when infection was well established (third passage), virus titer of the culture fluid was 1.5×10^6 pfu/ml.

The AKR-L1 virus was isolated from a spontaneously leukemic AKR mouse (12) and adapted to growth in tissue culture; the titer was 10^7 pfu/ml in SC-1 cells.

Assay of infectious virus. Titrations of cell-free virus were done with the SC-1 mouse cell line using the standard XC plaque procedure (11). For quantitation of cells which became virus producers at various times following exogenous infection or IdUrd induction, the UV-ME test was used (13, 14).

Induction of endogenous virus from AKR-2B cells. AKR-2B cells were induced with IdUrd, as previously described (8, 9, 15).

Assay for group-specific (gs) antigens. Cells were stained for gs antigens utilizing the direct immunofluorescence test, or p30 antigens were determined by radioimmunoassay by Dr. W. D. Parks.

Virion-associated reverse transcriptase. The virion-associated reverse transcriptase activity of supernatant fluids was measured as described previously (15).

Interferon. Interferon, a generous gift of Dr. K. Paucker, was prepared and purified as described (8); the preparation used had a specific activity 5×10^7 units/mg of protein.

RESULTS AND DISCUSSION

Our results indicate that, in the case of AKR leukemia virus, exogenous, IdUrd-induced endogenous and chronic MLV infections are all comparably sensitive to interferon. The patterns of results observed with these three types of infection are summarized in Table 1. With all three infections, the amount of infectious virus in culture fluids was markedly reduced by interferon, and the effect was temporary. Thus, the MLV infection or induction by IdUrd was not aborted in interferon-treated cells; when the antiviral effect decayed, MLV production commenced.

In general, there was no difference in the effect of interferon on the acute exogenous and endogenous infection. There was proportionate reduction in the virus infectivity and reverse transcriptase activity in culture fluids. The fact that the number of virus-producing cells after exogenous infection or

TABLE 1. The effect of interferon on MLV infection

	Degree of inhibition by interferon [a]			
	Acute exogenous infection	Induction of endogenous virus	Chronic infection	Chronic infection (literature)
Culture fluids				
Infectious virus	++	++	++	++
Virus particles [b]	++	++	+	++ [c,d]
Cells				
Cells producing infectious virus (UV-resistant infectious centers)	++	++		
Virus particles [e]	++		-	- [d]
gs antigen (p30)	-	-	-	- [c]

[a] ++ = > 100-fold inhibition; + = 2- to 10-fold inhibition; - = less than 2-fold inhibition.

[b] By reverse transcriptase activity.

[c] Friedman and Ramseur (18).

[d] By ^{3}H-uridine incorporation; Billiau et al. (19); van Griensven et al. (21).

[e] By electron microscopy.

IdUrd induction was reduced, as well as the quantity of released virus, indicates that interferon not only prevents the virus release from infected cells, but blocks virus replication at a point prior to the assembly of infectious virions. Although the interferon in these two infections produced a general inhibition of formation of virus particles, it appeared to have little effect on the synthesis of gs antigen. Under the conditions where virion production was inhibited 20- to 600-fold, gs antigen synthesis was reduced less than two-fold. These observations indicate that the inhibition of MLV production by interferon is not due to an overall inhibition of synthesis of virus-specific proteins, but represents a block in virus maturation.

Interferon treatment also inhibited the production of infectious MLV by chronically infected AKR-2B cells. However, the nature of the interferon effect on the late stages of virus synthesis in the chronically infected cells may not be identical in all respects to that on the acute infections. In this case, we observed a disproportionate decrease in infectivity (100-fold), as compared to production of virus particles (as measured by reverse transcriptase activity and by electron microscopy, two- to eightfold) in culture fluids.

Thus, in this system, in contrast to its action on most other viruses, interferon does not block MLV-specific protein synthesis or prevent the establishment of infection either by exogenous MLV or following IdUrd-induced activation of the endogenous genome. Rather, in these systems, interferon appears to inhibit some later step(s) in the virus replicative cycle involving the assembly of infectious virions.

The failure of interferon to inhibit the establishment of MLV infection by exogenous virus indicates that there is no interferon-sensitive step required for the synthesis of the DNA (provirus) copy of the MLV genome, or for the integration of the provirus into the cellular genome. Furthermore, the failure of interferon to block gs (p30) antigen synthesis in chronic infection and following IdUrd induction of the endogenous AKR-MLV genome indicates that the transcription of at least a portion of the integrated provirus into mRNA and the translation of that mRNA into protein is not affected by interferon treatment. It is possible, however, that interferon does block the transcription or translation of other portions of the provirus genome, and that the inhibition of virus production observed in interferon-treated cells results from the absence of one or more viral proteins other than p30.

The observations on chronic infection are somewhat at variance with other reported studies (Table 1). Friedman and Ramseur found that in interferon-treated AKR-2B cells chronically infected with AKR virus, there is a marked inhibition of virus production and a simultaneous accumulation of viral p30 protein in the cells; however, there was no disproportion between ineffectivity and reverse transcriptase activity in these experiments. On the other hand, Billiau et al. (19,20) found that in both JLSV5 cells (cells derived from the spleen and thymus of Balb/c mice and chronically infected with Rauscher MLV) and in C3H mouse embryo cells chronically infected with Kirsten MSV, interferon inhibited virus production without altering the number of cell-associated virus particles; they interpreted these findings as indicating that the effect of interferon was not on maturation, but on release of virus from the cell surface. Our data are most compatible with the report of van Griensven et al. (21), who found that interferon treatment of JLSV5 cells led to the production of incomplete virions lacking part of the MLV genome. Some of the discrepancies in the results obtained in these MLV and MSV cell systems may be related to differences in the interferon preparations used, in the virus-cell systems studied, or in experimental design.

Although the exact mechanism of interferon's antiviral action is still unclear, studies with viruses other than oncornaviruses have consistently shown that when interferon inhibits virus replication, it inhibits the synthesis of all detectable virus-specific proteins (22-24). Thus, the transcription of at least a portion of the integrated provirus into mRNA and its translation to gs antigens (p30) in interferon-treated cells is in sharp contrast to results obtained in other virus systems. The possibility that some other portion of the provirus genome is not transcribed or translated in interferon-treated cells cannot be completely eliminated; however, this would require postulating polycistronic transcription or translation of the viral genome, in which one cistron is sensitive to interferon, whereas another is resistant. Thus, our findings are difficult to interpret in terms of current models of interferon effect (e.g., general inhibition of translation or transcription of viral genomes), and suggest a unique mode of interferon action in this system.

Finally, it should be pointed out that it is conceivable that the interferon effect observed does not involve only inhibition of viral genome expression, through the synthesis of an antiviral protein. Interferon could also be affecting cell physiology, such as altering cell membrane properties which then may interfere with the complex process of viral assembly. It has been recently shown by several laboratories (25-27) that high concentrations of interferon can affect growth of both normal and tumor cells, affect cloning efficiency of these cells, and change the expression of the H-2 antigens on mouse lymphocytes. All these effects could be explained by direct modification of the cell surface by interferon. It is, therefore, conceivable that the observed inhibition in virus assembly or maturation reflects changes in the properties of plasma membranes caused by interferon which are so small or so slow that they have not been observed by other means as yet.

SUMMARY

The effect of purified mouse interferon on the replication of AKR MLV in a clonal line of AKR cells was studied, with emphasis on comparing the effect of interferon on the replication of exogenous virus, activation of endogenous virus by IdUrd, and production of virus by chronically infected cells. It was found that interferon inhibited replication of virus in all three systems. Interferon did not abort exogenous infection or virus induction by IdUrd, but only delayed appearance of infectious virus. Virus production by chronically infected cells was also suppressed in the presence of interferon; however, after removal of interferon, rapid recovery of virus production occurred. Under conditions where interferon treatment inhibited virus yield, as measured both by infectious virus and virion-associated reverse transcriptase activity, no significant inhibition of synthesis of virus-specific (gs) antigen was observed.

These results indicate that, unlike its effect on the majority of lytic viruses, interferon does not inhibit MLV by a general inhibition of viral protein synthesis; rather, it appears to inhibit one or more of the later steps in MLV replication which occur after the expression of viral gs antigen.

REFERENCES

1. Oxman, M. N. (1973): Interferon, tumors and tumor viruses. In: Interferons and Interferon Inducers, edited by N. B. Finter, pp. 391-480. North Holland Publishing Co., Amsterdam, London.
2. Fitzgerald, G. R. (1969): The effect of interferon on focus formation and yield of murine sarcoma virus in vitro. Proc. Soc. Exp. Biol. Med., 130:960-965.
3. Sarma, P. S., Shiu, G., Baron, S., and Huebner, R. J. (1969): Inhibitory effect of interferon on murine sarcoma and leukemia virus infection in vitro. Nature, 223:845-846.

4. Peries, J., Canivet, M., Guillemain, B., and Boiron, M. (1968):
    Inhibitory effect of interferon preparations on the development of foci of
    altered cells induced in vitro by mouse sarcoma virus. J. Gen. Virol.,
    3:465-468.

5. Gresser, I., Coppy, J., Fontaine-Brouty-Boye, D., and Falcoff, R.
    (1967): Interferon and murine leukemia. Efficacy of interferon prepara-
    tions administered after inoculation of Friend virus. Nature, 215:174-
    175.

6. Hartley, J. W., and Rowe, W. P. (1966): Production of altered foci in
    tissue culture by defective Moloney sarcoma virus particles. Proc.
    Natl. Acad. Sci. (U.S.A.), 55:780-786.

7. Temin, H. M. (1969): Studies on carcinogenesis by avian sarcoma
    viruses; requirement for new DNA synthesis and for cell division.
    J. Cell. Physiol., 69:53-64.

8. Ogburn, C. A., Berg, K., and Paucker, K. (1973): Purification of
    mouse interferon by affinity chromatography on anti-interferon globulin
    sepharose. J. Immunol., 111:1206-1218.

9. Lowy, D. R., Rowe, W. P., Teich, N., and Hartley, J. W. (1971):
    Murine leukemia virus: High frequency activation in vitro by 5-iodeoxy-
    uridine and 5-bromodeoxyuridine. Science, 174:155-156.

10. Hartley, J. W., and Rowe, W. P. (1975): Clonal cell lines from a feral
    mouse embryo which lack host-range restrictions for murine leukemia
    virus. Virology, 65:128-134.

11. Rowe, W. P., Pugh, W. E., and Hartley, J. W. (1970): Plaque assay
    techniques for murine leukemia viruses. Virology, 42:1136-1139.

12. Hartley, J. W., Rowe, W. P., and Huebner, R. J. (1970): Host range
    restriction of murine leukemia viruses in mouse embryo cell cultures.
    J. Virol., 5:221-226.

13. Teich, N., Lowy, D. R., Hartley, J. W., and Rowe, W. P. (1973):
    Studies on the mechanism of induction of infectious murine leukemia
    virus from AKR mouse embryo cell lines by 5-iododeoxyuridine and
    5-bromodeoxyuridine. Virology, 51:163-173.

14. Pitha, P. M., Rowe, W. P., and Oxman, M. N. (1976): Effect of
    interferon on exogenous, endogenous and chronic murine leukemia virus
    infection. Virology, 70:324-338.

15. Pitha, P. M., Pitha, J., and Rowe, W. P. (1975): Lack of requirement
    of reverse transcriptase function for the activation of murine leukemia
    virus by halogenated pyrimidines. Virology, 63:568-572.

16. Svoboda, J., Chyle, P. P., Simkovic, D., and Hilgert, I. (1963):
    Demonstration of the absence of infectious Rous virus in rat tumor XC
    whose structurally intact cells produce Rous sarcoma virus when trans-
    ferred to chicks. Folia Biol. (Prague), 9:77-81.

17. Parks, W. P., and Scolnick, E. M. (1972): Radioimmunoassay of
    mammalian type C viral proteins; interspecies antigenic reactivities of
    the major internal polypeptide. Proc. Natl. Acad. Sci. (U.S.A.),
    69:1766-1770.

18. Friedman, R., and Ramseur, J. M. (1974): Inhibition of murine leukemia virus production in chronically infected AKR cells; a novel effect of interferon. Proc. Natl. Acad. Sci. (U.S.A.), 71:3542-3544.

19. Billiau, A., Edy, V. G., Sobis, H., and DeSommer, P. (1974): Influence of interferon on virus particle synthesis in oncornavirus carrier line. Evidence for a direct effect on particle release. Int. J. Cancer, 14:335-340.

20. Billiau, A., Sobis, H., and DeSommer, P. (1973): Influence of interferon on virus particle formation in different oncornavirus carrier cell lines. Int. J. Cancer, 12:646-653.

21. Van Griensven, L. J., Baudelaire, M. F., Peries, J., Emanoil-Ravicovitch, R., and Boiron, M. (1971): Studies on the biosynthesis of murine leukemia virus RNA. Some properties of Rauscher leukemia virus isolated from interferon treated JLSV cells. In: Lepetit Colloquia, Paris, pp. 143-145.

22. Metz, D. H., and Esteban, J. (1972): Interferon inhibits viral protein synthesis in L cells infected with vaccinia virus. Nature, 238:385-388.

23. Joklik, W. K., and Merigan, T. C. (1966): Concerning the mechanism of action of interferon. Proc. Natl. Acad. Sci. (U.S.A.), 56:558-565.

24. Jungwirth, C., Horak, I., Bodo, G., Lindner, J., and Schultze, B. (1972): The synthesis of poxvirus specific RNA in interferon treated cells. Virology, 48:59-70.

25. Gresser, I., Brouty-Boye, D., Thomas, M. T., and Macieira-Coelho, A. (1970): Interferon and cell division; inhibition of multiplication of mouse leukemia L1210 cells in vitro by interferon preparations. Proc. Natl. Acad. Sci. (U.S.A.), 66:1052-1053.

26. Lindahl-Magnusson, D., Leary, P., and Gresser, I. (1971): Interferon and cell division VI. Inhibitory effect of interferon on the multiplication of mouse embryo and mouse kidney cells in primary cultures. Proc. Soc. Exp. Biol. Med., 138:1044-1050.

27. Lindahl, P., Leary, P., and Gresser, I. (1973): Enhancement by interferon of the expression of surface antigens on murine leukemia L1210 cells. Proc. Natl. Acad. Sci. (U.S.A.), 70:2785-2788.

Control of Neoplasia by Modulation of the Immune System, edited by M. A. Chirigos. Raven Press, New York   1977.

EFFECTIVENESS OF EXOGENOUS MOUSE INTERFERON IN AKR LEUKEMIA

Julia P. Roboz, James F. Holland, and J. George Bekesi

Department of Neoplastic Diseases, Mount Sinai School of Medicine and Hospital of the City University of New York, New York, New York 10029

INTRODUCTION

We have previously reported partial success in the treatment of AKR leukemia-lymphoma with combined chemoimmunotherapy (1-3). Although the duration of remission in the treated mice depended on the modality of the therapy, relapse inevitably followed. Since the etiologic agent of the AKR leukemia is the Gross murine leukemia virus (4), the cause of the relapse is the reinduction of secondary lymphoma by the RNA virus which has not been eliminated in course of the therapy. In an attempt to eradicate the oncogenic virus in experimental animals, antiviral agents and interferon inducers have been applied in combination with or without cytoreductive therapy (3, 5-11). Although a certain degree of reduction of the viral titer was achieved by such combination therapy, the next logical step was to employ exogenous mouse interferon which has been shown to inhibit the multiplication and cellular transformation of many RNA viruses (12-18). We introduced interferon both prophylactically and therapeutically in various experimental protocols involving AKR mice. The MuLV titer, life-span, and changes in leukemic organ weights of the experimental animals were monitored.

MATERIALS AND METHODS

Animals

Eight- to twelve-week-old female AKR mice and female retired breeders of the AKR strain were supplied by Jackson Laboratories. The mice were kept in a room thermostatically controlled at 20 to 22°C and were allowed Purina Chow and tap water <u>ad libitum.</u>

Diagnosis of AKR Leukemia

Spontaneous leukemic AKR mice were selected from a colony of 3,500 to 4,000 female retired breeders. Clinical diagnosis of spontaneous leukemia was made with 95% accuracy by splenic and lymph node palpation, followed by leukocyte count. Animals were considered to be leukemic when their leukocyte counts were greater than $17,000/mm^3$ and had splenic and lymph node enlargement. At the time of diagnosis, the average splenic weight was 470 mg, the thymus 650 mg, and the leukocyte count $28,000/mm^3$. The normal spleen weight in nonleukemic AKR mice is 50 to 70 mg, and the normal thymus weight is 30 to 50 mg.

Production and Purification of Mouse Interferon

Interferon was produced at 20,000 units/ml in C-243 mouse tissue culture line infected with Newcastle disease virus (3). The culture fluid was centrifuged at 100,000 X g in a Beckman preparative ultracentrifuge for 2 hr at $4°C$ and concentrated approximately two and a half fold by an Amicon cell concentrator using a UM-2 membrane with an exclusion limit of 1,000 molecular weight. Twenty-five milliliters of the crude mouse interferon preparation (about 5×10^4 units/ml) were dialysed against 0.05 M sodium acetate buffer, pH 5.0, for 20 hr at $4°C$. Following dialysis, the sample was centrifuged and applied onto an Affi-Gel 202 (Bio Rad Laboratories) column (0.9 X 10 cm) which had been equilibrated for 24 hr with the same buffer (19). A flow rate of 17 ml/hr was maintained by means of an LKB peristaltic pump. After the breakthrough fraction the column was equilibrated with 0.02 M sodium phosphate buffer, pH 7.4. Finally, the column was eluted with 0.02 M sodium phosphate, 0.5 M sodium chloride buffer, pH 7.4. One-milliliter fractions were collected and were then assayed for both protein and interferon content.

Titration of Mouse Interferon

The titration of the purified interferon was performed by using L cells which had been cultured for 24 hr at $37°C$ in microtiter plates. Interferon samples were added in dilutions ranging from 1/10 to 1/500 in quadruplicate wells. After incubation for an additional 24 hr at $37°C$, the cultures were replaced with 10^{-6} dilution of the challenging vesicular stomatitis virus. The interferon titers were expressed as the reciprocal of the maximum dilution showing a 50% reduction of the cytopathic effect (CPE). The mouse interferon reference standard, indicated to have a titer of 12,000, had a titer of 9,000 by this method (20).

Prophylactic Therapy of MuLV-Infected AKR Mice with Purified Mouse Interferon

Eighty-five- to ninety-day-old female preleukemic AKR mice were randomized into four groups of 40 animals each. The control group received i.m. injections of mock interferon (0.4 mg of protein per injection) on the day of randomization and on days 3, 5, 7, and 9. Group 2 mice received 5×10^4 units of interferon, whereas group 4 mice were injected with 5×10^5 units of interferon per injection i.m. at the time of randomization and on days 3, 5, 7, and 9. In a second protocol, group 1 mice were treated with mock interferon i.m. at weekly intervals for 10 weeks plus two additional biweekly injections. The mice in group 2 received 2×10^5 units of interferon per injection at the same time sequence as the control group, totaling 2.4×10^6 units.

Interferon Therapy of Leukemic AKR Mice

For therapeutic evaluation of interferon, positively diagnosed spontaneous leukemic female AKR mice were used. The control group received i.m. injections of mock interferon on days 1, 2, 3, 4, 7, 10, and 15. Groups 2 and 3 were treated on the same days with 2×10^4 and 2×10^5 units of mouse interferon, respectively.

Determination of MuLV Titer

The MuLV titer in the pre- and postleukemic AKR mice were determined by obtaining a 2% extract of a short section (5 to 8 mm) of mouse tail from 10 individual animals in each group. The samples were obtained prior to the treatment, at the time of randomization, during the treatment, and at posttreatment periods. Each tail specimen was individually assayed as described by Rowe, Pugh, and Hartley (21). The MuLV titer is expressed per milliliter of 2% extract of a 5- to 8-mm section of AKR mouse tail.

RESULTS

Purification of Mouse Interferon

The crude mouse interferon was produced in C-243 mouse tissue line following infection with Newcastle disease virus (NDV). The preparation was subsequently subjected to affinity chromatographic purification using Affi-Gel 202. Figure 1 represents the affinity chromatography profile of mouse interferon. The breakthrough fraction (peak 1) represents about 98% of protein and less than 1% of interferon activity. The second peak, which was eluted with 0.02 M sodium phosphate, 0.5 M sodium chloride buffer, pH 7.4, contained 98% of the applied interferon. The specific activity of the purified interferon was 1.2×10^8 units/mg of protein. This relatively simple purification procedure resulted in 1,800- to 2,000-fold purification and a recovery of 95 to 99% of the applied crude mouse interferon.

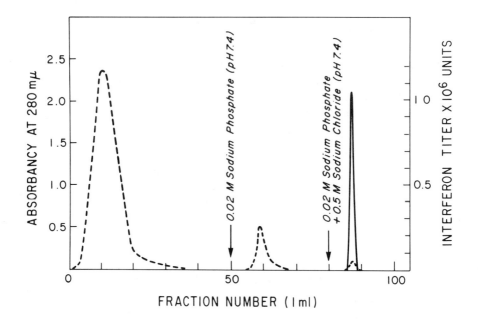

FIG. 1.   Purification of crude mouse interferon on an Affi-Gel 202 column.
Twenty-five milliliters of concentrated mouse interferon sample (5 X 10⁴
units/ml) were applied on Affi-Gel 202 column (0.9 X 10 cm) equilibrated
with 0.05 M sodium acetate buffer, pH 5.0.   The column was developed with
0.02 M sodium phosphate, pH 7.4, followed by a linear gradient of 0.02 M
sodium phosphate, 0.5 M sodium chloride, pH 7.4.   Protein — — — ;
interferon ——— .

Prophylactic Therapy of MuLV-Infected AKR Mice with Purified Mouse Interferon

Three-month-old female AKR mice were randomized into five groups of
40 animals each.   The effect of mouse interferon on MuLV in AKR mice was
tested by determining the viral titer prior to treatment and at 10, 30, and
80 days after the initiation of treatment.   For each time point the mean was
obtained from at least 10 individually assayed tail specimens in each experimental group using the XC focus-forming assay.   It is apparent from Figure
2 that there was no change in MuLV titer in experimental groups which received mock mouse interferon.   However, a profound effect was observed on
the viral titer of the group of animals which received 5 X 10⁵ or 5 X 10⁴ mouse
interferon.   Similar reduction of MuLV titer was observed when 2 X 10⁵ units
of interferon were injected at weekly intervals.   There was also a reduction
in the viral titer of animals receiving 5 X 10³ units of mouse interferon, but
to a lesser degree.   It is significant that the reduction of viral titer from
2,000 to less than 100 was not transient.   Animals tested 85 days after the
initiation of treatment showed no significant change in their viral titer as

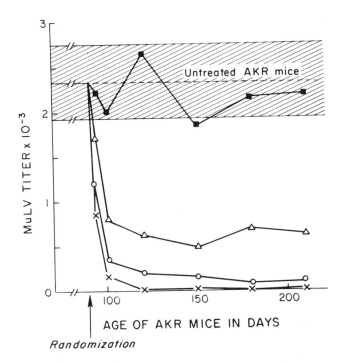

FIG. 2. Change of MuLV titer in preleukemic AKR mice after treatment with mouse interferon. Treatment of AKR mice was performed after randomization by injection of mock interferon or various dosages of interferon, i.p., on days 1, 3, 5, 7, and 9. MuLV titer is determined by the XC focus-forming assay and is expressed per milliliter of 2% extract of a short section of AKR mouse tails obtained from animals at days indicated. Mock interferon ━■━■━; interferon, 5 X 10^3 units X 5 ─△─△─; interferon, 5 X 10^4 X 5, ─○─○─; interferon, either 5 X 10^5 units on days 1, 3, 5, 7, and 9, or 2 X 10^5 units weekly X 9 and two biweekly injections (total dose 2.4 X 10^6 units) ─X─X─.

compared to the one obtained 4 days after initiation of the mouse interferon therapy. Figure 3 shows that the administration of mouse interferon in chronically infected preleukemic AKR mice had a direct effect on the appearance of primary spontaneous leukemia. The median life-span of AKR mice receiving mock interferon was about 36 weeks. At 47 weeks of age, only 10% of the animals remained alive in the control groups. All the animals in the control groups which died had primary lymphoma which was confirmed by autopsy, the average spleen weight being >400 mg and thymus >600 mg. Although the MuLV titer was drastically reduced in the group which received the highest concentration of mouse interferon (Fig. 2), animals still died at the same rate as the control group, but only 5 of 40 died of leukemia. The remaining animals showed marked signs of organ atrophy and wasting. In contrast, 50% of the animals which received 5 X 10^4 units of mouse interferon

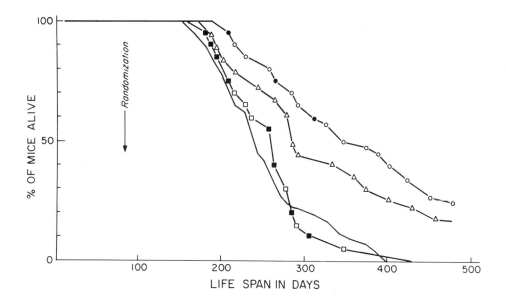

FIG. 3.   The effect of mouse interferon on the appearance of spontaneous leukemia in AKR mice.   Twelve-week-old preleukemic mice were random-ized into four groups of 20 mice each.   The control group received 2 mg of mock interferon injection on the day of randomization, then 3, 5, 7, and 9 days later ——; group 2 received 5×10^5 units of interferon at random-ization, then 3, 5, 7, and 9 days later —□—□—; group 3 received 5×10^4 units of interferon at randomization, then 3, 5, 7, and 9 days later —O—O—; group 4 received 5×10^3 units of interferon at randomization, then 3, 5, 7, and 9 days later —Δ—Δ—.   Open symbols, animals which died of tumor. Closed symbols, animals which died of organ atrophy.

were still alive at 48 weeks of age and only 2 animals of 8 which died showed any sign of organ atrophy.   Mouse interferon at 5×10^3 units also showed beneficial effect.

    In order to avoid organ atrophy and wasting of the treated animals which may be due to an overloading effect of the high dosage of mouse interferon administered within a short period of time, we have changed the frequency of treatment.   The injection schedules were changed from every second day to once a week, maintaining the same total dose of mouse interferon amounting to 2.4 to 2.5×10^6 units.   As shown in Fig. 4, with this treatment schedule organ atrophy and wasting were no longer apparent, but the appearance of primary lymphoma of AKR mice remained significantly delayed.

The Therapeutic Effectiveness of Purified Mouse Interferon

    As an extension of the prophylactic therapy of MuLV-infected AKR mice with interferon, we have examined whether or not interferon has antitumor activity in AKR mice diagnosed with spontaneous leukemia.   Leukemic AKR

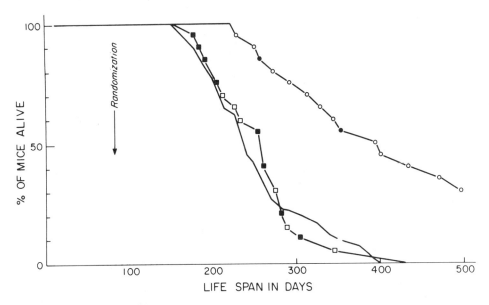

FIG. 4. Correlation between the frequency of interferon administration and its therapeutic efficacy in AKR mice. Twelve-week-old preleukemic mice were randomized into three groups of 20 mice each. The control group received 2 mg of mock interferon injection on the day of randomization, then 3, 5, 7, and 9 days later ———; group 2 mice were treated with 5 X 10^5 units of interferon at randomization, then 3, 5, 7, and 9 days later (total 2.5 X 10^6 units) —□—□—; group 3 mice were injected with 2 X 10^5 units of interferon at randomization then at weekly intervals X 9 plus two additional biweekly injections of interferon (total 2.4 X 10^6 units) —O—O—. Open symbols, animals which died of tumor. Closed symbols, animals which died of organ atrophy.

mice were randomized into three groups of 30 mice each. In group 1 each mouse was injected with 0.5 mg of mock interferon i.m. on days 1, 2, 3, 4, 7, 10, and 15. Groups 2 and 3 mice were injected with 2 X 10^4 or 2 X 10^5 units of interferon, respectively, on days 1, 2, 3, 4, 7, 10, and 15. The results of this study are summarized in Table 1. Interferon alone showed therapeutic value in the treatment of spontaneous leukemia in AKR mice. This effect appears to be dose related. There is greater reduction of the leukemic organ weights as well as a more prolonged survival duration of the animals which received 5 X 10^5 units of interferon per injection as compared to the control group or the group which was treated with 5 X 10^4 units of interferon.

TABLE 1. Increased survival time and reduction of tumor burden in leukemia AKR mice following multiple administration of exogenous mouse interferon

Treatment	Survival in days		Organ weight [a]			
			Thymus		Spleen	
	+SE	p [a]	mg	p [a]	mg	p [a]
Mock interferon	17.6 ± 2.4	—	475 ± 54	—	540 ± 51	—
2×10^4 units of interferon	24.4 ± 3.8	0.064	374 ± 60	0.19	335 ± 48	0.003
2×10^5 units of interferon	29.6 ± 5.2	0.018	335 ± 48	0.0032	255 ± 49	0.002

Group 1 mice received mock interferon; group 2 mice were treated with 2×10^4 mouse interferon; and group 3 mice were treated with 2×10^5 mouse interferon (i.m.) on days 1, 2, 3, 4, 7, 10, and 15.

[a] Significance between the group of AKR mice receiving mock interferon versus those treated with interferon.

DISCUSSION

The etiologic agent for spontaneous leukemia in AKR mice is the Gross leukemia virus (MuLV) (4). The effectiveness of purified mouse interferon was tested in an attempt to eradicate the virus in chronically infected AKR mice both in preleukemic stage and after positive diagnosis of the spontaneous disease. The viral titer was determined prior, during, and 10, 30, and 85 days after treatment with various dosages of purified mouse interferon. Based on the XC focus-forming assay utilizing mouse tail extracts, there was no change in the MuLV titer in experimental groups when the animals received saline or mock interferon. The viral titer was markedly decreased in animals which received interferon treatment, especially after multiple injections of 5×10^5 or 5×10^4 units interferon. The reduction of viral titer (2,000 to >100) was not a transient one, since the animals tested on day 85 showed no significant difference from their MuLV titer observed only 4 days after the initiation of the interferon therapy. The magnitude of MuLV titer reduction in AKR mice achieved by exogenous interferon is far greater than by combined cytoreductive therapy and virazole (ribavirin) with or without immunotherapy with syngeneic or allogeneic leukemic cells (1-3). There was a significant delay in the appearance of primary spontaneous leukemia in chronically infected AKR mice upon treatment with purified mouse interferon. The median life-span of the control group receiving mock interferon was 36 weeks. All control animals died of primary lymphoma, as confirmed by autopsy. AKR mice treated with the highest dose of interferon (five courses of 5×10^5 units of interferon) died at the same rate as animals given injections of mock interferon, but only 15 of 40 died of leukemia, the remaining ones showing marked signs of organ atrophy and wasting. However, 45% of the AKR mice treated with five doses of 5×10^4 units of interferon were still alive at 54 weeks of age, with only 8 animals of 22 which died showing any sign of organ atrophy.

Immunosuppressive side effects of higher dosage (5×10^5 units) of mouse interferon was effectively controlled when injection schedules were changed from every second day to once a week maintaining the same total dose of interferon. With the modified treatment schedule, wasting and organ atrophy of AKR mice were no longer apparent, MuLV titer was reduced from pretreatment level of 2.3×10^3 to 30, and the appearance of the primary spontaneous leukemia in AKR mice was significantly delayed. Thus, interferon when used under optimal conditions not only reduces the MuLV titer in the chronically infected AKR mice but also significantly delays the appearance of primary lymphoma.

Therapeutic and antiviral effect of mouse interferon was also demonstrated in AKR mice with spontaneous leukemia. Positively diagnosed leukemic mice treated with seven courses of 200,000 units of interferon had reduced leukemic organ weights, MuLV titers, and an increased life-span compared to those treated with mock interferon. The therapeutic effect of interferon was clearly dose related.

Our studies substantiate and further extend observations reported by several laboratories that interferon treatment appears to offer a certain degree of protection in animals infected with oncogenic viruses, and appears to inhibit the growth of some type of tumors (3, 8, 12–17, 22). Whether the increase in life span is due to the inhibitory effect of interferon on the leukemic proliferation alone, or whether it is the result of both cytocidal and antiviral activity is currently under investigation.

SUMMARY

Mouse interferon was produced in a C-243 mouse tissue culture line infected with Newcastle disease virus. Crude interferon was purified about 1,800- to 2,000-fold by the Affi-Gel 202 affinity chromatography technique. The specific activity of the purified interferon used for the preventive and therapeutic experiments in preleukemic and leukemic AKR mice was 1.2×10^8 units/mg of protein. Three-month-old preleukemic AKR mice were treated with saline, mock interferon, or various doses of purified mouse interferon. There was no change in the MuLV titer of AKR mice treated with saline or mock interferon. There was, however, a significant reduction in MuLV titers of 2,400 to less than 100 after multiple injections of 5×10^4 or 5×10^5 units of interferon. All mice treated with mock interferon developed spontaneous leukemia and at 12 months of age less than 10% remained alive. AKR mice treated with the highest concentration of interferon every second day showed reduced MuLV titer, but still died at the same rate as the control, not from leukemia, but from marked signs of wasting and organ atrophy. Changing the injection schedule of interferon treatment from every second day to once a week, maintaining the same total dose of interferon, produced no toxic side effects, reduced the MuLV titer, and significantly delayed the appearance of primary leukemia in AKR mice. Therapeutic and antiviral effect of mouse interferon alone was also demonstrated in AKR mice with spontaneous leukemia. The treatment resulted in a significant reduction of tumor load and substantial increase in the life-span of the treated leukemic AKR mice. Thus, exogenous mouse interferon, when used under optimal conditions, not only reduced the MuLV titer of the infected AKR mice and delayed the appearance of spontaneous leukemia but also exhibited both therapeutic and antiviral activity in diagnosed AKR mice with spontaneous leukemia.

ACKNOWLEDGMENTS

This work was supported in part by grant CA-1-5936-02 and NCI Special Cancer Virus Program Contract N01-CB-43879.

We thank Michael Ward for excellent technical assistance and Petra Mantia for the typing of this manuscript.

REFERENCES

1. Bekesi, J. G., and Holland, J. F. (1974): Combined chemotherapy and immunotherapy of transplantable and spontaneous murine leukemia in DBA/2 and AKR mice in investigation and stimulation of immunity in cancer patients. Recent Results Cancer Res., 47:357-369.

2. Bekesi, J. G., Roboz, J. P., Walter, L., and Holland, J. F. (1974): Stimulation of specific immunity against cancer by neuraminidase-treated tumor cells. Symposium on Neuraminidase. Behringwerke-Mitt., 55:309-321.

3. Bekesi, J. G., Roboz, J. P., Zimmerman, E., and Holland, J. F. (1976): Treatment of spontaneous leukemia in AKR mice with chemotherapy, immunotherapy, or interferon. Cancer Res., 36:631-639.

4. Gross, L. (1970): Mouse leukemia. In: Oncogenic Viruses, 24th ed., pp. 286-291. Pergamon Press, New York.

5. Pearson, J. W., Griffin, W., and Chirigos, M. A. (1969): Inhibition of sarcoma and leukemia viruses and a transplantable leukemia by a synthetic interferon inducer. Proc. Am. Assoc. Cancer Res., 10:68.

6. Sarma, P. S., Baron, S., Huebner, R. J., and Shiu, G. (1969): Inhibitory effect of a synthetic interferon inducer on murine sarcoma and leukemia virus infection in vitro. Nature, 224:604-605.

7. Meier, H., Myers, D. D., and Huebner, R. J. (1970): Statolon therapy of spontaneous viral-caused mouse tumors. Naturwissenschaften, 57(6):310.

8. Rhim, J. S., and Huebner, R. J. (1971): Comparison of the antitumor effect of interferon and interferon inducers. Proc. Soc. Exp. Biol. Med., 136(2):524-529.

9. Grossberg, S. E. (1972): The interferons and their inducers: Molecular and therapeutic considerations. N. Engl. J. Med., 287:122-128.

10. Kleinschmidt, W. J., Ellis, L. F., Van Frank, R. M., and Murphy, E. B. (1968): Interferon stimulation by a double stranded RNA of a mycophage of statolon preparations. Nature, 220:167-168.

11. Kleinschmidt, W. J., and Probst, G. W. (1962): The nature of statolon, an antiviral agent. Antibiot. Chemother., 12:298-309.

12. Sabashvill, M. K., and Furer, N. M. (1970): Effect of exogenous and endogenous interferons on the course of leukemia induced in mice by Friend virus. Antibiotiki, 15(1):52-55.

13. Gresser, I., Coppey, J., Fontaine-Brouty-Boye, D., Falcoff, E., Falcoff, R., Zagdela, F., Bourali, C., and Thomas, M. P. (1967): The effect of interferon preparations on Friend Leukemia in mice. In: Ciba Symposium on Interferon, edited by G. A. Wolstenholme and J. O'Connor, pp. 240-248. J. and A. Churchill, London.

14. Gresser, I., Falcoff, R., Fontaine-Brouty-Boye, D., Zagdela, F., Coppey, K., and Falcoff, E. (1967): Interferon and murine leukemia IV. Further studies on the efficacy of interferon preparations administered after inoculation of Friend virus. Proc. Soc. Exp. Biol. Med., 126:791-797.

15. Gresser, I., Fontaine-Brouty-Boye, D., Bourali, C., and Thomas, M. P. (1969): A comparison on the efficacy of endogenous, exogenous and combined endogenous-exogenous interferon in the treatment of mice infected with encephalomyocarditis virus. Proc. Soc. Exp. Biol. Med., 130:236-242.

16. Gresser, I., Maury, C., and Fontaine-Brouty-Boye, D. (1972): Mechanisms of the antitumor effect of interferon in mice. Nature, 239:167-168.

17. Rossi, G. B., Marchegiani, M., Matarese, G. P., and Gresser, I. (1975): Inhibitory effect of interferon on multiplication of Friend leukemia cells in vivo. J. Natl. Cancer Inst., 54:993-996.

18. Grossberg, S. E. (1973): The interferons and their inducers: Molecular and therapeutic considerations. N. Engl. J. Med., 287:13-19.

19. Davey, M. W., Sulkowski, E., and Carter, W. A. (1976): Purification and characterization of mouse interferon with novel affinity sorbents. J. Virol., 17:439-445.

20. Tilles, J. G., and Finland, M. (1968): Microassay for human and chick cell interferons. Appl. Microbiol., 16:1706-1707.

21. Rowe, W. P., Pugh, W. E., and Hartley, J. W. (1970): Plaque assay techniques for murine leukemia viruses. Virology, 42:1136-1139.

22. Carter, W. A., and De Clercq, E. (1974): Viral infection and host defense. Science, 186:1172-1178.

23. Gresser, I. (1972): Antitumor effects of interferon. Adv. Cancer Res., 16:97-140.

Control of Neoplasia by Modulation of the Immune System. edited by M. A. Chirigos. Raven Press, New York 1977.

SUPPRESSION OF ENDOGENOUS TYPE C RNA VIROGENE EXPRESSION IN MICE BY SEROTYPE-SPECIFIC VIRAL VACCINES: PROGRESS REPORT

*Robert J. Huebner, **Raymond V. Gilden, *William T. Lane, *Roy W. Trimmer, and *Paul R. Hill

*Laboratory of RNA Tumor Viruses, National Cancer Institute, Bethesda, Maryland 20014, and
**Flow Laboratories, Inc., Rockville, Maryland 20852

INTRODUCTION

High titers of virus in tissues of certain strains of crossbred and back-cross mice have been shown by Meier, Lilly, and Heiniger and their associates (1-3) to be correlated with relatively high incidences of spontaneous leukemias and other cancers occurring later in life. Should it be possible with serotype-specific viral vaccines or passive immunization to prevent naturally occurring cancers by suppressing specific endogenous virus expressions, the role of endogenous type C viruses as specific causes of spontaneous cancer would be established.

Viral vaccines and passively administered immunoglobulin (IgG) have been reported to successfully prevent leukemias in mice produced by horizontal transmission of Friend, Rauscher, Gross, and Kirsten leukemia viruses (4-8). In this chapter we report that administration of type-specific viral vaccines resulted in significant suppression of spontaneous type C virogene expressions in F_1's of normally high-virus-expressor crossbred mice. Successful prevention of spontaneous tumors would make feasible serious attempts to prevent cancers due not only to the endogenous viruses but perhaps also cancers induced by environmental carcinogens; in this context Whitmire and her associates described reductions of 3-methylcholanthrene (3MC)-induced sarcomas in C57BL mice immunized with low doses of live radiation leukemia virus (RADLV) (9,10).

MATERIALS, METHODS, AND PROCEDURES

Mice

AKR/J, C57L/J, and SWR/J mice were obtained from the Jackson Laboratory, Bar Harbor, Maine; the NIH Swiss mice from the National Institutes of Health; and the BALB/cCan mice from the Frederick Cancer Research Center (FCRC), Frederick, Maryland. F_1 progeny obtained by mating AKR males with C57L, SWR, NIH Swiss, and BALB/c females were selected because background information revealed quantitative correlations between natural type C virus expression early in life with high and low incidences of spontaneous leukemia and other cancers later in life (1, 2).

Vaccines

The Gross leukemia virus (GLV, passage A) used for preparation of inactivated vaccines was provided in 27th subculture by Dr. Janet Hartley of the National Institute of Allergy and Infectious Diseases. It was plaque purified and grown in NIH-3T3 mouse embryo cells. The vaccines produced by Flow, Inc. (Drs. R. Gilden and J. Olpin) and Electro-Nucleonics (Mr. John Lemp) represented 1,000-fold concentrate suspensions of clarified banded GLV inactivated with 1:1,000 final dilution formalin solution for approximately 6 days at 4° C and then frozen at N_2 temperatures. When it was found that the formalin vaccines contained small amounts of infectious virus, the formalin-treated vaccine preparations were further inactivated in the frozen state by ionizing radiation procedure[1] similar to that suggested by Dr. Jack Gruber, NCI (11). Subsequently Dr. George Shibley of the Frederick Cancer Research Center provided similar vaccine preparations which were inactivated by ionizing radiation only. The irradiated virus vaccines from each source were entirely comparable and interchangeable when used at optimum titers; no infectious virus was demonstrated in any of the irradiated products. In many of the preparations a final dilution of 0.05 M sodium citrate was added to help preserve intact virus particles (12). After inactivation by formalin and by ionizing radiation the vaccine potency remained stable in nitrogen storage for 6 months or more.

---

[1] Irradiation of the vaccine in frozen state in 2.0-ml vials was accomplished at the Armed Forces Radiobiology Research Institute, Bethesda, Maryland, through the courtesy of Major Fred C. Grey, Capt. Ronald Weitz, and Mr. Robert E. Carter. The procedure employed a 55 MeV, S band traveling wave electron linear accelerator (linac) using an electron beam with a nominal energy of 13 MeV at 5 m from the machine exit window. Total doses of 3×10^6 to 10^7 rads were given to samples frozen in dry ice or in N_2. Dosimetry measurements established that dose rates were $\pm 7\%$ of the center-fold dose. No radioactivation of the samples or vials was detected.

Potency of Vaccines

The potencies of the vaccine preparations were assayed before and after inactivation in two ways: (a) Aliquots of each batch were tested in the micro-titer complement fixation test for p30 antigen (13) before and after treatment with equal quantities of ether, the ether being exhausted in the cold before testing for p30. The most potent vaccines were those that before ether treatment gave CF titers of 1:128 to 1:256 and after treatment 1:2,048 or 1:4,096, thus establishing 8- to 32-fold release of p30 antigen and ensuring a high degree of viral particle integrity in each of the vaccine preparations used for immunization. Tests of aliquots of all vaccines selected for use revealed full retention of intact viral particles after formalin treatment and irradiation or after irradiation alone. (b) Viral envelope antigen titers were determined by complement fixation using vaccine-induced virus-neutralizing antisera from immunized weanling NIH Swiss mice (see below.)

Assays of Virus Expressions in Extracts of Tails of Mice

Tests for infectious virus in vaccinated and control mice were determined in the XC test by assays of 2% extracts of tail specimens for infectious virus at various intervals before and after immunization. The XC test of Klement et al. (14), later modified by Rowe et al. (15), utilizes the highly sensitive SC-1 wild mouse cell as the virus-permissive susceptible cell and the XC rat cell as the indicator cell; however, N- and B-type cells were also often used as susceptible cells in order to evaluate the relative sensitivity of the XC system. Standard positive N-type viruses were titrated as controls, thus helping to stabilize the sensitivity of the SC-1 and/or N-cells used in each test.

Tests for Neutralizing Antibody

Neutralizing antibody titers in sera of vaccinated and control mice were determined in the MSV focus reduction test (16) using MSV(GLV) and MSV(AKR) pseudotypes.

Vaccine Immunization Procedures

The active immunization vaccine studies were done in crossbred mice in which young females of the low-expressor strains (C57L, SWR, NIH Swiss, and BALB/c) were immunized three times at 14-day intervals with killed GLV or AKR virus vaccines, following which they were bred to AKR males. The pregnant mothers during midpregnancy, and the F_1 offspring at 10 days of age were challenged with concentrated live MSV(GLV) virus.[2] Both the live and killed immunizations were necessary in order to achieve significant long-term suppression of spontaneous virus in the tissues of the F_1 offspring.

TABLE 1. Representative log titers of ecotropic type C virus in tail extracts in F1 progeny of four categories of vaccinated and control crossbred mice

| Exp. no. | F1 cross | Vaccinated mice | | | | Exp. no. | Age (days) | Unvaccinated mice | | |
| | | Age (days) | No. of litters | Log titers | | | | No. of litters | Log titers | |
				Average	Range				Average	Range
876	SWR X AKR	41–58	12	$10^{1.9}$	$<10^{1.0}-10^{3.1}$	877	41–58	7	$>10^{4.6}$	$>10^{4.6}$
		309–321	3	$10^{4.1}$	$10^{3.9}-10^{4.4}$		309–321	2	$>10^{5.4}$	$>10^{5.4}$
045	C57L X AKR	30	9	$<10^{1.0}$	$<10^{1.0}$	046	30	7	$10^{4.2}$	$10^{4.1}-10^{4.6}$
		112–125	3	$10^{2.5}$	$10^{2.5}-10^{2.6}$		112–125	4	$10^{4.4}$	$10^{4.4}$
228	C57L X AKR	107–128	3	$10^{2.6}$	$10^{2.6}$	229	107–128	6	$>10^{4.6}$	$>10^{4.6}$
299	NIH X AKR	40	9	$10^{1.5}$	$10^{1.5}-10^{1.7}$	300	40	6	$10^{3.8}$	$10^{3.7}-10^{4.0}$
		80	2	$<10^{1.0}$	$<10^{1.0}$		80	2	$10^{4.9}$	$10^{4.9}$
259	BALB/c X AKR	76	10	$<10^{1.0}$	$<10^{1.0}$	260	76	8	$10^{2.8}$	$10^{1.5}-10^{4.1}$
		109–113	3	$10^{2.0}$	$10^{1.8}-10^{2.1}$		109–113	4	$10^{3.9}$	$10^{3.9}$

An additional procedure was added to the first experiment (#876, see Table 1). This procedure included five daily applications of 1% 3-methylcholanthrene on the skin of 5 litters each of both vaccinated and unvaccinated F_1 mice; the applications were given 4 weeks after the final immunization with live MSV(GLV). For additional details concerning the vaccine protocols see an earlier preliminary report (17).

RESULTS

The infectious virus titers in tail specimens of vaccinated and unvaccinated mice from four separate crossbred lines are shown in Table 1; the virus in each instance was shown to be ecotropic N-tropic AKR virus (18) and to be the product of the Akv-1 gene. Tails taken at 30 to 40 days generally contained less than $10^{1.0}$ or $10^{2.0}$ logs, whereas tail specimens of control mice at the same age averaged over $10^{4.0}$ logs. Since in many mice virus expressions seemed to be completely suppressed for long periods, some up to 80 days, it is possible that the vaccine effects were to totally suppress natural expressions of the Akv-1 gene in many normally positive cells; it is also possible that immune responses may have eliminated some cells which normally produce virus.

Comparative p30 virus expressions at 56 to 76 days postimmunization in spleens, thymuses, and tails in F_1 progeny of vaccinated and unvaccinated C57L X AKR mice are shown in Table 2. Virus titers were determined in the complement fixation test as well as in the XC infectious plaque test; both tests of each of the three tissues show significant differences in viral titers between vaccinated and control tissues. The virus expressions in the thymic tissue appeared to be lower than that found in tails and spleens.

Although the suppression of virus expression in tails, spleens, and thymuses at 40 to 50 days must be attributed to specific immune responses, all attempts to demonstrate antiviral (AKR) antibodies by complement fixing, viral neutralizing, and RIA[3] tests in the sera of the suppressed F_1 mice at 40 to 50 days were unsuccessful. The absence of antiviral antibodies may reflect complexes of viral antigen and antibody or this simply could be due to the low viral antigen levels in the tissues of the vaccinated mice; also, cell-mediated immune responses may have eliminated many if not most of the virus-producing cells in the F_1 mice.

---

[2] The live vaccine challenge, estimated to have sarcoma-inducing titers of 10^5 in normal newborn mice, did not produce sarcomas in any of the vaccinated pregnant females or in their progeny; all of a limited number of comparable unvaccinated control F_1's succumbed to sarcomas within 10 to 14 days after inoculations of MSV(GLV).

[3] The RIA tests were performed by Dr. James Ihle, Frederick Cancer Research Center.

TABLE 2. Virus expressions of individual spleens, thymuses, and tails in F_1 progeny of C57L X AKR mice at 56 to 76 days postimmunization

		Infectious virus titers[a]			
		Vaccinated		Controls	
Litter no.	Tissues	No. of plaques	Log titer	No. of plaques	Log titer
1	Spleen	1	$10^{1.0}$	440	$10^{3.6}$
	Thymus	4	$10^{1.6}$	87	$10^{2.9}$
	Tail	26	$10^{2.4}$	>1280	$>10^{4.1}$
2	Spleen	0	$<10^{1.0}$	>1280	$>10^{4.1}$
	Thymus	0	$<10^{1.0}$	65	$10^{2.8}$
	Tail	31	$10^{2.5}$	>1280	$>10^{4.1}$

Complement-fixing (CF) p30 antigen titers (reciprocal of final dilution)[b]

Litter no.	Tissues	Vaccinated Antigen titer	Controls Antigen titer
1	Spleen	<10	>80
	Thymus	<10	40
	Tail	10	>80
2	Spleen	<10	>80
	Thymus	<10	40
	Tail	10	>80

[a] In 10% extracts of specified tissues.

[b] Differences in twofold dilutions in CF corresponds approximately to single log difference in infectious virus log titers. Note: Tail specimens and spleens of controls express more virus than thymic tissues. CF tests represent reciprocal p30 antigen titers determined with use of standard MSV rat serum (R. Wilsnack, Huntingdon Research Center, Inc., Baltimore, Md.).

DISCUSSION

The significant suppression of endogenous type C oncornaviruses described in this and a previous report (17) suggests that immunological control of endogenous virogenes might well provide a feasible approach to the control or prevention of spontaneous cancer in mice and perhaps laboratory animals such as rats, hamsters, and cats known to have similar specific ecotropic type C viruses.

More recent extensions of these studies show that the combined killed and live vaccines provide equivalent suppression of virogenes in the progeny of AKR backcrosses to AKR males as well. This is fortunate since spontaneous tumors are known to occur earlier and more frequently in the AKR backcrosses than in F_1's. Also, previous studies of the C57L and BALB/c backcrosses to AKR mice by Meier and Lilly and their associates provided clear correlations between high and low virus titers early in life with correspondingly high or low incidences of cancer much later in life.

To date only the first experiment, #876, SWR X AKR (Table 1), has progressed sufficiently to provide a neoplastic incidence: Seven neoplasms occurred at 300 to 350 days of age in the unvaccinated group which received the 3MC application to the skin; these included 5 mice with lymphocytic leukemias, 1 with astrocytoma of the brain, and another with several adenomas of the lung. Leukemias were not observed by 350 days of age in the 3MC-treated vaccinated mice.[4] Although these differences in neoplastic incidences are interesting, they cannot at this point be regarded as more than that.

SUMMARY

Up to four logs of naturally expressed ecotropic type C virus were suppressed in the progeny of four different categories of normally high-virus-expressor crossbred mice following immunization with combined killed and live vaccines. Weanling females of low-expressor strains were immunized with radiation-inactivated banded GLV prior to pregnancy. Live Gross pseudotype sarcoma virus [MSV(GLV)] was given to the mothers during midpregnancy and to F_1 progeny at 10 days of age. Tests of tail extracts (2% w/v) taken from F_1 progeny at approximately 40 days of age showed natural viral titers generally exceeding 4.0 logs, whereas the vaccinated mice had viral titers varying from $< 10^{1.0}$ to $10^{2.0}$; at 100 to 300 days of age the latter still revealed virus titers significantly lower than the controls. Since previous natural history studies of crossbred mice have shown correlations between high and low virus expressions early in life with high and low incidences of leukemia and other cancers, reduced incidences of spontaneous cancer in the vaccine groups would not be unexpected.

---

[4] Tumor histopathology was performed by Dr. Bernard Sass, Microbiological Associates, Walkersville, Maryland.

REFERENCES

1. Meier, H., Taylor, B. A., Cherry, M., and Huebner, R. J. (1973):
   Host-gene control of type C RNA tumor virus expression and tumorigenesis in inbred mice. Proc. Natl. Acad. Sci. (U.S.A.), 70:1450-1455.
2. Lilly, F., Duran-Reynals, M., and Rowe, W. (1975): Correlation of
   early murine leukemia virus titer and H-2 type with spontaneous
   leukemia in mice of the BALB/c X AKR cross: A genetic analysis.
   J. Exp. Med., 141:882-889.
3. Heiniger, H. J., Huebner, R. J., and Meier, H. (1975): Effect of
   allelic substitutions at the hairless locus on endogenous ecotropic murine
   leukemia virus titers and leukemogenesis. J. Natl. Cancer Inst.
   (in press).
4. Friend, C., and Rossi, G. B. (1968): Transplantation immunity and the
   suppression of spleen colony formation by immunization with murine
   leukemia virus preparations (Friend). Int. J. Cancer, 3:523-529.
5. Fink, M. A., and Rauscher, F. J. (1964): Immune reactions to a
   murine leukemia virus. I. Induction of immunity to infection with virus
   in the natural host. J. Natl. Cancer Inst., 32:1075-1082.
6. Ioachim, H. L., Gimovsky, M. L., and Keller, S. E. (1973): Maternal
   vaccination with formalin-inactivated gross lymphoma virus in rats and
   transfer of immunity to offspring. Proc. Soc. Exp. Biol. Med.,
   144:376-379.
7. Kirsten, W. H., Stefanski, E., and Panem, S. (1974): Brief communication: An attenuated mouse leukemia virus. I. Origin and immunization. J. Natl. Cancer Inst., 52:983-985.
8. Hunsmann, G., Moennig, V., and Shaefer, W. (1975): Properties of
   mouse leukemia viruses. IX. Active and passive immunization of mice
   against Friend leukemia with isolated viral GP_{71} glycoprotein and its
   corresponding antiserum. Virology, 66:327-329.
9. Whitmire, C. E. (1973): Virus-chemical carcinogenesis: A possible
   viral immunological influence on 3-methylcholanthrene sarcoma
   induction. J. Natl. Cancer Inst., 51:473-478.
10. Lieberman, M., and Kaplan, H. S. (1959): Leukemogenic activity of
    filtrates from radiation-induced lymphoid tumors of mice. Science,
    130:387-388.
11. Gruber, J. (1970): Purification, concentration and inactivation of
    Venezuelan equine encephalitis virus. Appl. Microbiol., 20:427-432.
12. Moloney, J. B. (1960): Biological studies on a lymphoid-leukemia
    virus extracted from sarcoma 37. I. Origin and introductory
    investigations. J. Natl. Cancer Inst., 24:933-951.
13. Huebner, R. J., Rowe, W. P., Turner, H. C., and Lane, W. T.
    (1963): Specific adenovirus complement-fixing antigens in virus-free
    hamster and rat tumors. Proc. Natl. Acad. Sci. (U.S.A.), 50:379-389.
14. Klement, V., Rowe, W. P., Hartley, J. W., and Pugh, W. E. (1969):
    Mixed culture cytopathogenicity: A new test for growth of murine
    leukemia viruses in tissue culture. Proc. Natl. Acad. Sci. (U.S.A.),
    63:753-758.

15. Rowe, W. P., Pugh, W. E., and Hartley, J. W. (1970): Plaque assay techniques for murine leukemia viruses. Virology, 42:1136–1139.

16. Hartley, J. W., and Rowe, W. P. (1966): Production of altered cell foci in tissue culture by defective Moloney sarcoma virus particles. Proc. Natl. Acad. Sci. (U.S.A.), 55:780–786.

17. Huebner, R. J., Gilden, R. V., Lane, W. T., Toni, R., Trimmer, R. W., and Hill, P. R. (1975): Suppression of murine type C virogenes by type-specific oncornavirus vaccines. Prospects for prevention of cancer. Proc. Natl. Acad. Sci. (U.S.A.) (in press).

18. Chattopadhyay, S. K., Rowe, W. P., Teich, N. M., and Lowy, D. R. (1975): Definitive evidence that the murine C-type virus-inducing locus Akv-1 is viral genetic material. Proc. Natl. Acad. Sci. (U.S.A.), 72:906–910.

Control of Neoplasia by Modulation of the Immune System, edited by M. A. Chirigos. Raven Press, New York   1977.

EFFORTS TO CONTROL TYPE C VIRUS EXPRESSION IN WILD MICE

*Murray B. Gardner, **Vaclav Klement, *,[†]Brian E. Henderson, *John D. Estes, *Mary Dougherty, [††]John Casagrande, and [‡]Robert J. Huebner

*Department of Pathology, University of Southern California School of Medicine, Los Angeles, California 90033,
**Departments of Pediatrics and Microbiology, University of Southern California School of Medicine, Los Angeles, California 90033,
[†]University of Southern California Cancer Center, Los Angeles, California 90033,
[††]Department of Public Health, University of Southern California School of Medicine, Los Angeles, California 90033, and
[‡]Viral Carcinogenesis Branch, National Cancer Institute, Bethesda, Maryland 20014

INTRODUCTION

Most wild mice (Mus musculus) are resistant to cancer and show only a few lymphomas and tumors of other types after 2 years of age (1). Indigenous murine leukemia virus (MLV) expression is low in these mice except in those with lymphoma. However, wild mice from one particular trapping site in southern California, a squab farm near Lake Casitas (LC), have an earlier onset and an increased incidence of lymphoma with aging and show a high level throughout life of infectious (ecotropic) MLV expression (2). The major type C viral characteristics of LC wild mice are summarized in Table 1.

Although resembling AKR laboratory mice in terms of MLV infection early in life, presence of high-titered infectious virus in systemic distribution (3), and increased susceptibility to lymphoma, the LC wild mice differ in several important aspects. In LC mice the viruses constitute a new class of MLV (4), distinct in host range and envelope properties from AKR and other laboratory MLV strains. They replicate in B- rather than T-cell areas of the normal spleen (5), and the lymphomas arise from B- or "null"-cells rather than T-cells (6). The total cumulative incidence of lymphoma in LC

TABLE 1. Characteristics of LC wild mice

---

1. The high natural incidence of lymphoma is predictable by the high level of genetically determined ecotropic type C virus expression.
2. Type C virus causes lymphoma and, independently, a lower motor neuron disease.
3. In lymphoma-paralysis susceptible LC mice, infectious ecotropic virus is present early after birth and soon rises to high titers in viscera and sera. In resistant mice from other trapping areas, infectious virus expression is low, except in old mice with lymphoma.
4. In susceptible LC mice, a humoral immune to ecotropic virus is generally not detected, although general immune competence is probably normal.
5. The wild mouse viruses are a third major class of MLV characterized by a wide in vitro host range.
6. The ecotropic virus and associated diseases of LC mice can be controlled by genetic means.

---

mice is about 20% occurring from 12 to 35 months of age (7) as compared with >90% of T-cell lymphomas occurring by 12 months of age in AKR mice. Furthermore, the indigenous virus also causes a neurogenic type of lower limb paralysis in 11% of LC mice between 10 and 18 months of age (7,8), whereas this neurologic disease apparently does not occur in AKR mice. LC mice also develop an increased incidence of certain epithelial tumors in old age (7).

There appears to be an ineffective or deficient autogenous immune response to the indigenous MLV in LC mice although there is no evidence of a general defect in immune competence (9). As with all virus infections, many factors are involved in the host–virus interrelationship, obviating a 1:1 relationship of virus to disease, as evidenced by the observation that many LC mice, heavily infected with MLV, live long lives without developing lymphoma or paralysis (7). On the other hand, there is solid evidence (8,10) that the virus is the essential determinant of the lymphomatous and paralytic diseases to which LC mice show increased susceptibility. High levels of virus early in life clearly correlate with a predisposition to the paralytic disease (3). Although the LC mice are truly a feral outbred population and thus subject to considerable genetic variation (11), it is remarkable how stable these characteristics have remained over the past 5 years. Apparently these traits do not threaten the survival of these wild mice in their natural habitat and, under laboratory observation, the longevity of LC mice is, apart from lymphoma, paralysis, and epithelial tumors, comparable to other wild mice. LC mice, therefore, offer a unique and potentially informative naturally occurring animal model, perhaps more relevant to humans in this regard than are laboratory mice, for investigation of host-viral factors in the pathogenesis of cancer and paralysis and for attempts at disease prevention through antiviral measures. In this chapter we show that control of the LC MLV and related diseases is, indeed, possible by genetic means. A preliminary report of this observation has been made (12). We also show the futility of actively immunizing LC mice after the neonatal period with their indigenous virus. These findings indicate the necessity of suppressing MLV replication in LC mice by antiviral measures initiated either before or shortly after birth.

MATERIALS AND METHOD

Genetic Control of Type C Virus Expression in LC Wild Mice

Although the genetic control of type C virus and tumorigenesis has been well described (13-16) in crosses between high- and low-leukemia incidence strains of laboratory mice, this has not heretofore been done with wild mice. We therefore attempted to suppress LC virus expression by cross-breeding LC wild mice with the inbred laboratory mouse strain C57 B1/10 Snell (designated B10). The B10 mouse was selected because of its homozygosity for two nonlinked dominant alleles, $Fv-1^b$ and $MLv-1^b$, either of whose function might be expected to restrict virus expression in the hybrid progeny. Laboratory strains of MLV are classified according to their in vitro host range as N-, B-, or X (xeno)-tropic, depending on whether they grow preferentially in NIH Swiss or Balb/c embryo cells or replicate only in nonmurine cells (17, 18). B10 mice within the first year of life show a low incidence of both N- and B-tropic infectious virus (19) and also harbor an endogenous X-tropic viral genome (18). The virus isolates of LC wild mice have an unusually wide, so-called amphotropic, in vitro host range (4), duplicating that of the N-, B-, and X-tropic MLV laboratory strains. They are, however, N-tropic for murine cells; LC embryo cells in vitro are most susceptible to N-tropic virus. Thus, MLV activated or acquired before or shortly after birth can spread readily from cell to cell within individual LC mice (i.e., ecotropic behavior). The $Fv-1^b$ allele from the B10 parent should restrict the replication of N-tropic virus within the LC X B10 progeny (20), presumably by interfering with the integration or transcription of the proviral DNA (21). The $MLv-1^b$ allele, whose function is unknown, might restrict either N-, B-, or X-tropic expression in the progeny since this allele completely suppressed gs antigen expression in B10 crosses with the congenic resistant (58N) strain (22). In addition, B10 mice would contribute to the progeny the $H2^b$ allele which is unfavorable for leukemogenesis, presumably because of its association with an enhanced immune responsiveness (23).

Parental B10 mice, 6 months of age, were obtained from Jackson Laboratory, Bar Harbor, Maine, and reciprocally bred with newly trapped LC wild mice. Based on their weight of 10 to 15 g, the LC parental mice were estimated to be 4 to 6 months of age. The F_1 progeny were separated by sex at weanling age and raised in separate cages per individual litter. These mice were isolated for life-long observation from other wild mouse or rodent colonies. All ill, dead, or tumor-bearing mice were necropsied with microscopic examination and virologic study. The necropsy procedure and processing of tissues for histopathology and CF gs antigen testing have been reported (1, 2). The data on each mouse was coded, keypunched, and stored for computer analysis. Parental mice were splenectomized prior to breeding, and the segregated progeny from the various crosses were splenectomized at 6 to 8 weeks of age. All parental LC mice were positive and all parental B10 mice were negative for spleen gs antigen.

Spleen extracts (10%, w/v) were tested at 1:2 and 1:4 antigen dilutions for group-specific (gs) (p30) antigen by the complement-fixation (CF) test using a 1:20 dilution of rat sera pools (#30, #3490, #4918) prepared in Fisher rats bearing Moloney sarcoma virus (MSV) tumor transplants. The specificity of these sera was confirmed by comparison of CF reactions with guinea pig antisera to electrofocus-purified MLV p30 antigen (24).

For virus isolation, 0.1 ml of 10% tissue extracts (spleen, liver, tumor) frozen at $-70^\circ C$ for several weeks and previously tested for gs antigen by CF, and fresh 20% tail homogenates were assayed undiluted and at 10^{-1} dilution for induction of CF gs antigen (COMUL test) (25) on mouse (SC-1) and rabbit (SIRC) cells. SC-1 cells, kindly provided by Dr. J. Hartley (NIAID, NIH), are a cloned wild mouse embryo cell line which appear to lack both the $Fv-1^n$ and $Fv-1^b$ alleles and thus are equally susceptible to N-tropic and B-tropic viruses (26). SIRC cells are a rabbit cornea cell line (27) susceptible to the X-tropic viruses of laboratory mice and the amphotropic viruses from LC wild mice (4). Some of the cultures which were COMUL-negative at 21 days were blind-passed and retested after 42 days. Several of the virus isolates propagated in SC-1 cells were tested for their N- or B-tropism by infectivity titration (COMUL test) on NIH Swiss or Balb/c embryo cells.

Virus Immunization of LC Wild Mice

An indigenous type C virus (strain 292), isolated in NIH Swiss embryo cells from the pooled spinal cord extracts of three naturally paralyzed LC mice (8), was propagated in NIH Swiss embryo cells for use as a viral vaccine. The virus was purified and two vaccine preparations (#709 and #989) were made by Drs. R. Gilden and R. Toni at Flow Laboratories, Rockville, Maryland (28). The virus was treated at $4^\circ C$ for 72 hr with a 1:2,000 dilution of formalin; vaccine #709 was subsequently found to contain a small amount of residual live virus. The CF titer of these vaccines were, respectively, 1:32 and 1:128 untreated, and 1:256 and 1:1,024 after ether treatment. The vaccines were distributed in 2.0-ml quantities and stored in N_2.

Freshly trapped LC wild mice, weighing 5 to 15 g and assumed to average about 6 months of age, were inoculated intraperitoneally or intramuscularly with 0.25 ml of vaccine and 0.25 ml of complete Freund's adjuvant three or four times, 2 weeks apart. Other mice received 0.5 ml of vaccine without Freund's adjuvant, Freund's adjuvant alone, or saline diluent alone, by the same schedule. The mice were observed for 8 months and all were necropsied with microscopic study. For neutralization tests mice were prebled and rebled by retroorbital puncture 2 weeks after the final inoculation. The sera were diluted 1:5 in phosphate-buffered saline (PBS) and stored at $-20^\circ C$.

Attempts were also made to immunize LC mice by induction of regressing MSV sarcomas. Several pseudotype MSV sarcoma preparations were made with the LC strain 292 MLV (8) and with an immunologically closely related

MLV strain (1504E) (29) from another colony of wild mice. The MSV (292) and MSV (1504E) pseudotypes were prepared in vitro by rescue of the defective MSV genome from NRK cells nonproductively transformed by the Kirsten strain of MSV (30). The viruses titered $10^{3.8}$ to $10^{5.0}$ focus-forming units (FFU) per milliliter on NRK cells. LC mice of various ages, newborn to several weeks old, from our laboratory breeding colony, and young adults, newly trapped, were inoculated in the thigh muscle with 0.1 ml of virus at dilutions of 10^0 to 10^{-3}. Two or three repeat inoculations were given 2 weeks apart to many of the mice which failed to develop sarcomas following the initial inoculation. The mice were bled periodically by retroorbital puncture, the sera diluted 1:5 with PBS and stored at -20°C for neutralization tests. All mice were necropsied with microscopic study whether or not showing gross evidence of tumors.

The neutralization test (9) was a focus-reduction assay in which the MSV (292) virus, diluted to contain 30-60 FFU/0.2 ml, was mixed with an equal volume of serum dilution (after heating at 56°C for 30 min), incubated 1 hr at room temperature, and 0.4 ml of the mixture incubated per dish. This technique was also adapted to a semimicroassay (31) requiring only 0.025 or 0.05 ml of serum dilution. Reduction of the number of foci by ≥67% was considered as positive. As a positive control a goat antisera to 292 virus was used. This sera was furnished by Dr. R. Gilden and titered 1:640 in the MSV (292) neutralization test.

RESULTS

Genetic Control

The segregation of gs antigen expression in the different generations and crosses is shown in Table 2. In striking contrast to the high prevalence and titer of detectable spleen CF gs antigen in the LC parental (72.6% gs positive, 52.0% ≥ 1:4) and 6- to 8-week-old LC mice born in the laboratory (60.0% gs positive, 33.7% ≥ 1:4), there was an almost complete absence of detectable spleen gs antigen in the 4- to 6-week-old reciprocal B10 X LC F_1 hybrids (1.4% gs positive) and in the reciprocal F_1 and F_2 B10 backcrosses (2.1% gs positive). The negligible occurrence of detectable gs antigen at weanling age in the F_1 and B10 backcross progeny indicated a strongly dominant negative effect on this form of viral expression. This suppression of gs antigen appeared to be fairly long-lasting since this antigen was not detected by CF in 10% liver extracts from 23 F_1 hybrids and 93 F_1 backcross to B10 progeny observed an average of 7 months (range 3 to 10 months).

In the F_2 generation spleen gs antigen was found with an average of 9.6% (range 3.5 to 16.1% in the four reciprocal crosses) and, in the F_1 backcross to LC mice spleen gs antigen was found with an average of 28.1%. Although suggestive of a two-gene suppressive effect on gs antigen expression which would have predicted 7% gs antigen positive in the F_2 generation and 25% gs antigen positive in the LC backcross progeny, this is still open to question.

TABLE 2. Type C virus expression in crosses between LC wild mice and B10 inbred mice

Generation or cross	Spleen gs antigen (CF)[a]				Virus isolation[b]	
	1:2	Percent	≥1:4	Percent	Spleen gs positive	Spleen gs negative
Parental strains						
B10	0/97[c]		0/97			2/15
LC	239/329	72.6	171/329	52.0	7/9	
F1 generation[d]	2/164	1.4	0/164		1/4	1/20
F2 generation[d]	49/597	9.6	14/597	2.9	1/23	0/34
F1,2 backcross to B10[d]	6/288	2.1	3/288	1.2	1/6	0/14
F1 backcross to LC[d]	84/299	28.1	43/299	14.4	13/19	0/11
F1 laboratory bred LC X LC	57/95	60.0	32/95	33.7	3/4	

[a] Spleens were removed from parental LC and B10 mice at 4 to 6 months of age and from progeny mice at 6 to 8 weeks of age. Ten percent extracts were tested by CF at 1:2 and 1:4 antigen dilution with a 1:20 dilution of rat sera pools (MSV 30, 3490, 4918) prepared in Fisher rats bearing Moloney sarcoma virus tumor transplants. The specificity of these sera was confirmed by comparison with guinea pig antisera to electrofocus-purified MLV p30 antigen.

[b] Virus isolation was done on either 10% spleen extracts collected at 6 to 8 weeks of age and stored at -70°C for several months or on fresh 20% tail homogenates collected at 6 to 12 months of age, not necessarily from the same individual mice. 0.1 ml of spleen extract or tail homogenate were assayed undiluted for induction of CF gs (p30) antigen after 21 days (COMUL test) on wild mouse SC-1 and rabbit SIRC cells.

[c] Number positive/number tested.

[d] Figures are pooled for the different reciprocal matings making up each of these crosses.

A greater prevalence of spleen gs antigen was observed in backcross matings with LC females as compared with LC males (average 40.9 vs. 22.3%).

Virus was recovered in both SC-1 and SIRC cells from most of the gs positive spleens and tails (23 of 31) tested from the parental and laboratory bred LC mice and from the F_1 backcross to LC progeny (Table 2). By contrast, virus was recovered in only SC-1 cells from just 6 of 116 total assays from spleens and tails of parental B10 and F_1, F_2, and B10 backcross progeny, including a sample from those few mice in these groups whose spleen extracts were weakly positive (1:2) for CF gs antigen. In no instance was virus isolated on SIRC and not on SC-1 cells. Thus, infectious amphotropic virus was readily recovered from spleen or tail only of LC or backcross LC mice which had high-titered spleen gs antigen and none of the isolates were of the X-tropic class. Suppression of gs antigen expression in B10 X LC hybrids was clearly correlated with a suppression of infectious MLV production.

The frequency of spontaneous lymphomas and paralysis observed in parental and B10 X LC F_1 hybrids is shown in Table 3. Since our previous observations (7) showed that field-trapped LC mice do not begin to develop lymphoma or paralysis until about 12 months of age, i.e., after 6 months of laboratory observation, we calculated the frequency of lymphoma and paralysis in the parental and F_1 hybrid mice in terms of mouse-months of observation after reaching 12 months of age (assuming that mice caught in the field were 6 months of age). However, none of the parental or hybrid mice have yet reached beyond 2 years of age. In the parental LC mice this incidence was 15 lymphomas per 1,148 mouse-months (1.3%). By contrast, in the F_1 hybrids only 5 lymphomas were found per 1,449 mouse-months (0.3%), a statistically significant difference ($p = 0.01$). Similarly, in the F_1 and F_2 backcrosses to B10, no lymphomas have yet occurred despite 919 mouse-months of observation (data not shown). The paralytic disease has not been observed in any of the F_1 hybrids or $F_{1,2}$ backcrosses to B10. The average age at diagnosis of lymphoma in the parental LC mice was about 16 months, whereas in the F_1 hybrids the average age at lymphoma diagnosis was about 23 months. Apparently in the F_1 hybrids lymphoma has been significantly reduced in incidence and delayed in onset, and paralysis has been essentially eliminated.

Type C virus was isolated on SC-1 but not on SIRC cells from 3 of the 5 spontaneous lymphomas occurring in F_1 hybrid mice (Table 4). Virus was recovered only after blind passage on SC-1 cells, suggesting a much lower titer than that present in LC lymphomas. Two of these isolates appeared N-tropic, the other not yet determined. Each of the tumors from which virus was recovered was strongly positive ($\geq 1:8$) for CF gs antigen, and the two lymphomas yielding no virus were both negative for CF gs antigen. At weanling age none of these 5 tumor-bearing F_1 mice had had detectable spleen CF gs antigen. Interestingly, the two lymphomas from which virus was not isolated were distinctly different histopathologically from the typical LC lymphoma pattern. They were of histiocytic type and involved only liver and mesenteric lymph nodes. Two of the lymphomas, from which N-tropic virus was isolated, resembled LC lymphomas in being poorly differentiated and of more generalized distribution with leukemia. The remaining

TABLE 3. Incidence of spontaneous lymphoma and paralysis in parental and B10 X LC F$_1$ hybrids

Generation or cross [a]	Number lymphomas/number mouse-months of observation [b]	Percent		Number paralysis/number mouse-months of observation [b]	Percent
Parental strains					
B10	0/735			0/735	
LC	15/1148 [c]	1.3		6/1148 [d]	0.5
F$_1$ generation	5/1449 [e]	0.3	p = 0.01	0/1449	

[a] Parental B10 mice were splenectomized at 6 months of age. Parental LC mice were splenectomized soon after trapping. Their actual age was not known, but based on their weights of 10 to 15 g, they were estimated to be 4 to 6 months of age. F$_1$ mice were splenectomized at 6 to 8 weeks of age.

[b] After reaching 12 months of age.

[c] Average observation period at diagnosis 11 months; range 5 to 19 months.

[d] Average observation period at diagnosis 10 months; range 4 to 18 months.

[e] Average age at diagnosis 23 months; range 20 to 26 months.

TABLE 4. Type C virus expression in spontaneous lymphomas developing in B10 X LC F_1 hybrids

Cross	Mouse number	Sex	Age (months)	Lymphoma type [a]	Spleen CF gs antigen (1:2) 6-8 weeks	Tumor CF gs antigen at necropsy	Virus isolation [b]
(B10 X LC) F_1	9,365	Female	22	WD	Negative	Positive ($\geq$1:8)	Positive
	9,369	Female	23	PD	Negative	Positive ($\geq$1:8)	Positive (N-tropic)
	13,295	Female	18	H	Negative	Negative	Negative
(LC X B10) F_1	9,385	Male	19	PD	Negative	Positive ($\geq$1:8)	Positive (N-tropic)
	9,377	Female	24	H	Negative	Negative	Negative

[a] WD = well differentiated, involving only mesenteric lymph nodes and uterus; PD = poorly differentiated and general-ized, involving only mesenteric lymph nodes and uterus; H = histiocytic involving only liver and lymph nodes.

[b] COMUL assay on SC-1 and SIRC cells; virus was isolated only on SC-1 cells.

lymphoma was also different from the LC lymphomas in being better differentiated and confined to the mesenteric lymph nodes and uterus. Thus, of the
5 lymphomas in F_1 hybrids, only 2 appeared similar to the LC lymphomas in
their pathologic and virologic features.

Three epithelial tumors, a breast carcinoma, a lung adenoma, and an
adrenal adenoma have also been observed in F_1 hybrids, each from an LC
mother. These occurred after latent periods of 12, 27, and 25 months, respectively. Virus was not isolated from the breast tumor, the only one
tested. The breast tumor and adrenal adenoma were free of detectable CF
gs antigen, and all 3 mice were negative at weaning age for spleen CF gs
antigen. Among the parental LC mice, the only epithelial tumor observed so
far was a lung adenoma after a latent period of 15 months.

Virus Immunization

The lack of induction of specific viral neutralizing antibody or of lymphoma
and paralysis prevention following attempted immunization of young adult LC
mice with their indigenous MLV is shown in Table 5. MSV (292) neutralizing
antibody (>1:10) was not detected in 50 vaccinated or 18 control LC mice, and
neither lymphoma nor paralysis were abated. There was no histopathologic
evidence of glomerulonephritis or other immunogenic disease in the vaccine
recipients.

Attempts to immunize LC mice by induction of regressing MSV (292) or
MSV (1504E) sarcomas were also unsuccessful (Table 6). The incidence of
sarcomas was low (36%), even in young LC mice, the latent periods were
prolonged (6 to 8 weeks), the sarcomas inevitably progressively growing, and
lymphomas were often induced either alone or concomitant with sarcoma.
Neutralization of MSV (292) was found at a 1:10 serum dilution in only 2 of 38
sera tested from this group of mice.

DISCUSSION

Our findings show that control of type C virus expression and the related
diseases, lymphoma and paralysis, can be accomplished by genetic means in
wild mice. The suppression of gs antigen and infectious type C virus expression in the F_1 hybrids and B10 backcross progeny up to 24 months of age is
quite convincing and seems to be correlated during that time with a significant
reduction in the incidence of lymphoma and paralysis. Furthermore, most
of the lymphomas in the F_1 hybrids differed from LC lymphomas in their
gross and microscopic appearance and in their lack of high-titered N- or
amphotropic LC virus. Observation of these hybrid mice beyond 2 years of age
will show if this LC virus suppressive effect is long-lasting.

One precautionary note in the interpretation of the disease incidence data
is the possible influence of splenectomy at weaning age on susceptibility to
lymphoma and paralysis. We know that the spleen is a major site of virus
replication in young LC mice and that it is early involved in the pathogenesis
of the lymphomatous disease (2). Therefore, removing the spleens of hybrid

TABLE 5. Lack of lymphoma-paralysis prevention and of specific neutralizing antibody in LC wild mice actively immunized as young adults with indigenous type C virus

Treatment group	Number of mice in test [a]	Number of lymphomas	Average latent period (months)	Number paralysis	Average latent period (months)	Neutralizing antibody [b]
Formalinized virus [c]	198	7	7.0	4	8.0	0/50 [d]
Freund's adjuvant	197	7	6.4	4	7.1	0/8
Saline	219	7	7.1	4	6.8	0/10

[a] This includes mice surviving ≥3 months after inoculation. The mice were recently trapped and, based on a weight of 10 to 15 g, were assumed to be about 4 to 6 months of age. The experiment was terminated after 8 months.

[b] Serum, diluted 1:10, tested for MSV (292) focus reduction on NRK cells. Positive neutralization indicates ≥67% focus reduction.

[c] The vaccines, prepared by Dr. R. Gilden at Flow Laboratories, were formalin-treated virus strain (292), isolated from the pooled spinal cord extracts of three naturally paralyzed LC wild mice. Several different vaccine schedules were followed.

[d] Number positive/number tested.

TABLE 6. Attempts to immunize LC wild mice by induction of regressing MSV sarcomas[a]

Age	Number inoculated	Number of sarcomas[b]	Latent period	Number of lymphomas[c]	Latent period	Number of sarcomas and lymphomas[c]	Latent period	Neutralizing antibody[d]
NB — 2 weeks	70	12	6-8 weeks	7	3-7 months	13	1-8 months	1/27[e]
Young adult	62	6	6-8 weeks	1	4 months	3	2-4 months	1/11

[a] Mice were inoculated intramuscularly once or more with several different MSV (292) or MSV (1504E) virus preparations.

[b] All sarcomas were progressively growing.

[c] Lymphomas were generally of histiocytic type in liver and spleen and distinctly different from the naturally occurring lymphomas in older LC wild mice.

[d] Sera, diluted 1:10 and inactivated at 56°C for 30 min, were tested for MSV (292) focus reduction on NRK cells. Positive neutralization indicates ≥67% focus reduction.

[e] Number positive/number tested.

mice at 6 to 8 weeks of age may contribute a nongenetic factor to the reduction in lymphoma and paralysis. This would presumably not be as evident in the parental LC mice splenectomized after 4 months of age. To resolve this question we are currently following intact laboratory-bred parental and F_1 hybrid progeny, both of known age, into old age for virus expression and incidence of disease. For virus expression we have developed a new semi-microassay technique (31), which avoids splenectomy, by detecting and titering infectious virus in serum or tail clips based on induction of fluorescent foci in SC-1 cells.

The ratio of detectable spleen gs antigen in the reciprocal F_2 crosses (9.6%) and F_1 backcrosses to LC (23.3%) suggests a two-gene suppressive effect on virus expression which would predict 7% gs antigen positive in the F_2 generation and 25% gs antigen positive in the F_1 backcrosses to LC. However, the gene segregation analysis is clouded by the prominent maternal effect observed in the F_1 to LC backcross. The greater prevalence of spleen gs antigen found in backcross matings with LC females (average 40.9%) as compared with LC males (22.3%) suggests either a positive maternal influence on virus expression by epigenetic spread of virus to offspring from the heavily infected LC productive tract (3) and milk (32), or a negative maternal effect presumably from neutralizing antibody passed to their offspring by the viral-antigenically stimulated hybrid mothers (14). The absence of detectable infectious virus in almost all of the F_1 hybrids tested, and the inability to detect high-titered viral antibody in these mice by neutralization or radioimmunoassay (Dr. J. Ihle, personal communication) (although these tests are still quite preliminary), argue against a negative maternal effect, whereas the readily accomplished transmission of LC virus to foster-nursed susceptible laboratory mice (33) favors a positive LC maternal effect from the epigenetic transmission of milk-borne virus. Other evidence against maternal passage of viral neutralizing antibody is the lesser degree of litter variation in spleen gs antigen expression in backcross progeny of hybrid mothers as compared with backcross progeny of the LC mothers (data not shown). If maternal antibodies were suppressing virus expression, one might expect greater protection of later litters than of early litters, which was not seen. The natural maternal transmission of MLV by milk in some inbred lines of mice (19) and following experimental MLV inoculation of low-leukemia-incidence laboratory mice (34) has been well documented. However, Rowe and Hartley (14) and Lilly et al. (15) favored the alternative interpretation in their analysis of Balb/c X AKR F_1 backcrosses, namely a negative maternal influence, presumably antiviral antibody, in backcrosses with the hybrid mothers.

One major gene responsible for the suppression of LC virus in the B10 X LC hybrids must be the $Fv-1^b$ allele, since the Fv-1 locus has been shown to be the major determinant of virus expression and spontaneous leukemia in hybrids with AKR and other high-leukemia $Fv-1^n$ laboratory mouse strains (14,15). The mechanism of this protection is at the intracellular level, involving a block in replication and cell-to-cell spread of LC MLV (21). Whether or not the $MLv-1^b$, the $H2^b$ and closely associated immune response alleles or other as yet unidentified genes from B10 mice contribute to the suppression of virus and lymphoma in the LC hybrids and their mechanism of action will require a more extensive genetic analysis and further correlations among virus, immunologic status, and tumors in individual parental and progeny mice in the different segregating crosses. The H2^b type has been shown to exert a favorable influence on the occurrence of virus-induced lymphoma in laboratory mice (23), presumably by an effect on the immunologic defense mechanism rather than on early MLV expression. It will be interesting to see if there will also be any effect on the incidence of epithelial tumors in the aging hybrid mice and whether this can be related to an enhanced immune response to specific viral or tumor antigens.

Our total experience now shows that most LC mice are heavily infected with MLV shortly after birth (3) and lack, in adulthood, an effective immune response to this virus (9). This clearly accounts for our early failure to protect young adult LC mice against naturally occurring lymphoma or paralysis or to induce specific neutralizing antibody by active immunization with their indigenous MLV. Efforts to immunize LC mice by induction of regressing MSV pseudotype sarcomas in the first few weeks after birth were also unsuccessful. The low incidence and prolonged latent period of inducible MSV sarcomas might, as in AKR mice (35), have a genetic basis. The inevitably progressive growth of induced sarcomas, the frequent induction of lymphomas, and the lack of detectable neutralizing antibody are consistent with an unchecked proliferation of helper virus in the face of an ineffective immune response to this virus.

It should now be evident that effective attempts to control MLV expression in LC mice must be instituted before or no later than the neonatal period. Since the MLV replicates preferentially in the B- or humoral effector cell areas of the normal LC spleen, it is imperative that, for control of virus spread and ultimate disease, secondary infection of these cells must be limited until immunocompetence to this virus can possibly be achieved. With this purpose in mind we are currently attempting to protect LC mice by restricting MLV replication and, possibly, primary virogene expression in the newborn period using passive immunization with viral antisera (goat anti-292 immunoglobulin) until the mice reach an immunocompetent age when active viral immunization will be initiated. A better understanding of the natural history of this virus and of the opportunities for its control in wild mice will, hopefully, guide our approach toward the ultimate suppression of similar human diseases by exploitation of specific type C viral genetic or immune mechanisms.

SUMMARY

LC wild mice have a high incidence of spontaneous lymphoma and lower limb paralysis, both caused by a high level of type C virus infection present soon after birth. Virus was suppressed and lymphoma and paralysis largely prevented in the hybrid progeny of crosses between LC wild mice and C57 black 10 Snell (B10) inbred mice. The Fv-1^b allele from the B10 mice was probably one major gene responsible for this effect, although analysis of virus expression in segregating F$_2$ and LC backcross progeny suggested a suppressor effect from an additional gene(s). Attempts to actively immunize LC mice after the neonatal period with their indigenous murine leukemia virus and to prevent lymphoma and paralysis were not successful, apparently because of relative tolerance to this virus.

ACKNOWLEDGMENTS

We thank Mr. Angel Chiri and Mrs. Teresa Zavala for technical assistance, Mr. Michael Hejjas for preparation of data for computerization, and Miss Ann Dawson for preparation of the manuscript. The work described in this report was supported by contract number NO1 CP 53500 with the National Cancer Institute. This research involved animals maintained in animal care facilities fully accredited by the American Association for Accreditation of Laboratory Animal Care.

REFERENCES

1. Gardner, M. B., Henderson, B. E., Rongey, R. W., Estes, J. D., and Huebner, R. J. (1973): Spontaneous tumors of aging wild house mice. Incidence, pathology, and C-type virus expression. J. Natl. Cancer Inst., 50:719-734.
2. Gardner, M. B., Henderson, B. E., Estes, J. D., Menck, H., Parker, J. C., and Huebner, R. J. (1973): Unusually high incidence of spontaneous lymphomas in wild house mice. J. Natl. Cancer Inst., 50:1571-1579.
3. Gardner, M. B., Klement, V., Officer, J. E., McConahey, P., Estes, J. D., and Huebner, R. J. (1975): Type C virus expression in lymphoma-paralysis prone LC wild mice. J. Natl. Cancer Inst. (in press).
4. Rasheed, S., Gardner, M. B., and Chan, E. (1976): Amphotropic host range of naturally occurring wild mouse leukemia viruses. J. Virol., 19:13-18.
5. Brown, J. C. (1975): Unpublished observations.
6. Blankenhorn, E. P., Gardner, M. B., and Estes, J. D. (1975): Immunogenetics of a thymus antigen in lymphoma-prone and lymphoma-resistant colonies of wild mice. J. Natl. Cancer Inst., 54:665-672.
7. Gardner, M. B., Henderson, B. E., Estes, J. D., Rongey, R. W., Casagrande, J., Pike, M., and Huebner, R. J. (1976): The epidemiology and virology of C-type virus-associated hematological cancers and related diseases in wild mice. Cancer Res., 36:574-581.
8. Gardner, M. B., Henderson, B. E., Officer, J. E., Rongey, R. W., Parker, J. C., Oliver, C., Estes, J. D., and Huebner, R. J. (1973): A spontaneous lower motor neuron disease apparently caused by indigenous type-C RNA virus in wild mice. J. Natl. Cancer Inst., 51:1243-1254.
9. Klement, V., Gardner, M. B., Henderson, B. E., and Ihle, J. (1976): Inefficient humoral immune response of lymphoma-prone wild mice to persistent leukemia virus infection. J. Natl. Cancer Inst. (in press).

10. Henderson, B. E., Gardner, M. B., Gilden, R. V., Estes, J. D., and Huebner, R. J. (1974): Prevention of lower limb paralysis by neutralization of type-C RNA virus in wild mice. J. Natl. Cancer Inst., 53:1091-1092.

11. Lewontin, R. C. (1974): The Genetic Basis of Evolutionary Changes. Columbia University Press, New York.

12. Gardner, M. B., Klement, V., Henderson, B. E., Meier, H., Estes, J. D., and Huebner, R. J. (1976): Genetic control of type C virus of wild mice. Nature, 259:143-145.

13. Taylor, B. A., Meier, H., and Myers, D. D. (1971): Host-gene control of C-type RNA tumor virus: Inheritance of the group-specific antigen of murine leukemia virus. Proc. Natl. Acad. Sci. (U.S.A.), 68:3190-3194.

14. Rowe, W. P., and Hartley, J. W. (1972): Studies of genetic transmission of murine leukemia virus by AKR mice. II. Crosses with Fv-1^b strains of mice. J. Exp. Med., 136:1286-1301.

15. Lilly, F., Duran-Reynals, M. L., and Rowe, W. P. (1975): Correlation of early murine leukemia virus titer and H-2 type with spontaneous leukemia in mice of the BALB/c X AKR cross: A genetic analysis. J. Exp. Med., 141:882-889.

16. Meier, H., Taylor, B. A., Cherry, M., and Huebner, R. J. (1973): Host-gene control of type C RNA tumor virus expression and tumorigenesis in inbred mice: Highly predictable association between endogenous viral expression in early life and tumorigenesis with advancing age. Proc. Natl. Acad. Sci. (U.S.A.), 70:1450-1455.

17. Hartley, J. W., Rowe, W. P., and Huebner, R. J. (1970): Host-range restrictions of murine leukemia viruses in mouse embryo cell cultures. J. Virol., 5:221-225.

18. Levy, J. A. (1973): Xenotropic viruses: Murine leukemia viruses associated with NIH Swiss, NZB, and other mouse strains. Science, 182:1151-1153.

19. Melief, C. J. M., Lowe, S., and Schwartz, R. S. (1975): Ecotropic leukemia viruses in congenic C57B1 mice: Natural dissemination by milk-borne infection. J. Natl. Cancer Inst., 55:691-698.

20. Pincus, T., Rowe, W. P., and Lilly, F. (1971): A major genetic locus affecting resistance to infection with murine leukemia viruses. II. Apparent identity to a major locus described for resistance to Friend leukemia virus. J. Exp. Med., 133:1234-1241.

21. Sveda, M. M., Fields, B. N., and Soeiro, R. (1974): Host restriction of Friend leukemia virus; fate of input virion RNA. Cell, 2:271-277.

22. Taylor, B. A., Meier, H., and Huebner, R. J. (1973): Negative genetic control of the group-specific antigen of murine leukemia virus. Nature (New Biol.), 241:184-185.

23. Lilly, F., and Pincus, T. (1973): Genetic control of murine viral leukemogenesis. Adv. Cancer Res., 17:231-277.

24. Gilden, R. V., Oroszlan, S., and Huebner, R. J. (1971): Coexistence of intraspecies and interspecies specific antigenic determinants on the major structural polypeptide of mammalian C-type viruses. Nature (New Biol.), 231:107-108.

25. Hartley, J. W., Rowe, W. P., Capps, W. I., and Huebner, R. J. (1965): Complement fixation and tissue culture assays for mouse leukemia viruses. Proc. Natl. Acad. Sci. (U.S.A.), 53:931-938.

26. Hartley, J. W., and Rowe, W. P. (1975): Clonal cell lines from a feral mouse embryo which lack host-range restrictions for murine leukemia viruses. Virology, 65:128-134.

27. Benveniste, R. E., Lieber, M. M., and Todaro, G. J. (1974): A distinct class of inducible murine type C viruses which replicate in the rabbit SIRC cell line. Proc. Natl. Acad. Sci. (U.S.A.), 71:602-606.

28. Huebner, R. J., Gilden, R. V., Lane, W. T., Toni, R., Trimmer, R. W., and Hill, P. R. (1975): Suppression of type C RNA virogenes by type specific oncornavirus vaccines. Proc. Natl. Acad. Sci. (U.S.A.) (in press).

29. Gardner, M. B., Officer, J. E., Rongey, R. W., Charman, H. P., Hartley, J. W., Estes, J. D., and Huebner, R. J. (1973): C-type RNA tumor virus in wild house mice (Mus musculus). In: Unifying Concepts of Leukemia, Bibl. Haemat. No. 39, edited by R. M. Dutcher and L. Chieco-Bianchi, pp. 335-344. Karger, Basel.

30. Klement, V., Nicolson, M. O., and Huebner, R. J. (1971): Rescue of the genome of focus forming virus from rat non-productive lines by 5'-bromodeoxyuridine. Nature (New Biol.), 234:12-14.

31. Klement, V., Dougherty, M. F., Bryant, M. L., Diaz, B. B., and Zavala, T. (1975): Semi-microassay for murine leukemia-sarcoma viruses: Application for viruses negative in XC test. Appl. Microbiol. (submitted).

32. Rongey, R. W., Hlavackova, A., Lara, S., Estes, J. D., and Gardner, M. B. (1973): Types B and C RNA virus in breast tissue and milk of wild mice. J. Natl. Cancer Inst., 50:1581-1589.

33. Gardner, M. B., Chiri, A., Dougherty, M. F., Klement, V., and Huebner, R. J.: Epigenetic maternal transmission of leukemia virus in wild mice. J. Natl. Cancer Inst. (submitted).

34. Law, L. W. (1966): Transmission studies of a leukemogenic virus, MLV, in mice. Natl. Cancer Inst. Monogr., 22:267-285.

35. Colombatti, D., Collavo, D., Biasi, G., and Chieco-Bianchi, L. (1975): Genetic control of oncogenesis by murine-sarcoma virus Moloney pseudotype. I. Genetics of resistance in AKR mice. Int. J. Cancer, 16:427-434.

Control of Neoplasia by Modulation of the Immune System, edited by M. A. Chirigos. Raven Press, New York 1977.

IMMUNOLOGICAL RESPONSES WITH TILORONE — UPDATE

H. Megel, A. Raychaudhuri, and J. P. Gibson

Merrell-National Laboratories, Division of Richardson-Merrell, Inc., Cincinnati, Ohio 45215

INTRODUCTION

At the last conference,[1] we described studies that confirmed and extended the observation of Hoffman, Ritter, and Krueger (1) that tilorone hydrochloride [2,7-bis(2-diethylaminoethoxy)fluoren-9-one dihydrochloride] enhanced antibody production. We reported that tilorone hydrochloride enhanced antibody production of the IgM and of the IgG classes in mice (2) and of the IgE class in rats (2). The compound was also shown to serve as an adjuvant for influenza vaccine in guinea pigs when injected at the same site or when the vaccine and tilorone were injected at different sites (3). The effect of tilorone on antibody production has been subsequently confirmed (4).

We also reported that tilorone markedly suppressed a variety of cell-mediated immune responses (2,3): It suppressed paralysis induced in the experimental allergic encephalomyelitis model in Lewis rats and this effect persisted for as long as 4 weeks depending on dose. We demonstrated that tilorone was effective prophylactically and, to a slightly lesser extent, therapeutically, in reducing the paw edema associated with adjuvant arthritis. It suppressed the tuberculin skin reaction in rats and guinea pigs when used prophylactically to prevent the initiation of the response, or therapeutically to suppress an established skin reaction. Wildstein (5) also reported that skin and heart allografts were prolonged in tilorone-treated rats.

We went on to show that tilorone, when given for a period of 11 consecutive days, increased the wet and dry spleen weights in mice (3). All these phenomena on humoral and cell-mediated immune responses could be

---

[1] Conference on Modulation of Host Immune Resistance in the Prevention or Treatment of Induced Neoplasias, December 9-11, 1974, Bethesda, Maryland.

explained if one were to assume that tilorone selectively suppressed the T-lymphocyte while increasing the number of B-lymphocytes. For the past year, we have continued to gather support for this concept. We shall report on the effect of tilorone in still another model of cell-mediated immunity — the local graft-versus-host (GVH) response in Lewis X Brown-Norway hybrid rats. We shall also show the selective action of tilorone on T-lymphocytes using other systems — the athymic nude mouse and by immunofluorescence techniques.

EXPERIMENTAL

GVH

The effect of tilorone on the local GVH reaction in Lewis X Brown-Norway hybrid rats was studied (6) using the procedure as described by Levine (7). Parent donor Lewis rats were treated with tilorone orally at doses of 100 mg or 250 mg/kg for 1, 2, or 3 consecutive days. The effects of hydrocortisone (25 mg/kg, s.c.) and cyclophosphamide (25 mg/kg, p.o.) administered for 3 days were also studied. Control rats received no treatment. All rats were killed 24 hr after the last dose of compound. The spleens of the donor rats were removed and single-cell suspensions were prepared. A volume of 0.05 ml of the spleen cell suspensions was injected into the hind paws of recipient hybrid rats. The recipient rats were killed 7 days following cell transfer and the popliteal lymph nodes were removed and weighed. A statistically significant decrease in the weights of the popliteal lymph nodes of the experimental groups compared with the control groups was indicative of a suppressed GVH response.

The data shown in Table 1 indicate that when the donors were treated with three daily doses of 100 mg/kg tilorone orally, a statistically significant decrease ($p < 0.05$) in the popliteal lymph nodes weight was seen in all studies. One or two days of treatment with this dose resulted in popliteal lymph node weights that were less than those of the control but not statistically significant from the control. When the dose of tilorone was increased to 250 mg/kg, p.o., a decrease in the GVH reaction was seen after a single dose and generally to a greater extent if the donor rats were treated for 2 or more days. Hydrocortisone, given subcutaneously for three daily doses, sufficient to cause a marked thymus involution, had no effect on the GVH response. The lack of effect with hydrocortisone was expected in view of the recent evidence by Cohen, Fischback, and Claman (8,9) that hydrocortisone does not influence immunocompetent T-lymphocytes in the GVH model. Cyclophosphamide, as expected (10), significantly suppressed the GVH response.

Effect on Peripheral Lymphocytes of Nude Athymic Mice

To determine more specifically the effect of tilorone on the T-lymphocyte subpopulations, tilorone was studied in the nude athymic mice (homozygous nu/nu) which lack functional thymus tissue and therefore can be considered to

TABLE 1. Effects of tilorone on the local graft–versus–host reaction (6)

Treatment of donor	No. of days treated	Popliteal lymph node weight (mg) mean + SD No. of spleen cells $\times 10^7$/footpad:		
		2.5 Exp. 1	5.0 Exp. 2	12.5 Exp. 3
Control (no treatment)	—	48 ± 17	51 ± 21	141 ± 68
Tilorone 100 mg/kg p.o.	1	—	—	87 ± 66
	2	—	—	111 ± 43
	3	—	26 ± 3[a]	60 ± 39[a]
Tilorone 250 mg/kg, p.o.	1	20 ± 8[b]	—	72 ± 23
	2	18 ± 4[c]	—	66 ± 34[a]
	3	29 ± 9[c]	21 ± 5[a]	25 ± 6[b]
Hydrocortisone 25 mg/kg	3	40 ± 12	—	—
Cyclophosphamide 25 mg/kg, p.o.	3	—	21 ± 6[a]	—

[a] $p < 0.05$.
[b] $p < 0.01$.
[c] $p < 0.001$.

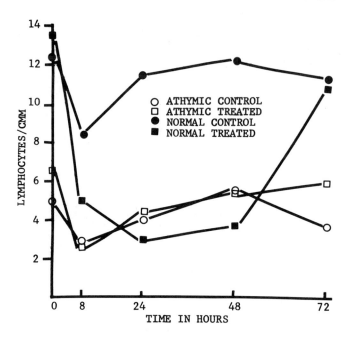

FIG. 1.   Effect of oral tilorone hydrochloride administration (100 mg/kg) on the peripheral lymph counts of athymic and phenotypically normal mice (n = 5).   From Gibson et al. (11).

be devoid of T-lymphocytes (11).   This model system would also be of use in the elaboration of the role of T-lymphocytes on interferon production. Athymic nude mice (homozygous nu/nu) and phenotypically normal litter mates (nu/+) of mixed sex were separated into four groups each containing 5 animals.   One group of normal mice and one group of athymic mice were given tilorone at a dose of 100 mg/kg by gavage.   Similar groups of athymic and normal mice were given water and served as controls.   Blood samples were collected from the tail of each mouse before dosing and at 8, 24, 48, and 72 hr after dosing.   Total and differential white blood cell counts were made on the blood of individual mice and the mean peripheral lymphocyte counts were calculated.

Lymphocyte counts for each group during the course of the study are shown in Fig. 1.   Initial pretreatment lymphocyte counts were lower in the athymic mice than in the phenotypically normal mice.   A mild reduction in the lymphocyte count occurred 8 hr after dosing in all groups, an effect frequently noted in studies of this type and attributed to the stress of handling and dosing the mice.   Following the administration of tilorone to the normal group of mice, a striking lymphopenia was observed 8 hr after the single oral dose. This persisted for 48 hr, with the peripheral lymphocyte counts returning to control levels at 72 hr.   In contrast, no lymphopenia occurred in the athymic group following tilorone administration.   The results strongly suggest that tilorone selectively suppresses the T-lymphocyte.

TABLE 2. Serum antiviral activity induced by a 150 mg/kg oral dose of tilorone hydrochloride in normal and athymic mice (11)

Dose group	No. of samples tested [a]	Geometric mean titer [b]	(95% confidence interval)
Phenotypically normal	3	< 25	—
Phenotypically normal tilorone-treated	5	1,600	(1,032-2,477)
Nude athymic vehicle control	2	<25	—
Nude athymic tilorone-treated	3	1,007	(634-1,600)

[a] Pooled samples containing the serum of 2 to 6 mice each.

[b] Dilution producing 50% reduction in plaque forming units.

Effect on Serum Antiviral Activity of Nude Athymic Mice

To determine whether the antiviral response following tilorone treatment could be attributed to "interferon" released from the T-lymphocyte, normal and athymic mice were given tilorone at a single dose of 150 mg/kg by gavage and the mice were sacrificed 18 hr later, the approximate time when maximal serum antiviral activity was previously observed. The sera were evaluated for the presence of antiviral activity in vitro against vesicular stomatitis virus by the plaque reduction assay on L-929 cells. Athymic and normal mice not receiving tilorone were used as additional controls. The results shown in Table 2 indicate that tilorone did induce serum antiviral activity in normal and in athymic mice when compared with their respective controls not receiving compound. The response of the athymic mice was very distinct despite their lack of T-lymphocytes; however, there is a suggestion that the T-lymphocyte may have contributed to the serum antiviral activity.

Effect on B- and T-Subpopulations of Lymphocytes

Our next objective was to describe more directly the effect of tilorone on the B- and T-subpopulations of lymphocytes in blood and in spleen as a function of time using the fluorescein-conjugated antimouse IgG antiserum prepared in rabbits (12).

Adult female CF_1 mice, 18 to 24 g, were given tilorone by gavage at a dose of 100 mg/kg orally for 1, 2, 3, and 9 consecutive days. Control mice received the methylcellulose vehicle. All groups of mice were killed 24 hr after the last dose by exsanguination from the retroorbital sinus. A white blood cell count and a differential count were made for each blood sample and the remainder was used to isolate the leukocytes by layering approximately 0.5 ml of blood over 0.75 ml of separation fluid consisting of 1 volume of Isopaque and 2-1/2 volumes of 6% Dextran. After the blood was layered on the separation fluid and passed into it, the leukocyte-enriched plasma fraction was removed and the red blood cells were lysed by the addition of 0.75% ammonium chloride. After additional washings and centrifugation with Hank's balanced salt solution supplemented with 5% inactivated fetal calf serum, the leukocyte suspension was filtered through a loosely packed glass wool column to remove the red blood cell debris and any adherent cells. After centrifugation, the packed cells were resuspended in a drop of the Hank's balanced salt solution and 0.1 ml of a fluorescein-conjugated antimouse IgG antiserum was added and incubated in an ice bath for 30 min. The leukocytes were washed to remove the excess fluorescein conjugated antiserum and the packed cells resuspended in 0.1 ml of salt solution. A drop of the suspension was sealed under a glass cover slip for counting the number of fluorescent cells and the total number of cells. Another drop was taken for a differential count.

The effects of tilorone on the total leukocyte, lymphocytes, and granulocytes counts are shown in Fig. 2. Tilorone caused a marked reduction in the total white blood count 24 hr after the first dose, which was still depressed at 3 days but returned to control levels at 9 days. Leukopenia was primarily a result of a lymphocyte depletion since the granulocytes were not substantially different from the control levels. These results confirm those previously reported by Zbinden and Emch (13) and Levine, Gibson, and Megel (14) on the effect of tilorone on the peripheral leukocytes.

The effect of tilorone on the B-lymphocyte population of peripheral blood is shown in Table 3. Since a differential count was made, these data were corrected for the numbers of granulocytes which ranged from 5 to 20%. The results are reported as the incidence of immunoglobulin-bearing fluorescent B-lymphocytes in percent. A striking increase in the percent B-lymphocytes was observed in the peripheral blood of the tilorone-treated mice compared with controls at all the time periods.

A summary table was reconstructed from the available data to reflect changes by tilorone on the absolute numbers of lymphocytes and on the absolute numbers of B-lymphocytes in terms of cells per cubic millimeter (Table 4). The effect on T-cells and the other subpopulations of lymphocytes that may exist in peripheral blood such as Null cells or K-cells were obtained by difference. The data show a marked lymphopenia at 1 and 3 days after tilorone administration, reaching control levels at 9 days. Tilorone caused a slight, but statistically significant, depletion of B-cells 24 hr after the first dose; however, a highly significant increase of B-cells was noted on the third day and ninth day equivalent to a 1.3- and 2.5-fold increase over control levels, respectively. Conversely, tilorone markedly depleted the remaining cells, which we shall refer to as T-cells, at 24 hr, and these cells

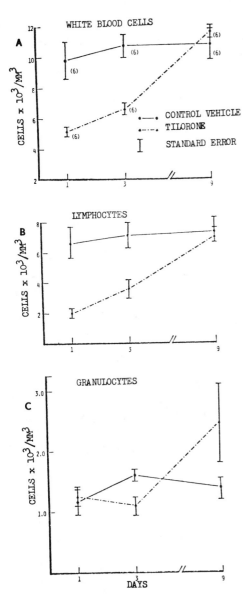

FIG. 2. **A**, Effect of tilorone on the number of white blood cells; **B**, on the absolute number of lymphocytes; and **C**, on the number of granulocytes per cubic millimeter following 1, 3, and 9 daily doses at 100 mg/kg, p.o. From Raychaudhuri and Megel (12).

remained depressed during the 9-day period. There is a suggestion, however, that the T-cells were higher on the ninth day as compared to the first and third days. These results suggest that, after the initial depletion of lympho-cytes which are predominantly the T-cells, these T-cells are subsequently replaced by B-cells in the return of the lymphocyte to control levels.

TABLE 3. Effect of continuous daily administration of tilorone on the incidence of Ig-bearing lymphocytes (B-cells) in the peripheral blood of mice (12)

No. of days of tilorone administration	Percent of Ig-bearing lymphocytes mean + SD	
	Vehicle control	Tilorone 100 mg/kg, p.o.
1	31.2 ± 4.7 (5)	72.8 ± 6.6[a] (6)
2	34.9 ± 4.6 (5)	82.8 ± 11.8[a] (6)
3	31.5 ± 2.7 (6)	83.0 ± 16.5[a] (5)
9	36.6 ± 7.6 (6)	84.9 ± 8.4[a] (6)

[a] $p < 0.001$.

($\boxtimes$) = number of mice per group.

Effect on Spleen Weights of Nude Athymic Mice

We previously reported that tilorone at 100 mg/kg orally significantly increased wet and dry weights of spleen after 11 consecutive daily doses (3). To determine whether the T-lymphocyte plays a role in this phenomenon, phenotypically normal mice and athymic nude mice were given tilorone at a dose of 100 mg/kg orally for 11 days (12). The mice were killed 24 hr after the last dose and the spleens were weighed. Two such experiments were performed. In both studies, tilorone increased spleen weights in normal mice whereas decreases in spleen weights were observed in the athymic nude mice (Table 5).

Effect on B-Lymphocytes in Spleens

The incidence of B-lymphocytes in spleens of adult female CF_1 mice was determined after 1, 3, and 9 consecutive daily doses of tilorone (12). A differential count, made on an aliquot of spleen suspension, indicated that 90 to 95% of the cells in the tilorone-treated and vehicle-treated groups were lymphocytes. The results indicated the percent of B-lymphocytes following tilorone treatment was not different from control values after one dose but was significantly increased after the third and ninth doses (Table 6).

TABLE 4. Effect of tilorone on Ig-bearing lymphocytes (B-cells) in the peripheral blood of mice — summary (12)

Treatment	No. of days of tilorone administration	Lymphocytes X 10^3/mm^3 mean $\pm$ SD		
		Total lymphocytes	B-cells	T-cells and others
Control	—	7.08 ± 2.02	2.31 ± 0.7	4.73 ± 1.34
Tilorone 100 mg/kg, p.o.	1	1.97 ± 0.45 [c]	1.43 ± 0.33 [b]	0.54 ± 0.12 [c]
	3	3.60 ± 0.75 [c]	2.99 ± 0.62 [a]	0.61 ± 0.12 [c]
	9	7.08 ± 1.48	6.01 ± 1.26	1.07 ± 0.22 [c]

[a] $p < 0.05$.
[b] $p < 0.01$.
[c] $p < 0.001$.

TABLE 5.   Effect of continuous daily administration of tilorone on
the spleen weight of nude mice (12)

Type of mouse	Spleen weight (mg) mean $\pm$ SD	
	Exp. 1	Exp. 2
Phenotypically normal	76.2 $\pm$ 17.8 (12)	109.7 $\pm$ 17.1 (6)
Phenotypically normal tilorone-treated	115.4 $\pm$ 46.5[a] (10)	143.4 $\pm$ 38.5 (5)
Nude athymic vehicle control	90.1 $\pm$ 36.4 (9)	136.7 $\pm$ 35.8 (6)
Nude athymic tilorone-treated	64.1 $\pm$ 16.8[a] (7)	110.3 $\pm$ 26.0 (5)

[a] $p < 0.05$.

($\boxtimes$) = number of mice per group.

TABLE 6.   Effect of continuous daily administration of tilorone on the
incidence of Ig-bearing lymphocytes (B-cells) in spleens of mice (12)

No. of days of tilorone administration	Percent of Ig-bearing lymphocytes mean $\pm$ SD	
	Vehicle control	Tilorone 100 mg/kg, p.o.
1	40.8 $\pm$ 4.6 (6)	43.2 $\pm$ 4.2 (6)
3	42.9 $\pm$ 4.9 (6)	56.4 $\pm$ 8.2[a] (6)
9	42.2 $\pm$ 0.67 (3)	58.9 $\pm$ 6.4[b] (8)

[a] $p < 0.01$.
[b] $p < 0.001$.

($\boxtimes$) = number of mice per group.

DISCUSSION

We have shown in this "Update" that tilorone suppresses the local GVH response in rats — another model of cell-mediated immunity — and that this effect appears to be by the selective suppression of the T-lymphocyte. The latter was shown by the effect of the compound in inducing lymphopenia in phenotypically normal mice but not in nude mice which do not have a thymus and are considered to be devoid of T-lymphocytes. It was also demonstrated that the induction of serum antiviral activity was not completely dependent on the T-lymphocyte.

The effect of tilorone on the T- and B-subpopulations of lymphocytes in peripheral blood and in spleen were more directly shown using fluorescein-conjugated antimouse IgG. The results with the conjugated antiserum substantiated the selective depletion of T-lymphocytes following tilorone, but the most striking finding was the replacement of the T-lymphocyte in peripheral blood with the B-lymphocyte during the time following the initial lymphopenia when the lymphocytes were returning to control levels.

Continued administration of tilorone increased the weight and, from preliminary studies, the cellularity of the spleen and also the percent of B-lymphocytes in spleen. This effect on spleen weight was not observed in the athymic nude mice, suggesting that the T-cell may be in some way responsible for this phenomenon. The effect of tilorone on peripheral blood and the morphological changes induced in spleen agree with the functional effects already reported for the compound — namely, the ability of tilorone to enhance B-cell populations responsible for antibody production and to suppress a variety of cell-mediated immune responses.

REFERENCES

1. Hoffman, P. F., Ritter, H. W., and Krueger, R. F. (1972): _Advances in Antimicrobial and Antineoplastic Chemotherapy._ Urban and Schwarzenburg, Munich.

2. Megel, H., Raychaudhuri, A., Goldstein, S., Kinsolving, C. R., Shemano, I., and Michael, J. G. (1974): Tilorone: Its selective effects on humoral and cell-mediated immunity. _Proc. Soc. Exp. Biol. Med._, 145:513-518.

3. Megel, H., Raychaudhuri, A., Shemano, I., and Gibson, J. P. (1976): Immunological responses with tilorone. _Fogarty International Center Proceedings_, U.S. Government Printing Office, Washington, D. C. (in press).

4. Diamantstein, T. (1973): Stimulation of humoral immune response by tilorone. _Immunology_, 24:771-775.

5. Wildstein, A., Stevens, L. E., and Hashim, G. (1976): Skin and heart allograft prolongation in tilorone treated rats. _Transplantation_, 21:129-132.

6. Megel, H., Raychaudhuri, A., and Thomas, L. L. (1976): Effect of tilorone on the local graft-vs.-host reaction in rats. _Transplantation_, 21:81-83.

7. Levine, S. (1968): Local and regional forms of graft-versus-host disease in lymph nodes. Transplantation, 6:799-802.

8. Cohen, J. J., Fischbach, M., and Claman, H. N. (1970): Hydrocortisone resistance of graft vs. host activity in mouse thymus, spleen, and bone marrow. J. Immunology, 105:1146-1150.

9. Cohen, J. J., and Claman, H. N. (1971): Hydrocortisone resistance of activated initiator cells in graft versus host reactions. Nature, 229: 274-275.

10. Whitehouse, M. W., Levy, L., and Beck, F. J. (1973): Effect of cyclophosphamide on a local graft-vs.-host reaction in the rat: Influence of sex, disease, and different dosage regimens. Agents Actions, 3:353-360.

11. Gibson, J. P., Megel, H., Camyre, K. P., and Michael, J. G. (1976): Effect of tilorone hydrochloride on the lymphoid and interferon responses of athymic mice. Proc. Soc. Exp. Biol. Med., 151:264-266.

12. Raychaudhuri, A., and Megel, H. (1976): The effect of tilorone on immunoglobulin-bearing lymphocytes (B-cells) in peripheral blood and spleens of mice. J. Reticuloendothel. Soc., 20:127-134.

13. Zbinden, G., and Emch, E. (1972): Effect of tilorone HCl, an oral interferon-inducer on leukopoiesis in rats. Acta Haematol., 47:49-58.

14. Levine, S., Gibson, J. P., and Megel, H. (1974): Selective depletion of thymus dependent areas in lymphoid tissue by tilorone. Proc. Soc. Exp. Biol. Med., 146:245-248.

Control of Neoplasia by Modulation of the Immune System, edited by M. A. Chirigos. Raven Press, New York 1977.

POTENTIATION OF A TUMOR CELL VACCINE BY PYRAN COPOLYMER

Stephen J. Mohr and Michael A. Chirigos

Laboratory of RNA Tumor Viruses, National Cancer Institute, National Institutes of Health, Bethesda, Maryland 20014

INTRODUCTION

There are a large number of agents capable of modulating the host immune response to neoplasia, and pyran copolymer (NSC-46015) has been one of the most effective in our hands. Pyran is a polyanionic copolymer of divinyl ether and maleic anhydride and is a well-known interferon inducer (1). It is also capable of preventing the oncogenesis induced by several different murine leukemia viruses (2,3) and, in addition, is of therapeutic benefit against several experimental murine neoplasias (4,5). Moreover, we have recently reported good activity using pyran as an adjuvant following cytoreductive chemotherapy (6). Several investigators have reported that pyran can stimulate the antitumor activity of macrophages (7-9), and this activity probably accounts for much of pyran's beneficial effect.

Using rather simple in vivo studies, we have been able to demonstrate that pyran is indeed a strong stimulator of antitumor immunity (10). Furthermore, this immunity was specifically directed against the tumor in question. The technique used to show this involved a tumor vaccine which was applied in a suboptimal manner so that little immunity was induced. However, when vaccination was combined with pyran, a striking potentiation of the vaccine in the form of antitumor immunity to subsequent challenge was produced.

MATERIALS AND METHODS

Animals

Adult, male B6D2F1 and CD2F1 mice were obtained from the Mammalian Genetics and Animal Production Section, Drug Research and Development, National Cancer Institute, NIH, Bethesda, Maryland. Animals were 6 to 8 weeks of age and weighed 25 g and were housed in plastic cages with Purina laboratory chow and water ad libitum.

421

Tumors

The L1210 leukemia has been carried in the transplantable ascites form in
B6D2F1 mice over 80 generations in our laboratory. The LSTRA leukemia
was established by the inoculation of Balb/c mice with Moloney leukemia
virus and has been carried in the transplantable ascites form in CD2F1 mice
for over 180 generations. Cells were diluted in Eagles minimal essential
media, and viability was determined with trypan blue.

Drugs

Pyran copolymer (NSC-46015) and the other pyrans of varying intrinsic
viscosity were supplied by Hercules Research Center, Wilmington, Delaware.
They were dissolved in sterile physiologic saline, and the pH was adjusted to
7.0 with sodium hydroxide. Tilorone hydrochloride was supplied by Merrell-
National Laboratories, Cincinnati, Ohio, and levamisole was supplied by
Janssen Pharmaceutica, Beerse, Belgium. Polyriboinosinic-polyribocytidylic
acid (poly I:C) and polyriboadenylic-polyribouridylic acid (poly A:U) were
purchased from the P-L Biochemical Company, Milwaukee, Wisconsin. These
drugs were dissolved in sterile physiologic saline as well, and all drugs were
administered intraperitoneally to the mice in an injection volume equal to 1%
of their body weight.

Vaccine Preparation

L1210 or LSTRA ascites cells were adjusted to a concentration of 5.0 X
10^7 cells/ml in Eagles minimal essential media and inactivated by exposure
to 5,000 R X-radiation. Vaccination was done by the intraperitoneal injection
of 10^7 cells 7 days before live tumor challenge. At no time did the vaccine
produce systemic leukemia. Animals receiving both vaccine and drug treatment received the vaccine 1 to 2 hr after the drug in a separate injection. If
the vaccine and drug were given mixed, this was done by physically mixing
the two agents 30 min before injection.

RESULTS

Potentiation of Tumor Vaccine by Pyran

The result of administering pyran copolymer on the day of tumor vaccination is shown in Table 1. Vaccination with L1210 or pyran treatment alone did
not significantly alter the response of the animals to subsequent challenge.
However, if pyran and vaccine were both given 7 days before challenge, a
markedly enhanced resistance was seen, with about 45% of the animals resistant to 10^4 L1210 cells and the remainder having a marked increase in
their average survival time. Furthermore, almost 90% of the animals were
still resistant 70 days later on rechallenge with 10^5 cells.

TABLE 1. Potentiation of L1210 vaccine by pyran (B6DF1 mice)

+/- L1210 vaccine (10^7 cells, i.p., day -7)	+/- L1210 challenge (10^4 cells, i.p., day 0)	+/- Pyran copolymer (25 mg/kg, i.p., day -7)	Survivors [a] Total	Average [b] survival time (days ± SE)	Rechallenge [c] survivors/total
+	-	-	112/112	>70	0/52
-	+	-	0/119	10.8 ± 0.1	
+	+	-	0/122	11.1 ± 0.2	
-	+	+	0/121	12.4 ± 0.1	
+	+	+	57/126	27.9 ± 1.3	31/34

[a] Animals scored for survival 70 days after L1210 challenge.

[b] Calculated from the individual days of death of animals dying from systemic leukemia.

[c] Animals rechallenged with 10^5 L1210 cells on day 70.

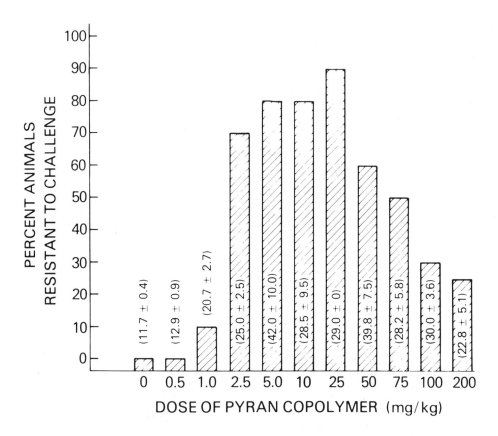

FIG. 1. Effect of pyran dosage on vaccine potentiation. B6D2F1 mice were given 10^7 cells/mouse of X-radiated (5,000 R) L1210 vaccine, i.p., on day -7. They were also given varying doses of pyran on a mg/kg basis, i.p., in a separate injection on day -7. Subsequent live tumor challenge was done with 10^4 L1210 cells, i.p., on day 0, and 70 days later the number of survivors was determined to give the percent resistant to challenge. The average survival time ± standard error of those animals dying of systemic leukemia is indicated parenthetically inside the vertical bars. There were 10 animals/ group and 2 animals died of drug toxicity in the 200-mg/kg group.

Effect of Pyran Dose

Having demonstrated that concomitant administration of pyran and vaccine resulted in a synergistic response in which the inadequate immunization with L1210 vaccine was strongly improved by pyran, we looked to see if the experimental variables initially chosen were really optimal. To determine the effective dose range of pyran, all other conditions were held constant and the dose of pyran given with vaccine was varied over a wide range. That pyran has a widely effective dosage range in this system is evident in Fig. 1. Doses less than 1.0 mg/kg were ineffective, and doses over 100 mg/kg were

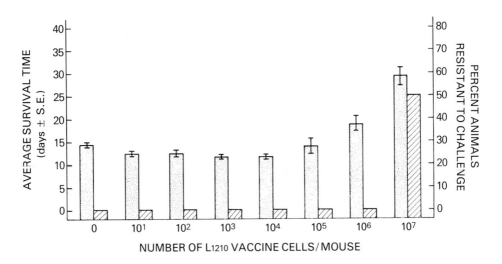

FIG. 2.   Effect of vaccine dosage on its potentiation by pyran.   B6D2F1 mice were given pyran copolymer, 25 mg/kg, i.p., on day -7.   They were also given varying doses of X-radiated (5,000 R) L1210 vaccine, i.p., on day -7. Subsequent live tumor challenge was done with 10^4 L1210 cells, i.p., on day 0, and 70 days later the number of survivors was determined to give the percent resistant to challenge (shown by the hatched bars).   The average survival time ± standard error of those animals dying from systemic leukemia is shown by the open bars.   There were 10 animals/group.

somewhat toxic.   The dose of 25 mg/kg seemed optimal and therefore was used in subsequent studies.

Effect of Vaccine Dose

We next sought to establish the minimal effective dose of vaccine, keeping the other variables constant.   In Fig. 2, it is apparent that no enhancement of vaccine occurred at cell doses less than 10^6 cells/mouse.   At that dose there was a slight increase in the average survival time, but 10^7 cells/mouse were necessary to produce a large number of animals resistant to challenge and a longer average survival time among those that were not resistant. Hence, the amount of antigen present at the time of pyran therapy was critical for vaccine potentiation to occur.

Effect of Timing of Pyran Injection in Relation to Vaccination

Since it seemed that the amount of L1210 vaccine present at the time of pyran therapy greatly affected the results, one would expect the efficacy of pyran therapy to diminish the longer after vaccination it is given because natural host processing would be steadily reducing the antigenic mass available for pyran's activity.   This was found to be true in a study where the

TABLE 2. Effect of time of pyran therapy on L1210 vaccine potentiation (B6D2F1 mice)

Day of pyran therapy (25 mg/kg, i.p.)	+/- L1210 vaccine (10^7 cells, i.p., day -7)	+/- L1210 challenge (10^4 cells, i.p., day -0)	Average survival time (days $\pm$ SE)	Survivors[a] Total
–	+	–	>70	10/10
–	–	+	10.3 $\pm$ 0.3	0/10
–	+	+	12.0 $\pm$ 0.7	0/10
Day –10	+	+	14.0 $\pm$ 0.8	0/10
Day –9	+	+	13.3 $\pm$ 0.4	0/10
Day –8	+	+	17.8 $\pm$ 1.8	2/29
Day –7	+	+	26.5 $\pm$ 2.3	13/30
Day –6	+	+	23.8 $\pm$ 3.5	8/20
Day –5	+	+	25.4 $\pm$ 3.5	1/9
Day –3	+	+	17.6 $\pm$ 1.1	1/10

[a] Survivors scored for survival on day 70 after live L1210 challenge.

TABLE 3. Effect of pyran dosage route on potentiation of L1210 vaccine (B6D2F1 mice)

+/- L1210 vaccine (10⁷ cells, i.p., day -7)	+/- L1210 challenge (10⁴ cells, i.p., day 0)	+/- Pyran route [a] (25 mg/kg, day -7)	Survivors [b] Total	Average [c] survival time (days ± S.E.)
+	-	-	10/10	>40
-	+	-	0/15	10.1 ± 0.2
+	+	-	0/15	10.3 ± 0.2
-	+	+ - i.p.	0/15	12.2 ± 0.1
+	+	+ - i.p.	7/20	21.4 ± 0.7
+	+	+ - i.p.-mixed	16/20	27.5 ± 1.6
+	+	+ - s.c.	0/20	11.1 ± 0.3
+	+	+ - i.d.	0/20	11.8 ± 0.5
+	+	+ - i.v.	0/19	12.4 ± 0.4
+	+	+ - p.o.	0/20	10.2 ± 0.2
+	+	+ - i.m.	0/20	11.8 ± 0.7

[a] Route: i.p. = intraperitoneally, s.c. = subcutaneously, i.d. = intradermally, i.v. = intravenously, p.o. = orally, i.m. = intramuscularly, i.p.-mixed = pyran and vaccine mixed together and given intraperitoneally.

[b] Animals scored for survival 40 days after L1210 challenge.

[c] Calculated from the individual days at death at animals dying from systemic leukemia.

TABLE 4. Comparative activity of several drugs in potentiation of L1210 vaccine (B6D2F1 mice)

Drug (i.p., day -7)	+/- L1210 vaccine (10^7 cells, i.p., day -7)	+/- L1210 challenge (10^4 cells, i.p., day 0)	Average survival time (days ± SE)	Survivors[a] Total
Saline control	+	-	>70	20/20
Saline control	-	+	11.0 ± 0.2	0/20
Saline control	+	+	10.4 ± 0.3	0/20
Pyran copolymer (25 mg/kg)	-	+	12.0 ± 0.2	0/20
Pyran copolymer (25 mg/kg)	+	+	20.6 ± 2.1	8/19
Poly I:C (200 µg/mouse)	-	+	10.6 ± 0.2	0/20
Poly I:C (200 µg/mouse)	+	+	10.2 ± 0.5	0/20
Poly A:U (300 µg/mouse)	-	+	10.8 ± 0.3	0/20
Poly A:U (300 µg/mouse)	+	+	10.2 ± 0.2	0/20
Levamisole (10 mg/kg)	-	+	10.1 ± 0.2	2/20
Levamisole (10 mg/kg)	+	+	10.2 ± 0.2	0/20

| Tilorone HCl (25 mg/kg) | − | + | 11.2 ± 1.2 | 0/20 |
| Tilorone HCl (25 mg/kg) | + | + | 10.2 ± 0.3 | 1/9 |

[a] Animals were scored for survival 70 days after live L1210 challenge.

time of pyran injection was varied from several days prior to vaccination to several days afterward. As can be seen in Table 2, optimal effects in the form of vaccine potentiation are obtained only if pyran is given on the same day as vaccine or 24 hr afterward. Since pyran has no effect if given more than 24 hr prior to vaccination, it would seem that the pyran effect in this model only lasts approximately 1 day.

Effect of Pyran Route of Administration

It appeared that pyran and the antigen must be present at the same time, and therefore we tested whether mixing the two agents might improve the results. At the same time, several other different routes of pyran adminis-tration were tested, the vaccine always being given intraperitoneally. In Table 3 it is clear that pyran was ineffective by any route other than intra-peritoneal injection. Furthermore, the act of mixing the pyran and vaccine prior to inoculation did seem to have an advantage over giving the two agents in separate injections a few hours apart.

Comparison of Pyran to Other Drugs

Table 4 shows the results of testing several other compounds of known immunological activity against pyran for vaccine potentiating properties. No significant effect was seen with any of the other agents tried in comparison to pyran in this particular model system.

Effect of the Molecular Weight of Pyran

The preparation of pyran used in all of the preceding studies is that en-titled NSC-46015. It was originally formulated for clinical tests and has had the most widespread usage. It consists of a mixture of long and short polymers of divinyl ether and maleic anhydride. Several other pyran prep-arations were available, and these polymers were of more uniform size. In Fig. 3 the relationship between intrinsic viscosity, which is an indirect measure of molecular weight, and biological activity in the form of vaccine potentiation is shown. It is readily apparent that as the molecular weight in-creased, so did the activity. The dose of pyran used here was 5 mg/kg be-cause at higher doses the differential effect of molecular weight was less apparent. Although those pyran compounds with a higher intrinsic viscosity tended to be more effective, all the preparations had significant activity.

Specificity of the Vaccine Potentiation by Pyran

Because of the very strongly increased resistance to challenge provided by the addition of pyran to the L1210 tumor vaccine, we were curious to see if this treatment might protect against a different tumor challenge. If it did, then pyran would have nonspecifically augmented the antitumor immunity of

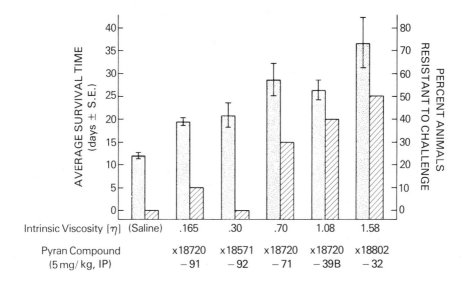

FIG. 3. Relationship of vaccine potentiation to pyran intrinsic viscosity. B6D2F1 mice were given 10^7 cells/mouse of X-radiated (5,000 R) L1210 vaccine, i.p., on day -7. On the same day they were also given 5 mg/kg of the different pyran compounds indicated or saline, i.p. Intrinsic viscosity [η], an indirect measure of molecular weight, was determined as the polyelectrolyte run as the sodium salt in 0.5 M NaCl. For comparison, NSC-46015 has an intrinsic viscosity of 0.76 and a molecular weight about 18,000. Animals were scored for resistance to challenge of 10^4 live L1210 tumor cells on day 0 and are shown by the hatched bars. Average survival time ± standard error of those animals dying from systemic leukemia is shown by the open bars. There were 10 animals/group.

the animal. This was not the case, however, and therefore pyran was acting synergistically with the vaccine to produce a specific resistance directed toward the vaccinating cell type alone (Table 5). In this experiment, the CD2F1 mouse was used to accommodate both the L1210 and the LSTRA murine leukemias. The LSTRA leukemia was sensitive to pyran pretreatment alone, but best effects were with combined vaccine and pyran treatments as was the case with L1210. The cross challenge, however, shows that those animals that were protected against LSTRA challenge could not reject the L1210 leukemia and the reverse was also true. Hence the high degree of resistance conferred was directed only toward that cell type used in the vaccine.

TABLE 5. Specificity of vaccine potentiation by pyran (CD2F1 mice)

Vaccine cell type (10^7 cells, i.p., day −7)	Challenge cell type (10^4 cells, i.p., D0)	+/− Pyran (25 mg/kg, day −7)	Survivors [a] Total	Average [b] survival time (days ± SE)
LSTRA	—	—	12/12	>70
L1210	—	—	12/12	>70
—	LSTRA	—	0/12	11.2 ± 0.3
—	L1210	—	0/12	10.2 ± 0.2
LSTRA	LSTRA	—	1/11	14.0 ± 0.9
L1210	L1210	—	0/12	13.0 ± 0.6
—	LSTRA	+	1/12	17.5 ± 0.3
—	L1210	+	0/12	11.0 ± 0.2
LSTRA	LSTRA	+	7/12	15.4 ± 0.7
L1210	L1210	+	12/12	>70
LSTRA	L1210	—	0/12	10.1 ± 0.1
LSTRA	L1210	+	0/12	11.5 ± 0.3
L1210	LSTRA	—	0/12	10.7 ± 0.4
L1210	LSTRA	+	0/12	16.5 ± 0.3

[a] Animals scored for survival 70 days after live tumor cell challenge.

[b] Calculated from the individual days of death of animals dying from systemic leukemia.

DISCUSSION

We have shown that pyran can strongly augment the immunity to tumor challenge induced by a suboptimal application of tumor vaccine. Furthermore, this immunity was still present 70 days after initial tumor challenge (Table 1). Although the in vitro studies to determine the mechanisms and cell types involved with this potentiation have not been completed, it is clear that those cells involved with long-term memory have been activated by pyran and vaccine. It is likely that pyran's effects on macrophages are also involved with this potentiation phenomenon.

The wide range of effective doses for pyran (see Fig. 1) confirms earlier findings (6) and indicates that drug toxicity can be avoided without losing good effect. Possibly the reason for this is that pyran was given at the optimal time. The requirement for a high antigenic load at the time of pyran therapy is indicated in Fig. 2 and clearly demonstrated in Table 2. Furthermore, pyran's immediate effect does not seem to be long-lasting, so that if it is given too soon before antigen presentation its beneficial effect is lost. This critical effect of timing may allow one to see good effects at lower drug doses and probably should be kept in mind when pyran or other drugs are being used to modulate host immune responses in other tumor systems.

It was quite apparent that pyran was ineffective if given by any route other than intraperitoneal (Table 3). Possibly the vaccine and the pyran must physically be in the same space for immunopotentiation to occur. The increased beneficial effect of mixing the two agents partially supports this view. However, pyran may be denatured or not absorbed at all if given by some of the other routes.

This may partially explain why some of the other drugs tested in comparison to pyran were inactive in this system. Certainly other doses and routes would be necessary to completely rule out any activity. Also, levamisole has been reported in this meeting to primarily augment depressed immune responses back toward normal. This system of vaccine potentiation involved normal, immunologically competent animals and pyran-stimulated immune responses far above normal. Hence, the mechanism of action of these other drugs is probably different than that of pyran and therefore they show little activity in this particular model system.

The relationship of activity to the molecular weight of pyran is interesting in that similar results have been reported when pyran was used as an adjuvant to chemotherapy of an established tumor (6). In addition, molecular weight has an influence on the ability of pyran to induce interferon and on its toxicity (11). A similar phenomenon has also been observed for the polyriboinosinic acid moiety of poly I:C (12), and the meaning of this relationship is being further investigated. Because both compounds are polyanions, the effects they produce may be related to the amount of negative charge present on the molecule.

The fact that potentiation was specific for the cell type used as the vaccine is significant. Pyran when used alone is a nonspecific stimulator of macrophage activity (9), and this was reflected in its activity alone against the LSTRA tumor. However, as a result of combination with a specific antigenic mass, pyran's potentiating effect was specifically directed. To test how sensitive this specificity really is, one would need to use two extremely similar yet different tumors in cross-reactivity tests. The L1210 tumor is poorly antigenic, requiring multiple immunizations to achieve even a slight degree of immunity (13), whereas LSTRA is highly immunogenic due to the presence of the Moloney viral antigen. Hence the potentiated immune system could easily distinguish between these two rather dissimilar ascites tumors.

Vaccination potentiation, with respect to a nononcogenic virus, was originally reported by Campbell and Richmond (14). We have extended this finding to neoplastic cells, and similar types of results have been reported for BCG (15), C. parvum (16), and endotoxin (17). Our results suggest that pyran might have application in those situations where biological immune stimulation, currently in clinical practice, is not possible or potentially harmful.

SUMMARY

Pyran copolymer (NSC-46015) was shown to strongly potentiate the immunity to subsequent tumor challenge induced by suboptimal tumor vaccination. This potentiation was dose-dependent on pyran and vaccine and required the simultaneous administration of both agents. Optimal results were achieved by mixing the vaccine and pyran prior to inoculation, and the intraperitoneal route of pyran injection was the only effective method. Other agents such as poly I:C, poly A:U, tilorone, and levamisole were ineffective in this system. However, pyrans of differing intrinsic viscosities were all significantly active, although better activity tended to correlate with higher molecular weight. Finally, the highly potentiated immunity was shown to be specific for the vaccinating cell type.

REFERENCES

1. Merigan, T. C. (1967): Induction of circulating interferon by synthetic anionic polymers of known composition. Nature, 214:416-417.
2. Chirigos, M. A., Turner, W., Pearson, J., and Griffin, W. (1969): Effective antiviral therapy of two murine leukemias with an interferon-inducing synthetic carboxylate copolymer. Int. J. Cancer, 4:267-278.
3. Hirsch, M. S., Black, P. H., Wood, M. L., and Monaco, A. P. (1972): Effects of pyran copolymer on oncogenic virus infections in immuno-suppressed hosts. J. Immunol., 108:1312-1318.
4. Morahan, P. S., Munson, J. A., Baird, L. G., Kaplan, A. M., and Regelson, W. (1974): Antitumor action of pyran copolymer and tilorone against Lewis lung carcinoma and B-16 melanoma. Cancer Res., 34:506-511.
5. Sandberg, J., and Goldin, A. (1971): Use of first generation transplants of a slow growing solid tumor for the evaluation of new cancer chemotherapeutic agents. Cancer Chemother. Rep., 55:233-238.

6. Mohr, S. J., Chirigos, M. A., Fuhrman, F. S., and Pryor, J. W. (1975): Pyran copolymer found to be an effective adjuvant to chemotherapy against a murine leukemia and solid tumor. Cancer Res., 35:3750-3754.

7. Harmel, R. P., Jr., and Zbar, B. (1975): Tumor suppression by pyran copolymer: Correlation with production of cytotoxic macrophages. J. Natl. Cancer Inst., 54:989-992.

8. Kapila, K., Smith, C., and Rubin, A. A. (1971): Effect of pyran copolymer on phagocytosis and tumor growth. J. Reticuloendothel. Soc., 9:447-450.

9. Kaplan, A. M., Morahan, P. S., and Regelson, W. (1974): Induction of macrophage-mediated tumor-cell cytotoxicity by pyran copolymer. J. Natl. Cancer Inst., 52:1919-1923.

10. Mohr, S. J., Chirigos, M. A., Smith, G. T., and Fuhrman, F. S. (1976): Specific potentiation of L1210 vaccine by pyran copolymer. J. Natl. Cancer Inst., 36:2035-2039.

11. Breslow, D. S., Edwards, E. I., and Newberg, N. R. (1973): Divinyl ether-maleic anhydride (pyran) copolymer: The effect of molecular weight on biological activity. Nature, 246:160-162.

12. Mohr, S. J., Brown, D. G., and Coffey, D. S. (1972): Size requirement of polyinosinic acid for DNA synthesis, viral resistance, and increased survival of leukemic mice. Nature (New Biol.), 240:250-252.

13. Chirigos, M. A., Thomas, L. B., Humphreys, S. R., Glynn, J. P., and Goldin, A. (1964): Therapeutic and immunological response of mice with meningeal leukemia (L1210) to challenge with antifolic-resistant variant. Cancer Res., 24:409-415.

14. Campbell, C. H., and Richmond, J. Y. (1973): Enhancement, by two carboxylic acid interferon inducers, of resistance stimulated in mice by foot-and-mouth disease vaccine. Infect. Immun., 7:199-204.

15. Hawrylko, E. (1975): Immunopotentiation with BCG: Dimensions of a specific antitumor response. J. Natl. Cancer Inst., 54:1189-1197.

16. Scott, M. T. (1975): Potentiation of the tumor-specific immune response by coryne-bacterium parvum. J. Natl. Cancer Inst., 55:65-72.

17. Prager, M. D., Ludden, C. M., Mandy, W. J., Allison, J. P., and Kitto, G. B. (1975): Brief communication: Endotoxin-stimulated immune response to modified lymphoma cells. J. Natl. Cancer Inst., 54:773-775.

Control of Neoplasia by Modulation of the Immune System, edited by M. A. Chirigos. Raven Press, New York 1977.

TUMORICIDAL EFFECT IN VITRO OF PERITONEAL MACROPHAGES FROM MICE TREATED WITH PYRAN COPOLYMER

Richard M. Schultz, Michael A. Chirigos, Stephen J. Mohr, and Wilna A. Woods

Viral Biology Branch, National Cancer Institute, National Institutes of Health, Bethesda, Maryland 20014

INTRODUCTION

In recent years, considerable evidence has accumulated from both in vivo and in vitro studies which suggests that mononuclear phagocytes are prominent effectors in transplantation and tumor immunity. Evans (1) observed that many macrophages are present in syngeneic solid tumors and that their content was correlated with the magnitude of the host's antitumor immune response. Tevethia and Zarling (2) demonstrated that cooperation of macrophages with immune lymphoid cells was essential for rejection of SV40-transformed cells in inbred Balb/c mice. Hanna et al. (3) noted that the protective effect afforded by living Mycobacterium bovis, strain BCG, was contingent on a greater influx of histiocytes into the tumor. Moreover, most agents which potentiate host antitumor resistance stimulate the reticuloendothelial compartment; activated macrophages having the ability in vitro to recognize and nonspecifically destroy target cells with abnormal growth properties can be recovered from animals infected with intracellular parasites such as BCG (4,5) and Toxoplasma gondii (6-8), as well as mice treated with agents such as endotoxin (9), killed Corynebacterium parvum (10,11), polyinosinic-polycytidylic acid (9), and pyran copolymer (12). Indeed, macrophages may be essential for successful immunotherapy of cancer.

There appear to be two distinct mechanisms whereby macrophages inhibit or destroy tumor target cells in vitro (Table 1): (a) Through cooperation with sensitized thymus-derived lymphocytes, the resultant "armed" macrophage can rapidly lyse tumor cells in an immunologically specific manner in both allogeneic (8,13-16) and syngeneic (9,17-19) systems; (b) macrophages can become "activated" by several pathways to nonspecifically inhibit DNA synthesis in neoplastic cells (7,8,20-23). Although the exact mechanisms

TABLE 1. Classification of cytotoxic macrophages

Designation	Immunologic specificity	Trigger	Mode of action
Armed	Specific; directed to histo-compatibility and tumor-associated antigens (thymus requirement)	(a) SMAF from T-cell (b) Cytophilic Ab	Inhibition of DNA synthesis Rapid lysis
Activated	Nonspecific; cells with ab-normal growth properties more susceptible	(a) Immune macrophage with specific antigen in vitro or in vivo (b) Endotoxin (c) Polyinosinic–polycytidylic acid (d) Lymphokine released from immune lymphoid cells (different from SMAF) (e) Pyran copolymer	Inhibition of DNA synthesis

are unknown, the destruction of target cells by macrophages results primarily from a nonphagocytic cell-to-cell contact independent of complement (12, 13, 21, 23).

We previously monitored several in vitro parameters of the immune response of CD2F1 mice to a leukemia allograft during pyran copolymer-induced tumor enhancement. Although pyran was capable of augmenting specific macrophage reactivity to a high degree, significantly fewer macrophages infiltrated the tumor allograft. Therefore, a critical factor in the enhanced allograft survival appeared to be the capacity to mobilize sufficient macrophages at the tumor site. This chapter characterizes the effects of pyran on both specific and nonspecific macrophage-mediated cytotoxicity in tumor allograft immunity.

MATERIALS AND METHODS

Mice

Male CD2F1 and C57B1/6 mice, 6 to 8 weeks old, were obtained from the Mammalian Genetics and Animal Production Section of the National Institutes of Health, Bethesda, Maryland. Male athymic nude (nu/nu) mice were supplied by the Animal Breeding Farms at the Frederick Cancer Research Center, Frederick, Maryland.

Tumors

MBL-2 ($H2^b$[C57B1/6], Moloney murine leukemia virus-induced) and L1210 ($H2^d$[DBA/2], nonviral induced) murine leukemia cells were used both for immunization and as target cells. For allograft studies, 1.0×10^7 MBL-2 or L1210 ascites tumor cells were inoculated subcutaneously into the right inguinal region of CD2F1 ($H2^d$) or C57B1/6 mice, respectively.

Pyran Copolymer

Pyran copolymer (NSC-46015) was dissolved in 0.9% NaCl, adjusted to pH 7.0 by addition of 1 N NaOH, and given intraperitoneally at 1% body weight.

Cell Cultures

MBL-2 and L1210 target cells were maintained as suspension cultures in RPMI-1640 medium supplemented with 20% heat-inactivated fetal bovine serum, 100 μg/ml of gentamicin solution, 0.075% $NaHCO_3$, and 10 mM HEPES buffer (RPMI-FBS).

Labeling Target Cells

1.0×10^7 Viable cells were resuspended in 2 ml of RPMI-FBS containing $200\,\mu$Ci of $Na_2{}^{51}CrO_4$. The mixture was then incubated at $37^\circ C$ in a CO_2 incubator for 90 min with occasional shaking. After incubation, the cells were pelleted by centrifugation and washed four times with 30-ml volumes of medium. Specific activity was maintained between 0.1 and 0.3 cpm/cell.

Preparation of Peritoneal Macrophages

Peritoneal exudates were harvested from mice by intraperitoneal injection of 5 ml of Hank's balanced salt solution (HBSS) containing 2 units heparin/ml. Within 10 min after injection, the mice were sacrificed and the peritoneal exudate was collected by paracentesis. Exudates from 5 mice in each group were pooled, washed once in 30 ml of HBSS, and resuspended in 10 ml of RPMI-FBS. Peritoneal macrophages were purified by adherence in 100 X 20 mm tissue culture dishes. The adhering cells were gently scraped with a soft rubber policeman into RPMI-FBS, adjusted to 5×10^6 viable cells/ml RPMI-FBS, and kept in an ice bath prior to use to prevent adherence. Representative preparations of purified peritoneal adherent cells were stained with Giemsa stain; >95% of the cells had morphologic characteristics of macrophages.

Chromium-51 Release Test for Cellular Cytotoxicity

Suspensions of ^{51}Cr-labeled target cells were diluted to contain 1.0×10^5 cells/ml. 10^4 cells in 100-μl aliquots were plated with an automatic repeating dispenser (Hamilton Co., Reno, Nevada) into wells of No. 3040 Microtest II Plates (Falcon Plastics, Oxnard, California). One-hundred microliter aliquots containing the appropriate concentrations of peritoneal macrophages were added to quadruplicate wells. Effector-to-target cell ratios were maintained at 50:1 except when otherwise noted in text. Spontaneous release was determined from wells which contained only target cells. The plates were incubated at $37^\circ C$ for 16 hr in a 5% CO_2-in-air atmosphere. Following this incubation, the plates were centrifuged (1,000 rpm for 10 min), and radioactivity was measured in the cell-free supernatant. One-hundred microliters of supernatant fluid from each well was placed into a disposable vial and counted in a Beckman Biogamma Spectrometer.

$$\text{Percent specific } ^{51}\text{Cr release} = \frac{\text{cpm}_E - \text{cpm}_N}{\text{cpm}_M} \, 100$$

where cpm_E = counts per minute released in the presence of test effector cells − spontaneous release; cpm_N = counts per minute released in the presence of normal mouse effector cells − spontaneous release; cpm_M = maximum release − spontaneous release.

Estimation of Tumor Macrophage Content

The entire mass of a subcutaneously growing MBL-2 allograft was excised, minced with scissors, washed twice with HBSS, and suspended in 0.1% trypsin solution (Grand Island Biological Co., Grand Island, New York). The tumor fragments were stirred continuously by a magnetic stirring device at room temperature for 1 hr. The fragments were then allowed to settle and the cell suspension was removed, centrifuged, and washed with HBSS. The percentage of macrophages was determined by the method of Evans (1).

RESULTS

Specificity of Macrophage-Mediated Cytotoxicity

Previous studies in our laboratory have shown that peritoneal macrophages possess heightened tumoricidal activity when taken from mice which receive a subcutaneous inoculation of 1 X 10^7 allogeneic leukemia cells. This response peaks approximately on day 12 in both the L1210 and MBL-2 allograft-bearing hosts. By utilizing criss-cross cytotoxicity tests, we have found that this tumoricidal action is immunologically specific (Table 2). Macrophages taken from MBL-2 tumor-bearing mice kill MBL-2, but not L1210 target cells; whereas with L1210 tumor-bearing mice the converse is true. Preliminary experiments in our laboratory have demonstrated that normal macrophages can be rendered specifically cytotoxic towards leukemia cells following incubation with immune peritoneal or splenic lymphocytes.

Influence of Pyran Copolymer on Macrophage-Mediated Cytotoxicity

We studied the effect of pyran treatment on macrophage reactivity from nonsensitized, athymic nude (nu/nu) mice. Pyran, when administered at 25 mg/kg, was found to morphologically and functionally activate macrophages from nontumor-bearing animals (Fig. 1). Macrophages were weakly cytotoxic for MBL-2 cells at 6 days after pyran inoculation. Macrophages collected from normal CD2F1 mice treated with pyran copolymer were stimulated in a similar manner.

To test if specific macrophage-associated cytotoxicity could be similarly enhanced by pyran treatment, mice bearing MBL-2 allografts were treated with pyran copolymer and monitored for macrophage-mediated cytolytic activity. The specific macrophage reactivity was highly potentiated by pyran treatment (Fig. 2).

Requirement for Direct Contact for Macrophage-Mediated Cytotoxicity

To determine if soluble factors from "armed" or pyran-activated macrophages were cytotoxic to MBL-2 target cells, peritoneal macrophages were admixed with MBL-2 tumor cells and incubated under similar conditions as in the test for cellular cytotoxicity. After 24 hr of incubation, supernatant

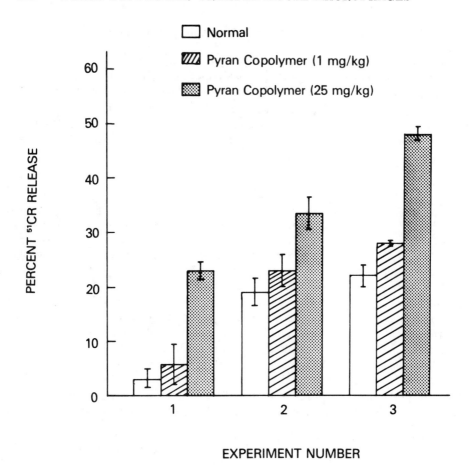

FIG. 1. Effect of pyran copolymer on the cytotoxic activity of purified normal macrophages from nude (nu/nu) mice to MBL-2 target cells. Pyran treatment was administered i.p. 6 days prior to harvesting the peritoneal exudate. Experiments involved 5 mice/group each.

fluids from these cultures were tested for their cytotoxic potential against MBL-2 cells using the standard chromium-51 release technique for measuring cellular immunity; in no instance was significant killing observed. Therefore, the tumoricidal activity of peritoneal macrophages does not appear to be attributable to soluble factors elaborated into the culture medium, but probably requires cell-to-cell contact between macrophage effector and target cells.

Effect of Varying Effector-to-Target Cell Ratios

We looked at the effect of varying numbers of armed or pyran-activated, armed macrophages on cytolysis of a constant number of target cells.

TABLE 2. Specificity of macrophage-mediated cytotoxicity

Immunization[a]	Target cells	Percent specific ^{51}Cr release[b] mean + standard error	
		Days after tumor inoculation	
		Day 12	Day 14
MBL-2 allograft in CD2F1 mice	MBL-2	39 ± 1	17 ± 2
	L1210	-2 ± 1	0 ± 3
L1210 allograft in C57B1/6 mice	MBL-2	-11 ± 2	-4 ± 2
	L1210	53 ± 3	30 ± 2

[a] Mice were inoculated subcutaneously with 1.0 X 10^7 ascites tumor cells on day 0.

[b] Peritoneal adherent cells were pooled from 5 mice and tested at an effector-to-target cell ratio of 50:1.

Macrophages were harvested from CD2F1 mice 12 days after a subcutaneous inoculation of 1 X 10^7 MBL-2 cells. Varying numbers of peritoneal macrophages from normal, MBL-2 tumor-bearing, and pyran-treated MBL-2 tumor-bearing mice were reacted against a constant number of ^{51}Cr-labeled MBL-2 target cells to give final effector-to-target cell ratio of 100:1, 50:1, 10:1, 5:1, and 1:1. When 1 X 10^4 target cells were challenged with varying numbers of armed or activated-armed macrophages, the level of cytolysis increased markedly as the ratio of macrophages to target cells was increased (Fig. 3). Armed macrophages gave elevated cytotoxicity over normal macrophages at only 100:1 and 50:1 ratios. In contrast, cytolysis effected by a modest majority (5:1) of pyran-activated, armed macrophages was highly significant.

Influence of Pyran Copolymer on Macrophage Content of Tumor Allograft

We have attempted to measure the concentration of macrophages at the allograft site early after pyran administration by the method of Evans (1). At 11 days of allograft growth, tumors contained 16% macrophages. In contrast, tumors taken from pyran-treated mice contained only 1% macrophages. Thus, pyran copolymer in certain treatment modalities appears to interfere with the normal mobilization of macrophages into the tumor allograft.

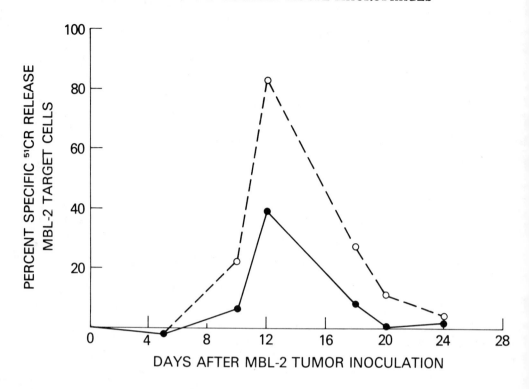

FIG. 2. Effect of pyran copolymer on the cytotoxic activity of purified peritoneal macrophages from MBL-2 tumor-bearing CD2F1 mice to MBL-2 target cells. Mice were inoculated subcutaneously with 1.0×10^7 ascites tumor cells on day 0. Pyran was administered intraperitoneally at 25 mg/kg on day 6 (O). Tumor-bearing mice which did not receive drug served as controls (●). The figures are means obtained from quadruplicate samples. The standard error never exceeded ±3%.

DISCUSSION

The specific cytotoxic action of macrophages from allograft-bearing mice has been demonstrated by several investigators (13, 18, 24). This cytotoxicity results from an initial cooperation between macrophages and immune lymphoid cells (14, 17) and requires direct contact between macrophage and target cell (13). Pyran copolymer has previously been shown to activate macrophages to nonspecifically destroy cells with abnormal growth properties through a thymus-independent process (12). We similarly found that pyran activates macrophages in athymic nude mice to lyse allogeneic leukemia cells. By analyzing the kinetics of the in vitro interaction between pyran-activated, armed macrophages and allogeneic tumor cells, we found that pyran markedly potentiates the specific tumoricidal action of armed macrophages. These cells were extremely efficient effectors of target cell cytolysis even at a 5:1 effector-to-target cell ratio.

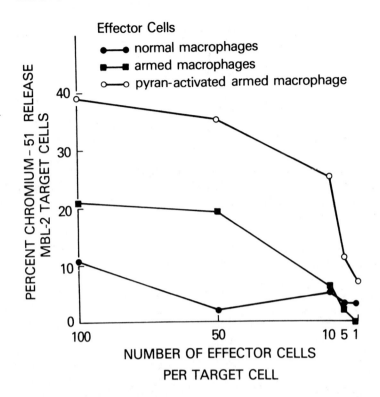

FIG. 3. Effect of varying numbers of armed or pyran activated–armed macrophages on cytolysis of a constant number of target cells. Macrophages were harvested from CD2F1 mice 12 days after a subcutaneous inoculation of 1.0×10^7 MBL-2 cells. Pyran copolymer was administered intraperitoneally at 25 mg/kg on day 6 after tumor inoculation. The figures are means obtained from quadruplicate samples.

The presence of large numbers of macrophages in allografts or syngeneic tumor grafts offers the most compelling evidence that they play a major role in the rejection reaction. Evans (1) showed that tumors with high immunogenicity have a corresponding high macrophage content. Macrophages appear to be drawn to a tumor as part of the immune reaction; soluble mediators such as migration inhibition factor (MIF) and macrophage chemotactic factor from sensitized lymphocytes have been implicated in this process. Pearsall and Weiser (16) showed that when silica treatment was given prior to or as late as 6 days after grafting, extensive macrophage destruction was observed and the survival of the SaI tumor allograft was prolonged. Similarly, BCG is most effective when inoculated directly into the tumor (3). Not only does macrophage activation result, but a chronic inflammatory reaction of the delayed-hypersensitivity type occurs. This granulomatous reaction is characterized by an intense migration of histiocytes into the tumor bed. We found that the presence of macrophages in the tumor allograft correlated with allograft rejection. Because macrophage-mediated cytotoxicity requires close contact between target cell and macrophage, the major limitation of the macrophage effector arm of the immune response is cell concentration at the tumor site.

Pyran copolymer has previously been demonstrated to increase the histio-cytic infiltration into the Lewis lung carcinoma in mice (26). Contrary to this, we have found a decrease in the macrophage content of tumor allografts from mice treated with pyran despite the macrophages being more reactive in vitro. The reason for these contrasting results, other than different mouse strains and target cells used, is not known, although it may be dependent on the time of pyran treatment in relationship to the existing tumor load. Because the decrease in macrophage infiltrate in MBL-2 tumors corresponded with tumor allograft enhancement, perhaps pyran may be more beneficially used in combination with agents which provoke a delayed hypersensitivity reaction at the tumor site (25). By these means, more pyran-activated macrophages would reach the tumor site. Local passive transfer experiments are presently being conducted to clarify the clinical usefulness of these pyran-activated macrophages.

SUMMARY

Pyran copolymer weakly activates macrophages to nonspecifically lyse tumor target cells through a thymic-independent process. Macrophages can acquire specific cytotoxicity against a tumor allograft by cooperation with immune lymphoid cells. Pyran treatment in the tumor-bearing host works synergistically with the developing antitumor immune response to markedly augment specific macrophage reactivity. Macrophage stimulation by pyran requires 6 days in either the tumor or nontumor-bearing host. Macrophage-mediated cytotoxicity is not mediated by the elaboration of cytotoxins into the culture medium. Pyran copolymer in certain treatment modalities interferes with the normal mobilization of macrophages into a tumor allograft, and this failure in macrophage infiltration is associated with allograft enhancement.

REFERENCES

1. Evans, R. (1972): Macrophages in syngeneic animal tumors. Transplantation, 14:468-473.
2. Tevethia, S. S., and Zarling, J. M. (1972): Participation of macrophages in tumor immunity. Natl. Cancer Inst. Monogr., 35:279-282.
3. Hanna, M. G., Snodgrass, M. J., Zbar, B., and Rapp, H. J. (1972): Histopathology of Mycobacterium bovis (BCG)-mediated tumor regression. Natl. Cancer Inst. Monogr., 35:345-357.
4. Cleveland, R. P., Meltzer, M. S., and Zbar, B. (1974): Tumor cytotoxicity in vitro by macrophages from mice infected with Mycobacterium bovis strain BCG. J. Natl. Cancer Inst., 52:1887-1894.

5. Hibbs, J. B. (1974): Heterocytolysis by macrophages activated by Bacillus Calmette-Guérin: Lysosome exocytosis into tumor cells. Science, 184:468-471.
6. Droller, M. J., and Remington, J. S. (1975): A role for the macrophage in in vivo and in vitro resistance to murine bladder tumor cell growth. Cancer Res., 35:49-53.
7. Hibbs, J. B., Lambert, L. H., and Remington, J. S. (1972): Control of carcinogenesis: A possible role for the activated macrophage. Science, 177:998-1000.
8. Krahenbuhl, J. L., and Remington, J. S. (1974): The role of activated macrophages in specific and nonspecific cytostasis of tumor cells. J. Immunol., 113:507-516.
9. Evans, R. (1973): Macrophages and the tumour bearing host. Br. J. Cancer, 28:Suppl., 1, 19-24.
10. Ghaffar, A., Cullen, R. T., and Woodruff, M. F. A. (1975): Further analysis of the antitumor effect in vitro of peritoneal exudate cells from mice treated with Corynebacterium parvum. Br. J. Cancer, 31:15-24.
11. Halpern, B., Fray, A., Crepin, Y., Platica, O., Lorinet, A. M., Rabourdin, A., Sparros, L., and Isac, R. (1973): Corynebacterium parvum, a potent immunostimulant in experimental infections and in malignancies. In: Immunopotentiation, edited by G. E. W. Wolstenholme and J. Knight, pp. 217-233. Associated Scientific Publishers, New York.
12. Kaplan, A. M., Morahan, P. S., and Regelson, W. (1974): Induction of macrophage-mediated tumor-cell cytotoxicity by pyran copolymer. J. Natl. Cancer Inst., 52:1919-1921.
13. Den Otter, W., Evans, R., and Alexander, P. (1972): Cytotoxicity of murine peritoneal macrophages in tumour allograft immunity. Transplantation, 14:220-226.
14. Evans, R., and Alexander, P. (1972): Mechanism of immunologically specific killing of tumour cells by macrophages. Nature, 236:168-170.
15. Pels, E., and Den Otter, W. (1974): The role of a cytophilic factor from challenged immune peritoneal lymphocytes in specific macrophage cytotoxicity. Cancer Res., 34:3089-3094.
16. Pearsall, N. N., and Weiser, R. S. (1968): The macrophage in allograft immunity. I. Effects of silica as a specific macrophage toxin. J. Reticuloendothel. Soc., 5:107-120.
17. Evans, R., and Alexander, P. (1970): Cooperation of immune lymphoid cells with macrophages in tumour immunity. Nature, 228:620-622.
18. Loveren, H. V., and Den Otter, W. (1974): In vitro activation of armed macrophages and the therapeutic application in mice. J. Natl. Cancer Inst., 52:1917-1919, 1974.
19. Loveren, H. V., and Den Otter, W. (1974): Macrophages in solid tumors. 1. Immunologically specific effector cells. J. Natl. Cancer Inst., 53:1057-1060.
20. Hibbs, J. B. (1973): Macrophage nonimmunologic recognition: Target cell factors related to contact inhibition. Science, 180:868-870.
21. Hibbs, J. B. (1974): Discrimination between neoplastic and non-neoplastic cells in vitro by activated macrophages. J. Natl. Cancer Inst., 53:1487-1492.

22. Keller, R. (1973): Cytostatic elimination of syngeneic rat tumor cells in vitro by nonspecifically activated macrophages. J. Exp. Med., 138:625-644.

23. Krahenbuhl, J. L., and Lambert, L. H. (1975): Cytokinetic studies of the effects of activated macrophages on tumor target cells. J. Natl. Cancer Inst., 54:1433-1437.

24. Lohmann-Matthes, M. L., Schipper, H., and Fischer, H. (1972): Macrophage-mediated cytotoxicity against allogeneic target cells in vitro. Eur. J. Immunol., 2:45-49.

25. Bernstein, I. D., Thor, D. E., Zbar, B., and Rapp, H. J. (1971): Tumor immunity: tumor suppression in vivo initiated by soluble products of specifically stimulated lymphocytes. Science, 172:729-731.

26. Snodgrass, M., Kaplan, A. M., and Morahan, P. (1974): Histopathological study of the antitumor action of pyran copolymer against Lewis lung carcinoma. J. Reticuloendothel. Soc., 16:11a.

Control of Neoplasia by Modulation of the Immune System, edited by M. A. Chirigos. Raven Press, New York 1977.

MACROPHAGE-MEDIATED TUMOR RESISTANCE

Page S. Morahan and Alan M. Kaplan

Departments of Microbiology and Surgery, MCV/VCU Cancer Center, Virginia Commonwealth University, Richmond, Virginia 23298

INTRODUCTION

Activated macrophages have been proposed as major effectors of tumor resistance induced by immunotherapy with immunopotentiators such as BCG, C. parvum, and pyran (1-4). However, most studies have concentrated on one tumor system and one immunopotentiator. In order to determine if activated macrophages are a common effector of immunopotentiator action, we have examined the role of macrophages in tumor resistance induced by two diverse immunopotentiators, the biological vaccine C. parvum and the synthetic polyanion pyran. To demonstrate further the general nature of macrophage activation in immunotherapy, we examined therapy with the two drugs against two different tumor systems, the Lewis lung carcinoma and a methylcholanthrene-induced sarcoma. Although the two immunopotentiators are not identical in their activity, the results are consistent with activated macrophages playing a prominent role in immunotherapy with C. parvum and pyran against both tumors.

MATERIALS AND METHODS

Mice. C57B1/6 mice were obtained from Jackson Laboratories, Bar Harbor, Maine, and from National Laboratory Supply, Indianapolis, Indiana.

Drugs. Pyran copolymer, lot XA124-177, was obtained from Hercules, Inc., Wilmington, Delaware. The drug was solubilized in 0.15 N NaCl and brought to pH 7.2. The killed vaccine of Corynebacterium parvum was obtained from Burroughs Wellcome, Triangle Research Park, North Carolina. Trypan blue was prepared as originally described by Hibbs (4); for some experiments trypan blue was obtained from Dr. John Hibbs, VA Hospital, Salt Lake City, Utah. Silica (Dorentruper No. 12) was suspended in balanced salt solution.

Tumors. The Lewis lung carcinoma and a methylcholanthrene-induced sarcoma (MCA 2182) have been maintained in our laboratory by continuous s.c. passage of 1 mm^3 fragments in mice. The tumors were periodically shown to be free from lactic dehydrogenase virus. For some experiments, tumors were trypsinized and mice were inoculated with various doses of viable tumor cells, either intramuscularly or into the footpad. Tumor size was measured as previously described by Attia and Weiss (5).

Statistical analysis. Statistical analysis was performed using Student's t-test.

Depletion of thymus-derived lymphocytes. Young adult mice (5 to 6 weeks old) were thymectomized by aspiration, irradiated with 900 rads 2 weeks later, and reconstituted within 2 hr with an i.v. inoculation of 10^7 syngeneic bone marrow cells. Mice were maintained on acidified, chlorinated water to inhibit pseudomonas growth. Thymus depletion was shown by lack of phyto-hemagglutinin-induced blastogenesis of spleen cells and lack of thymus at autopsy.

Tumor immunity studies. For assessment of transplantation immunity, mice were implanted s.c. with tumors, the primary tumor surgically excised on day 7, 10, or 14, and the mice remaining tumor-free at approximately 60 days were rechallenged with graded doses of homologous or heterologous tumor. For assessment of humoral immunity, mice were bled at 7, 14, 21, and 28 days after s.c. tumor implantation. The serum was tested against homologous and heterologous tumors by the indirect fluorescent technique for the appearance of tumor-specific fluorescence. Fluoroscein-conjugated rabbit anti mouse IgG or IgM was used as the developing serum. No non-specific fluorescent staining occurred when the sera were used to stain preparations of live cells.

RESULTS

Characterization of the Lewis Lung Carcinoma

The Lewis lung carcinoma is derived from a tumor that spontaneously oc-curred in C57B1/6 mice (6). The tumor rapidly metastasizes from a s.c. implant (7). By day 14 after tumor implantation, the tumor metastasized in approximately 80% of the mice. However, mice bearing the Lewis lung carcinoma did not develop concomitant immunity (Table 1) or tumor-specific transplantation resistance (Table 2). Indeed, the growth of the tumor in mice depleted of thymus-derived lymphocytes was significantly delayed as compared to control animals (Table 3). These results indicated that thymus-derived lymphocytes may enhance tumor growth, as has been proposed by Umiel and Trainin (8) for another line of this tumor. Although there is little evidence for cellular protective immunity toward the tumor, mice bearing the primary tumor did exhibit an IgM humoral response. This antibody has not shown any complement dependent tumor cytotoxicity. IgG was not detected; however, the antibody could have been adsorbed by the tumor or have been present as IgG-tumor complexes. In mice depleted of macrophage function by treatment with trypan blue (4 mg s.c. the day before implantation and

TABLE 1. Lack of concomitant immunity to Lewis lung carcinoma[a]

| Days after initial s.c. tumor | Tumor incidence in mice challenged i.m. | |
	At various days after tumor implantation	In normal mice
3	10/10	4/4
7	9/9	4/4
10	6/6	3/3

[a] Mice were implanted s.c. with Lewis lung carcinoma on the right flank. On 3, 7, and 10 days later, these tumor-bearing mice and normal mice were injected i.m. on the left flank with 10^5 Lewis lung cells. The incidence of the i.m. tumors on day 30 after the initial s.c. tumor implant was then calculated. There was no significant difference in the time of appearance or the growth rates of the i.m. tumors in animals bearing a s.c. tumor as compared to i.m. tumors in control animals.

TABLE 2. Lack of tumor-specific transplantation immunity to Lewis lung carcinoma demonstrated by rechallenge[a]

Day of tumor removal	Mean survival time $\pm$ SE
Control	34.6 $\pm$ 1.5
Day 7	30.1 $\pm$ 2.2
Day 10	29.2 $\pm$ 2.1
Day 14	33.3 $\pm$ 0.5

[a] Mice were implanted s.c. with Lewis lung carcinoma and all tumors were surgically excised on day 7, 10, or 14. Normal mice and mice surviving until day 60, who showed no local tumor recurrence, were rechallenged i.m. with 10^5 Lewis lung carcinoma cells, and the mean survival time $\pm$ standard error was calculated.

TABLE 3. Growth of Lewis lung carcinoma in normal mice and mice deprived of T-cells [a]

| Experiment no. | Mean survival time + SE | |
	Normal	TxBM
1	22.5 + 2.2	36.2 + 1.1 (s)
2	34.0 + 2.0	38.6 + 1.8
3	29.1 + 1.4	36.6 + 1.3 (s)
4	30.3 + 2.1	40.3 + 2.9 (s)
5	28.5 + 1.9	44.4 + 3.7 (s)

[a] 1-mm^3 Pieces of Lewis lung tumor were transplanted s.c. into normal or TxBM mice. TxBM = thymectomized, lethally irradiated, bone marrow reconstituted mice. (s) = $p < 0.05$.

1 mg s.c. per week thereafter) or silica (40 mg i.p. 2 hr before implantation and 10 to 20 mg i.p. per week thereafter) the Lewis lung carcinoma grew slightly faster than in control animals. At days 18 to 28 tumor growth was two to three times greater than in controls, suggesting that macrophages may play a role in the natural resistance of the host to this tumor. The Lewis lung carcinoma appears comparable to many human tumors in its rapid metastasis to the lung and to its weakly immunogenic character, providing a pertinent tumor model in which to study immunotherapy.

Characterization of the Methylcholanthrene-Induced Sarcoma MCA 2182

In contrast to the Lewis lung carcinoma, we have shown that MCA 2182-bearing animals do develop tumor-specific transplantation resistance (2). In addition, the animals responded with an IgM humoral immune response similar to that observed toward the Lewis lung carcinoma. This immunogenic tumor does not metastasize readily (2).

Involvement of Macrophages in Immunopotentiator-Induced Resistance Against the Lewis Lung Carcinoma

We have previously shown that peritoneal macrophages recovered from mice treated with pyran or C. parvum were selectively cytotoxic in vitro for Lewis lung tumor cells and not for syngeneic mouse embryo cells (9). These results indicated that the immunopotentiators had the potential for inhibiting tumor growth through activated macrophages, but did not provide direct

TABLE 4. Inhibition of Lewis lung carcinoma growth in vivo by
activated peritoneal cells[a]

Preincubation treatment of Lewis lung cells	Tumor incidence (positive/total)	MST $\pm$ SE of tumor-positive mice
Alone	10/10	43.4 $\pm$ 3.5
Normal PEC	10/10	43.0 $\pm$ 2.9
Glycogen PEC	10/10	45.1 $\pm$ 1.9
Pyran PM	3/10	67.7 $\pm$ 19.1
C. parvum PEC	0/10	Alive at day 86

[a] Lewis lung cells were mixed with peritoneal exudate cells (PEC) or adherent peritoneal cells (PM) at a 10:1 ratio in vitro for 30 min at 36°C, the mixture then inoculated i.m. into mice, and the tumor incidence and mean survival time calculated.

evidence for macrophage involvement in the antitumor effects observed in vivo. Several other lines of evidence have more directly implicated activated macrophages in pyran- or C. parvum-induced resistance against the Lewis lung tumor.

With regard to inhibition of s.c. Lewis lung tumor growth by systemic i.p. administration of pyran, we have previously demonstrated that there is a prominent histiocytic infiltrate at the periphery of the s.c. tumor implant as well as around the pulmonary metastases in pyran-treated animals (10). Activated macrophages could be recovered from the peritoneal cavity of pyran-treated animals bearing the tumor, indicating that activated macrophages were present systemically in the mouse (10). Moreover, by using a transplantation assay as previously described (11), activated macrophages inoculated with tumor cells were demonstrated to inhibit the growth of Lewis lung cells in vivo (Table 4). Normal or glycogen-stimulated macrophages had no tumor inhibitory activity. The tumor-free survivors of these experiments were rechallenged with the homologous tumor and showed no transplantation resistance.

Although systemic i.p. or i.v. administration of C. parvum was ineffective in retarding growth of the s.c. Lewis lung implant (2), intralesional treatment with C. parvum into tumor growing in the footpad was effective in producing complete regressions in a small proportion of the animals (12). In a typical experiment, 17% of the mice showed complete regression of the tumors (Fig. 1). In this experiment the other mice showed an accelerated tumor growth rate, but this was not consistently observed. C. parvum activated macrophages were also effective in inhibiting Lewis lung growth

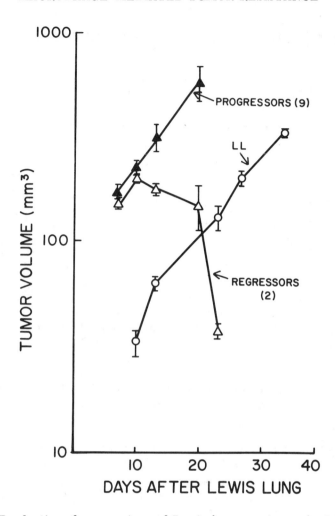

FIG. 1. Production of regressions of Lewis lung carcinoma by intralesional
C. parvum. Mice were injected with 2 X 10^4 tumor cells in the footpad, and
treated intralesionally with 70 mg/kg of C. parvum on day 3. Tumor size
was measured in individual mice, and plotted as the mean volume $\pm$ standard
error. The number of mice in parentheses indicates the number of mice in
each group. O——O = untreated mice (39.2 $\pm$ 3.0 days MST); $\triangle$——$\triangle$ =
C. parvum-treated mice which showed complete tumor regression (>60
days MST); $\blacktriangle$——$\blacktriangle$ = C. parvum-treated mice which showed no regression
(27.1 $\pm$ 2.4 days MST). A similar percentage of regressions (18%) was
produced in a larger experiment involving 70 tumor-bearing mice treated
with C. parvum.

in vivo (Table 4). Thus, macrophages appear likely to be involved in
C. parvum-induced resistance against the Lewis lung tumor.

TABLE 5. Inhibition of MCA 2182 sarcoma growth in vivo by activated peritoneal cells [a]

Preincubation treatment of MCA 2182 cells	Tumor incidence positive/total
Alone	9/9
Normal PEC	9/10
Glycogen PEC	10/10
C. parvum PEC	3/15

[a] MCA 2182 tumor cells were mixed in vitro for 30 min at 36°C with peritoneal exudate cells (PEC) at a 10:1 ratio before i.m. inoculation into mice, and the tumor incidence was calculated at day 40.

Involvement of Macrophages in C. parvum-Induced Resistance Against the MCA 2182 Sarcoma

Intralesional C. parvum treatment of mice bearing the MCA 2182 sarcoma in the footpad can produce complete regressions in a large percentage of the mice (12). That this inhibitory effect on the primary tumor is due to activated macrophages has been shown in a number of experiments. Inoculating C. parvum-activated peritoneal exudate cells with tumor cells reduced tumor incidence from 100% in control animals to 20% in the C. parvum-MCA 2182 group (Table 5). When mice were depleted of functional macrophages by treatment with trypan blue, a macrophage inhibitor, the tumor regressions induced by C. parvum in normal mice were reduced from 24% to 3% (Table 6). Thymus-derived lymphocytes did not appear to be essential for the immunopotentiator effect. When mice were depleted of thymus-derived lymphocytes by thymectomy, irradiation, and bone marrow reconstitution, intralesional treatment with C. parvum at high doses was as effective as in normal mice, although the drug was less effective at lower doses than in normal mice (Table 6).

DISCUSSION

We have previously shown that immunotherapeutic treatment of tumor-bearing mice with either the synthetic immunopotentiator, pyran, or the biological immunopotentiator, C. parvum, was effective in producing complete regressions or inhibition of solid tumor growth (12, 13). Systemic treatment of mice i.p. with pyran was effective in inhibiting the growth of s.c. implants of either the metastasizing, weakly immunogenic Lewis lung

TABLE 6. Effect of trypan blue or T-cell depletion on C. parvum-induced
regression of MCA 2182

	Regressors/total	
	Normal mice	Trypan blue-treated mice [a]
Treatment to inhibit macrophages		
Control	0/10 (0%)	0/8 (0%)
C. parvum	12/50 (24%)	1/37 (2.7%)
	Normal mice	TxBM mice [b]
Treatment to deplete T-cells		
Control	0/10 (0%)	0/10 (0%)
C. parvum, 70 and 35 mg/kg	16/20 (80%)	16/20 (80%)
C. parvum, 17.5, 8.8, 4.4, and 2.2 mg/kg	23/37 (62%)	15/40 (38%)

[a] Normal or trypan blue-treated (150 mg/kg on day 0 and 37.5 mg/kg
twice weekly thereafter) mice were inoculated with 5 X 10^4 MCA 2182 cells on
day 0, and on day 3 C. parvum was inoculated intralesionally. The data was
pooled over a dose range of C. parvum from 4.4 mg/kg to 70 mg/kg.

[b] Normal or TxBM mice were inoculated with 5 X 10^4 MCA 2182 cells on
day 0, and on day 3 the appropriate dose of C. parvum was inoculated intralesionally. The data with the indicated C. parvum doses were pooled as
shown because there were no significant differences in the regressions produced between the groups with 70 or 35 mg/kg or among the groups receiving
17.5, 8.8, 4.4, or 2.2 mg/kg.

carcinoma or the immunogenic but nonmetastasizing MCA 2182 sarcoma;
the drug was more effective against the Lewis lung carcinoma (2). Although
systemic i.p. or i.v. treatment with C. parvum was not effective in inhibiting
tumor growth, the drug was effective when administered intralesionally;
C. parvum was more effective against the MCA 2182 sarcoma than the Lewis
lung tumor (12). The difference may be related to the rapidity with which the
Lewis lung carcinoma metastasizes.

   Macrophages activated by treatment with either immunopotentiator appear
to be important effectors of the tumor resistance produced by these agents.
Both pyran and C. parvum-activated peritoneal cells were shown to inhibit
the growth of the tumors in vivo in a transplantation assay. Depletion of
mice of functional macrophages with trypan blue treatment abolished the
ability of C. parvum to produce regressions of the MCA 2182 sarcoma, indicating that macrophages are an essential component of the resistance induced

by C. parvum. These results are similar to those of Hibbs (4), who demonstrated that trypan blue abolished BCG protection. McBride has also recently reported that the antitumor action of C. parvum against another fibrosarcoma is reduced by treatment with gold salts, a macrophage toxin (personal communication).

Conversely, depletion of mice of thymus-derived lymphocytes did not markedly alter the tumor inhibitory activity of high doses of C. parvum, suggesting that T-lymphocytes are not essential for C. parvum-induced resistance against the primary tumor. These data are in accord with observations that T-cells are not necessary for activation of macrophages by pyran (9) or C. parvum (14). Several investigations have indicated that T-cells are not required for the antitumor effects of C. parvum. Treatment of mice with antilymphocyte serum did not alter the protective effect of prophylactic i.p. C. parvum against the ascitic Meth A tumor (15). Adult thymectomy, lethal irradiation, and bone marrow reconstitution did not significantly alter the tumor inhibitory effects of systemic i.p. C. parvum against the s.c. growth of either a fibrosarcoma or mammary carcinoma (16). Scott has also investigated the effects of thymectomy, irradiation, and bone marrow reconstitution on C. parvum therapy against the weakly immunogenic and nonmetastasizing P815 mastocytoma. Depletion of T-cells did not alter the transient antitumor effects of systemic i.v. C. parvum treatment (17). However, such T-cell depletion completely abolished the antitumor effect of intratumor C. parvum treatment. C. parvum inhibited tumor growth and produced complete regressions in approximately 50% of the animals in normal mice, while neither inhibiting tumor growth nor producing regressions in T-depleted mice (18). The differences observed among these diverse tumor systems emphasize the necessity for comparative studies of immunomodulators in several tumor systems. It is evident that different mechanisms of action are involved, depending on the particular tumor, route, and schedule of immunomodulator treatment. However, in the majority of systems it appears as if the antitumor effects of C. parvum do not require T-cells, but do require macrophages.

Thus, in two distinct tumor systems, and with two diverse immunomodulators, activated macrophages appear to be common effectors of antitumor resistance.

SUMMARY

Macrophages are implicated as important effectors of the resistance induced against solid tumors by two diverse immunopotentiators: the biological vaccine, Corynebacterium parvum, and the synthetic polyanion, pyran. Analogous results were observed with a weakly immunogenic but rapidly metastasizing tumor, Lewis lung carcinoma, and an immunogenic but nonmetastasizing methylcholanthrene-induced sarcoma, MCA 2182. Intraperitoneal inoculation of either drug activated peritoneal macrophages which were selectively cytotoxic for tumor cells in vitro. Inoculation of activated macrophages with tumor cells in vivo also inhibited tumor cell growth. Other evidence for the involvement of activated macrophages in pyran-induced resistance against the Lewis lung carcinoma has come from the observations of a prominent histiocytic infiltrate at the periphery of the tumor in pyran-treated mice as compared to control tumor-bearing mice, and from the ability to recover activated macrophages from the peritoneal cavity of tumor-bearing mice treated with pyran. In addition, treatment of mice with the macrophage inhibitors trypan blue or silica caused an increase in the growth of the Lewis lung carcinoma, suggesting that macrophages are involved in the natural resistance of the host to this tumor. Trypan blue treatment markedly reduced the ability of C. parvum to induce regressions of the MCA 2182 sarcoma, whereas depletion of thymus derived lymphocytes did not affect the ability of high doses of C. parvum to induce tumor regressions. These data suggest that macrophages are also intimately involved in C. parvum-induced regressions, whereas the thymus is not involved in the immunopotentiator-induced resistance against the growth of the primary tumor.

ACKNOWLEDGMENTS

This research was supported by U.S. Public Health Service grant CA-1537 and contract CB-43877. P.S.M. is a U.S. Public Health Service Research Career Development Awardee, AI 70863. The authors thank J. A. Munson, S. C. Johnson, and S. Bulgin for their excellent technical assistance.

REFERENCES

1. Bast, R. C., Zbar, B., Borsos, T., and Rapp, H. J. (1974): BCG and cancer. N. Engl. J. Med., 290:1413-1420.
2. Morahan, P. S., and Kaplan, A. M. (1976): Macrophage activation and antitumor activity of biologic and synthetic agents. Int. J. Cancer, 17:82-89.
3. Bomford, R., and Olivotto, M. (1974): The mechanism of inhibition by C. parvum on the growth of lung nodules from intravenously injected tumor cells. Int. J. Cancer, 14:226-235.
4. Hibbs, J. B. (1975): Activated macrophages as cytotoxic effector cells. I. Inhibition of specific and nonspecific tumor resistance by trypan blue. Transplantation, 19:77-81.
5. Attia, M. A. M., and Weiss, D. W. (1966): Immunology of spontaneous mammary carcinoma in mice. Cancer Res., 26:1787-1800.
6. Sugiura, K., and Stock, C. C. (1955): Studies in a tumor spectrum. Cancer Res., 15:38-45.
7. Mayo, J. G. (1972): Biologic characterization of the SC implanted Lewis lung tumor. Cancer Chemother. Rep., 3:325-330.
8. Umiel, T., and Trainin, N. (1974): Immunological enhancement of tumor growth by syngeneic thymus-derived lymphocytes. Transplantation, 18:244-250.
9. Kaplan, A. M., Morahan, P. S., and Regelson, W. (1974): Induction of macrophage-mediated tumor-cell cytotoxicity by pyran copolymer. J. Natl. Cancer Inst., 52:1919-1923.

10. Snodgrass, M. J., Morahan, P. S., and Kaplan, A. M. (1975): Histopathology of host response to Lewis lung carcinoma: Modulation by pyran. J. Natl. Cancer Inst., 55:455-462.

11. Zarling, J. M., and Tevethia, S. S. (1973): Transplantation immunity to simian virus 40-transformed cells in tumor bearing mice. J. Natl. Cancer Inst., 50:137-148.

12. Morahan, P. S., and Kaplan, A. M. (1976): Paradoxical effects of immunopotentiators in antitumor and antitumor virus treatment. J. Infect. Dis., 133:A249-A255.

13. Morahan, P. S., Munson, J. A., Baird, L. G., Kaplan, A. M., and Regelson, W. (1974): Antitumor action of pyran copolymer and tilorone against Lewis lung carcinoma and B-16 melanoma. Cancer Res., 34:506-511.

14. Bomford, R., and Christie, G. H. (1975): Mechanisms of macrophage activation by Corynebacterium parvum. II. In vivo experiments. Cell. Immunol., 17:150-155.

15. Castro, J. E. (1974): Antitumor effects of Corynebacterium parvum in mice. Eur. J. Cancer, 20:121-127.

16. Woodruff, M., Dunbar, N., and Ghaffar, A. (1973): The growth of tumors in T-cell deprived mice and their response to treatment with Corynebacterium parvum. Proc. Roy. Soc. Lond., 184:97-102.

17. Scott, M. T. (1974): Corynebacterium parvum as a therapeutic antitumor agent in mice I. Systemic effects from intravenous injection. J. Natl. Cancer Inst., 53:855-860.

18. Scott, M. T. (1974): Corynebacterium parvum as a therapeutic antitumor agent in mice II. Local injection. J. Natl. Cancer Inst., 53:861-865.

Control of Neoplasia by Modulation of the Immune System, edited by M. A. Chirigos. Raven Press, New York 1977.

MACROPHAGE REGULATION OF TUMOR CELL GROWTH AND MITOGEN-INDUCED BLASTOGENESIS

Alan M. Kaplan, Lynn G. Baird, and Page S. Morahan

Departments of Surgery and Microbiology and Division of Medical Oncology, MCV/VCU Cancer Center, Medical College of Virginia, Richmond, Virginia 23298

INTRODUCTION

Recent evidence indicates that macrophages play an important regulatory role in the proliferation of both normal and neoplastic cells. Synthetic reticuloendothelial stimulants such as polyacrylic acid-maleic anhydride, pyran, and polyriboinosinic-polycytidylic acid, and biologic reticuloendothelial stimulants such as Mycobacterium bovis, Corynebacterium parvum, and Toxoplasma gondii, are known to enhance macrophage function as well as to induce resistance to tumor growth (1-6). Macrophages from animals treated with these biological or chemical stimulants have been demonstrated to be selectively cytostatic and/or cytotoxic for tumor cells while demonstrating quantitatively less cytotoxicity for normal cells (1,2,4,6). Moreover, macrophages have been shown to inhibit mitogen-induced blastogenesis (7-9). We have also recently reported that normal or activated mouse peritoneal exudate cells (PEC) could inhibit the proliferation of normal spleen cells in response to either B- or T-cell mitogens (10).

Although macrophages can exert a regulatory effect on normal and neoplastic target cell proliferation in vitro, there is much controversy concerning the mechanism of regulation by this population of cells. Certain data suggest that macrophage target cell contact is required for tumoricidal activity, whereas several other lines of evidence have suggested that supernatants from activated macrophages can be cytotoxic for normal or tumor cells as well as inhibit mitogen-induced blastogenesis of normal lymphoid cells (11-13). Keller (14) and others (15-17) have presented evidence that soluble factors secreted from macrophages can substitute for cells in the modulation of cell proliferation in vitro. Waldman and Gottlieb (7) also demonstrated a soluble mediator, but the factor was only about 10% as effective as the macrophages themselves in inhibiting lymphocyte proliferation. In contrast, Parkhouse and Dutton (8) and Hersh and Harris (9) found that cell-to-cell contact was required for modulation of proliferation to occur.

The present studies concerning the mechanisms of regulation of cell proliferation were undertaken to compare the regulatory effects of normal and activated macrophages on both tumor cell growth and mitogen-induced blastogenesis.

MATERIALS AND METHODS

Mice

Adult (C57B1/6 X DBA/2) F_1 mice (BDF_1) or C57B1/6 mice were used in all experiments, and within a single experiment all mice were matched for sex and age.

Culture Medium and Cell Lines

Culture medium used was Eagle's minimum essential medium with Earle's balanced salt solution, 2x essential amino acids, vitamins, 100 U penicillin/ml, 100 µg streptomycin/ml, and 20% heat-inactivated fetal bovine serum (EMEM). The target cells included the murine Lewis lung carcinoma and C57B1/6J secondary mouse embryo cells.

Spleen Cell Suspensions

Mice were sacrificed by cervical dislocation, the spleens removed and cell suspensions prepared by forcing the spleens through 200-mesh stainless steel screens. Cells were washed three times in RPMI 1640 medium, counted, and suspended to the desired concentration.

Peritoneal Exudate Cells (PEC)

Cells were obtained from the peritoneal cavities of untreated, glycogen-treated, C. parvum-treated, or pyran-treated mice by washing twice with 4 ml of RPMI 1640. Normal PEC were obtained from either untreated mice or mice treated with type II oyster glycogen (Sigma G-8751, 0.5 ml of a 2.5% solution, i.p.) 5 days previously, a regimen which has been found to increase cell numbers without activating macrophages to kill tumor cells. In the experiments discussed in this chapter, PEC obtained from either untreated or glycogen-treated mice responded identically and will both be referred to as normal PEC. Activated macrophages are defined as macrophages which are cytotoxic to tumor cells in vitro but not to normal cells (2). Activated PE macrophages were obtained from mice given a single injection of 25 mg/kg of pyran copolymer or 17.5 mg/kg of C. parvum i.p. 7 days prior to harvesting. Histologic examination of smears from normal or pyran-treated mice revealed that the peritoneal exudate from normal mice contained 60% macrophages and 40% small lymphocytes, whereas that from pyran-treated mice contained 70% macrophages and 30% small lymphocytes.

In some experiments, adherent PEC were used. These were obtained by plating PEC in microtiter plates or Petri plates for 2 hr at 37°C in RPMI 1640 containing 10% human plasma or fetal bovine serum. The plates were then washed extensively with RPMI to remove nonadherent cells and the adherent cells harvested by gentle scraping with a rubber policeman.

Enzyme Treatment of PEC

In some experiments, PEC were treated with various enzymes before use in culture. PEC at a concentration of 2×10^6 cells/ml were incubated in 500 μg/ml of either β-galactosidase (0.32 U/mg protein, Sigma #G-1875), neuraminidase, Clostridium perfringens type V (0.12 U/mg protein, Sigma #N-2876), or type VI (2.1 U/mg protein, Sigma #N-3001) or pronase (Calbiochem #53702) for 30 min at 37°C. Before addition to spleen cell cultures, the cells were then washed three times and viabilities were found by trypan dye exclusion to be >95%.

Blastogenic Assay

Our assay for in vitro lymphocyte blastogenesis has been described in detail elsewhere (10). Briefly, a microtiter assay system was used to measure ^{3}H-thymidine incorporation into DNA after stimulation by mitogens. The T- and B-cell blastogenic responses of spleen cells in the presence of PEC were determined using phytohemagglutinin (PHA, Burroughs Wellcome) and lipopolysaccharide (LPS, Difco, E. coli, lipopolysaccharide, 0111:B4), respectively. When spleen cells were cultured in the presence of PEC, the total number of cells per culture was kept constant by using mitomycin-C (50 μg/ml, Sigma #M-0503)-treated normal spleen cells as filler cells. Cultures were incubated in RPMI 1640 supplemented with 9% fresh frozen human plasma in an atmosphere of 5% CO_2 and 95% air for 48 hr, at which time 2.0 μCi of ^{3}H-thymidine (New England Nuclear, sp. act. 1.9 Ci/mmole) were added and incubation was continued for an additional 24 hr. The cultures were then harvested and samples were counted in a liquid scintillation spectrometer.

Data were evaluated either as: (a) peak response in counts per minute, or (b) percent inhibition of the response compared to cultures without PEC. Values for peak counts per minute were the peak response of the entire dose-response curve for a given mitogen regardless of the concentration of mitogen. Values for percent inhibition were calculated using the following formula:

$$\text{percent inhibition} = 100 \times \left[1 - \frac{\text{(peak response with PEC)}}{\text{(peak response without PEC)}} \right]$$

Assay for Cytotoxicity by Release of ^{125}IUDR

Lewis lung carcinoma or secondary mouse embryo fibroblasts (1 X 10^4 cells/0.2 ml) were incubated in microtest plate wells (Falcon 3040) for 2 to 3 hr, after which the medium was removed and 0.01 to 0.02 μCi of ^{125}IUDR was added in new medium to give incorporation of approximately 200 to 500 cpm/well at 24 hr. Peritoneal exudate cells, either 4 X 10^5 or 2 X 10^5 in 0.2 ml (giving a final PE cell to target cell ratio of 20:1 or 10:1, respectively) were then added to the ^{125}IUDR-labeled target cells. Replicates of four to eight wells were used for each point. At various times during incubation, the supernatants were removed, and the amount of ^{125}IUDR determined by counting in a deep-well γ-scintillation counter. The plates were then fixed with 70% methanol, sprayed with clear plastic (Colony Paint Co., Baltimore, Maryland), the individual wells cut out with a band saw, and counted to determine the amount of ^{125}IUDR incorporated into the target cells. The percent cytotoxicity was determined by the following calculation:

$$\text{percent cytotoxicity} = 100 - \left(\frac{\text{cpm target cells}}{\text{cpm supernatant} + \text{cpm target cells}} \text{ X } 100 \right)$$

Assay for Cytostasis

The assay for cytostasis was done essentially as described for the ^{125}IUDR cytoxicity assay except that the target cells were not prelabeled with isotope. At various times after the addition of PE cells from normal, C. parvum-, or pyran-treated mice, the wells were pulsed for 1 hr with 0.2 μCi of ^{125}IUDR in EMEM with 10^{-6} M fluordeoxyuridine to inhibit thymidylate synthetase activity (18). After incubation for 1 hr, the supernatants with ^{125}IUDR were removed, the wells washed, and the plates handled as above.

RESULTS

Inhibition of Blastogenesis by Activated or Nonactivated PEC

We have previously shown that the blastogenic response of spleen cells removed from animals pretreated with pyran was inhibited compared to the response of normal spleens, and that removal of glass adherent spleen cells partially restored the blastogenic response to normal (10).

To investigate more readily the role of the adherent cell, or macrophage, as a regulator of lymphoid proliferation, we utilized a system in which activated or normal peritoneal exudate cells (PEC) were added to normal spleen cells and the blastogenic response of this mixed population determined. The addition of either activated or normal PEC to normal spleen cells inhibited blastogenesis of both T- and B-lymphocytes (Fig. 1). Although both populations of PEC were inhibitory, activated PEC were found to have greater inhibitory activity than normal PEC. Blastogenesis in response to LPS was consistently found to be more sensitive to inhibition by either activated or normal PEC than the response to PHA.

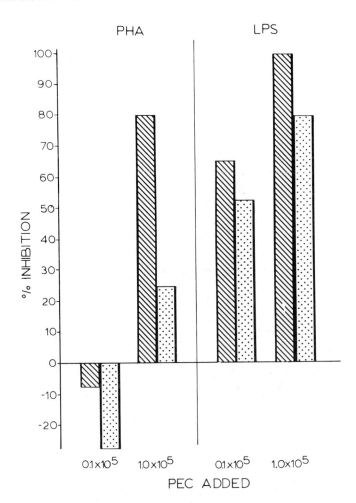

FIG. 1. Inhibition of blastogenesis as a function of the number of normal or activated PEC added to cultures of normal spleen cells. Each well contained 5 X 10⁵ normal spleen cells, the indicated number of PEC, and the appropriate number of mitomycin-C-treated spleen cells to give a total of 7 X 10⁵ cells/well. Percent inhibition was calculated from the peak response of the entire dose-response curve for a given mitogen. Values of negative inhibition indicate enhancement of blastogenesis. Hatched-activated PEC; stippled-normal PEC.

Inhibition of Blastogenesis by Adherent PEC

In order to determine whether the adherent or nonadherent subpopulation of PEC was responsible for the inhibition of blastogenesis of normal spleen cells, PEC were plated in microtest wells and allowed to adhere for 2 hr. The wells were then washed extensively with RPMI to remove nonadherent cells. Normal spleen cells, mitogen, and plasma were then added to these cultures in

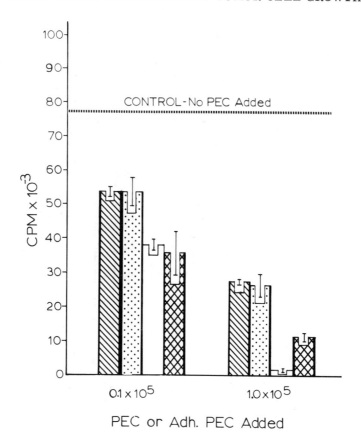

FIG. 2. Inhibition of the blastogenic response to LPS as a function of total PEC and the adherent PEC concentration. Each well contained 5 X 10^5 normal spleen cells, 0.1 or 1.0 X 10^5 PEC, and an appropriate number of mitomycin-C-treated spleen cells to give a total of 7 X 10^7 cells/well. In the case of adherent PE cells the number on the abscissa refers to the numbers of PEC added before adherence and washing. Only 10 to 20% of the cells initially plated remained after vigorous washing before addition of lymphocytes. Values for counts per minute are the peak response of the entire dose-response curve for LPS and represent the mean of three replicate cultures. The bars represent $\pm$SE. Hatched-normal PEC; stippled-normal adherent PEC; open-activated PEC; cross-hatched-activated adherent PEC.

the usual concentrations. Control cultures contained unseparated PEC rather than adherent PEC. The blastogenic response to LPS was inhibited by both activated and normal adherent PEC (Fig. 2). The curves obtained with normal PEC and normal adherent PEC were quite comparable, as were the curves obtained for activated PEC and activated adherent PEC. The greater inhibitory capacity of unseparated PEC may be due to the fact that the number of adherent PEC remaining after washing was only 10 to 20% of the number of unseparated PEC added to comparable wells. This decreased number of adherent cells also may explain the finding that no increase in inhibition of blastogenesis was observed following enrichment for macrophages by adherence.

The Effect of Enzymatic Treatment of PEC on Their Ability to Inhibit Blastogenesis

In an attempt to determine whether a specific glycoprotein or protein macrophage surface component was required for inhibition of blastogenesis, PEC were treated with various enzymes prior to their addition to cultures of normal spleen cells. Untreated control PEC were incubated at the same cell concentration in RPMI instead of the specificied enzyme. PEC were washed three times following treatment to remove excess enzyme, and all PEC preparations were found to be >95% viable by trypan blue exclusion. Untreated activated PEC inhibited the blastogenic responses to PHA and LPS by 95% and 94%, respectively (Table 1). Treatment of PEC with β-galactosidase had no effect on the inhibition of the LPS response, although a slight decrease in inhibition was seen in the PHA response. In contrast, treatment of PEC with Cl. perfringens neuraminidase type V decreased the PEC-mediated inhibition of both PHA and LPS responses to 25 to 30%. When PEC were treated with both neuraminidase and β-galactosidase (data not presented), the PEC inhibited to the same extent as those treated with neuraminidase alone.

Because neuraminidase type V is contaminated with a small amount of protease (0.030 U/mg protein), it became important to determine whether the release from inhibition was the result of protease or neuraminidase activity. Therefore, PEC were treated with type VI (which has less protease activity, 0.003 U/mg enzyme) or pronase before their addition to culture. The purer type VI enzyme had no effect on the inhibition of the response to LPS, although inhibition of the response to PHA was significantly reduced from 95% to 56% after enzyme treatment of PEC. Pronase treatment also decreased the inhibition of activated PEC and, as with type VI neuraminidase, pronase had a greater effect on the response to PHA than LPS. The response to LPS was reduced from 94% to 48% inhibition after pronase treatment, whereas the response to PHA was actually enhanced by 63% compared to control cultures without PEC. Similar results were obtained when normal PEC treated with these enzymes were cultured with normal spleen cells. Therefore, it seems that pronase and, to a lesser extent, neuraminidase can remove macrophage surface components which are required for macrophage-mediated inhibition of lymphocyte proliferation.

Inhibition of Tumor Cell Division in Vitro by Activated Peritoneal Exudate Cells

We have previously shown that pyran- or C. parvum-activated macrophages are selectively cytotoxic for tumor cells as compared to normal cells, and that cytotoxicity was a delayed event occurring between 24 and 48 hr after

TABLE 1.   The effect of enzymatic treatment of PEC on their ability to inhibit blastogenesis

Enzyme treatment of PEC[b]	Normal spleen ± activated PEC[a]			
	PHA		LPS	
	Counts per minute[c]	Percent inhibition	Counts per minute[c]	Percent inhibition
No PEC added (control)[d]	124,244	—	43,586	—
None	5,818	95	2,588	94
β-Galactosidase	14,972	88	2,729	94
Neuraminidase (type V)	94,397	24	31,039	29
Neuraminidase (type VI)	54,667	56	4,359	90
Pronase	202,518	-63[e]	22,665	48

[a] 5×10^5 Normal spleen cells cultured with 0.5×10^5 mitomycin-C-treated normal spleen cells and 1.5×10^5 activated PEC.

[b] 2×10^6 PEC/ml were treated with 500 μg/ml of the designated enzyme for 30 min at $37°C$. PEC which received no enzyme treatment were similarly incubated in RPMI 1640. All cells were washed three times and viabilities determined before addition to culture.

[c] Counts per minute given for peak response of complete dose-response curve of mitogen.

[d] 5×10^5 Normal spleen cells cultured with 2×10^5 mitomycin-C-treated normal spleen cells.

[e] Negative inhibition denotes enhancement.

the introduction of macrophages to cultured tumor cells (2,19). However, the selectivity of normal and/or activated macrophages for tumor cell cytostasis is as yet undefined.

Both Lewis lung cells alone and Lewis lung cells incubated with normal PEC continued to grow, as measured by incorporation of ^{125}IUDR over the 48-hr test period (Table 2). In contrast, Lewis lung cells incubated with C. parvum-activated peritoneal exudate cells at a ratio of 20:1 showed a 68% inhibition of DNA synthesis at 6 hr. By 24 hr after the addition of pyran-activated peritoneal exudate cells, DNA synthesis was inhibited by >98% by

TABLE 2. Pyran- and C. parvum-activated peritoneal exudate cell-mediated inhibition of DNA synthesis in Lewis lung and secondary mouse embryo cells

Target cells	Peritoneal cell addition	Incorporation of ^{125}IUDR (cpm $\pm$ SE) [a]		
		6 hr	24 hr	48 hr
Lewis lung	None	$3,172 \pm 68$	$5,591 \pm 361$	$12,347 \pm 613$
	Normal PEC	$2,368 \pm 86$	$3,035 \pm 236$	$7,323 \pm 425$
	Pyran PEC	$2,064 \pm 77$	89 ± 22	25 ± 15
	C. parvum PEC	$1,023 \pm 54$	89 ± 17	3 ± 2
Mouse embryo	None	375 ± 25	393 ± 87	425 ± 168
	Normal PEC	222 ± 15	185 ± 34	228 ± 120
	Pyran PEC	262 ± 12	28 ± 6	6 ± 4
	C. parvum PEC	158 ± 6	38 ± 13	1 ± 2

[a] Normal, C. parvum-, or pyran-activated PEC were added to 18-hr subconfluent monolayers of target cells at a 20:1 PEC-to-target cell ratio, and the cells pulsed at various times for 1-hr intervals with ^{125}IUDR. After 1 hr the cells were washed, fixed with methanol, the wells cut out, and the amount of ^{125}IUDR incorporated determined by counting in a γ-scintillation spectrometer.

either C. parvum- or pyran-activated macrophages. Inhibition of DNA synthesis in the presence of activated peritoneal exudate cells was maintained throughout the 48-hr test period.

In contrast to the results which have previously demonstrated that activated PEC were not cytotoxic to labeled normal target cells (2, 19), activated PEC were cytostatic to both tumor and normal cells. Both pyran- and C. parvum-activated macrophages, at a ratio of 20:1 macrophages:mouse embryo cells, caused a 92% reduction in the uptake of ^{125}IUDR at 24 hr after the addition of macrophages to the mouse embryo cells. Comparable results have been obtained with WI-38 human lung fibroblasts (Kaplan and Morahan, unpublished observations).

DISCUSSION

Previous work done by us (10) and others (7, 8, 14, 16) has demonstrated that the addition of normal or activated PEC to cultures of normal mouse spleen cells inhibited the blastogenic response of the lymphocytes to both T- and B-lymphocyte mitogens. The current experiments in which nonadherent PEC were removed prior to culture with normal spleen cells indicated that the adherent subpopulation of PEC was responsible for the suppression of blastogenesis. Similarly, the removal of adherent spleen cells from either normal or pyran-treated mice caused an enhancement of blastogenesis when compared to unseparated spleen cells (Baird and Kaplan, unpublished observations).

Although significant inhibition of blastogenesis could be obtained with normal PEC, activated PEC were found to be more efficient suppressor cells. The blastogenic response of normal spleen cells to LPS appeared to be more sensitive to inhibition by PEC than the comparable responses to PHA. Furthermore, enzymatic treatment of PEC before their addition to culture was more effective in reducing the PEC-mediated inhibition of blastogenesis of normal spleen cells to PHA than to LPS. The differential inhibition of T- and B-cell blastogenesis by PEC could be due to: (a) qualitative differences in subpopulations of PEC which inhibit T- and B-lymphocytes, or (b) differential sensitivities of B- and T-lymphocytes toward the same inhibitory adherent cell or macrophage.

Macrophage regulation of lymphocyte proliferation is well documented in the current literature. Both inhibition (7, 8, 10, 14, 16, 17, 20) and enhancement (9, 13, 21) of lymphocyte proliferation have been reported in various systems and the outcome may be dependent on the macrophage-to-lymphocyte ratio in culture (7, 14). The present data are in agreement with this concept, because we demonstrated enhancement of the PHA response at low PEC concentrations and inhibition of the PHA response at high PEC concentrations (Fig. 1).

Several lines of evidence from our laboratory indicate that cell-to-cell contact rather than a soluble mediator is responsible for inhibition of blastogenesis in this system (22): (a) Supernatant materials harvested from PEC cultures were capable of producing only minimal inhibition of blastogenesis compared to lesser numbers of intact PEC; and (b) in experiments in which PEC were present for only part of the culture period rather than the entire time, 80 to 90% inhibition of the response could still be obtained. These cultures were washed thoroughly at the time of removal of PEC, and thus a soluble mediator would have been removed unless it had become irreversibly bound to the lymphocyte surface. This is unlikely in view of the work done by others (7, 13, 14) who reported that their soluble factors act reversibly. (c) The strongest evidence in favor of cell-to-cell contact as a requisite of inhibition of lymphoid proliferation are those experiments in which pretreatment of PEC with various enzymes before addition to culture reduced the inhibition of blastogenesis. Treatment with a highly purified preparation of Cl. perfringens neuraminidase was able to partially reduce the inhibition of the response to PHA while having no effect on the response to LPS. Pronase treatment, in contrast, was able to reduce the PEC-mediated inhibition of the response to both PHA and LPS, although it was more effective in the response to PHA. These results indicate that protein or glycoprotein components on the surface of the macrophage are necessary for inhibition of blastogenesis to occur and are inconsistent with the presence of a soluble inhibitor.

We have previously demonstrated that macrophage-mediated cytotoxicity was a delayed event (19). The kinetics of cytotoxicity in vitro in the ^{125}IUDR release assay were consistent with cell death occurring after 24 hr and primarily by 48 hr. The delayed occurrence of cytoxocity of ^{125}IUDR-labeled tumor cells explains the inability of Keller (15) to detect ^{51}Cr release from labeled tumor target cells cultured with macrophages for only 12 hr. Cytotoxicity was tumor cell-selective (as opposed to antigen-specific) because pyran-activated macrophages demonstrated little cytotoxicity against normal mouse embryo fibroblasts (1, 2, 4, 23).

In the present report, cytostasis of tumor cell growth, as measured by inhibition of ^{125}IUDR incorporation into DNA of the target cells, could be detected by 6 hr after incubation with activated macrophages. Cytostasis was produced by macrophages activated by the synthetic immunomodulator, pyran, or the biologic immunomodulator, C. parvum. Experiments using mouse embryo fibroblasts or WI-38 cells (Kaplan and Morahan, unpublished observations) as target cells indicated that activated macrophages were equally cytostatic for normal and tumor target cells. In most other reports of macrophage-mediated cytostasis, only tumor cells were used as target cells (24-26). Although more recent data suggest that the regulatory or cytostatic effect of macrophages may be partially dependent on the rate of proliferation of target cells (15), the data presented here indicate that both a relatively rapidly proliferating tumor line (Lewis lung) and relatively slowly growing fibroblasts (secondary mouse embryo cells and WI-38 cells) are subject to macrophage cytostasis. Thus, although selectivity exists for macrophage-mediated tumor cell cytotoxicity, there does not appear to be tumor-versus-normal selectivity of activated macrophage-mediated cytostasis.

It is possible that cytostasis may be a general nonspecific property of activated macrophages, whereas the eventual cytotoxic event is selective for tumor cells. If cytostasis is actively maintained for a long enough period, it may result in irreversible cell death: The ultimate specificity of cytotoxicity may be due to differential tumor-versus-normal cell sensitivity to prolonged inhibition of DNA synthesis or to differential sensitivities at the cell membrane. Alternatively, a separate cytotoxic event may require approximately 24 to 48 hr to occur. This would be consistent with the results of Keller (25), who demonstrated that activated macrophage-tumor cell contact had to be maintained for 24 hr to get irreversible cytostasis in tumor cells. Moreover, Keller (15) demonstrated an inhibited cloning efficiency for tumor but not normal cells after 72 hr of contact with macrophages.

Tumor cytostasis and/or cytotoxicity was dependent on the presence of macrophages activated by either synthetic agents such as pyran copolymer or biologic agents such as C. parvum. Glycogen-stimulated macrophages were neither cytostatic nor cytotoxic, and these results are consistent with other reports which indicate that, in the mouse, macrophages cytotoxic for tumor cells cannot be activated by glycogen, starch, protease peptone, or thioglycollate (23). However, although thioglycollate-stimulated macrophages are not cytotoxic or cytostatic to tumor cells, they can inhibit the replication of vaccinia virus in mouse embryo fibroblasts (Morahan and Glasgow, unpublished observations). Moreover, as we have demonstrated, both normal and activated macrophages can be inhibitory to mitogen-induced blastogenesis.

These results are consistent with the concept that the ultimate regulatory effect of macrophages on either tumor cell growth or lymphocyte blastogenesis depends primarily on target cell susceptibility and the state of differentiation of the macrophage. Normal peritoneal macrophages, or glycogen, thioglycollate-, pyran-, or C. parvum-elicited peritoneal macrophages differ quantitatively and/or qualitatively in their ability to inhibit lymphocyte blastogenesis, viral replication, or tumor cell growth. Whether these functional differences are representative of different steps in a common differentiation pathway or represent separate classes of macrophages is at present unknown.

SUMMARY

Syngeneic mouse macrophages activated by the immunopotentiator, pyran copolymer, inhibited the blastogenic response of mouse lymphocytes to B- and T-cell mitogens. This could be demonstrated by the removal of adherent cells from the spleens of pyran-treated mice or by the addition of peritoneal macrophages from pyran-treated mice to cultures of normal lymphocytes. Similar, but less striking inhibition was demonstrated with normal macrophages, suggesting a regulatory role for macrophages in lymphoproliferation. Pretreatment of macrophages with either pronase or Cl. perfringens neuraminidase before their addition to cultures of normal spleen cells resulted in a decrease in inhibition of the blastogenic response.

Activated peritoneal macrophages from mice treated with pyran copolymer or C. parvum have previously been shown to be cytotoxic to ^{125}IUDR-labeled Lewis lung tumor cells but not to normal secondary mouse embryo fibroblasts or WI-38 human lung fibroblasts. In contrast, activated macrophages were cytostatic to both normal cells and tumor cells. Cytotoxicity was shown to be a delayed event, whereas cytostasis could be detected within 6 hr after the introduction of macrophages to cultured tumor cells. These results are consistent with a separate mechanism for macrophage-mediated tumor cell cytostasis and cytotoxicity.

ACKNOWLEDGMENTS

This research was supported in part by U. S. Public Health Service grants CA 1537 and AI 11561 and contract CB-43877. P. S. M. is a recipient of U. S. Public Health Service Research Career Development Award AI 70863.

REFERENCES

1. Hibbs, J. B., Jr., Lambert, L. H., Jr., and Remington, J. S. (1971): Resistance to murine tumors conferred by chronic infection with intracellular protozoa, Toxoplasma gondii and Besnoitia jellisoni. J. Infect. Dis., 124:587-592.

2. Kaplan, A. M., Morahan, P. S., and Regelson, W. (1974): Induction of macrophage-mediated tumor-cell cytotoxicity by pyran copolymer. J. Natl. Cancer Inst., 52:1919-1923.

3. Parr, I., Wheller, E., and Alexander, P. (1973): Similarities of the antitumor action of endotoxin, lipid A and double stranded RNA. Br. J. Cancer, 27:379-389.

4. Holterman, O. A., Klein, E., and Casale, G. P. (1973): Selective cytotoxicity of peritoneal leucocytes for neoplastic cells. Cell. Immunol., 9:339-352.

5. Ghaffar, A., Cullen, R. T., Dunbar, N., and Woodruff, M. F. A. (1974): Anti-tumor effect in vitro of lymphocytes and macrophages from mice treated with Corynebacterium parvum. Br. J. Cancer, 29:199-205.

6. Cleveland, R. P., Meltzer, M. S., and Zbar, B. (1974): Tumor cytotoxicity in vitro by macrophages from mice infected with Mycobacterium bovis strain BCG. J. Natl. Cancer Inst., 52:1887-1895.

7. Waldman, S. R., and Gottlieb, A. A. (1973): Macrophage regulation of DNA synthesis in lymphoid cells: Effect of a soluble factor from macrophages. Cell. Immunol., 9:142-156.

8. Parkhouse, R. M. E., and Dutton, R. W. (1966): Inhibition of spleen cell DNA synthesis by autologous macrophages. J. Immunol., 97:663-669.

9. Hersh, E. M., and Harris, J. E. (1968): Macrophage-lymphocyte interaction in the antigen-induced blastogenic response of human peripheral blood leukocytes. J. Immunol., 100:1184-1194.

10. Baird, L. G., and Kaplan, A. M. (1975): Immunoadjuvant activity of pyran copolymer. I. Evidence for direct stimulation of T-lymphocytes and macrophages. Cell. Immunol., 20:167-176.

11. Currie, G. A., and Basham, C. (1975): Activated macrophages release a factor which lyses malignant cells but not normal cells. J. Exp. Med., 142:1600-1605.

12. Pincus, W. B. (1967): Formation of cytotoxic factor by macrophages from normal guinea pigs. J. Reticuloendothel. Soc., 4:122-139.

13. Unanue, E. R., Calderon, J., and Kiely, J. M. (1975): Secretion by macrophages of two molecules modulating cell proliferation. In: Immune Recognition, edited by A. S. Rosenthal, pp. 555-570. Academic Press, New York.

14. Keller, R. (1975): Major changes in lymphocyte proliferation evoked by macrophages. Cell. Immunol., 17:542-551.

15. Keller, R. (1974): Modulation of cell proliferation by macrophages: A possible function apart from cytotoxic tumor rejection. Br. J. Cancer, 30:401-415.

16. Opitz, H. G., Niethammer, D., Lemke, H., Flad, H. D., and Huget, R. (1975): Inhibition of ^{3}H-thymidine incorporation of lymphocytes by a soluble factor from macrophages. Cell. Immunol., 16:379-388.

17. Nelson, D. A. (1973): Production by stimulated macrophages of factors depressing lymphocyte transformation. Nature, 246:306-307.

18. Cohen, A. M., Burdick, J. F., and Ketchum, A. S. (1971): Cell mediated cytotoxicity: An assay using ^{125}I-iododeoxyuridine labelled target cells. J. Immunol., 107:895-898.

19. Kaplan, A. M., Walker, P. L., and Morahan, P. S. (1975): Tumor cell cytotoxicity versus cytostasis of pyran activated macrophages. Fogarty International Center Proceedings, No. 28. U.S. Government Printing Office, Washington, D. C. (in press).

20. Calderon, J., Williams, R. T., and Unanue, E. R. (1974): An inhibitor of cell proliferation released by cultures of macrophages. Proc. Natl. Acad. Sci. (U.S.A.), 71:4273-4277.

21. Seeger, R. C., and Oppenheim, J. J. (1970): Synergistic interaction of macrophages and lymphocytes in antigen-induced transformation of lymphocytes. J. Exp. Med., 132:44-63.

22. Baird, L. G., and Kaplan, A. M. (1976): Macrophage mediated inhibition of lymphocyte blastogenesis. In: Leukocyte Membrane Determinants Regulating Immune Reactivity, edited by V. P. Eijsvoogel, D. Roos, and W. P. Zeijlemaker, p. 361. Academic Press, New York.

23. Hibbs, J. B., Lambert, L. H., and Remington, J. S. (1972): In vitro nonimmunologic destruction of cells with abnormal growth characteristics by adjuvant activated macrophages. Proc. Soc. Exp. Biol. Med., 139:1049-1052.

24. Keller, R., Keist, R., and Ivatt, R. J. (1974): Functional and biochemical parameters of activation related to macrophage cytostatic effects on tumor cells. Int. J. Cancer, 14:675-683.

25. Keller, R. (1974): Mechanisms by which activated normal macrophages destroy syngeneic rat tumor cells in vitro. Immunology, 27:285-298.

26. Keller, R. (1973): Cytostatic elimination of syngeneic rat tumor cells in vitro by nonspecifically activated macrophages. J. Exp. Med., 138:625-644.

Control of Neoplasia by Modulation of the Immune System, edited by M. A. Chirigos. Raven Press, New York 1977.

GLUCAN-INDUCED ENHANCEMENT IN HOST RESISTANCE TO EXPERIMENTAL TUMORS

*Nicholas R. Di Luzio, *,**Ernesto O. Hoffmann, *James A. Cook, †William Browder, and †,‡ Peter W. A. Mansell

*Departments of Physiology and †Surgery, Tulane University School of Medicine,
**Department of Pathology, L.S.U. School of Medicine,
New Orleans, Louisiana 70112, and
‡Department of Surgery, Royal Victoria Hospital, Montreal, Canada

INTRODUCTION

In contrast to the rather wide variety of defense mechanisms available to the body to protect itself against invading bacteria or viruses, the defense mechanisms which are now known to exist to protect man against malignant cell populations are much more limited in nature. It is generally agreed that host defense mechanisms against neoplastic cells involve two predominant cell populations, the macrophage and the lymphocyte, and that the interaction of these cells and their component populations, which form the basis of humoral and cell-mediated immunity, are critical events in determining eventual outcome of tumor growth and proliferation.

Although in the past major emphasis has been placed on the role of lymphocytes, and particularly the T-lymphocyte, as killer cells (1-4), increasing evidence is being provided that the major determinant to tumor growth and proliferation is the macrophage. Activated macrophages, in contrast to lymphocytes (5), possess the ability to kill tumor cells in vitro at what might be considered physiological macrophage:tumor cell ratios (6). Additionally, the macrophage content of tumors has been demonstrated to influence tumor immunogenicity as well as metastases (5). In support of this concept, it has been demonstrated that the administration of activated macrophage populations, either within the primary tumor site (7) or intravenously (8), can markedly affect the growth of the tumor and the dissemination of tumor cells. The intralesional administration of a variety of agents which possess the ability to mobilize and activate macrophages into tumor to where changes occur in tumor cell:macrophage populations contributes to the destruction of malignant cell populations in both experimental animals (9,10) and man (11-14).

Although it is becoming increasingly evident that macrophages play an important role in host defense against neoplasia, the specific mechanism is not fully ascertained. It appears that a dysfunctional state of the macrophage population such as impaired macrophage surveillance (15) or a limitation in number of host macrophages (5,16) may be two critical physiological determinants to the growth of malignancy.

In view of the unique role the reticuloendothelial system (RES) plays in maintaining the purity of the internal environment, numerous attempts have been made during the past 20 years to develop pharmacological agents which possess the ability to enhance specifically the functional activity of this unique system and thus define the dimensions of RES function. The accent on pharmacological agents was required because of the inability to produce a deficiency syndrome by surgical excision of the RES and the questionable nature of RES blockade as a functional entity. At the present time there are a limited number of biological and/or pharmacological agents which possess the ability to enhance specifically the functional activity of this system (17, 18), and relatively few that fulfill criteria proposed for a desirable macrophage stimulant (17).

Among one of the first agents employed in an attempt to delineate the physiological and immunological role of the RES was zymosan (19). Zymosan was the name given by Pillemer and Ecker (20) to a yeast cell wall fraction which had the property of inactivating the third component of the complement and adsorbing properdin. This cell wall preparation, derived from Saccharomyces cerevisiae, was initially demonstrated to be an effective RE stimulant by Benacerraf and Sebestyen (19).

Zymosan is a complex yeast cell wall fraction consisting of protein, lipid, and complex polysaccharides, namely mannan and glucan (21). Di Carlo and Fiore (22) reported that the composition of the yeast cell wall on a dry basis was approximately 58% glucan and 18% mannan. Glucan comprises the inner cell wall with mannan comprising the outer cell wall (23). Since the observations of Benacerraf and Sebestyen (19), zymosan has been uniformly demonstrated to produce marked stimulation of the RES. These events include enhancement in phagocytosis, increased rate of intracellular degradation of phagocytized particulates, increased resistance to certain infections, elevation in properdin levels, enhanced humoral immunity, and inhibition or regression of certain experimental tumors (24-28).

In view of the profound biological activities produced by the administration of zymosan, studies were initiated in our laboratory in the late 1950s to isolate the component of zymosan which possessed the specific ability to initiate activation and proliferation of the RES and thereby increase a variety of host defense mechanisms. In an extensive study of various components present in zymosan, we reported in 1961 that the active RE stimulant in zymosan was glucan (29). Glucan has been characterized as a polyglucose consisting of a chain of gluco-pyranose units united by a β (1 → 3) glucosidic linkage (30) (Fig. 1). In addition, a minor β (1 → 6) glucan component has also been

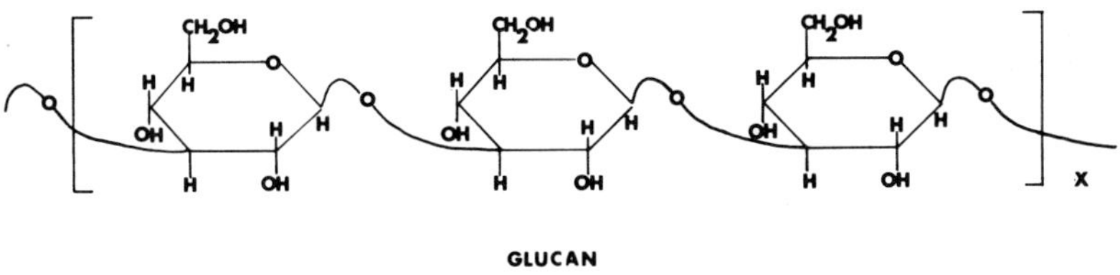

GLUCAN

FIG. 1. Structural formula for yeast glucan, which has a proposed molecular weight of about 6,500 (30).

recently reported (31). The latter component of yeast glucan has been found to be inactive relative to macrophage activation (32).

The current clinical immunotherapeutic experimental procedures are heavily dependent on the use of such nonspecific immunostimulants as Bacillus Calmette-Guerin (BCG) and Corynebacterium parvum. These agents clearly have a number of disadvantages which relate directly to their bacterial nature, antigenic qualities, the inability of standardization, infectious complications, unknown metabolites, and the fact that the immunostimulant is an unknown molecular entity (33-35). Jones, McBride, and Weir (36) demonstrated that macrophages from mice which have been injected with anerobic coryneform organisms possess cytotoxicity to normal cells. In view of the experimental clinical use of C. parvum, the possible problem of C. parvum initiating macrophage killing of normal cells may be a matter of concern and a possible contributory factor to its toxicity.

In studies conducted in our laboratory to define the influence of macrophage activation on tumor growth, it was observed that the simultaneous subcutaneous administration of glucan with Shay myelogenous leukemia cells significantly inhibited growth of the tumor (37). In subsequent preliminary clinical studies involving three types of metastatic lesions, the intralesional administration of glucan produced, in all cases studied, a prompt and striking reduction in the size of the lesion (7) in five to ten days. Regression of the glucan-injected tumor was associated with necrosis of the malignant cells and a pronounced monocytic infiltrate.

Because glucan appeared to offer distinct advantages (7,14,16,17,38) over most other currently employed forms of immunotherapy which make use of viable organisms, this chapter reviews our studies on the utilization of glucan in the prevention and treatment of Shay myelogenous leukemia tumor.

To define further the importance of the number and function of host macrophages in resistance in neoplasia, and the role of tumor macrophage number and function with regard to growth and dissemination of the malignant cells, studies were conducted in which varying concentrations of glucan-activated peritoneal macrophages were added to tumor cells at the time of transplantation. The influence of altered tumor-macrophage cell ratios on growth and dissemination of the tumor was ascertained.

Although intralesional glucan was effective in producing regression of various types of tumors in man (7) and in the rat leukemia model (16), in view of the allogeneic nature of the acute myelogenous leukemia tumor, additional studies were conducted evaluating the tumor-inhibitory effect of glucan in two syngeneic mouse tumor models. The common ancestry of various rat strains may limit genetic dissimilarity of the employed rat tumor system, as Palm and Wilson (39) point out that the 52 existing inbred rat strains are virtually all descendants of the original Wistar colonies.

Our composite experimental studies denote that glucan activation of macrophages, either before or after tumor cell transplantation, significantly modified the course of the malignancy in both the rat and mouse models. Additionally, the growth as well as dissemination of tumor cells from the primary site appears to be regulated by the number of macrophages which exist within the primary tumor site.

MATERIALS AND METHODS

Long Evans hooded rats, 3 to 4 weeks old, were employed as hosts for the Shay chloroleukemia tumor (40). Because certain features of the tumor, particularly with respect to its veroperoxidase content, as well as its virulence (41-42), have changed since it was first isolated by Shay et al. in 1951 (40), we have designated the tumor as the Shay myelogenous leukemia tumor (16) rather than chloroleukemia.

The Shay myelogenous leukemia tumor was specifically selected as the tumor of choice in view of our previous studies on the role of recognition factors in controlling macrophage surveillance of malignant cells (43-45) and the desire to have the circulating leukemia cells exposed to the fixed macrophage populations which are readily activated by glucan. The rapid dissemination of the tumor cells from the primary site also allows evaluation of the effectiveness of therapy on the secondary as well as the primary lesions. The increased susceptibility of the leukemic rats to bacterial infection (Fig. 2) also effectively permits an evaluation of macrophage activation on enhanced bacterial susceptibility, an important facet of human neoplastic disease.

Two syngeneic mouse tumors were also employed, the adenocarcinoma BW10232 and melanoma B16, spontaneous tumors of C57BL/6J mice which were first delineated in 1958 and 1954, respectively (Jackson Laboratory, Bar Harbor, Maine). Lung metastases occur in the former, whereas metastases to lung, spleen, and liver occur in the latter.

Tissue specimens from control and experimental animals were fixed in buffered formalin (4%) for 24 hr and embedded in paraffin. Six-micron sections were stained with hematoxylin and eosin. The specimens were evaluated without knowledge of the mode of treatment.

Glucan was prepared from Active Dry Yeast (Standard Brands, Inc., New York) by a modification of the method of Hassid, Joslyn, and McCready (30). The yield of glucan approximates 6%. The particulate glucan, which averaged about 1 to 2 μ in size (14) was suspended in a 5% dextrose and water solution and sterilized prior to use.

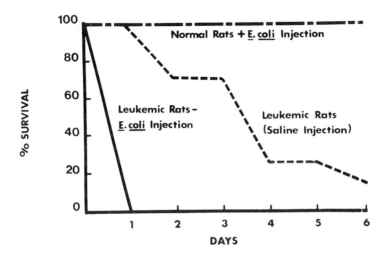

FIG. 2.   Mortality pattern of normal and leukemia rats following intravenous injection of viable E. coli (1 X 10^9/100 g). E. coli was injected 8 days following the intravenous injection of 5 X 10^6 leukemic cells/100 g.   No mortality was manifested in normal rats following E. coli administration, whereas 100% mortality was observed within 24 hr in leukemia rats.   This enhancement in mortality occurred at a time when there was not a significant elevation in circulating levels of leukocytes.   The mortality observed following E. coli administration in the leukemia group is also distinctly different from the mortality pattern resulting from leukemia alone.   This preliminary study had 10 rats/group.

RESULTS

The influence of the simultaneous administration of glucan on growth of 20 X 10^6 subcutaneously implanted myelogenous leukemia cells is presented in Table 1.   In agreement with previous observations (37), the administration of glucan significantly decreased tumor growth.   Because glucan when injected subcutaneously in normal rats produced a profound monocytic infiltrate due to its chemotactic nature, the inhibition of tumor growth probably reflects an alteration in tumor cell:macrophage ratio in favor of the latter cell.   In preliminary studies undertaken to evaluate this possibility, it was observed that the administration of glucan intralesionally produced a 76% increase in the number of tumor macrophages 12 hr after glucan was administered.   At 24 hr the enhancement in tumor macrophage content was no longer present, however, suggesting that activation of macrophages by glucan may be an important feature of glucan inhibition of tumor growth.

In an effort to determine whether glucan may be used as a treatment modality following the administration of leukemia cells, rats were transplanted with 5 X 10^6 Shay myelogenous leukemia cells intravenously.   One to five days following transplantation, glucan was administered in 5% glucose intravenously

TABLE 1. Influence of subcutaneous implant of glucan (4 mg) on growth of Shay myelogenous leukemia cells [a]

Group	No.	Body weight	Tumor weight (g)
Saline	42	128 ± 2	10.1 ± 1.1
Glucan	42	132 ± 5	4.6 ± 0.9

[a] Tumor weight was determined 10 days posttransplantation of 20×10^6 cells. Values are expressed as means $\pm$ standard error.

in the amount of 0.2 mg daily. Control animals were injected with isotonic glucose. As can be noted (Fig. 3), significant enhancement in survival was observed in the glucan-treated group. Additionally, the development of leukemia at early intervals following leukemia cell transplant was identical in the glucan- and the dextrose-treated group. However, leukocyte levels rapidly normalized in the glucan group, denoting rejection of the leukemic cell transplant. There were no recurrences of leukemia in any of the survivors in the glucan-treated group. When surviving glucan-treated rats were rechallenged with 40×10^6 tumor cells subcutaneously on day 30, immunity to the leukemic cells appeared to have occurred as tumor rejection was

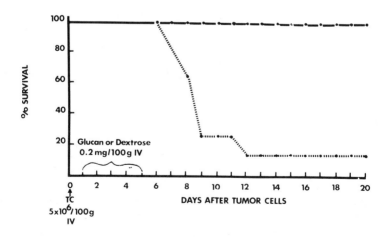

FIG. 3. Influence of glucan on survival of rats which received 5×10^6 Shay myelogenous leukemic cells/100 g intravenously. Glucan (0.2 mg) in dextrose (0.8 mg) or 1 mg of dextrose was given daily on days 1 to 5.

TABLE 2. Inhibitory influence of glucan on growth of adenocarcinoma
BW 10232

| Group | No. | Weight (g) | |
		Body	Tumor
Glucose	8	25 $\pm$ 1.5	4.21 $\pm$ 0.41
Glucan	10	20 $\pm$ 0.6	0.98 $\pm$ 0.15

0.5 X 10^6 Tumor cells injected subcutaneously on day 0. Glucan (0.2 mg,
i.v.)/glucose injections on days 1, 6, 10, and 15. Killed on day 20. Values
are expressed as means $\pm$ standard error.

manifested. The average weight of the tumor on day 11 was 18.3 g in the control group and 0.7 g in the "glucan-immune" group. Histologically, the
tumor in the latter group was composed of connective tissue and macrophages
with no viable tumor cells detected.

The influence of glucan administered intravenously on the growth of the
adenocarcinoma and melanoma mouse tumors is presented in Tables 2 and 3.
Glucan in the amount of 0.2 mg/mouse, or glucose, was administered days 1,
6, 10, and 15 following the subcutaneous injection of 0.5 X 10^6 adenocarcinoma tumor cells. The animals were killed at day 20 and tumor weight
ascertained. The adenocarcinoma experiment was terminated at this time,
because 20% of the control group died as a result of pulmonary metastasis.
At this time there were no deaths in the glucan-treated group. In essential
agreement with observations employing the Shay myelogenous leukemia model,
the glucan-treated mice showed a 76% inhibition of growth in the adenocarcinoma tumor at day 20 (Table 2). Likewise, a rather comparable mean 69%
inhibition of tumor growth was observed in the mice injected subcutaneously
with 1 X 10^6 melanoma cells and treated with glucan in an identical fashion
(Table 3).

In an effort to evaluate further the importance of tumor macrophages to
the growth of the primary tumor, as well as to its dissemination, the
myelogenous leukemic cells were administered to normal rats either alone or
in the presence of varying concentrations of glucan activated peritoneal macrophages. As can be noted in Table 4, a significant inhibition of tumor weight
was observed, particularly when macrophage:tumor cell ratios approximated
1:1. In addition to the inhibition of tumor growth as reflected by the weight
of the tumor, distinct histological changes were noted in liver, lung, and
spleen, as well as in the tumor of the animals bearing tumor implants with
varying macrophage populations (16,38).

In the control groups which received tumor cells alone, liver showed a
heavy infiltrate of tumor cells which compressed and displaced parenchymal
cells (Fig. 4). A heavy infiltrate of tumor cells, particularly in the red pulp,

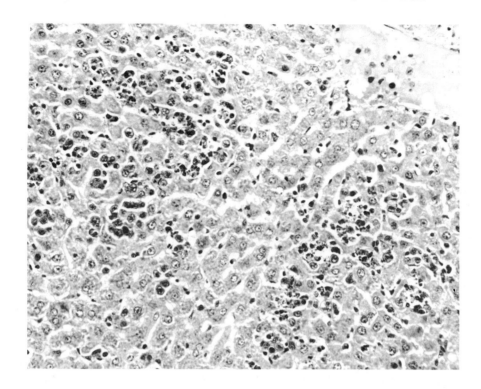

FIG. 4. Liver from a control rat injected with 20 X 10^6 tumor cells sub-cutaneously shows a heavy infiltrate of tumor cells wherein hepatocytes are completely replaced by tumor cells. The animal was killed on day 10 after tumor cell transplantation. (H&E, X250.)

was also observed in the spleen. In the tumor itself, which was character-ized by the presence of myeloblastic cells, limited areas of necrosis and hemorrhage were observed. A relatively small number of mononuclear cells were present.

In the group that received tumor cell:macrophage implants at the ratio of 10:1, the infiltrate of tumor cells in the liver was not as prominent and there appeared to be significant foci of tumor cells undergoing necrosis. The tumor infiltrate of lung was quite extensive, as was that of spleen. The tumor presented irregularities in necrosis and hemorrhage and a mild in-filtrate of vacuolated macrophages.

In the animals which received tumor cells:macrophages in the ratio of 2:1, the liver showed a significant decrease in tumor cells and indeed in some livers only a few tumor cells were present. The infiltrate of tumor cells in the lung was characterized as mild to absent. Tumor infiltration of the spleen was significantly reduced compared to the control group.

The most prominent histological findings were observed in those animals which received macrophages and tumor cells in the ratio of 1:1. In this

TABLE 3. Inhibitory influence of glucan on growth of melanoma B16

| Group | No. | Weight (g) | |
		Body	Tumor
Glucose	7	21 ± 0.28	1.26 ± 0.25
Glucan	9	20 ± 0.72	0.39 ± 0.08

1×10^6 Tumor cells injected subcutaneously on day 0. Glucan (0.2 mg, i.v.) given on days 1, 6, 10, and 15. Killed day 21. Values are expressed as means $\pm$ standard error.

TABLE 4. Influence of addition of glucan-induced peritoneal macrophages[a] on growth of Shay acute myelogenous leukemia tumor in rats

Group	Tumor cells $(\times 10^6)$	Peritoneal macrophages added $(\times 10^6)$	Tumor weight (g)
Control	20	—	5.9 ± 0.66
Experimental-A	20	2	2.9 ± 0.71[b]
Experimental-B	20	10	2.3 ± 0.63[b]
Experimental-C	20	20	2.4 ± 1.10[b]

[a] Peritoneal macrophages were obtained 4 days following the intraperitoneal administration of 10 ml of a 0.5% suspension of glucan. Tumor cells and glucan-activated macrophages were administered subcutaneously.

The groups number 5 to 7 rats. Tumor weights were ascertained on day 10. Values are expressed as means $\pm$ standard error.

[b] $p < 0.05$.

group the presence of tumor cells in liver was judged to be slight to absent (Fig. 5). When tumor cells were present they appeared to be undergoing destruction by the mononuclear population. The lung appeared normal and the spleen, relative to degree of tumor infiltrates, was characterized as mild to absent. The tumor presented more extensive areas of necrosis and hemorrhage and had a moderate infiltrate of vacuolated mononuclear cells.

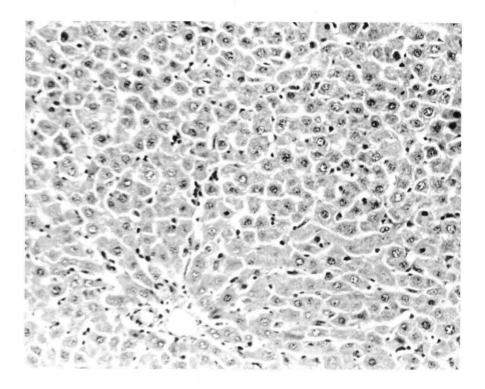

FIG. 5. Liver of an animal that received tumor cells and glucan stimulated macrophages (1:1 ratio) possesses essentially normal structure with prominent Kupffer cells and an absence of disseminated tumor cells. Day 10 postinjection. (H&E, X250.)

These findings denote that by increasing tumor macrophage population and enhancing the ratio of macrophages to tumor cells, a decreased dissemination of malignant cells occurred in association with a more extensive necrosis of the primary lesion (16,38).

To ascertain the degree of antitumor action of glucan, studies were undertaken in which the first injection of glucan was made on the seventh day following tumor cell administration, at which time a mean tumor weight of 4.6 g was established (Table 5). The control group showed a mean 303% increase in tumor weight by day 11. No significant difference was noted in the group injected with glucan subcutaneously. A significant 50% inhibition of tumor growth was observed in the group which received glucan intravenously. The infiltration of liver by tumor cells, which was significant by day 7, was decreased in both glucan-treated groups, with the most effective decrease in hepatic tumor cell infiltrate occurring in the intravenously treated group.

Further studies were also conducted in which survival as well as tumor growth was established in control and glucan-treated rats in which glucan treatment began at day 5 (Figs. 6 and 7). The mean tumor weights on day 7, 12, and 17 were 5.9, 23.1, and 13.8, respectively, in the control group.

TABLE 5. Comparative influence of intravenously or subcutaneously
administered glucan on growth of the acute myelogenous tumor in rats

Group	Day	No. of rats	Weight (g)	
			Body	Tumor
Control I	7	16	132 ± 3.0	4.55 ± 0.29
Control II	11	9	141 ± 3.1	18.34 ± 2.18
Glucan IV	11	11	132 ± 5.5	9.07 ± 1.16
Glucan SQ	11	10	148 ± 3.8	21.29 ± 2.99

All rats received 40 X 10^6 cells subcutaneously on day 0. The initial
group (control I) was killed on day 7 to establish degree of tumor growth.
Glucan (4 mg) was administered intravenously or subcutaneously on day 7.
Control rats received glucose subcutaneously. Control II and glucan-treated
rats were killed on day 11 and tumor weight ascertained. Values are expressed as means ± standard error.

In marked contrast, the weights of tumor in the glucan-treated groups were
2.9, 4.0, and 2.5 at the same times. (Fig. 6). Thus, significant inhibition
of primary tumor growth was achieved by glucan.

The survival of the glucan-treated group was significantly enhanced over
the control group (Fig. 7). In the surviving population no deaths from tumor
recurrence were observed even though no further glucan injections were
made after the 15 day posttumor cell transplantation. Complete regression
of the primary tumor was observed in the 16 surviving rats, which have now
been followed for 4 months following the initial tumor cell injection. Thus,
glucan administered when significant body tumor burden exists can markedly
modify the course of experimental leukemia.

Studies were also undertaken to provide an evaluation of the comparative
effectiveness of BCG and glucan in the myelogenous leukemia rat model. As
shown in Fig. 8, compared to the 100% mortality observed in the control
group, BCG effectively enhanced survival. However, the 33% survival was
significantly less than the 100% survival noted in the glucan-treated group.
Because routes of administration were different and equivalent doses cannot
be established, the greater survival of the glucan group over the BCG-treated
group must be viewed at the present time with a certain degree of reservation.

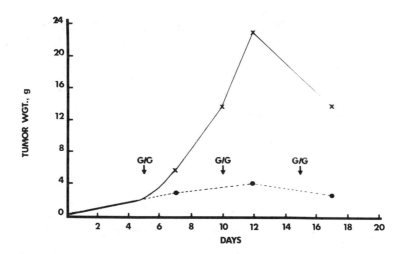

FIG. 6. Influence of intravenous glucan (4 mg) administration on days 5–10–15 on growth of the leukemic tumor. The growth of the subcutaneously injected tumor cells was rapidly arrested and indeed reversed in the glucan-treated group (●——●) relative to the glucose-treated group (X——X). Each point is a mean of 3 to 6 rats. The apparent decrease in tumor weight at day 17 in the control group is due to the prolonged survival of the rats with lower-weight tumors and does not reflect a rejection event.

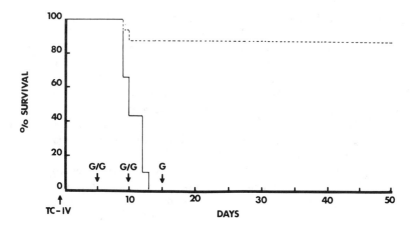

FIG. 7. Comparative survival of glucan- or glucose-treated animals following the administration of 20 X 10⁶ leukemic cells subcutaneously. The control group is composed of 9 rats and the glucan-treated group of 18 rats.

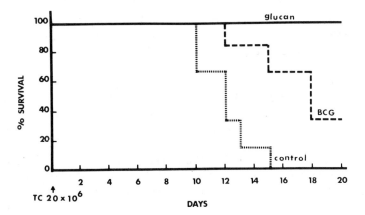

FIG. 8. Comparative influence of pretreatment of glucan or BCG on survival of Long-Evans rats following the subcutaneous administration of Shay myelogenous leukemia cells. Agents were administered -7, -5, -3, and on day 0. 0.1 ml of BCG (Glaxo Research, Ltd.) were given intraperitoneally. Glucan (2 mg) was given intravenously. Tumor cells (20 X 10[6]) were injected subcutaneously on day 0. Six rats comprised each group.

DISCUSSION

Jacobsen (46, cited also in 47, 48) may well have been the first to advance the reticuloendothelial theory of malignancy. Jacobsen proposed that the predicated increased incidence of cancer may well be a result of the decreased incidence of acute bacterial infections. Jacobsen concluded (a) "that the evidence tends to support the hypothesis that the reticuloendothelial system, when sufficiently active (as when stimulated by one or a number of acute infectious processes), may attain in a measure the ability to cope with neoplastic diseases in a similar if not identical manner, and (b) that the present increase in malignant morbidity is due to the decreased resistive powers of the reticuloendothelial system occasioned by the lessened incidence of exposure to and infection of the general public with those diseases which were widely endemic before the advent of modern public health methods." Jacobsen also noted (a) "that as acromegaly is regarded as a disease of the pituitary so should cancer be regarded as a disease of the reticuloendothelial system, and (b) that the hope of prevention, if not the treatment of cancer, lies in vaccinotherapy with markedly antigenic substances" (46). Thus, the concept of nonspecific immunotherapy and the possible role of reticuloendothelial dysfunction as a factor in malignancy was advanced approximately 40 years ago. Indeed, the conclusions of the editorial (46), that "further studies on the effect of powerfully antigenic substances in inoperable malignant conditions or as a postoperative measure in attempting to combat recurrence seem to be indicated in the light of the accumulated evidence, " are as pertinent today as when they were written.

It has now been amply demonstrated that macrophages, particularly those which are activated either specifically or nonspecifically, have the ability to destroy malignant cells predominantly by as yet an undefined contact lysis mechanism which requires the presence of viable macrophages (6,36,49-52). Krahenbuhl and Lambert (50) observed that activated macrophages had an enhanced ability to inhibit DNA synthesis in tumor cells. Direct contact between macrophages and target cells was required for cytostasis (50,51). The mechanism by which macrophages exert their cytotoxic effect on tumor cells is not as yet established. One possibility is the antimicrobial myeloperoxidase-hydrogen peroxide-halide system. Employing four different assays of cytotoxicity, a cytotoxic effect of this antimicrobial system was demonstrated by Clark et al. (53) on mouse ascites lymphoma cells. The comparative contribution of the lysosomal system (54) and the peroxidase system to the tumor cell-killing ability of macrophages is as yet to be defined.

Haskill, Proctor, and Yamamura (55) evaluated the composition of tumor cell populations in rat sarcomas. Employing enzymatically or mechanically dispersed tumor cell preparations, various cell fractions were obtained by velocity sedimentation procedures. The major nontumor host cell population was the macrophage, with remaining cells being granulocytes and lymphocytes. Indeed, in their studies, host cells were approximately 95% macrophages, 3% polymorphonuclear leukocytes, and 1.5% lymphocytes. The macrophage population was found to be extremely potent at killing tumor cells. Indeed, the tumor macrophage possessed greater killing ability than normal peritoneal macrophages. It appears on this basis that the host response to these specific tumors was predominantly macrophage-mediated. Haskill et al. (55) found that although macrophages appear to be capable of proliferating within the tumor, in vitro studies indicate that the presence of tumor cells inhibited the proliferative ability of macrophages. The importance of the tumor-inhibitory effect on macrophage proliferation to the growth and establishment of a solid tumor remains to be established. Whether glucan-enhanced activation and proliferation of macrophages may overcome any inhibitory action of the tumor on macrophage effector cells remains to be ascertained.

Our composite studies indicate that tumor macrophage populations play a significant role in determining the degree at which tumor cells disseminate to peripheral sites.. This finding is confirmation of the observations of Birbeck and Carter (56), who predicated a difference in behavior of a metastatic and nonmetastatic lymphoma due to variations in intratumor host macrophage populations. The previous studies of Gershon, Carter, and Lane (57) also add to the concept that failure of macrophage mobilization and activation intralesionally contributes significantly to the dissemination of tumor cells. Gershon et al. (57) observed that sinus histiocytosis which resulted in the region of a nonmetastasizing lymphoma were absent in lymph nodes draining a metastasizing lymphoma. The clinical importance of such observations may be denoted by the studies of Baum et al. (58). These investigators studied macrophage phagocytic activity in patients with breast cancer. Baum et al. (58) reported that as long as the macrophage response of the host remained intact, the tumor remained localized to the breast and underlying muscle. In those individuals in whom the tumor disseminated to lymph nodes and beyond, profound impairments were seen in macrophage function. These studies contribute further to an appreciation of the potential importance of macrophages as determinant cells in tumor cell dissemination.

Keller (59) has demonstrated that activated peritoneal macrophages rapidly and effectively eliminate syngeneic tumor cells in vitro. Keller's studies indicated effector:target cell ratios of 10:1 and 5:1 as well as a pronounced inhibition of thymidine incorporation of tumor cells at macrophage: target cell ratios of 1:1. In the present study, employing an in vivo system, we observed that dissemination of leukemic cells from the primary subcutaneous site to liver, lung, and spleen was effectively inhibited when macrophages were added to establish tumor cell:macrophage ratios at 2:1 and 1:1. These ratios of tumor cells to macrophages are physiologically based on the studies of Eccles and Alexander (60). Eccles and Alexander have reported that a high macrophage content of the tumor was associated with decreased metastases whereas, conversely, mouse tumors which possess low macrophage content showed increased dissemination (60).

Eccles and Alexander (61) have also indicated the existence of a monocytic defect in tumor induced "anergy." Immunological competence was restored in rats possessing tumor implants by the administration of peritoneal macrophages, but not lymphocytes. Eccles and Alexander (61) suggested that the resulting immunological anergy which develops as the tumor grows is due to the fact that the tumor competes for the available blood monocytes. Eccles and Alexander concluded that the state of anergy in association with tumor development may not be a failure of immunological recognition or reactivity, but may be due to the unavailability of monocytes to fulfill their role as modulators of immunological events. It is therefore possible, by increasing the availability of macrophages through our mechanisms of glucan-induced macrophage proliferation and activation, that immunological competence can be maintained in the presence of tumor cells. Preliminary studies in our laboratory have supported this postulate.

It is evident on the basis of our experimental and clinical studies (7, 11, 14) that glucan provides a unique means to initiate an enhancement of host resistance to neoplasia by macrophage activation and proliferation with a resulting significant increase in level of host resistance. It is obvious that the ability to induce a functional macrophage population within the tumor mass, which has the ability to kill neoplastic cells selectively, would be of significant clinical importance. These activated macrophages would not only tend to function to eliminate neoplastic cells, but in vivo events associated with macrophage antigen processing and initiation of both T- and B-cell responsiveness would also contribute to a decrease in tumor cell dissemination. This concept is well supported by the findings of Vorbrodt et al. (62-64). Vorbrodt et al. (62) have reported that during X-ray therapy of human skin cancers, macrophages were found to be actively engaged in tumor cell destruction. Intimate contact between "invading macrophages" and cancer cells with concomitant formation of cytoplasmic bridges and fusion zones were frequently observed following radiation therapy. In a subsequent investigation to pursue this finding, Vorbrodt et al. (63) demonstrated that radiation of macrophage and tumor cells in culture was associated with macrophage activation, increase in lysosomes and phagolysosomes, as well as associated macrophage adherence to cancer cells and the presence of phagocytized cancer cells. Vorbrodt et al. (64) suggested that X-irradiation of the tumor cells results in alteration in the tumor cell membrane which promotes adhesion and contact between the macrophage and the tumor cell and, in an as yet unknown fashion, leads to degeneration of the tumor cell and phagocytosis of the cell by the macrophages. Close juxtaposition of cell membranes of glucan-activated macrophages and human tumor cells have also been observed (14). Glucan particulates were readily identifiable in human macrophages at early intervals following intralesional administration (7,11,14).

The antitumor effects of yeast glucan are clearly evident by present and past experimental studies (16,25,26,38), as well as previous clinical endeavors (7). Glucans obtained from a variety of other sources have also been demonstrated to have antitumor activity in various experimental systems. Sakai et al. (65) have compared the antitumor action of certain glucans against the sarcoma 180-in ascites form and attempted to relate antitumor action to chemical structure. Those glucans possessing a linear β 1→3 linked D glucose structure were most effective. Glucans composed of alpha-configurations were ineffective. With the exception of a tendency for a slight loss in body weight, no other ill effects were observed in the glucan-treated groups.

Singh et al. (66) reported that antitumor action of a scleroglucan derived from Sclerotium glucanicum. This glucan possesses a chain of (1→3) β-D-glucopyranosyl units with every third or fourth unit carrying a (1→6) β-D-glucopyranosyl group. Singh et al. indicated that scleroglucan did not show toxic effects in the test animals. The absence of overt toxicity of various glucans may be of future significance in their consideration as immunostimulants. Chihara et al. (67) have reported that the glucans which are very effective in modifying tumor growth in experimental animals were ineffective in modifying growth of tumor cell cultures, noting that the action is host-mediated and not directly cytocidal. When our yeast glucan preparation was incubated with tumor cells in vitro, no direct cytotoxicity was manifested, supporting the observation of Chihara et al. (67) that the antitumor effect of glucan is host-mediated.

Dennert and Tucker (68) have reported that Lentinan, a linear β 1,3 glucan obtained from the mushroom lentiusedodes, possesses pronounced antitumor activity. Antitumor effect was found in normal, but not in neonatally thymectomized mice, indicating that an intact T-cell system was a prerequisite for the demonstrated antitumor effect of lentinan. It remains to be established whether yeast glucan is a T-cell adjuvant and whether its antitumor activity is mediated through the specific proliferation and activation of macrophages or by a concurrent enhancement in T-cell populations and function. However, the mechanism by which lentinan exerts its antitumor activity is not clear, because macrophage stimulation or enhancement in cell or humoral immunity has not been observed (60). One postulated mechanism is that lentinan may exert its antitumor effect by stimulation of histamine or serotonin (69).

An area which as yet remains essentially unexplored is the influence of specific macrophage stimulants not only on the effectiveness of chemotherapeutic agents but also on the alteration of responsiveness of tumor-bearing animals to bacterial and viral challenges. The previous studies of Sokoloff et al. (70) may well be significant in denoting effectiveness of combined macrophage activation and chemotherapy. Sokoloff et al. (70) reported that zymosan administered to mice bearing sarcoma 180 and Ehrlich carcinoma transplants considerably increased the tumor oncolytic effect of mitomycin D, while reducing its toxicity. Further studies will be required to determine whether effectiveness of glucan in controlling tumor growth can be enhanced by antineoplastic agents and, similarly, whether it will be possible to reduce the required dose of chemotherapeutic agents by glucan or other such macrophage stimulants and thus reduce problems of drug toxicity.

There is little question, in view of the diverse reports of various investigators, that glucans derived from various sources, but possessing a $1 \rightarrow 3$ β-configuration, have significant antitumor activity against a variety of tumors in diverse animal species, including man. It is obvious that glucan is a unique agent not only relative to its ability to activate host defense mechanisms, including those directed against malignant and nonmalignant allogeneic and xenogeneic cells (71), but also as a chemically defined agent employable in evaluation of the concept of immunotherapy and immunoprophylaxis. Additionally, glucan appears to be nonantigenic in nature, because the plasma obtained from glucan-treated mice (three injections of 2.2 mg over 5 days) produced no aggregation of glucan particles, suggesting the absence of agglutinating antibodies. Azuma, Kimura, and Tamamura (72) also reported that glucan isolated from Aspergillus fumigatus was not antigenic as reflected by immunodiffusion and precipitation reactions or by expression of cell-mediated immunity.

It is generally presently considered that immunotherapy, as exemplified by the employment of BCG, is effective only against a small number of tumor cells which approximate 10^5 cells. In the present study involving two animal species and three different tumors, initial numbers of tumor cells injected were on the order of 10^6. In the acute myelogenous leukemia model we have also found it possible to reverse the tumor state completely when glucan is injected on days 5 to 7 after tumor cell transplantation. At this time the primary tumor is 2 to 3% of body weight, and considerable metastasis has already occurred to liver, lung, and spleen. The effectiveness of glucan in this situation may be due not only to its ability to initiate production of monocytes in prodigious numbers, but also to its nonviable state, because the use of viable organisms and the induction of septicemia presents to the organism the choice of diverting macrophages from tumor target cells to control the infectious episode induced in the host. Indeed, in view of the apparent significant role that macrophages play in controlling tumor growth and dissemination, facilitation of tumor growth under instances of BCG therapy may well reflect the diversion of the macrophage population from what should be their primary dedication, namely the destruction of tumor cells within the internal environment, to an attempt to control the infectious episode. Although further studies will be essential to evaluate these possibilities, the potential danger of employing living, still partially pathogenic bacteria has also been stressed by Weiss (73). Israel et al. (74) also questioned the concept that immunotherapy can be effective only in so-called minimal residual disease, because they observed tumor regression induced by daily C. parvum injections in 40% of their patients with disseminated malignancies. It therefore appears that appropriate stimulation of the RES and/or the lymphoreticular system can be effective against large numbers of tumor cells.

The ability of glucan-activated macrophages to induce necrosis of tumor cells and inhibit growth and metastasis of various experimental tumors raises the question of specificity of response, which is of major significance in view of the observation of Jones et al. (36). In our previous studies (71), it was observed that the administration of glucan prior to bone marrow transplantation was associated with acceptance of syngeneic bone marrow cells, but nonacceptance of allogeneic or xenogeneic bone marrow. Indeed, there appeared to be a definitive relationship between the state of activation of the RES induced by glucan and survival of the animals to radiation injury by allogeneic bone marrow transplantation. More important, the administration of glucan to radiation chimeras was associated with 100% mortality of animals bearing allogeneic or xenogeneic grafts, but not of syngeneic grafts. These studies indicate that the activation of macrophages by glucan is associated not only with the destruction of malignant cells, but also of normal cells which are "non-self" cells. Our findings demonstrate that glucan possesses a unique ability to activate the RES in expression of enhanced phagocytosis, chemotaxis, enhanced humoral, and cellular immunity and increased ability to initiate the destruction of both normal, nonmalignant allogeneic cells, and perhaps more important, malignant cells.

Lymphocytic stimulation of macrophages may be one mechanism by which macrophages and lymphocytes cooperate in the mediation of cellular cytotoxicity. Fidler (8) demonstrated that activation of mouse macrophages in vitro by supernatants obtained from the interaction of tumor cells and lymphocytes resulted in inhibition of pulmonary metastases. It is entirely possible that the large number of mediators released by stimulated lymphocytes initiate macrophage events which render the macrophage pronouncedly cytotoxic to tumor cells. Fidler demonstrated that the factors capable of activating mouse macrophages were initiated from lymphocytes that were sensitized to tumor cells. The activating factor, once released, rendered syngeneic, allogeneic, or xenogeneic macrophages cytotoxic to tumor cells both in vitro and in vivo. Fidler also reported that cytotoxic macrophages do not kill normal cells but are specifically directed to the malignant cell population. It is clear that macrophages when rendered cytotoxic may occupy a major role in defense mechanisms against neoplasia.

Piessens, Churchill, and David (75) reported that normal guinea pig macrophages, when incubated with mediator-rich lymphocyte supernatants, become cytotoxic for line 1 hepatoma and MCA-24 fibrosarcoma cells. Cytotoxicity was not observed toward normal syngeneic cell types. Thus, macrophage-mediated cytotoxicity induced by unrelated antigens is directed toward malignant cells. In a further investigation of macrophage-lymphocyte interactions, Wahl et al. (76) observed that lymphokine production by guinea pig lymph node and spleen cells required macrophages for thymus-dependent antigens and mitogens. In contrast, B-cell stimulants which also induce the synthesis of lymphokines were macrophage-independent. These findings demonstrate that macrophages play an essential role in lymphocyte activation. The role of nonspecific activation of macrophages by glucan and the possible proliferation and activation of T- and B-lymphocytes must be established in the appreciation of the mechanism of inhibition of tumor growth and dissemination by glucan. Holtermann et al. (77) also reported that human monocytes possess cytotoxicity toward human osteosarcoma and reticulum cell sarcoma cells in vitro. Increased monocytotoxicity was induced by lymphocyte supernatant fluids from nonspecifically stimulated human lymphocytes. Thus, the activation of monocytes by lymphokines is an increasingly important facet of tumor cell rejection mechanisms and must be ascertained in our tumor systems.

Calderon et al. (78) have demonstrated that culture fluids obtained from peritoneal macrophages contained a fraction which stimulated lymphocyte proliferation and influenced B-cell differentiation. Thus, a macrophage product possesses the ability to produce T-cell proliferation and activation of B-cells. Calderon also reported that the culture fluid also contained a low-molecular-weight inhibitor of DNA and protein synthesis. This factor may be the agent responsible for the observation of Keller whereby macrophages may regulate the unorthodox proliferative events of normal cells (79).

The present studies establish the importance of macrophages as host defense cells against the growth of various tumor cells, as well as the importance of macrophages in determining dissemination of malignant leukemic cell populations. The use of glucan as a nonspecific host defense stimulus appears to merit further investigative effort not only in the area of neoplasia, but in other disease states, because Elinov et al. (80) reported that glucan prepared from Rhodatorula glutinin induced interferon production and protected mice against influenza virus. It can also be anticipated that through a delineation of the role of macrophages in tumor cell destruction, as well as the further evaluation of the role of macrophage populations of tumors to tumor growth and dissemination, an appreciation of host defense mechanisms against neoplastic states will be forthcoming.

SUMMARY

In an effort to evaluate the role of macrophages in tumor growth and dissemination, studies were conducted on the influence of the macrophage stimulant, glucan, and/or glucan-activated macrophages on growth and dissemination of acute myelogenous tumor cells in rats. Additionally, the influence of glucan administration on the growth of the mouse melanoma and adenocarcinoma tumor model was ascertained. Glucan, which induced proliferation and activation of macrophages and is profoundly chemotactic in nature, inhibited tumor growth and promoted survival when given to rats either before or after tumor cell administration. The most effective route of administration was intravenous, whereas subcutaneous administration at a nontumor site produced minimal change on the primary tumor but was effective in reducing metastases. Glucan also reversed tumor growth and metastases when administered to rats when the primary tumor was 2 to 3% of body weight and when tumor infiltration of liver, lung, and spleen had already occurred, suggesting that immunostimulants can be effective in modifying neoplasia when tumor burden exceeds minimal states. To assess further the importance of tumor macrophage on growth and dissemination of tumor cells, studies were undertaken in which 20 X 10^6 tumor cells were transplanted subcutaneously alone or with varying numbers of glucan-activated peritoneal macrophages. A significant reduction in primary tumor growth was observed in the presence of the added macrophage population which established initial tumor:macrophage ratios of 10:1, 2:1, and 1:1. Significant inhibition of liver, lung, and spleen metastasis was also observed, with the most pronounced inhibition of metastasis occurring in the groups where macrophage tumor ratios were 1:2 or 1:1. Facilitation of tumor growth was never observed in glucan-treated animals. These studies demonstrate that glucan, a potent nonspecific immunostimulant, has distinct advantages over the currently employed bacterial agents and should be of significant value in evaluating various concepts of immunotherapy. Activated macrophages appear to be key cells in the regulation of the internal environment against malignant cell populations as an intrinsic phase of the neoplastic process appears to be an inadequate number and function of host and tumor macrophages.

REFERENCES

1. Rosenau, W., and Moon, H. D. (1961): Lysis of homologous cells by sensitized lymphocytes in tissue culture. J. Natl. Cancer Inst., 27:471-483.
2. Wilson, D. B. (1965): Quantitative studies on the behavior of sensitized lymphocytes in vitro. I. Relationship of the degree of destruction of homologous target cells to the number of lymphocytes and to the time of contact in culture and consideration of the effects of isoimmune serum. J. Exp. Med., 122:143-166.
3. Perlmann, P., and Holm, G. (1969): Cytotoxic effects of lymphoid cells in vitro. Adv. Immunol., 11:117-193.
4. Hellstrom, K. E., and Hellstrom, I. (1974): The role of cell-mediated immunity in control and growth of tumors. Clin. Immunobiol., 2:233-264.
5. Kumar, S., and Taylor, G. (1973): Specific lymphocytotoxicity and blocking factors in tumours of the central nervous system. Br. J. Cancer, (Suppl. 1)28:135-141.
6. Keller, R. (1973): Cytostatic elimination of syngeneic rat tumor cells in vitro by nonspecifically activated macrophages. J. Exp. Med., 138:625-644.
7. Mansell, P. W. A., Ichinose, H., Reed, R. J., Krementz, E., McNamee, R., and Di Luzio, N. R. (1975): Macrophage-mediated destruction of human malignant cells in vivo. J. Natl. Cancer Inst., 54:571-580.
8. Fidler, I. J. (1974): Inhibition of pulmonary metastasis by intravenous injection of specifically activated macrophages. Cancer Res., 34: 1074-1078.

9. Zbar, B., Bernstein, I., Tanaka, T., and Rapp, H. J. (1970): Tumor immunity produced by the intradermal inoculation of living tumor cells and living Mycobacterium bovis (strain BCG). Science, 170:1217-1218.

10. Hanna, M. G., Jr., Zbar, B., and Rapp, H. J. (1972): Histopathology of tumor regression after intralesional injection of Mycobacterium bovis. II. Comparative effects of vaccinia virus, oxazolone, and turpentine. J. Natl. Cancer Inst., 48:1697-1707.

11. Mansell, P. W. A., and Di Luzio, N. R. (1976): In vivo destruction of human tumour by glucan activated macrophages. In: Role of Macrophages in Neoplasia, edited by Mary Fink. Academic Press, New York (in press).

12. Morton, D. L., Eilber, F. R., Malmgren, R. A., and Wood, W. C. (1970): Immunological factors which influence response to immunotherapy in malignant melanoma. Surgery, 68:158-164.

13. Bornstein, R. S., Mastrangelo, M. J., Sulit, H., Chee, D., Yarbro, J. W., Prehn, L., and Prehn, R. T. (1973): Immunotherapy of melanoma with intralesional BCG. Natl. Cancer Inst. Monogr., 39:213-220.

14. Mansell, P. W. A., Di Luzio, N. R., McNamee, R., Rowden, G., and Proctor, J. W. (1976): Recognition factors and non-specific macrophage activation in the treatment of neoplastic disease. In: Immunotherapy of Cancer, edited by H. Friedman and C. M. Southam. New York Academy of Science (in press).

15. Di Luzio, N. R. (1975): Role of heat-labile opsonins and recognition factors in host defense mechanisms. In: Microbiology — 1975, edited by D. Schlessinger, pp. 206-208. American Society for Microbiology, Washington, D. C.

16. Di Luzio, N. R., McNamee, R., Jones, S., Lassoff, S., Sear, W., and Hoffmann, E. (1976): Inhibition of growth and dissemination of Shay myelogenous leukemic tumor in rats by glucan and glucan activated macrophages. In: Proceedings of the VII International Congress of the Reticuloendothelial Society, edited by M. Escobar. Plenum Press, New York (in press).

17. Di Luzio, N. R. (1976): Pharmacology of the reticuloendothelial system — Accent on glucan. In: Proceedings of the VII International Congress of the Reticuloendothelial Society, edited by M. Escobar. Plenum Press, New York (in press).

18. Schmidtke, J. R., and Simmons, R. L. (1974): Experimental models of tumor immunotherapy. Clin. Immunobiol., 2:265-285.

19. Benacerraf, B., and Sebestyen, M. M. (1957): Effect of bacterial endotoxins on the reticuloendothelial system. Fed. Proc., 16:860-867.

20. Pillemer, L., and Ecker, E. E. (1941): Anticomplementary factor in fresh yeast. J. Biol. Chem., 137:139-142.

21. Northcote, D. H., and Horne, R. W. (1952): The chemical composition and structure of the yeast cell wall. Biochem. J., 51:232-236.

22. Di Carlo, F. J., and Fiore, J. V. (1958): On the composition of zymosan. Science, 127:756-757.

23. Mundkur, B. (1960): Electron microscopical studies of frozen-dried yeast. Exp. Cell Res., 20:28-42.
24. Cutler, J. L. (1960): The enhancement of hemolysin production in the rat by zymosan. J. Immunol., 84:416-419.
25. Diller, I. C., and Mankowski, Z. T. (1960): Response of sarcoma 37 and normal cells of the mouse host to zymosan and hydroglucan. Acta Un Int. Cancer, 16:584-587.
26. Mankowski, Z. T., Diller, I. C., and Nickerson, W. J. (1958): The action of hydroglucan on experimental mouse tumors. Proc. Am. Assoc. Cancer Res., 2:324.
27. Old, L. J., Clarke, D. A., Benacerraf, B., and Goldsmith, M. (1960): The reticuloendothelial system and the neoplastic process. Ann. N. Y. Acad. Sci., 88:264-280.
28. Thiele, E. H. (1974): Induction of host resistance in different mouse strains. Proc. Soc. Exp. Biol. Med., 146:1067-1070.
29. Riggi, S. J., and Di Luzio, N. R. (1961): Identification of a reticulo-endothelial agent in zymosan. Am. J. Physiol., 200:297-300.
30. Hassid, W. Z., Joslyn, M. A., and McCready, R. M. (1941): The molecular constitution of an insoluble polysaccharide from yeast, Saccharomyces cerevisiae. J. Am. Chem. Soc., 63:295-298.
31. Bacon, J. S. D., Farmer, V. C., Jones, D., and Taylor, I. F. (1969): The glucan components of the cell wall of baker's yeast (Saccharomyces cerevisiae) considered in relation to its ultrastructure. Biochem. J., 114:557-567.
32. Sear, W., Strickland, J., and Di Luzio, N. R. (1976): Unpublished observations.
33. Pinsky, C. M., Hirshaut, Y., and Oettgen, H. F. (1973): Treatment of malignant melanoma by intratumoral injection of BCG. Natl. Cancer Inst. Monogr., 39:225-228.
34. Aungst, C. W., Sokal, J. E., and Jager, B. V. (1975): Complications of BCG vaccination in neoplastic disease. Ann. Intern. Med., 82:666-669.
35. Sparks, F. C., Silverstein, J. F., and Hunt, J. S. (1973): Complications of BCG immunotherapy in patients with cancer. N. Engl. J. Med., 289:827-830.
36. Jones, J. T., McBride, W. H., and Weir, D. M. (1975): The in vitro killing of syngeneic cells by peritoneal cells from adjuvant-stimulated mice. Cell. Immunol., 18:375-383.
37. Di Luzio, N. R. (1975): Macrophages, recognition factors and neoplasia. In: The Reticuloendothelial System: International Academy of Pathology Monograph, chap. 5, pp. 49-64. Williams and Wilkins Co., Baltimore.
38. Di Luzio, N. R., McNamee, R., Jones, E., Cook, J. A., and Hoffmann, E. O. (1976): The employment of glucan and glucan activated macrophages in the enhancement of host resistance to malignancies in experimental animals. In: Role of Macrophages in Neoplasia, edited by Mary Fink. Academic Press, New York (in press).
39. Palm, J., and Wilson, D. B. (1974): The ag-B locus of rats: A major histocompatibility complex. In: Immunobiology of Transplantation, edited by F. H. Bach, pp. 75-79. Grune & Stratton, New York.

40. Shay, H., Gruenstein, M., Marx, H. E., and Glazer, L. (1951): The development of lymphatic and myelogenous leukemia in Wistar rats following gastric instillation of methylcholanthrene. Cancer Res., 11:29-34.

41. Lapis, K., and Benedeczky, I. (1967): Electron microscopic study of Shay chloroleukemia. Cancer Res., 27:1544-1564.

41. Handler, E. E., and Handler, E. S. (1970): Experimental leukemias: Model systems for the study of hematopoiesis. In: Regulation of Hematopoiesis, edited by A. S. Gordon, vol. 2, chap. 47, pp. 1273-1296. Appleton-Century-Crofts, New York.

43. Di Luzio, N. R., Miller, E. R., McNamee, R., and Pisano, J. C. (1972): Alterations in plasma recognition factor activity in experimental leukemia. J. Reticuloendothel. Soc., 11:186-197.

44. Di Luzio, N. R., McNamee, R., Miller, E. F., and Pisano, J. C. (1972): Macrophage recognition factor depletion after administration of particulate agents and leukemia cells. J. Reticuloendothel. Soc., 12:314-323.

45. Di Luzio, N. R., McNamee, R., Olcay, I., Kitahama, A., and Miller, R. H. (1974): Inhibition of tumor growth by recognition factors. Proc. Soc. Exp. Biol. Med., 145:311-315.

46. Jacobsen, C. (1934): Chronic irritation of the reticuloendothelial system — A hindrance to cancer. Arch. Dermatol. Syph., 169:562-576.

47. Erysipelas and prodigiosus toxins (Coley) (1934): Editorial. J. Am. Med. Assoc., 103:1070-1071.

48. Nauts, H. C., Fowler, G. A., and Bogatko, F. H. (1953): Review of influence of bacterial infections and of bacterial products (Coley's toxins) on malignant tumors in man; critical analysis of 30 inoperable cases treated by Coley's mixed toxins in which diagnosis was confirmed by microscopic examination selected for special study. Acta Med. Scand., (suppl. 276)145:1-103.

49. Ghaffar, A., Cullen, R. T., and Woodruff, M. F. A. (1975): Further analysis of the anti-tumor effect in vitro of peritoneal exudate cells from mice treated with Corynebacterium parvum. Br. J. Cancer, 31:15-24.

50. Krahenbuhl, J., and Lambert, L. H., Jr. (1975): Cytokinetic studies of the effects of activated macrophages on tumor target cells. J. Natl. Cancer Inst., 54:1433-1437.

51. Boyle, M. D. P., and Ormerod, M. G. (1975): The destruction of allogeneic tumour cells by peritoneal macrophages from immune mice: Purification of lytic effector cells. Cell. Immunol., 17:247-258.

52. Meltzer, M. S., Tucker, R. W., and Breuer, A. C. (1975): Interaction of BCG-activated macrophages with neoplastic and nonneoplastic cell lines in vitro: Cinemicrographic analysis. Cell. Immunol., 17:30-42.

53. Clark, R. A., Klebanoff, S. J., Einstein, A. B., and Fefer, A. (1975): Peroxidase H$_2$O$_2$ halide system: Cytotoxic effect on mammalian tumor cells. Blood, 45:161-170.

54. Hibbs, J. B. (1973): Macrophage nonimmunologic recognition: Target cell factors related to contact inhibition. Science, 180:868-870.

55. Haskill, J. S., Proctor, J. W., and Yamamura, Y. (1975): Host responses within solid tumors. I. Monocytic effector cells within rat sarcomas. J. Natl. Cancer Inst., 54:387-393.

56. Birbeck, M. S. C., and Carter, R. L. (1972): Observations on the ultrastructure of two hamster lymphomas with particular reference to infiltrating macrophages. Int. J. Cancer, 9:249-257.

57. Gershon, R. K., Carter, R. L., and Lane, N. J. (1967): Studies on homotransplantable lymphomas in hamsters. IV. Observations on macrophages in the expression of tumor immunity. Am. J. Pathol., 51:1111-1133.

58. Baum, M., Sumner, D., Edwards, H., and Smythe, P. (1973): Macrophage phagocytic activity in patients with breast cancer. Br. J. Surg., 60:899-900.

59. Keller, R. (1973): Evidence for compromise of tumour immunity in rats by a non-specific blocking serum factor that inactivates macrophages. Br. J. Exp. Pathol., 54:298-305.

60. Eccles, S. A., and Alexander, P. (1974): Macrophage content of tumours in relation to metastatic spread and host immune reaction. Nature, 250:667-669.

61. Eccles, S. A., and Alexander, P. (1974): Sequestration of macrophages in growing tumours and its effect on the immunological capacity of the host. Br. J. Cancer, 30:42-49.

62. Vorbrodt, A., Hliniak, A., Krzyzowska-Gruca, S., and Gruca, S. (1972): Ultrastructural studies on the behaviour of macrophages in the course of X-ray therapy of human skin cancer. Acta Histochem., 43:270-280.

63. Vorbrodt, A., Grabska, A., Krzyzowska-Gruca, S., and Gruca, S. (1973): Cytochemical and ultrastructural studies on the contact formation between macrophages and irradiated cancer cells in vitro. Folia Histochem. Cytochem., 11:357-358.

64. Vorbrodt, A., Grabska, A., Krzyzowska-Gruca, S., and Gruca, S. (1973): The formation of contacts between macrophages and neoplastic cells. Folia Histochem. Cytochem., 11:185-190.

65. Sakai, S., Takada, S., Kamaskua, T., Momoki, Y., and Sugayama, J. (1968): Antitumor action of some glucans: Especially on its correlation to their chemical structure. Gann, 57:507-512.

66. Singh, P. P., Whistler, R. L., Tokuzen, R., and Nakahara, W. (1974): Scleroglucan, an antitumor polysaccharide from Sclerotium glucanicum. Carbohydrate Res., 37:245-247.

67. Chihara, G., Hamuro, J., Maeda, Y. Y., Arai, Y., and Fukuoka, F. (1970): Fractionation and purification of the polysaccharides with marked antitumor activity, especially lentinan from Lentinus edodes (Berk.) sing. (an edible mushroom). Cancer Res., 30:2776-2781.

68. Dennert, G., and Tucker, D. (1973): Antitumor polysaccharide lentinan— A T cell adjuvant. J. Natl. Cancer Inst., 51:1727-1729.

69. Maeda, Y. Y., Hamuro, J., Yamada, Y. O., Ishimura, K., and Chihara, G. (1973): The nature of immunopotentiation by the anti-tumor polysaccharide lentinan and the significance of biogenic amines in its action. In: Immunopotentiation (Ciba Foundation Symposium), pp. 259-286. Elsevier, North-Holland.

70. Sokoloff, B., Toda, Y., Fujisawa, M., Enomoto, K., Saelhof, C., Bird, L., and Miller, C. (1961): Experimental studies on mitomycin C. 4. Zymosan and the RES. Growth, 25:249-263.

71. Wooles, W. R., and Di Luzio, N. R. (1964): Inhibition of homograft acceptance and homo- and hetero-graft rejection in chimeras by reticuloendothelial system stimulation. Proc. Soc. Exp. Biol. Med., 115:756-759.

72. Azuma, I., Kimura, H., and Yamamura, Y. (1968): Purification and characterization of an immunologically active glycoprotein from Asperigillus fumigatus. J. Bacteriol., 96:272-273.

73. Weiss, D. W. (1975): In: Immunobiology of Tumor-Host Relationships, edited by R. T. Smith and M. Landy, pp. 327-330. Academic Press, New York.

74. Israel, L., Edelstein, R., Depierre, A., and Dimitrov, N. (1975): Daily intravenous infusions of Corynebacterium parvum in twenty patients with disseminated cancer: A preliminary report of clinical and biologic findings. J. Natl. Cancer Inst., 55:29-33.

75. Piessens, W. F., Churchill, W. H., Jr., and David, J. R. (1975): Macrophages activated in vitro with lymphocyte mediators kill neoplastic but not normal cells. J. Immunol., 114:293-299.

76. Wahl, S. M., Wilton, J. M., Rosenstreich, D. L., and Oppenheim, J. J. (1975): The role of macrophages in the production of lymphokines by T and B lymphocytes. J. Immunol., 114:1296-1301.

77. Holtermann, O. A., Djerassi, I., Lisafeld, B. A., Elias, E. G., Papermaster, B. W., and Klein, E. (1974): In vitro destruction of tumor cells by human monocytes. Proc. Soc. Exp. Biol. Med., 147:456-459.

78. Calderon, J., Kiely, J-M., Lefko, J. L., and Unanue, E. R. (1975): The modulation of lymphocyte functions by molecules secreted by macrophages. I. Description and partial biochemical analysis. J. Exp. Med., 142:151-164.

79. Keller, R. (1974): Modulation of cell proliferation by macrophages: A possible function apart from cytotoxic tumour rejection. Br. J. Cancer, 30:401-415.

80. Elinov, H. P., Vitovskaya, G. A., Aksencv, O. A., Ageeva, O. N., and Agnaeva, A. E. (1972): M "polysaccharide" glucan-I-II isolated from "yeast" Rhodotorula glutinis i.v. induction "interferon" prophylaxis aginst exp. "infection respiration" with influenza-virus Ao-PR8 mouse. Biokhimiya, 37:590-593.

Control of Neoplasia by Modulation of the Immune System, edited by M. A. Chirigos. Raven Press, New York 1977.

ASSESSMENT OF POLYNUCLEOTIDES AS STIMULATORS OF IMMUNITY TO SYNGENEIC TUMORS

*O. J. Plescia, **G. Cavallo, **A. Pugliese, **G. Forni, and **S. Landolfo

*Waksman Institute of Microbiology, Rutgers— The State University of New Jersey, New Brunswick, New Jersey 08903, and **Institute of Microbiology, University of Turin, Turin, Italy

INTRODUCTION

The concept of immune surveillance of cancer, coupled with evidence of tumor-specific transplantation antigens, has generated interest in immunotherapy as a measure of controlling cancer. The development of an autochthonous tumor to a clinical stage may be regarded as evidence of a breakdown in immune surveillance or of a weakly antigenic tumor. For this reason, the current focus is primarily on immunostimulating agents that act nonspecifically to activate immunocytes and to increase their efficiency against weakly antigenic tumors.

The success of this form of immunotherapy depends on our ability to discover potentially effective immunostimulating drugs and to optimize their use, either through an understanding of their mode of action or by methodical experimentation. Several such drugs have already been uncovered that show promise.

Our own study centers on double-stranded polyribonucleotides as immunostimulatory agents. As reported last year at the first of these Conferences (1), and as published elsewhere (2,3), the effects of these agents varies depending on their concentration, route of administration, and, most important, the time of their administration relative to antigen. They act synergistically with antigen, and therefore are immunostimulating only if they are given concomitantly and are in close proximity to antigen. It so happens that double-stranded polyribonucleotides, such as polyadenylic-polyuridylic acid (poly A:U) and polyinosinic-polycytidylic acid (poly I:C), tend to bind to cells, including tumor cells, and in this form they seem able to enhance the immunogenicity of the cells to which they are bound. The cellular immune response of C57B1/6J strain mice to allogeneic DBA/2J mastocytoma cells is significantly increased by pretreating the tumor cells with poly A:U (1,3).

The next step in exploiting polyribonucleotides as immunostimulating agents was to test them in a syngeneic mouse tumor system, using poly I:C-treated tumor cells as immunogen. The tumor used was a transplantable mammary adenocarcinoma that developed spontaneously in the BALB/c strain mouse. Tumor immunity was assessed in terms of resistance of the immunized mice to a challenge of viable untreated tumor cells, in terms of the percent of animals failing to develop a tumor and the percent of animals surviving the challenge. Also, the lymph nodes of immunized animals were assayed for cytotoxic effector cells, and their sera were analyzed for cytotoxic antibodies. Poly I:C-treated tumor cells proved significantly more immunogenic than untreated cells, an indication that simple binding of polyribonucleotides to immunogenic tumor cells may be an expedient manner of using them as immunostimulatory agents.

RESULTS

Tumor Resistance Induced by Poly I:C-Treated Tumor Cells

Preparation of Cells

ADK-it tumor cells (5×10^6) were suspended in 1.0 ml of minimum essential medium (MEM) containing 500 µg of poly I:C and incubated at 37° C for 20 min. This suspension was then diluted 1/1,000, to be used for immunization. Tumor cells, suspended in MEM without poly I:C, were used as a control preparation for the effect of poly I:C, and normal liver cells treated with poly I:C were used as a control for tumor cells.

Immunization of Syngeneic BALB/c Mice

Randomized groups of 20 mice each were inoculated subcutaneously with 0.2 ml of the above preparations of cells. Each animal received 1×10^3 cells, and 0.1 µg of poly I:C if it had been added to the preparation. An additional group of mice was inoculated with 0.1 µg of poly I:C, and no cells, to test the effect of poly I:C by itself. It should be noted that the tumor cells, though viable, did not induce a neoplasia because of the limited number of cells inoculated.

Challenge of Immunized Mice

Eight days following immunization, each group of mice was divided into subgroups and challenged with viable ADK-it tumor cells, ranging in number from 2.5×10^4 to 2.0×10^5. The challenge cells, like the immunizing cells, were also inoculated subcutaneously, but at a distant site, and their ability to take and grow was monitored. Failure of the challenge cells to develop into a neoplasia is regarded as evidence of tumor immunity.

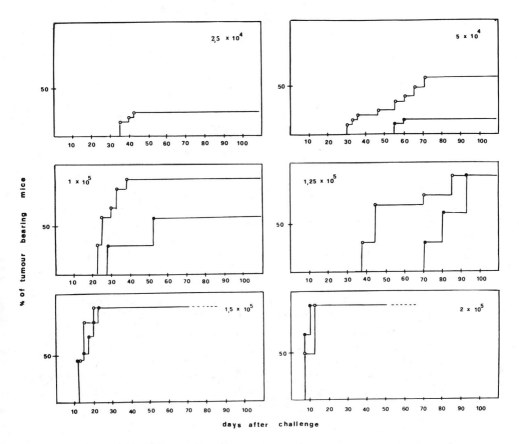

FIG. 1. Poly I:C as a stimulator of immunity to syngeneic tumor cells. Groups of 20 BALB/c mice were immunized with syngeneic ADK-it tumor cells (O) or with poly I:C-treated tumor cells (●). Eight days later they were challenged with viable ADK-it cells, ranging in number from 2.5 X 10[4] to 2 X 10[5], and resistance was measured in terms of positive take of the challenge tumor cells (percent of mice in each group developing a growing tumor).

From the results, shown in Fig. 1, it is clear that poly I:C was effective in increasing the immunogenicity of syngeneic tumor cells. Mice immunized with poly I:C-treated tumor cells resisted moderate challenges of viable tumor cells; fully 100% of these mice were resistant to a challenge of 2.5 X 10[4] cells, and 50% were resistant to 1 X 10[5] tumor cells that produced a 100% take in mice immunized with nontreated tumor cells. Moreover, poly I:C by itself, and poly I:C-treated liver cells, induced no significant tumor resistance (results not shown).

Immunity of the above groups of mice was also assessed in terms of their survival after challenge. The results, shown in Fig. 2, are graphed as the percent of animals that died in each group as a function of the time after

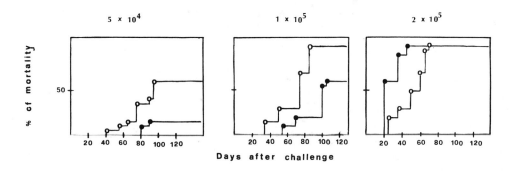

FIG. 2.   Resistance of BALB/c mice, immunized with ADK-it tumor cells
(O) or with poly I:C-treated cells (●).   Groups of 20 mice each were challenged with viable ADK-it tumor cells 8 days after immunization, and their
resistance was measured in terms of survival.

challenge.   Again it is evident that immunization with poly I:C-treated tumor
cells, compared with control untreated cells, afforded a significant measure
of resistance, but it was dependent on the challenge load.   The experimental
group of mice challenged with 2×10^5 tumor cells, a lethal dose, had a
median survival time of 20 days, whereas the median survival time of the
control group was 50 days.   Thus, depending on the challenge dose, one sees
evidence of both resistance and enhancement as a result of immunization with
tumor cells treated with poly I:C.

Analysis of Lymph Node Cells and Sera of Immunized Mice

Eight days after immunization of groups of mice with ADK-it tumor cells
or poly I:C-treated cells, these mice were sacrificed to obtain their axillary
and mesenteric lymph nodes, and from these were prepared suspensions of
lymph node cells.   A group of normal nonimmunized mice was used as control.   These lymph node cells were tested for cytotoxicity against ADK-it
target cells, according to the microtiter tumor cell colony inhibition assay
system of Hellström et al. (4).   Lymph node cells from mice immunized
with poly I:C-treated tumor cells were significantly more active than those
from mice immunized with untreated cells in inhibiting the development of
tumor cell colonies (53% vs. 28%).

The sera from the above groups of animals were tested for cytotoxic antibodies, in terms of the trypan blue dye exclusion test, and for ADK-it cell-
binding immunoglobulins, by indirect immunofluorescence.   In no instance
were tumor-specific antibodies directly demonstrable in response to immunization with tumor cells, poly I:C-treated or not.

There was evidence, however, of factors in the sera of mice immunized
with poly I:C-treated tumor cells that enhanced the cytotoxicity of lymph
node cells from this same group of mice (Fig. 3), but these same sera

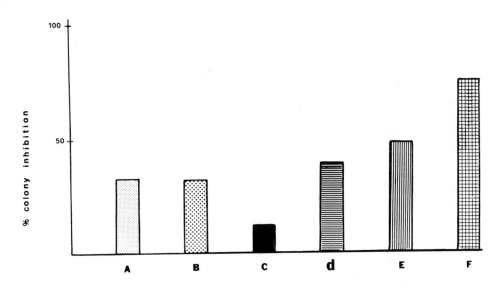

FIG. 3. Analysis of lymph node cells, from BALB/c mice immunized with ADK-it tumor cells or with poly I:C-treated cells, for cytotoxicity by the tumor cell colony inhibition assay. To in vitro cultures of ADK-it tumor cells were added: lymph node cells from mice immunized with ADK-it cells (A), lymph node cells from ADK-it immunized mice plus normal mouse serum (B), lymph node cells from ADK-it immunized mice plus serum from poly I:C-ADK-it immunized mice (C), lymph node cells from poly I:C-ADK-it immunized mice (D), lymph node cells from poly I:C-ADK-it immunized mice plus normal mouse serum (E), lymph node cells from poly I:C-ADK-it immunized mice plus serum from poly I:C-ADK-it immunized mice (F).

blocked the cytotoxicity of lymph node cells from mice immunized with untreated ADK-it tumor cells (Fig. 3). The test for these serum factors was that of Hellström and Hellström (5).

DISCUSSION

Mice immunized with ADK-it syngeneic tumor cells treated with poly I:C, compared with those immunized with untreated tumor cells, are significantly more resistant to challenge with the same tumor, measured in terms of take of the challenge tumor and survival of the challenged mice. This increased resistance correlated with the increased cytotoxicity of lymph node cells from these immunized mice. Essentially the same results were obtained with the MOPC-460 tumor, a chemically induced plasma cell tumor line of the BALB/c strain (unpublished results).

It would appear, therefore, that the immunostimulating potential of poly I:C can be realized by the simple expedient of adding the poly I:C to a suspension of tumor cells and letting it bind to the cell surface. That the poly

I:C does bind to the cell surface is evident from the reactivity of washed poly I:C-treated tumor cells with fluorescein-labeled antibody to poly I:C (unpublished results).

The addition of poly I:C directly to tumor cells, instead of administering it systemically, has several advantages. Relatively small amounts, of the order of 1 μg, may be used, thus minimizing the risk of any generalized toxicity of the drug to the host. It also assures the presence of the poly I:C at the locus and time of interaction between tumor cells and host immunocytes. This is a major consideration because the double-stranded polyribonucleotides, such as poly I:C and poly A:U, act synergistically with antigen (2).

These results confirm and extend a prior study, showing that a double-stranded polyribonucleotide in association with tumor cells enhances the cellular immune response of allogeneic strain mice to the histocompatibility antigens, and perhaps even the tumor-specific antigens, of the tumor cells (3).

Clearly, double-stranded polyribonucleotides (poly A:U and poly I:C) in association with tumor cells can increase significantly the immunogenicity of tumor cells even in syngeneic hosts, resulting in increased tumor immunity. Even this increased immunity, however, was inadequate in the face of a relatively large tumor load (cf. Figs. 1 and 2), and poly I:C-treated tumor cells were therapeutically ineffective in syngeneic tumor-bearing hosts once the tumor had become established (unpublished results). It should also be emphasized that in this study poly I:C-treated tumor cells proved effective in immunizing normal immunologically competent mice. There is no assurance that immunologically depressed mice would be equally responsive, an important consideration because of increasing evidence that cancer patients and experimental tumor-bearing animals tend to be immunologically depressed (6, 7). Any optimism should therefore be tempered until it can be established that polynucleotides, and indeed any immunostimulating agent, can potentiate effective immunity to a syngeneic tumor in tumor-bearing or immunodepressed hosts.

SUMMARY

The double-stranded polyribonucleotides, poly A:U and poly I:C, are immunomodulators. They act to stimulate the immune response if given together with antigen during the initiation of the response, and to suppress the response if given separately during the proliferative phase. Also, high doses of polynucleotides tend to be inhibitory, and should therefore be avoided.

Both poly A:U and poly I:C tend to bind to mammalian cells, including tumor cells, providing a convenient means of adding an optimal amount of polynucleotide to stimulate the immune response to cellular antigens. Thus, treatment of ADK-it tumor cells (a mammary adenocarcinoma cell line) with poly I:C significantly increased their immunogenicity in syngeneic BALB/c strain mice, measured as increased resistance of immunized mice to a challenge of viable homologous tumor cells and increased cytotoxicity of their lymph node cells. However, even this increased resistance afforded by poly I:C was inadequate to cope with a large, but not unreasonable, number of challenge cells. Specific immunization with polynucleotide-treated tumor cells may therefore be expected to be effective prophylactically, but to have limited value therapeutically. If the tumor load can be reduced by surgery, or any other means, this type of immunization might be able to contain any remaining primary cancer tissue and to prevent the development of metastases.

REFERENCES

1. Plescia, O. J. (1976): Cyclic AMP and immune responses: Role of poly A:U. Fogarty International Center Proceedings, No. 28, U.S. Government Printing Office, Washington, D.C. (in press).

2. Plescia, O. J., Yamamoto, I., and Shimamura, T. (1975): Cyclic AMP and immune responses: Changes in the splenic level of cAMP in response to antigen. Proc. Natl. Acad. Sci. (U.S.A.), 72:888-892.

3. Morris, C. (1974): Poly A:U as a stimulator of cell-mediated immunity. Ph.D. thesis, Rutgers University.

4. Hellström, I., Hellström, K. E., Sjögren, H. O., and Warner, G. A. (1971): Demonstration of cell-mediated immunity to human neoplasms of various histological types. Int. J. Cancer, 7:1-16.

5. Hellström, K. E., and Hellström, I. (1974): Lymphocyte-mediated cytotoxicity, and blocking serum activity to tumor antigens. Adv. Immunol., 18:209-277.

6. Plescia, O. J., Smith, A. H., and Grinwich, K. (1975): Subversion of the immune system by syngeneic tumors and the role of prostaglandins. Proc. Natl. Acad. Sci. (U.S.A.), 72:1848-1852.

7. Kersey, J. A., Spector, B. D., and Good, R. A. (1975): Immunodeficiency and cancer. Adv. Cancer Res., 18:211-230.

Control of Neoplasia by Modulation of the Immune System, edited by M. A. Chirigos. Raven Press, New York 1977.

CLINICAL TRIALS OF POLYRIBOINOSINIC-POLYRIBOCYTIDYLIC ACID (POLY I: C) AND POLY I: C/POLY-L-LYSINE IN PATIENTS WITH LEUKEMIA OR SOLID TUMORS

Arthur S. Levine, Peter G. Pushkas, and Hilton B. Levy

Pediatric Oncology Branch, National Cancer Institute; and the Laboratory of Viral Diseases, National Institute of Allergy and Infectious Disease, National Institutes of Health, Bethesda, Maryland 20014

The synthetic double-stranded polynucleotide, polyriboinosinic polyribocytidylic acid (poly I:C), is an extremely effective inducer of interferon in cells of many mammalian species in vitro (1, 2), including cells of human origin. In addition to its efficacy in the prevention and treatment of certain lytic viral infections in animal cells in vitro and in vivo (1-4), poly I:C in multiple doses has been shown to be effective in inhibiting the growth of various transplantable rodent tumors, both those apparently occurring spontaneously and those known to be induced virally (5-7). The demonstrated antitumor activity of poly I:C in certain animals may relate to one or a combination of the following activities: (a) induction of interferon; (b) a nonspecific adjuvant in augmenting humoral and cell-mediated immunity; and (c) effects on cell membranes and the synthesis of RNA, protein, and polyribosomes (8). Poly I:C is an effective antitumor agent in the mouse, but antitumor activity does not correlate with serum levels of interferon in this species (9).

The possibility that at least some human tumors may be virus-induced, together with the demonstrated antitumor effect in rodents, prompted a phase I-II trial of poly I:C in patients with malignancy. We wished to determine: (a) if doses of poly I:C that were nontoxic in dogs and monkeys are also nontoxic in man; (b) if the doses, schedules, and routes of administration employed in this study would induce interferon concentration of sufficient magnitude so that this antiviral protein could be detected in the serum and CSF; and (c) if poly I:C has antitumor activity in man. Detailed findings in this study have been presented elsewhere (21).

Twenty-six patients with various solid tumors, 9 patients with acute leukemia, and 2 patients with chronic myelogenous leukemia received poly I:C while hospitalized at the Clinical Center of the National Institutes of

509

Health. All patients had tumors which had become refractory to established anticancer therapy. Poly I:C was administered intravenously to 31 patients in 38 separate trials; 4 additional patients received one trial of poly I:C intramuscularly, and 2 patients received one trial of poly I:C by inhalation from a bedside nebulizer. The 38 intravenous trials of poly I:C were administered by three schedules. In 28 trials (schedule A) the drug was given in doses of 0.3 to 75 mg/m^2 on day 0 and daily from day 7 to a maximum of 35 days (the drug was given for at least 3 weeks in 20/28 trials). In 5 trials (schedule B), poly I:C was administered every other day for 6 to 9 doses. Finally, 5 trials consisted of intravenous poly I:C daily for 3 to 8 days (schedule C). Within the intravenous dose range of 0.3 to 75.0 mg/m^2, there were 11 dose levels, separated by progressively larger increments. A minimum of 3 trials were conducted at each dose level. Determinations of interferon titers in serum and CSF were performed at times 0, 3, 6, 12, and 24 hr in relation to the first dose of poly I:C on day 0 and the second dose (usually on day 7). During days 3 to 6, interferon levels were determined once daily, whereas from day 7 to the termination of treatment, assays were performed twice weekly 3 hr after administration of poly I:C (10).

The most frequently encountered toxicity in this study was fever, which occurred in 66% of the trials. The mean peak temperature elevation was 1.5°C, and this peak usually occurred 6 to 12 hr following drug administration; fever persisted for 24 to 36 hr. There was no correlation between the development of fever and the induction of detectable serum interferon. Slight prolongation of the thrombin time and a small increase in fibrin split products were noted in 59% of the trials. Modest elevations of liver enzymes (SGOT and SGPT) were detected in 25% of the trials within 10 to 25 days after initiation of treatment, but we observed no other liver function abnormalities that could be related to treatment. These enzymes reverted to pretreatment levels before or at the cessation of treatment. There was no relationship between the dose of poly I:C and elevation of the liver enzymes. Toxic manifestations severe enough to result in termination of the drug trial occurred in only 3 instances. One patient had clear laboratory evidence of disseminated intravascular coagulation, and 2 patients had moderately severe hypersensitivity reactions temporally related to the administration of poly I:C. These reactions were characterized by bronchospasm, chest and flank pain, and pedal edema.

In 63% of the 38 intravenous trials, we detected > 10 ref. units/ml of interferon in response to poly I:C, but mean interferon titers were low as compared with those observed in rodent studies (5) or in some natural viral infections of man (11). The correlation between the dose of poly I:C and the mean peak serum interferon level was not linear. There appeared to be a threshold dose of 1 mg/m^2 below which no serum interferon was induced, but even at higher dose levels, there was a very broad range of interferon titers, suggesting individual variation in response to this drug, or its metabolism. At the highest doses employed ($\geq$ 50 mg/m^2), induction of serum interferon was poor.

Measurable levels of interferon were not found in the CSF in any patient. Furthermore, inhalation or intramuscular administration of poly I:C did not result in detectable levels of serum interferon. Peak titers of serum interferon in response to single intravenous doses of poly I:C over the entire dose range were achieved at approximately 24 hr, and interferon was not detectable by 48 hr. Following a 6-day rest period (schedule A), all patients except one had significantly lower peak serum interferon titers in response to a second dose of intravenous poly I:C than to their first dose. Moreover, repeated daily administration of poly I:C at a given dose level resulted in a hyporesponsive state in which serum interferon could not be detected.

No patient in this study had a clinical response to treatment with poly I:C at any dose level or by any schedule or route of administration. Moreover, 65% of the patients with solid tumors and 100% of the patients with leukemia had signs of progressive disease while receiving poly I:C.

To summarize, poly I:C in doses of 0.3 to 75 mg/m^2 was administered to patients with malignant disease without untoward toxicity. Fever was the most common side effect encountered. Transient elevation of liver enzymes and coagulation abnormalities had been anticipated on the basis of earlier studies in monkeys and dogs (12). The ability of poly I:C to induce measurable, albeit low, serum titers of interferon in humans was demonstrated in this study as well as in previous reports (13-17). In all of these studies, the peak serum interferon level attained has been independent of the dose of poly I:C administered over a broad dose range. The disappointingly low levels of serum interferon induced in humans by poly I:C have been explained by the observation that there are present in human serum nucleases capable of rapidly degrading polynucleotides (18). This hydrolytic capacity is lacking in species which respond to poly I:C with the induction of high interferon titers (19).

In this study and others (13,14), poly I:C in multiple intravenous doses of up to 2.5 mg/kg does not appear to be an effective single agent in the treatment of patients with large tumor burdens. This lack of efficacy is not necessarily explained by failure of induction of high interferon titers. Poly I:C is an effective antitumor agent in the mouse, but antitumor activity does not correlate with serum levels of interferon in this species (9). Moreover, inhibition of tumor growth and viral replication are demonstrable in mice during the "hyporesponsive" state (serum interferon not detectable) associated with daily administration of poly I:C (19). On the other hand, hydrolysis of poly I:C (e.g., by human serum) prior to administration in the rabbit inhibits pyrogenicity, interferon induction, and the antitumor effect (5-8).

It is possible that a poly I:C preparation which would resist rapid degradation in human serum and therefore be capable of inducing consistently high levels of interferon might be a more useful antitumor agent whether or not interferon per se is the antitumor principle. For this reason, phase I-II studies are currently underway in patients with malignancy using a stabilized poly I:C/poly-L-lysine compound which resists enzymatic degradation by nucleases in human serum, and has been shown to be an effective inducer of interferon in vivo in subhuman primates (20).

Poly I:C/poly-L-lysine is a soluble complex of high-molecular-weight poly I:C and low-molecular-weight poly-L-lysine in 0.5% carboxymethylcellulose. The rate of hydrolysis of this complex by RNase or by primate (human or monkey) serum is five- to tenfold slower than the rate for poly I:C. During incubation with human serum, hydrolysis of the complex is barely detectable for the first hour. The increased stability of the complex is also indicated by its increased resistance to thermal denaturation. In 0.1 SSC, the T_m for poly I:C is 49°C, and that of the complex is 87° C. The poly-L-lysine complex is at least as good an inducer of interferon in mice as poly I:C, or perhaps a bit better. In chimpanzees and rhesus monkeys, administration of poly I:C has never induced serum or tissue interferon, but these animals have responded to the i.v. administration of the poly-L-lysine complex with peak titers of 100 to 7,500 units of interferon/ml of serum. Peak titers are obtained about 8 hr after injection, and detectable levels are sometimes found after 48 hr (20).

The low molecular weight of the lysine (2,000 to 4,000 daltons) is probably not restrictively antigenic, as might be the case with poly-D-lysine (MW 180,000). Toxicologic studies indicate that the poly-L-lysine derivative is no more toxic than the parent compound (unpublished observations). The LD_{50} in mice is approximately 50 mg/m^2, and in rats, the LD_{50} is approximately 150 mg/m^2. Below 50 mg/m^2, there is no significant toxicity in any species. Rhesus monkeys have been given 36 mg/m^2 of the drug daily for 6 days and then every other day for the following 2 weeks with no apparent toxicity nor gross pathology. Higher doses have, however, been associated with abnormal liver function tests. In all animals studied, the complex has been pyrogenic. Rhesus monkeys have been protected against Simian hemorrhagic fever virus using the poly-L-lysine complex (20; unpublished observations). The drug has been given (3 mg/kg, i.v.) 8 hr before an LD_{100} challenge of the virus and the dose repeated seven times during the next 2 weeks. All untreated monkeys were dead within 8 days; 3 of the 4 treated animals developed no disease. The fourth showed transient evidence of disease, but on further treatment, these symptoms disappeared. This is the first reported control of a systemic virus disease in a subhuman primate by an interferon inducer. Similar treatment has been administered to monkeys inoculated with yellow fever virus, and again, prophylaxis of clinical disease has been complete. Studies on the efficacy of poly I:C/poly-L-lysine as an antitumor agent in animals are incomplete. The agent has not been effective in L1210 leukemia. However, the parent poly I:C also showed no activity in L1210, although it was notably effective in animals with solid tumors.

Clinical trials of this complex are underway in patients with leukemia and various solid tumors at the National Cancer Institute. The objective of these initial phase I-II trials is to determine human toxicology, interferon induction, and antitumor effect. The complex is administered intravenously; after the initial dose, no drug is given for 1 week, and the drug is then given daily for the following 2 weeks. The initial dose employed was 0.5 mg/m^2, and six trials have been completed. No untoward toxicity has been experienced, other than pyrogenicity, and significant levels of serum interferon have been induced at a dose level of 7.5 mg/m^2. The poly-L-lysine complex has also been employed in initial clinical trials by M. Lerner (personal communication), who administered the drug i.v. as an antiviral agent in patients with St. Louis encephalitis or generalized zoster infection, and reports significant levels of

interferon induction in the 7.5 to 10 mg/m^2 dose range. There is not yet
sufficient data for us to comment on clinical antitumor or antiviral efficacy
of poly I:C/poly-L-lysine.

SUMMARY

Polyriboinosinic:polyribocytidylic acid (poly I:C), an interferon inducer,
was administered in multiple doses of 0.3 to 75 mg/m^2 to 37 patients with
solid tumors or leukemia. There were 44 separate drug trials, comprised of
various schedules and routes of administration. Toxicities encountered in
this study included fever, transient elevation of hepatocellular enzymes,
minimal laboratory evidence of coagulation abnormalities, and hypersensitivity
reactions. These toxic manifestations did not relate to dose level nor magnitude of interferon induction. Poly I:C, administered intravenously, induced
low serum concentrations of interferon in most trials, but the correlation
between drug dose and peak interferon titer was not linear. No patients experienced an objective tumor response to the administration of poly I:C, and
the majority of patients had progression of their disease while receiving the
drug.

Clinical trials of poly I:C/poly-L-lysine are underway in tumor patients.
This complex resists hydrolysis by primate serum and is able to induce high
serum concentrations of interferon in subhuman primates, unlike poly I:C.

ACKNOWLEDGMENTS

Portions of this report have been extracted from R. A. Robinson,
V. T. DeVita, H. B. Levy, S. Baron, S. P. Hubbard, and A. S. Levine: A
phase I-II trial of multiple-dose polyriboinosinic-polyribocytidylic acid
(poly I·poly C) in patients with leukemia or solid tumors, J. Natl. Cancer
Inst. (in press).

REFERENCES

1. Field, A. D., Tytell, A. A., Lampson, G. P., and Hilleman, M. (1967):
    Inducers of interferon and host resistance: II. Multistranded synthetic
    polynucleotide complexes. Proc. Natl. Acad. Sci. (U.S.A.), 58:1004–
    1010.
2. Hilleman, M. R. (1968): Interferon induction and utilization. J. Cell
    Physiol., 71:43–59.
3. Hill, D. A., Baron, S., Levy, H. B., Bellanti, J., Buckler, C. E.,
    Canellos, G., Carbone, P., Chanock, R. M., Devita, V., Guggenheim,
    E., Homan, E., Kapikian, A. Z., Kirschstein, R. L., Mills, J.,
    Perkins, J. C., Van Kirk, J. E., and Worthington, M. (1971): Clinical
    studies of induction of interferon by polyinosinic·polycytidylic acid. In:
    Perspectives in Virology, Vol. VII, edited by M. Pollard, pp. 198–222.
    Academic Press, New York.

4. Hill, D. A., Baron, S., Perkins, J. C., Worthington, M., Van Kirk, J. E., Mills, J., Kapikian, A. Z., and Chanock, R. M. Evaluation of an interferon inducer in viral respiratory diseases. JAMA, 219:1179-1184.

5. Levy, H. B., Law, L. W., and Rabson, A. S. (1969): Inhibition of tumor growth by polyinosinic-polycytidylic acid. Proc. Natl. Acad. Sci. (U.S.A.), 62:357-361.

6. Sarma, P. S., Shiu, G., Neubauer, R. H., Baron, S., and Huebner, R. J. (1969): Virus induced sarcoma of mice. Inhibition by a synthetic polyribonucleotide complex. Proc. Natl. Acad. Sci. (U.S.A.), 62:1046-1051.

7. Levy, H. B., Law, L. W., and Rabson, A. S. (1969): Third International Symposium on Interferon, Lyon, France, January 1969.

8. Levy, H. B., Asofsky, R., Riley, F., Garapin, H., Cantos, H., and Adamson, R. (1970): The mechanism of the antitumor action of poly I·poly C. Ann. N.Y. Acad. Sci., 173:640-648.

9. Weinstein, A. J., Gazdar, A. S., Sims, H. L., and Levy, H. B. (1971): Lack of correlation between interferon induction and anti-tumor effect of poly I·poly C. Nature (New Biol.), 231:53-54.

10. Oie, H. B., Buckler, C. E., Uhlendorf, C. P., Hill, D. A., and Baron, S. (1972): Improved assays for a variety of interferons. Proc. Soc. Exp. Biol. Med., 140:1178-1181.

11. Murphy, B. R., Baron, S., Chalhub, E. G., Uhlendorf, C. P., and Chanock, R. M. (1973): Temperature-sensitive mutants of influenza virus. IV. Induction of interferon in the nasopharynx by wild-type and a temperature-sensitive recombinant virus. J. Infect. Dis., 128:488-493.

12. Adamson, R. H., Fabro, S., Homan, E. R., O'Gara, R. W., and Zendzian, R. P. (1970): Pharmacology of polyriboinosinic: Polyribocytidylic acid, a new antiviral and antitumor agent. Antimicrob. Agents Chemother., 1969:148-152.

13. Young, C. W. (1971): Interferon induction in cancer. Med. Clin. North Am., 55:721-728.

14. Hilleman, M. R., Lampson, G. P., Tytell, A. A., Field, A. K., Nemes, M. M., Krakoff, I. H., and Young, C. W. (1971): Double stranded RNA's in relation to interferon induction and adjuvant activity. In: Biological Effects of Polynucleotides, edited by R. F. Beers and W. Braun, pp. 27-44. Springer-Verlag, New York.

15. Mathe, G., Amiel, J. L., and Schwarzenberg, L. (1970): Remission induction with poly I·poly C in patients with acute lymphoblastic leukemia. Rev. Eur. Etudes Clin. Biol., 15:671.

16. Sodemann, C. P., Malchow, H., and Schmidt, M. (1972): Die wirkung von polyinosin-polycytidyl-saure (poly I·poly C) auf die remission-szeit von akuten leukamien erwachsenen. In: Sonderdruck ans Leukamie, edited by R. Gross and J. van de Loo, pp. 557-561. Springer-Verlag, Berlin.

17. McIntyre, R. O. (1975): Observations on the use of poly I·poly C in the treatment of human leukemia. Report of the International Workshop on Interferon in the Treatment of Cancer, New York, March 31-April 2, 1975, p. 49.

18. Nordlund, J., Wolff, S., and Levy, H. B. (1970): Inhibition of biological activity of polyinosinic-polycytidylic acid by human plasma. Proc. Soc. Exp. Biol. Med., 133:439-444.

19. Baron, S., Dubuy, H., Buckler, C. E., Johnson, M., and Worthington, M. (1971): Factors affecting the interferon response of mice to poly-nucleotides. In: Biological Effects of Polynucleotides, edited by R. F. Beers and W. Braun, pp. 45-54. Springer-Verlag, New York.

20. Levy, H. B., Baer, G., Baron, S., Buckler, C. E., Gibbs, C. J., Iadarola, M. J., London, W. T., and Rice, J. (1975): A modified polyriboinosinic-polyribocytidylic acid complex that induces interferon in primates. J. Infect. Dis., 132:434-439.

21. Robinson, R. A., Devita, V. T., Levy, H. B., Baron, S., Hubbard, S. P., and Levine, A. S. (1976): A phase I-II trial of multiple-dose polyriboinosinic-polyribocytidylic acid (poly I·poly C) in patients with leukemia or solid tumors. J. Natl. Cancer Inst. (in press).

Control of Neoplasia by Modulation of the Immune System, edited by M. A. Chirigos. Raven Press, New York 1977.

ROLE FOR POLYNUCLEOTIDES AS INHIBITORS OF ENDONUCLEASE ACTIVITY

Timothy P. Karpetsky, Philip A. Ilieter, and Carl C. Levy

Enzymology and Drug Metabolism Section, Laboratory of Pharmacology,
Baltimore Cancer Research Center, Division of Cancer Treatment,
National Cancer Institute, National Institutes of Health,
Baltimore, Maryland 21211

INTRODUCTION

The widespread occurrence of relatively long tracts of polyadenylic acid (poly A) at the 3' termini of RNAs from eukaryotic (1-4), from viral (5), and from bacterial sources (6,7) has prompted a great deal of speculation on the role of the polynucleotide in cellular metabolism. It has been suggested, for example, that poly A at the terminus of heterogeneous nuclear RNA (hnRNA) in eukaryotic cells facilitates the transport of that material through the nuclear envelope. The recent discovery (6,7), however, of poly A tracts at the 3' termini of prokaryotic RNAs has raised serious questions, if not about the validity, then at least about the universality of this type of role for the polynucleotide.

Recently a protective function for poly A has been suggested (8,9), a suggestion which was based on the observation that poly A, much like the other purine homopolymer, polyguanylic acid (poly G), is a potent, yet reversible, inhibitor of a number of bacterial and mammalian endonucleases (8-13). The function alluded to is in accord, moreover, with a large body of evidence from many biological systems, which indicates that the functional stability of mRNA is dependent on the presence of a 3' terminal poly A sequence (5,14-18). Because all the endonucleases studied, irrespective of source, are inhibited by poly A, it would appear that the mechanism of inhibition is probably quite general and is not dependent on the individual enzyme examined. Although control of RNase activity by poly A constitutes an important regulatory system, certain other naturally occurring polynucleotides may act as inhibitors of this enzyme as well. For example, we have isolated from Citrobacter sp., a complex consisting of RNase and DNA. The inhibition of

517

RNase activity induced by this polydeoxynucleotide is similar to poly A-induced inhibition in several respects such as modulation by ionic strength or polyamine concentration. Therefore, in selecting an endonuclease to serve as a model in elucidating the possible mechanism of poly A inhibition, a bacterial ribonuclease (RNase) isolated from Citrobacter sp. was chosen for two reasons: first, because the Citrobacter enzyme, having been studied extensively (8, 11, 12), has several well-known properties, any change in which can be used as a guide to measure the effects of polynucleotide inhibitors; and second, because the enzyme has bound to it, a polydeoxynucleotide which acts as a potent inhibitor of RNase activity.

In addition to the control of RNase activity induced by poly A or by the endogenous DNA inhibitor, this chapter considers several other factors which regulate the hydrolysis of RNA by the Citrobacter enzyme. These factors are not restricted to the Citrobacter enzyme, but are found in several endonucleases and include the thermal inactivation of RNase and polyamine effects on the activity of the enzyme.

MATERIALS

Trypsin, pronase, RNase A, and Sephadex products were obtained from Sigma Chemical Company, St. Louis, Missouri. The polyamine hydrochlorides, also purchased from Sigma, were recrystallized twice from ethanol-water. RNase T_1, DNase I, and DNase II were obtained from Worthington Biochemical Corp., Freehold, New Jersey.

The exonuclease from rat ascites tumor was isolated according to the procedure of Lazarus and Sporn (19).

All synthetic polynucleotides were obtained from Miles Laboratories, Elkhart, Indiana.

METHODS

Purification of Citrobacter Ribonuclease

The methods used in extraction of the enzyme have been detailed elsewhere (11). Studies involving the enzyme-inhibitor complex were conducted with preparations carried through the gel filtration stage to retain the endogenous polynucleotide inhibitor. Thermal inactivation studies and measurements of thermodynamic parameters were performed on enzyme purified through the heat step stage. The enzyme, at this stage of purification, is homogeneous with respect to protein.

Assay of Citrobacter Nuclease

The standard assay system (1 ml) contained $0.5\,\mu$mol of polyuridylic acid (poly U), $100\,\mu$mol of Tris-HCl buffer (pH 7.2 at 37°C), and enzyme. After incubation of the reaction mixture for 5 min at 37°C, the reaction was terminated by the addition of 1 ml of 12% perchloric acid containing 20 mM lanthanum nitrate. Upon cooling in an ice bath for 20 min, the cloudy mixture was clarified by centrifugation and the acid-soluble nucleotides released during the course of the reaction were measured at 260 nm (12). An enzyme unit is defined as that amount of enzyme activity required to increase the absorbance at 260 nm 0.1 absorbance units under the conditions of the assay.

Ionic Strengths

Ionic strengths of potassium phosphate buffer, pH 7.2, were calculated from the salt composition of the buffer and dissociation constants (20). The method of Bates and Bower (21) was used to determine ionic strengths of Tris-HCl buffer solutions.

Determination of the Apparent Rate Constant (k_{app}) for Inactivation

A solution (0.9 ml) consisting of 8 units of heat step stage Citrobacter RNase and 100 μmol of Tris-HCl buffer (pH 7.2 at 37°C) was incubated at 37°C for a fixed interval of time, after which 0.5 μmol of polyuridylic acid (poly U) was added (final volume 1 ml) and enzyme activity measured. All determinations were in duplicate, utilizing, in most cases, five different presubstrate addition incubation times. It was noted that the maximum incubation time prior to addition of substrate need not exceed 1 hr, because the loss of enzyme activity was such that an accurate value of k_{app} could be obtained within that time from the slope of the linear ln ($\Delta A_{260\ nm}$) versus time of preincubation plot.

Thermodynamic Parameters

The activation energy, E_a, was determined directly from the slope of the ln k_{app} versus l/T (°K) plot (least-squares fit). The other constants ($\Delta H^{\ddagger}$, $\Delta G^{\ddagger}$, and $\Delta S^{\ddagger}$) were obtained from E_a and k_{app}, using the method Eyring and Stearn (22).

RESULTS

Isolation and Characterization of the Endogenous Polynucleotide Inhibitor

The Citrobacter RNase, at an early stage of its purification (11), is eluted after gel filtration, at a position in the elution profile which suggests a molecular weight in excess of 100,000. When the enzyme was carried through the remaining steps of the purification procedure (i.e., DEAE-cellulose chromatography, heating, and affinity chromatography), the molecular weight of the protein was estimated as approximately 25,000 (11). Accompanying the decrease in size of the enzyme, there is a large increase in specific activity, suggesting that a large-sized inhibitor was lost prior to the last stages of purification. Gel electrophoresis of enzyme preparations from either the heat step or affinity chromatography stages indicated the presence of a single protein band in each gel. The enzymes migrated with similar Rf's in each gel and, on elution from unstained gels, had similar physical characteristics (11). These data suggest that at the heat step stage of purification, the enzyme exists as a homogenous protein.

Although the characterization of the inhibitor is the subject of a separate paper, in essentials the procedure outlined below was followed. After repeated extraction of the EI complex with phenol, the inhibitor remains in the aqueous phase and is not attacked by proteolytic enzymes. There is no loss of inhibitory activity after exhaustive treatment of the inhibitor with either RNase A or RNase T1. In addition, the inhibitor is not digested by treatment with an ascites tumor exonuclease, an enzyme known to have a strong predilection for polyadenylic acid residues (19). Rapid hydrolysis of the inhibitor, with concomitant loss of inhibitory activity, is induced by either DNase I or DNase II. It appears, then, that the endogenous inhibitor probably represents a heterogenous group of polydeoxynucleotides.

Because there is no one inhibitor as such, but rather an array of naturally occurring inhibitory polydeoxynucleotides, studies of the interaction between the enzyme and this substance is probably best accomplished by using the entire biological entity, i.e., the array of polydeoxynucleotides bound to the enzyme.

Inhibition of Citrobacter RNase by Endogenous Inhibitor

Because the inhibition of the Citrobacter RNase by the endogenous substance was found to be sensitive to changes in ionic strength (μ), this property was used as a probe in studying the relationship between the enzyme and its bound polynucleotide. With various concentrations of Tris-HCl buffer (pH 7.2 at 37°C) as the fixed variable, a Hofstee plot [v versus v/(S)] yielded a series of lines with a common intercept on the v axis but with slopes dependent on ionic strength (Table 1). The pattern of this plot is characteristic for competitive inhibition (20). However, ionic strength is the fixed variable rather than inhibitor concentration which, in the case at hand, is kept constant throughout. The slopes of the lines from this plot (Table 1) are defined (23) as $-K_m [1 + (inhibitor)/K_i]$. Enzyme activity and K_m do not vary significantly with changes in ionic strength over the region studied, using preparations of the RNase free of inhibitor (I). Thus, because both the inhibitor concentration and K_m are fixed, K_i must vary with changes in ionic strength to account for the large changes in the slopes of the lines in the Hofstee plot. To test this contention, use was made of the relationship $K_i = K_{i_0} \cdot 10^{-1.04 Z_E Z_I \sqrt{\mu}}$, where K_{i_0} is the thermodynamic dissociation constant of the enzyme-inhibitor complex (EI complex) and Z_E and Z_I are the charges on the enzyme and inhibitor, respectively, involved in the formation of the EI complex (24, 25). A relationship between the slopes of the isoionic lines of the Hofstee plot and the square root of ionic strength may be expressed as Equation (1).

TABLE 1. Endogenous inhibition of Citrobacter ribonuclease: Variation of the slope of the Hofstee plot [v versus v/(S)] with ionic strength

Ionic strength (μ) of Tris-HCl buffer (pH 7.2 at 37°C)	Slope of v versus v/(S) plot (mM)
0.020	-4.15
0.032	-1.93
0.044	-1.16
0.060	-0.65
0.108	-0.20
0.160	-0.15

The reaction mixture (1.0 ml) contained 13 units of Citrobacter RNase bound to the endogenous inhibitor (see text). Tris-HCl (pH 7.2 at 37°C) was added to give the ionic strengths listed in the table. For each ionic strength assays were performed utilizing 0.15, 0.20, 0.25, 0.35, 0.50, 0.75, and 1.0 μmol of poly U as substrate. After incubation at 37°C for 5 min, enzyme activity was measured as described under Methods.

$$-\log\left(\frac{-\text{slope}}{K_m} - 1\right) = \log\frac{K_i}{(I)} = -1.04 Z_E Z_I \sqrt{\mu} + \log\frac{K_{i_0}}{(I)} \tag{1}$$

Equation (1) predicts that by plotting $-\log[(-\text{slope}/K_m) - 1]$ versus $\sqrt{\mu}$, a straight line of slope $-1.04 Z_E Z_I$ should be obtained. A computer "best fit" of the data to Equation (1), using the MLAB program (26), yielded the following values: $Z_E Z_I = -9.1$ and $K_{i_0}/(I) = 1.4 \times 10^{-3}$ with $K_m = 1.34 \times 10^{-4}$ M and $V_m = 1.8$. These constants gave a fit to the data with a correlation coefficient > 0.99. Therefore, the origin of the strong dependence on ionic strength of the endogenous polydeoxynucleotide competitive inhibition of Citrobacter RNase is the large product of charges ($Z_E Z_I = -9.1$). The consequence of so large a product of charges is a very strong modulation of K_i by changes in ionic strength.

Inhibition by Poly A

It has been shown previously that purine homopolymers, such as poly A, inhibit a variety of endonucleases (8-13). Poly A-induced competitive inhibition of Citrobacter RNase was found to be strongly dependent on ionic strength. This modulation of enzyme activity by a polynucleotide inhibitor and ionic strength resembles the system described above whereby control of enzyme activity is exerted by an endogenous DNA inhibitor and ionic strength. However, is the inhibition of RNase induced by poly A and by the DNA inhibitor identical? Do the inhibitions induced by these different inhibitors respond in the same manner to reversal by increasing ionic strength? To answer these questions, a study of the dependence on changes in ionic strength of the competitive inhibition of poly A (11) in the presence of the endogenous inhibition was conducted. A method formally similar to that discussed in the last section was utilized but, in this case the concentration of the substrate (poly U) was maintained constant (5×10^{-4} M) and the poly A concentration was varied from 0 to 5×10^{-6} M. The data obtained was analyzed as a Dixon plot ($1/v$ versus poly A) having isoionic lines. The advantage of this treatment is that the vertical intercepts [Equation (2a)] for this two-inhibitor, doubly competitive system depend on the endogenous inhibitor (I_{endo} and $K_{i_{endo}}$), whereas the horizontal or poly A intercepts depend on both the endogenous inhibitor and exogenously added poly A ($K_{i_{poly\,A}}$). It is possible, therefore, by this procedure to check the results of the last section by examination of the $1/V$ intercepts and to find $Z_E Z_I$ for the

$$\text{(a)} \quad \frac{1}{V} \text{ intercept} = \frac{1}{V_m} \left\{ 1 + \frac{K_m}{(S)} \left[1 + \frac{(I_{endo})}{K_{i_{endo}}} \right] \right\}$$

$$\text{(b)} \quad \text{poly A intercept} = -K_{i_{poly\,A}} \left[1 + \frac{(S)}{K_m} + \frac{(I_{endo})}{K_{i_{endo}}} \right]$$

(2)

poly A-induced inhibition of RNase activity from the poly A intercepts simultaneously. In fact, the computer-selected "best-fit" values for the inhibition by homopolymeric poly A are $Z_E Z_I = -4.1$ and K_{i_0} (for poly A) = 8.6×10^{-9} M. Thus the dependence on changes in ionic strength of K_i for poly A is less [$Z_E Z_I = -4.1$] than that for the naturally occurring DNA inhibitor [$Z_E Z_I = -9.1$]. These data clearly indicate that the Debye-Hückel-Bronsted mechanism governing the ionic strength dependent reversal of polynucleotide-induced RNase inhibition is the same for poly A and the endogenous DNA inhibitor.

Reversal of Endogenous Inhibition by Spermidine

Previous work with a number of endonucleases indicated that the polyamine, spermidine, reverses inhibition of enzyme activity induced by purine homopolymers (8-13). Because the endogenous inhibitor is a polydeoxynucleotide, it might therefore be expected that spermidine would reverse the inhibition of Citrobacter RNase activity induced by this DNA. That this is the case is seen in Table 2, in that a large enhancement of RNase activity results from addition of spermidine to the enzyme-endogenous inhibitor complex. This effect is not due to an increase in ionic strength caused by

TABLE 2. Spermidine-induced reversal of endogenous inhibition of
Citrobacter ribonuclease

[Spermidine] X 10^4 M	Citrobacter RNase activity (ΔA_{260} nm)
0	0.18
1.2	0.20
2.4	0.26
3.6	0.38
4.8	0.52
6.0	0.48
25.0	0.49

The reaction mixture (1 ml) contained 0.3 μmol of poly U, 8 μmol of
potassium phosphate buffer (pH 7.1), and 46.2 units of Citrobacter RNase
bound to the endogenous inhibitor (see text). The amounts of spermidine
listed were added prior to incubation at 37° C for 5 min. Enzyme activity
was then measured as described under Methods.

increasing spermidine levels, because the concentrations of the polyamine
are too low to perturb significantly the total ionic strength.

Spermidine Effects on the Inactivation of Citrobacter RNase

The polyamine, spermidine, is known to bind to the Citrobacter RNase,
resulting in an enzyme-spermidine complex that maintains activity toward
substrate (12). However, it was also noted that the half-life of the enzyme
(37°C) is a function of spermidine concentration. This dependence of the
half-life of the enzyme ($t_{1/2}$) on spermidine concentration is seen in Table 3.
Clearly, the presence of spermidine slows down or even prevents the thermal
inactivation of this enzyme. These studies were conducted with the polyamine being present at all times. If the polyamine can bind to the endonuclease and prevent thermal inactivation, can spermidine also restore activity
to thermally inactivated RNase? This question was answered by first
incubating the enzyme without substrate such that a degree of thermal inactivation took place. Then, in quick succession, spermidine and poly U
were added and enzyme activity was measured. The results of this study
(Table 4) demonstrate that the restoration of activity to RNase subjected to
thermal inactivation is dependent on the concentration of spermidine added.

TABLE 3.   Modulation of thermal inactivation of Citrobacter ribonuclease
by spermidine

Spermidine (M)	k_{app} (sec^{-1})	$t_{1/2}$ (min)
0	9.1×10^{-4}	12.7
5×10^{-5}	3.1×10^{-4}	37.3
5×10^{-4}	6.0×10^{-5}	193.0
5×10^{-3}	No inactivation after 40 min	

The reaction mixture (0.9 ml) contained 100 µmol of Tris-HCl buffer (pH 7.2 at 37°C), 8.4 units of Citrobacter RNase purified through the heat step stage (11) and the concentrations of spermidine listed. After incubation (37°C) for a fixed interval of time, 0.5 µmol of poly U was added (final volume, 1.0 ml) and, following incubation at 37°C for 5 min, enzyme activity was determined and the apparent rate constant for inactivation (k_{app}) calculated as described under Methods.

TABLE 4.   Spermidine-dependent restoration of enzyme activity to
thermally inactivated Citrobacter ribonuclease

Time (sec)	Citrobacter RNase activity ($\Delta A_{260 nm}$)		
	Spermidine concentration		
	0	1.5×10^{-5} M	3.0×10^{-5} M
0	0.61	0.65	0.74
600	0.25	0.41	0.58
1,200	0.14	0.28	0.39
1,800	0.07	0.24	0.36
2,400	0.04	0.25	0.36

The reaction mixture (0.9 ml) containing 100 µmol of Tris-HCl buffer (pH 7.2 at 37°C) and 6.1 units of Citrobacter RNase, was incubated (37°C) for the times indicated. Spermidine and 0.5 µmol of poly U were then added. After incubation at 37°C for 5 min, enzyme activity was measured as described under Methods.

TABLE 5. Entropies of activation for the inactivation of
Citrobacter ribonuclease

	Tris-HCl (e.u./mole)		Potassium phosphate (e.u./mole)	
	10^{-2} M	7.7 X 10^{-2} M	1.15 X 10^{-2} M	7.85 X 10^{-2} M
$\Delta S^{\ddagger}$	-52	-53	-41	-23

The reaction mixture (0.9 ml) contained 8.4 units of Citrobacter RNase and the amounts of Tris-HCl (pH 7.2 at 37°C) or potassium phosphate (pH 7.1) buffer indicated. After incubation for a fixed interval of time, 0.5 μmol of poly U (0.1 ml) was added and following incubation at 37°C for 5 min, enzyme activity was determined and the apparent rate constant for inactivation (k_{app}) calculated as described under Methods. The incubation of enzyme prior to addition of substrate was carried out at seven temperatures in the region 18 to 48°C for each buffer. Although the pH of a Tris-HCl buffer changes with temperature, it was determined that k_{app} (37°C) does not vary in the pH region 6.6 to 7.6. The slope of the $\ln(k_{app})$ versus 1/(absolute temperature) plot yielded the activation energy. Other thermodynamic parameters were obtained as described under Methods.

Thermodynamics of Inactivation of Citrobacter RNase

The fact that spermidine can restore enzyme activity to Citrobacter RNase that has been thermally inactivated may be interpreted to mean that there is no gross conformational change of the enzyme on thermal inactivation. This would account for the ease and rapidity with which RNase activity is regained upon addition of the polyamine. To test this hypothesis, thermodynamic parameters for the thermal inactivation of Citrobacter RNase (free of the endogenous inhibitor) were determined under a wide variety of experimental conditions. The entropy of activation ($\Delta S^{\ddagger}$) for the inactivation reaction (enzyme → inactivated enzyme) was found to be consistently large and negative as seen in Table 5. This thermodynamic evidence supports the contention that there is not a gross configurational change in the enzyme as the Citrobacter RNase is thermally inactivated.

DISCUSSION

The mechanisms presented in this chapter, by which the activity of Citrobacter RNase may be regulated, are summarized in Fig. 1. The bottom half of the figure represents the inhibition of enzyme, whereas the top half deals with the thermal inactivation. The competitive inhibition of RNase by either an endogenous DNA inhibitor or by exogenously added poly A is

ACTIVE   INACTIVE

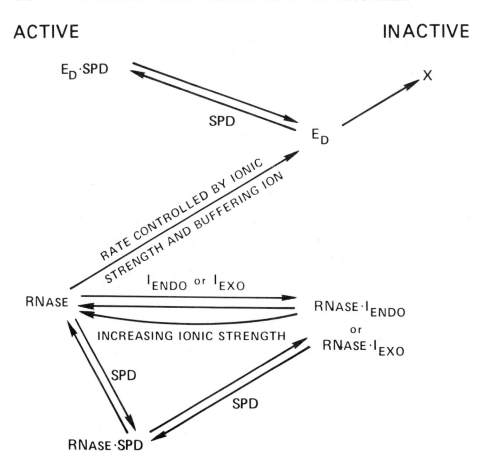

FIG. 1. Scheme for the regulation of Citrobacter ribonuclease activity. "Active" and "Inactive" indicate those enzyme forms with or without endonuclease activity. Abbreviations for the various enzyme forms are as follows: RNase (Citrobacter enzyme not bound to the endogenous inhibitor), RNase · I_{endo} or RNase · I_{exo} (RNase bound to endogenous inhibitor or exogenously added inhibitor (such as poly A, respectively), RNase· SPD (RNase bound to spermidine), E_D (thermally inactivated RNase), X (denatured RNase — not reversible by addition of spermidine), and E_D · SPD (E_D bound to spermidine).

strongly controlled by ionic strength. However, the electrostatic effect is more marked in the case of the endogenous inhibitor (as expressed by a greater absolute value of $Z_E Z_I$) than in poly A. The strength of this effect would be expected to vary with the base composition of the inhibitor. In addition, the double-stranded nature of the DNA inhibitor may also play a role in determining the dependence of inhibition on ionic strength. The fact that spermidine reverses the inhibition of RNase induced by the endogenous inhibitor was not unexpected, because it has been shown previously that the polyamine binds to the Citrobacter RNase (11,12) and causes reversal of polypurine inhibition in several endonuclease systems (8,9,13). This mechanism of reversal of inhibition is distinct from the ionic strength mechanism outlined above and might result presumably from a spermidine-induced change in enzyme conformation.

The modulation of RNase activity of polynucleotides, spermidine, and ionic strength has been proposed elsewhere (8,9). We believe that the mechanism of RNase modulation is not unique, but will occur with any endonuclease inhibited by poly A. As stated elsewhere, endonucleases from bacteria (10–12), from bovids, and from human sources (8,13) are inhibited by purine homopolymers. We predict that this mechanism will be operative (barring high concentrations of polyamine or salt) in any compartment where polynucleotides having 3' terminal tracts of poly A are processed by an endonuclease which is inhibited by homopolymeric poly A.

The Citrobacter model raises certain interesting questions. The enzyme will hydrolyze RNA or poly U rapidly (11), but in the presence of low concentrations of poly A, substrate degradation will not proceed. Thus, if the amount of poly A is progressively reduced relative to the amount of substrate, the rate of hydrolysis of the RNA increases. That this finding has biological significance is demonstrated by the fact that mRNAs from prokaryotes, having very short 3' terminal poly A tracts (6,7) are much shorter-lived than their eukaryotic counterparts which possess much longer 3' poly A segments. From another viewpoint, this type of mechanism offers a possible reason why large proteins consist of distinct subunits. Because tracts of poly A longer than 200 residues are unknown in mRNA, very large mRNAs coding for large proteins would have little protection from endonuclease activity. These large mRNAs would, therefore, be rapidly hydrolyzed because of poor inhibition of RNase activity stemming from the large ratio of the length of the nonpolyadenylated segment to the length of the 3' terminal poly A tract. One possible means of getting around this difficulty is to construct large proteins in polymeric subunits, the mRNAs for which would be adequately protected. After synthesis, the subunits would then be assembled into whatever size had been predetermined.

The thermal inactivation of Citrobacter RNase, presented in the upper half of Fig. 1, is yet another mechanism by which RNA levels may be regulated by RNase activity. The inactive, "storage," form of the RNase enzyme produced on thermal inactivation is converted to an active form by spermidine. Thus, there is a direct biochemical link between spermidine concentration and RNA levels, not only through the reversal of polynucleotide-mediated RNase inhibition, but also through the reactivation of enzyme activity as well. Although this facet of endonuclease regulation has not received as much attention as poly A-induced inhibition, the "storage" form concept of RNase activity is deserving of examination in other endonucleolytic systems.

SUMMARY

A naturally occurring DNA inhibitor bound to an endonuclease has been isolated from Citrobacter sp. The competitive inhibition of the RNase by this inhibitor was found to be extremely sensitive to small changes in ionic strength, more so than if homopolymeric poly A is used to induce inhibition. Changes in the concentration of the polyamine, spermidine, also regulate the inhibition caused by either of these polynucleotides. The rate of thermal inactivation of the enzyme is controlled by the level of spermidine present. Furthermore, the thermally inactivated form of the RNase serves to store endonucleolytic activity, because enzyme function is reactivated on the addition of spermidine. The combination of endogenous DNA inhibitor, polyamines, and thermal inactivation with reversibility induced by spermidine constitutes a system whereby fine regulation of ribonuclease activity, and hence RNA levels, can be readily achieved.

REFERENCES

1. Mendecki, J., Lee, S.-Y., and Brawerman, G. (1971): A polynucleotide segment rich in adenylic acid in the rapidly-labeled polyribosomal RNA component in mouse sarcoma 180 ascites cells. Proc. Natl. Acad. Sci. (U.S.A.), 68:1331-1335.
2. Kates, J. (1970): Transcription of the vaccinia virus genome and the occurrence of polyriboadenylic acid sequences in messenger RNA. Cold Spring Harbor Symp. Quant. Biol., 35:743-762.
3. Darnell, J. E., Wall, R., and Nakazato, H. (1971): An adenylic acid-rich sequence in messenger RNA of HeLa cells and its possible relationship to reiterated sites in DNA. Proc. Natl. Acad. Sci. (U.S.A.), 68:1321-1325.
4. Edmonds, M., Vaughn, H. M., and Nakazato, H. (1971): Polyadenylic acid sequences in the heterogeneous nuclear RNA and rapidly-labeled polyribosomal RNA of HeLa cells: Possible evidence for a precursor relationship. Proc. Natl. Acad. Sci. (U.S.A.), 68:1336-1340.
5. Spector, D. H., and Baltimore, D. (1974): Requirement of 3'-terminal poly(adenylic acid) for the infectivity of poliovirus RNA. Proc. Natl. Acad. Sci. (U.S.A.), 71:2983-2987.
6. Ohta, N., Sanders, M., and Newton, A. (1975): Poly(adenylic acid) sequences in the RNA of Caulobacter crescentus. Proc. Natl. Acad. Sci. (U.S.A.), 72:2343-2346.
7. Nakazato, H., Venkatesan, S., and Edmonds, M. (1975): Polyadenylic acid sequences in E. coli messenger RNA. Nature, 256:144-146.
8. Levy, C. C., Schmukler, M., Frank, J. J., Karpetsky, T. P., Jewett, P. B., Hieter, P. A., LeGendre, S. M., and Dorr, R. G. (1975): Possible role for poly(A) as an inhibitor of endonuclease activity in eukaryotic cells. Nature, 256:340-341.
9. Levy, C. C. (1975): Roles of RNases in cellular regulatory mechanisms. Life Sci., 17:311-316.

10. Frank, J. J., Hawk, I. A., and Levy, C. C. (1975): Polyamine activation of staphylococcal nuclease. Biochim. Biophys. Acta, 390: 117-124.

11. Levy, C. C., Mitch, W. E., and Schmukler, M. (1973): Effect of polyamines on a ribonuclease which hydrolyzes ribonucleic acid at uridylic acid residues. J. Biol. Chem., 248:5712-5719.

12. Levy, C. C., Hieter, P. A., and LeGendre, S. M. (1974): Evidence for the direct binding of polyamines to a ribonuclease that hydrolyzes ribonucleic acid at uridylic acid residues. J. Biol. Chem., 249:6762-6769.

13. Schmukler, M., Jewett, P. B., and Levy, C. C. (1975): The effects of polyamines on a residue-specific human plasma ribonuclease. J. Biol. Chem., 250:2206-2212.

14. Huez, G., Marbaix, G., Hubert, E., Leclercq, M., Nudel, U., Soreq, H., Salomon, R., Lebleu, B., Revel, M., and Littauer, U. Z. (1974): Role of the polyadenylate segment in the translation of globin messenger RNA in Xenopus oocytes. Proc. Natl. Acad. Sci. (U.S.A.), 71:3143-3146.

15. Soreq, H., Nudel, U., Salomon, R., Revel, N., and Littauer, V. S. (1974): In vitro translation of polyadenylic acid-free rabbit globin messenger RNA. J. Mol. Biol., 88:233-245.

16. Marbaix, G., Huez, G., Burny, A., Cleuter, Y., Hubert, E., Leclercq, M., Chantrenne, H., Soreq, H., Nudel, U., and Littauer, U. Z. (1975): Absence of polyadenylate segment in globin messenger RNA accelerates its degradation in Xenopus oocytes. Proc. Natl. Acad. Sci. (U.S.A.), 72:3065-3067.

17. Sheiness, D., Puckett, L., and Darnell, J. E. (1975): Possible relationship of poly(A) shortening to mRNA turnover. Proc. Natl. Acad. Sci. (U.S.A.), 72:1077-1081.

18. Wilt, F. (1973): Polyadenylation of maternal RNA of sea urchin eggs after fertilization. Proc. Natl. Acad. Sci. (U.S.A.), 70:2345-2349.

19. Lazarus, H., and Sporn, M. (1967): Purification and properties of a nuclear exoribonuclease from Ehrlich ascites tumor cells. Proc. Natl. Acad. Sci. (U.S.A.), 57:1386-1393.

20. Butler, J. H. (1964): Ionic Equilibrium — A Mathematical Approach, p. 441. Addison-Wesley, Reading, Mass.

21. Bates, R. G., and Bower, V. E. (1956): Alkaline solutions for pH control. Anal. Chem., 28:1322-1324.

22. Eyring, H., and Stearn, A. E. (1939): The application of the theory of absolute reaction rates to proteins. Chem. Rev., 24:253-270.

23. Hofstee, B. M. J. (1956): Graphical analysis of single enzyme systems. Enzymologia, 17:273-278.

24. Debye, P., and Hückel, E. (1923): Zur Theorie der Elektrolyte. Phys. Z., 24:185-206.

25. Webb, J. L. (1963): Enzyme and Metabolic Inhibitors, Vol. 1, p. 819. Academic Press, New York.

26. Knott, G. D., and Reece, D. K. (1972): MLAB: A civilized curve-fitting system. Proc. ONLINE 1972 Internatl. Conf., vol. 1, pp. 497-526. Brunel University, England.

Control of Neoplasia by Modulation of the Immune System, edited by M. A. Chirigos. Raven Press, New York 1977.

REVERSAL OF IMMUNODEPRESSION IN FRIEND LEUKEMIA VIRUS-INFECTED MICE BY AN RNA-RICH EXTRACT OF STATOLON

Preston A. Marx and E. Frederick Wheelock

Department of Microbiology, Thomas Jefferson University, Philadelphia, Pennsylvania 19107

INTRODUCTION

Much effort is currently being directed toward the development of effective immunotherapeutic agents for the treatment of human leukemia. Encouraging results have been obtained in animal leukemia model systems with BCG (1) and Levamisole (2), but clinical trials with these agents have produced only moderate success (1,3). The demonstration that synthetic polyribonucleotides have potent immunostimulatory properties (4,5) and tumor-suppressive effects in animals (6) raised high hopes for their effectiveness in man. However, extensive clinical trials with polyinosinic-polycytidylic acid (poly I:C) have produced little or no tumor-suppressive effects (7). More recently, polyadenylic-polyuridylic acid (poly A:U) has been used in clinical trials in patients with breast cancer as an extension of successful animal experiments in which its application in conjunction with surgery proved effective in treatment of mammary tumors in mice (8,9).

For several years we have been studying the immune-stimulatory and leukemosuppressive effects of statolon, an extract of the mycophage infected Penicillium stoloniferum. We have found that this extract abrogates Friend leukemia virus-induced immunodepression and macrophage dysfunction in all infected mice and results in complete suppression of erythroleukemia in 50 to 70% of infected mice (10-12). These clinically normal mice contain Friend leukemia virus (FLV) in a dormant state for many months. Erythroleukemia emerges in some mice late in life, but many mice remain normal for their entire life-spans. Other reports from this laboratory (13) indicate that statolon stimulates FLV-infected mice to mount a humoral immune response against both the Friend virion and Friend leukemic cells and that this immune response is essential for leukemosuppression. One of our goals has been to identify the active immune-stimulating factor in statolon. Such knowledge would be useful in determining the site and mechanism of action of statolon and would be required for future clinical studies in man.

Several studies suggest to us that double-stranded RNA (dsRNA) present in statolon may be responsible for suppression of erythroleukemia. In 1971 Pilch and Planterose from the Beecham Laboratories reported that treatment of FLV-infected mice with dsRNA isolated from P. stoloniferum mycophage suppressed splenomegaly and prolonged the survival in 80% of treated mice, with 20% of the mice remaining clinically normal for several weeks (14). Further studies from the Beecham Laboratories indicated that dsRNA from P. stoloniferum has immunostimulatory effects (15). We now report that the immune-stimulator and leukemosuppressive factor in statolon is contained in RNA-rich fractions of statolon that are sufficiently immunostimulatory to reverse immunodepression by FLV and suppress the disease.

MATERIALS AND METHODS

Mice

Female, DBA/2J mice, 6 to 8 weeks old, obtained from Jackson Memorial Laboratories, Bar Harbor, Maine, were used in all experiments.

Friend Leukemia Virus

Stocks of FLV were prepared as previously described (10). In all experiments mice were injected intraperitoneally (day 0) with 1,000 to 2,000 LD_{50} (50% leukemia-producing dose) in 0.2 ml volume.

Treatment of FLV-Infected Mice

Statolon (5.0 mg/mouse) or fractions derived from statolon were administered i.v. on day 3.

SDS-Phenol Extraction of Statolon

In all experiments statolon was hydrated as previously described (11). For fractionation, hydrated statolon was sonicated and then clarified by centrifugation at 100,000 X g for 90 min at 5°C in an SW50 rotor. The supernatant fraction, designated statolon supernatant in this chapter, was stored at -70°C until used for sodium dodecyl sulfate (SDS)-phenol extraction. Statolon supernatant was extracted three times with SDS and phenol as described (16). Briefly, statolon supernatant was diluted twofold with sterile distilled water and adjusted to 0.01 M sodium acetate (pH 5.0), 0.05 M NaCl, and 1% SDS with stock solutions. It was heated to 56°C for 1 min, and then extracted with an equal volume of phenol at 56°C for 1 min. The mixture was cooled to 0°C and the aqueous phase recovered after centrifugation of the mixture at 10,000 X g for 10 min at 5°C. The SDS-phenol extraction was repeated twice at 23°C. RNA was then precipitated from the aqueous phase with two volumes of ethanol at -23°C for 16 hr. For animal injection, statolon-derived precipitated RNA was recovered by centrifugation at 10,000 X g for 10 min at 5°C. The precipitate was washed twice with 95% ethanol, and residual ethanol was evaporated under a stream of filtered air. The precipitate was dissolved in SSC buffer (0.15 M sodium chloride and 0.015 M sodium citrate, pH 7.0), and injected intravenously into the mice.

Assay for Antibody Plaque-Forming Cells

All animals were immunized i.p. with 2×10^8 SRBC (day 4 with respect to FLV infection) and assayed for anti-SRBC antibody forming cells 4 days later. Spleens were examined for plaque-forming cells (PFC) against SRBC, employing the assay of Jerne and Nordin (17) as modified by Cunningham and Szenberg (18).

Assay for FLV Cytotoxic Antibody

FLV cytotoxic antibody was measured as previously described (19), with the following modification. The ^{51}Cr-labeled target cells for the assay were obtained from a continuous line of Friend leukemic cells (designated clone 745) derived by Friend et al. (20). These cells were kindly provided by C. Friend through the courtesy of the Institute of Medical Research, Camden, New Jersey.

RESULTS AND DISCUSSION

To learn whether the factor in statolon that restores immunocompetence in FLV leukemic mice is RNA, we extracted RNA by the SDS-phenol method and injected the extract into FLV-infected mice. The amount of RNA in the RNA-rich extract of statolon was adjusted so that it was equivalent to the amount of RNA in statolon supernatant. The results are presented in Table 1. The FLV-infected, untreated mice were eightfold immunodepressed as compared with normal controls. Both the statolon supernatant and the RNA-rich extract from statolon stimulated the immune response of FLV-infected mice to normal levels, whereas poly I:C had no such effect. The absorption ratio (A_{280}/A_{260}) of the RNA-rich extract was 0.5, indicating that the material is not significantly contaminated with protein. This experiment indicates that statolon-derived RNA is as potent an immunostimulant as statolon supernatant and more potent than poly I:C.

To determine whether the immunocompetence restoring RNA in statolon is double-stranded, we pretreated the RNA with RNAse A in either high ionic or low ionic strength buffer (1 X SSC vs. 0.1 X SSC). After RNAse treatment, the mixture was injected into FLV-infected mice as in the

TABLE 1. Restoration of immunocompetence to FLV-infected mice by
RNA-rich extracts derived from statolon

Experimental group [a]	Anti-SRBC PFC/10^6 nucleated cells	Percent control
Uninfected	84.6 ± 4.7	100
FLV infected	10.5 ± 5.7	12
FLV infected +		
statolon supernatant	97.2 ± 13.0	115
1 X RNA-rich extract	90.7 ± 15.7	107
Poly I:C (50 µg/mouse)	15.6 ± 10.7	18

[a] Five mice were in each group.

previous experiment. We reasoned that pretreatment with RNAse A should
diminish the immune stimulation in either salt solution if the RNA was
single-stranded, whereas immune stimulation by dsRNA should be diminished
by RNAse treatment only at low ionic strength. In these experiments untreated FLV-infected mice were tenfold immunodepressed, and mice treated
with statolon-derived RNA had about fivefold more anti-SRBC forming cells
than untreated controls. Only RNAse treatment in low salt diminished this
fivefold immune stimulation, confirming the double-strandedness of the RNA.

Results in the previous section suggested that statolon-derived RNA may
be FLV-leukemosuppressive. We found this to be the case. Mice were infected with FLV and treated with statolon-derived RNA 3 days after FLV
infection. Approximately 50% of treated mice suppressed the FLV infection,
and all mice with suppressed erythroleukemia contained high titers of antibody cytotoxic for Friend leukemic cells.   Thus, statolon-derived RNA
induces leukemosuppression to the same extent as previously observed with
unfractionated statolon (12).

The crude extract of Penicillium is not suitable for use in man because it
could cause serious allergic and other deleterious side effects. Purified
dsRNA, however, may be relatively free of these undesired properties.
This report establishes a link between the immunostimulatory and leukemosuppressive effects of statolon-derived dsRNA in FLV-infected mice.

ACKNOWLEDGMENTS

The technical assistance of Wilhelmina G. Marum is gratefully acknowledged. This research was supported by Public Health Service grant
CA-12461-04 from the National Cancer Institute.

REFERENCES

1. Bast, R. C., Jr., Zbar, B., Borsos, T., and Rapp, H. J. (1974): BCG and cancer. N. Engl. J. Med., 290:1458-1469.

2. Chirigos, M. A., Pearson, J. W., and Pryor, J. (1973): Augmentation of chemotherapeutically induced remission of a murine leukemia by a chemical immunoadjuvant. Cancer Res., 33:2615-2618.

3. Hirshaut, Y., Pinsky, C., Fried, J., and Oettgen, H. (1974): Trial of Levamisole as immunopotentiator in cancer patients. Proc. Am. Assoc. Cancer Res., 15:126.

4. Braun, W., and Nakano, M. (1967): Antibody formation: Stimulation by polyadenylic and polycytidylic acids. Science, 157:819-821.

5. Schmidtke, J. R., and Johnson, A. G. (1971): Regulation of the immune system by synthetic polynucleotides. I. Characteristics of adjuvant action on antibody synthesis. J. Immunol., 106:1191-1200.

6. Levy, H. B., Law, L. W., and Rabson, A. S. (1969): Inhibition of tumor growth by polyinosinic-polycytidylic acid. Proc. Natl. Acad. Sci. (U.S.A.), 62:357-361.

7. McIntyre, O. R.: personal communication.

8. Lacour, F., Spira, A., Lacour, J., and Prade, M. (1972): Polyadenylic-polyuridylic acid, an adjunct to surgery in the treatment of spontaneous mammary tumors in C3H-He mice and transplantable melanoma in the hamster. Cancer Res., 32:648-649.

9. Lacour, J. (1975): Trials with Poly A:Poly U as adjuvant therapy complementing surgery in randomized patients with breast cancer. In: Fundamental Aspects of Neoplasia, edited by A. A. Gottlieb, O. J. Plescia, and D. H. L. Bishops, pp. 229-232. Springer-Verlag, New York.

10. Weislow, O. S., Friedman, H., and Wheelock, E. F. (1973): Suppression of established Friend virus leukemia by statolon. V. Reversal of virus-induced immunodepression to sheep erythrocytes. Proc. Soc. Exp. Biol. Med., 142:401-405.

11. Levy, M. H., and Wheelock, E. F. (1975): Impaired macrophage function in Friend virus leukemia: Restoration by statolon. J. Immunol., 114:962-965.

12. Wheelock, E. F., Toy, S. T., Weislow, O. S., and Levy, M. H. (1974): Restored immune and nonimmune functions in Friend virus leukemic mice treated with statolon. Prog. Exp. Tumor Res., 19:369-389.

13. Wheelock, E. F., Toy, S. T., Caroline, N. L., Sibal, L. R., Fink, M. A., Beverley, P. C. L., and Allison, A. C. (1972): Suppression of established Friend virus leukemia by statolon. IV. Role of humoral antibody in the development of a dormant infection. J. Natl. Cancer Inst., 48:665-673.

14. Pilch, D. J. F., and Planterose, D. N. (1971): Effects on Friend disease of double-stranded RNA of fungal origin. J. Gen. Virol., 10:155-162.

15. Cunnington, P. G., and Naysmith, J. D. (1975): Naturally occurring double-stranded RNA and immune responses. I. Effects on plaque-forming cells and antibody formation. Immunology, 28:451-468.

16. Kingsbury, D. W. (1973): Cell-free translation of paramyxovirus messenger RNA. J. Virol., 12:1020-1027.

17. Jerne, N. K., and Nordin, A. A. (1963): Plaque formation in agar by single antibody-producing cells. Science, 140:405.

18. Cunningham, A. J., and Szenberg, A. (1968): Further improvements in the plaque technique for detecting single antibody-forming cells. Immunology, 14:599-600.

19. Toy, S. T., and Wheelock, E. F. (1975): In vitro depression of cellular immunity by Friend virus leukemic spleen cells. Cell. Immunol., 17:57-73.

20. Friend, C., Patuleia, M. C., and DeHarven, E. (1966): In: National Cancer Institute, Monograph No. 22 (Conference on Murine Leukemia), edited by M. A. Rich and J. B. Moloney, pp. 505-522. U.S. Government Printing Office, Bethesda, Md.

Control of Neoplasia by Modulation of the Immune System, edited by M. A. Chirigos. Raven Press, New York 1977.

SUPPRESSION OF FLV-INDUCED LEUKEMIA BY THIOGLYCOLLATE MEDIUM

Robert R. Strauss, Leony Mills, and Navin Patel

Department of Microbiology, Albert Einstein Medical Center, Philadelphia, Pennsylvania 19141

INTRODUCTION

It is well established that "activated" macrophages are selectively cyto-toxic to neoplastic target cells in tissue culture (1-6). Activation of these mononuclear phagocytes has been accomplished by in vivo infection of mice or guinea pigs with a variety of intracellular parasites such as bacteria or protozoa (7-11). Macrophage activation has been reported to be associated with a factor derived from lymphocytes (12,13). The cytotoxic effect of the "activated" macrophage appears to be independent of phagocytosis (14). It has been shown that cytotoxicity is preceded by adherence of the macrophage to the target tumor cell with subsequent transfer of lysosome-like granules from the macrophage to the target cell (14). Selective inhibition of macro-phage lysosomal enzyme activities also abolishes tumor cell cytotoxicity under these conditions (14).

Resident peritoneal macrophages or those elicited by intraperitoneal (i.p.) injection of sterile irritants do not possess the ability to kill tumor cells in vitro (3,6). Elicited macrophages have been shown to differ in both metabolic and bactericidal functions from resident and activated macrophages (15-17). We have found that peritoneal macrophages elicited in mice by a single i.p. injection of sterile thioglycollate medium have marked increases in both peroxidase and glucose-6-phosphate dehydrogenase (G6PD) activities. Moreover, treatment of these animals with thioglycollate medium also causes a significant reduction in splenomegaly associated with Friend leukemia virus (FLV) infection. These observations are the subject of this chapter.

537

MATERIALS AND METHODS

Female ICR or Balb/c mice weighing 20 to 25 g at the beginning of an experiment were used in these studies. ICR mice were purchased from Jackson Laboratories, Bar Harbor, Maine, and Balb/c mice were purchased from Cumberland View Farms, Clinton, Tennessee. Animals were housed in groups of 6 to 10 in plastic cages and allowed Purine mouse chow and water ad libitum.

Virus infection was by the i.p. route. ICR mice received 500 to 1,000 ID_{50} doses, whereas Balb/c animals were injected with 50 to 100 ID_{50} doses suspended in 0.5 ml of minimum essential medium (MEM). The FLV preparation used in these studies contained both leukemogenic and focus-forming agents but was free of LDH and LCM viruses (18).

Thioglycollate medium (Difco Laboratories, Detroit, Michigan) was prepared according to label. Sterile medium was administered by i.p. injection of 0.5 ml in all instances. The time of injection of thioglycollate relative to FLV infection varied with the experiment.

After specified time intervals for a given experiment, mice were killed by cervical dislocation. Peritoneal exudate (PE) cells were collected by lavage in sterile tissue culture medium either 199 or MEM. The cells were then washed by centrifugation twice at 50 X g for 10 min in the same medium. After recovery of PE cells, spleens were surgically removed, patted dry, and weighed. Spleen cell suspensions, relatively free of erythrocytes, were prepared by previously described procedures (19). Adherent cells, presumably phagocytes, were obtained by allowing PE cells or spleen cells suspended in tissue culture medium to adhere to the surface of sterile plastic petri dishes for 3 hr at 37°C in an atmosphere of 5% CO_2 in air. At this time, the nonadherent cells were removed by decantation, the cell sheet was washed three times with 37°C warmed medium, and the washed dishes were then chilled (4°C). Adherent cells were then collected by scraping with a sterile rubber policeman.

PE macrophage G6PD activity was determined in intact cells suspended in glycerin by measurement of NADP reduction at 340 nm in a Zeiss–Hitachi spectrophotometer (20). Peroxidase activity of whole-cell homogenates was assayed in the absence of sucrose by the color change of guaicol at 470 nm in the presence of H_2O_2 (21).

Virus content of spleen cell homogenates was assayed by the number of foci of transformed cells found in cultures of DB2 cells innoculated with serial dilutions of homogenates from infected mice.

The hemolytic assay for antibody plaque-forming cells (PFC) in agar gel was done essentially as described by Jerne and Nordin (22). Mice were immunized by i.p. injection of 0.5 ml of a 2% suspension of washed sheep erythrocytes (SRBC) purchased from Flow Laboratories, Rockville, Maryland. In vitro immunization of mouse splenocytes was done in Marbrook (23) chambers.

All chemicals used in this investigation were obtained from commercial sources and were of reagent grade.

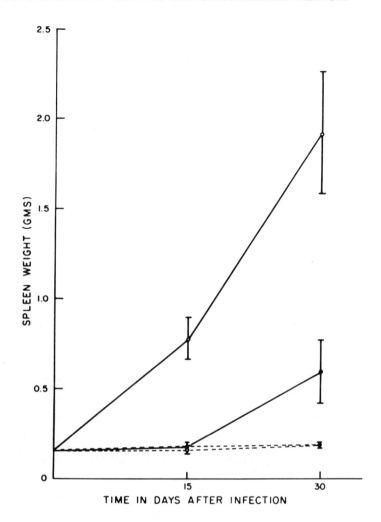

FIG. 1. Comparative splenomegaly in mice infected with FLV, with or without i.p. injection of sterile thioglycollate. Each point represents average spleen weight $\pm$ SE for 12 to 15 mice on days 15 or 30 after infection with FLV (solid line) or for uninfected control mice (broken line), either untreated (open circles) or given thioglycollate (filled circles) only.

RESULTS

The reports, confirmed by us, of increased metabolic activity including that of peroxidase in mouse peritoneal macrophages elicited by injection of thioglycollate medium led to experiments designed to determine the effect of such injections on FLV-induced leukemia in mice. The results of these experiments are shown in Fig. 1. The data depicted in the figure reveal that i.p. injection of this common bacterial growth medium 2 days before FLV

TABLE 1. Spleen weights of FLV-infected mice relative to time of
intraperitoneal injection of thioglycollate medium

FLV-infected	Time in days of thioglycollate infection relative to infection	No. of mice	Spleen wt. in mg $\pm$ SE	p Value relative to FLV
-	—	10	120 $\pm$ 112	—
+	—	12	728 $\pm$ 131	—
+	-7	8	365 $\pm$ 119	> 0.05
+	-4	4	399 $\pm$ 13	< 0.05
+	-3	4	325 $\pm$ 43	< 0.02
+	-2	11	375 $\pm$ 61	< 0.02
+	-1	4	368 $\pm$ 88	< 0.05
+	0	8	398 $\pm$ 60	< 0.05
+	+1	4	369 $\pm$ 113	< 0.05
+	+2	12	360 $\pm$ 96	< 0.05
+	+4	8	337 $\pm$ 37	< 0.01
+	+6	5	369 $\pm$ 37	< 0.02

Data obtained 15 days after FLV infection. p Values determined by
Student's t-test.

infection significantly reduces leukemia associated splenomegaly for up to
30 days. The effect of time of administration of thioglycollate medium relative to FLV infection on splenomegaly in ICR mice is presented in Table 1.
These data tend to indicate that i.p. injection of this sterile irritant may be
therapeutic as well as prophylactic. There is significant reduction of
splenomegaly when the growth medium is administered from 4 days before to
6 days after virus infection. The number of foci of transferred cells, an
observation associated with the number of virus particles, found in spleen
cell suspensions from thioglycollate treated mice is also markedly reduced
when compared to those from infected untreated animals. These results
are shown in Table 2. The data presented in Table 3 show that thioglycollate
treatment also inhibits splenomegaly induced by intravenous injection of up
to 5 X 10^6 nucleated spleen cells from untreated infected syngeneic mice.
    It is now firmly established that FLV infection suppresses the immune
response in mice (24). Administration of thioglycollate 2 days before FLV
infection partially reverses this phenomenon when sheep erythrocytes (SRBC)

TABLE 2. Enumeration of FLV-associated focus-forming agents of spleen cell homogenates from thioglycollate-treated mice [a]

Group	Spleen wt. (g) [b]	Foci/spleen [b]
Control	2.237	26,960
Thioglycollate -7 days [c]	1.185	625
Thioglycollate -2 days	0.272	23
Thioglycollate +2 days	0.931	6,800

[a] All data obtained 30 days after FLV infection.

[b] Values are averages for 2 to 3 spleens. Foci determined in monolayers of DB/2 cells.

[c] Time when thioglycollate was administered relative to FLV infection.

TABLE 3. Effect of thioglycollate treatment on splenomegaly after transfer of spleen cells from FLV-infected mice

Donor	Recipient	Spleen wt. of recipient (mg)
FLV + thioglycollate	None	468 ± 72
FLV	None	1,623 ± 260
FLV + thioglycollate	Thioglycollate	306 ± 25
FLV	Thioglycollate	782 ± 86

5×10^6 Spleen cells from mice infected with FLV 30 days earlier were injected intravenously into recipient animals. Intraperitoneal treatment with thioglycollate was 2 days before FLV infection. All values are expressed as the mean ± SE of mean for 5 animals/group.

are given in vivo (Table 4) or in vitro (Table 5). Trypan blue, a substance that is reported to be inhibitory to macrophage lysosomal enzymes (14,25), is shown on Table 6 to also be an immunosuppressive material. It can be seen from the data presented in Table 7 that trypan blue tends to increase FLV-associated splenomegaly. Pretreatment with thioglycollate abolishes this effect.

TABLE 4. Effect of thioglycollate treatment of mice on FLV-associated
in vitro immunosuppression to sheep erythrocytes

Group [a]	Thioglycollate [b]	Hemolytic PFCs per spleen [c]
Control	-	68,350
	+	30,117
FLV-infected	-	1,359
	+	20,083

[a] Groups of FLV-infected and normal control mice immunized i.p. with
0.5 ml of 2% sheep erythrocyte suspension 4 days prior to sacrifice.

[b] Treatment with thioglycollate, 0.5 ml, i.p., 2 days before infection
with FLV.

[c] Average number of plaque-forming cells (PFCs) for 6 to 8 spleens.

TABLE 5. Effect of in vivo thioglycollate treatment on in vitro
immunosuppression of mouse spleen cells

Group [a]	Thioglycollate [b]	Hemolytic PFCs per 10^6 cells [c]
Control	-	870
	+	1,078
FLV-infected	-	234
	+	758

[a] Spleen cell cultures from normal and FLV-infected mice. Animals
sacrificed 15 days after infection. Cultures immunized in vitro with washed
sheep erythrocytes.

[b] Mice injected i.p. with 0.5 ml of thioglycollate 2 days before FLV
infection.

[c] Average values for 3 cultures in duplicate per group.

TABLE 6.   Effect of trypan blue administration to mice on hemolytic plaque-forming cell response to sheep erythrocytes

Group	PFC/spleen[a]
Control[b]	101,979
0.5 mg of trypan blue[c]	73,448
1.0 mg of trypan blue	27,510
2.0 mg of trypan blue	16,192

[a] Values are averages of 5 animals per group.

[b] Animals were immunized by i.p. injection of 0.5 ml of 2% sheep erythrocytes 4 days before sacrifice.

[c] Trypan blue was injected i.p. immediately following immunization. The volume injected was 0.5 ml in all cases.

TABLE 7.   The effect of trypan blue and thioglycollate on FLV infection in Balb/c mice

Infection	Treatment	Spleen wt. (mg)[a]
+[b]	—	896.67 ± 177.34
+	Thioglycollate[c]	275.00 ± 57.26
+	Trypan blue[d]	1,246.25 ± 355.18
+	Thioglycollate and trypan blue	242.75 ± 10.80
−	Thioglycollate	177.50 ± 13.92
−	Trypan blue	188.75 ± 10.87
−	—	125.00 ± 4.56

[a] All values are expressed as the mean ± SE for 4 mice per group.

[b] Infection was 50 to 100 ID_{50} by the i.p. route. Mice were sacrificed 15 days after infection.

[c] Thioglycollate was given i.p. 2 days before infection.

[d] Trypan blue (1 mg/mouse) was injected i.p. immediately following FLV infection.

DISCUSSION

The marked increase in G6PD and peroxidase activities of peritoneal macrophages elicited in mice by i.p. injection of sterile thioglycollate medium tends to implicate these phagocytes in the inhibition of FLV-associated splenomegaly also seen following treatment with this bacterial culture medium. The flow of glucose through the hexose monophosphate shunt is controlled by G6PD (26). Inhibition of this enzyme causes a marked reduction in production of H_2O_2 (27). The combination of peroxidase, H_2O_2, and halide has been shown to be cidal to many different microorganisms including a variety of viruses (28, 29). The peroxidase-mediated antimicrobial system has also been reported to be able to kill both normal and malignant mammalian cells in culture (30, 31). The marked decrease in foci of transformed cells in cultures treated with spleen cell homogenates from thioglycollate-injected, FLV-infected mice tends to bear out this hypothesis. Because both FLV infection and thioglycollate treatment were by the peritoneal route, one could expect that elicited peritoneal macrophages might play a role in limiting the infection. However, we also observed that i.p. administration of thioglycollate also protected mice against intravenously injected spleen cells from leukemic animals of the same strain. This observation does not rule out a role for macrophages, because these cells are also found in the spleen. However, it has been reported that thioglycollate-elicited macrophages do not enhance ^{51}Cr release from target tumor cells in culture (3, 6).

The immunosuppressive effect of trypan blue coupled with its enhancement of FLV-associated splenomegaly would tend to involve the immune response in this viral leukemia. The observations that thioglycollate reverses both the FLV-associated immunosuppression and trypan blue enhancement of splenomegaly might indicate that thioglycollate is working via some effect on antibody synthesis. It is also well established that macrophages are involved in this humoral host defense mechanism (32).

Still another possible mechanism by which thioglycollate could be exerting its effect is through the enhanced production of interferon. It has been reported that mineral oil-elicited macrophages exhibit increased interferon production in culture (33). However, this antiviral substance could not account for all of the observed inhibition of splenomegaly because treatment with the sterile peritoneal irritant also protected against intravenous transfer of leukemic spleen cells.

Hence three possible mechanisms exist for the protective effect of thioglycollate against FLV-associated splenomegaly. Any combination, all three, or none may be involved. Additional experiments designed to test these hypotheses are in progress.

SUMMARY

Peritoneal macrophages elicited in ICR mice by injection of sterile thioglycollate medium exhibit markedly increased G6PD and peroxidase activities when compared to resident peritoneal cells from uninjected control animals.

Thioglycollate treatment of ICR mice also suppresses splenomegaly associated with Friend leukemia virus infection. This is accompanied by a reduced number of foci of transformed cells in cell cultures incubated with spleen cell homogenates from thioglycollate-treated, FLV-infected mice. Thioglycollate treatment is therapeutic as well as prophylactic. This treatment also partially reverses FLV-associated immunosuppression. Thioglycollate also reverses the proleukemic effects of trypan blue, an inhibitor of macrophage lysosomal enzymes that is immunosuppressive.

REFERENCES

1. Hibbs, John B., Jr., Lambert, L. H., Jr., and Remington, Jack S. (1972): Possible role of macrophage mediated nonspecific cytotoxicity in tumor resistance. Nature (New Biol.), 235:48-50.

2. Hibbs, John B. (1973): Macrophage nonimmunologic recognition: Target cell factors related to contact inhibition. Science, 180:868-870.

3. Hibbs, John B. (1974): Discrimination between neoplastic and non-neoplastic cells in vitro by activated macrophages. J. Natl. Cancer Inst., 53:1487-1492.

4. Holtermann, O. A., Casole, G. P., and Klein, E. (1972): Tumor cell destruction by macrophages. J. Med., 3:305-309.

5. Holtermann, O. A., Klein, E., and Casole, G. (1973): Selective cytotoxicity of peritoneal leukocytes for neoplastic cells. Cell. Immunol., 9:339-352.

6. Krahenbuhl, J. L., and Remington, J. S. (1974): The role of activated macrophages in specific and nonspecific cytostosis of tumor cells. J. Immunol., 113:507-516.

7. Gentry, L. O., and Remington, J. S. (1971): Resistance against cryptococcus conferred by introcellular bacteria and protozoa. J. Infect. Dis., 123:22-31.

8. Keller, R., and Jones, V. E. (1971): Role of activated macrophages and antibody in inhibition and enhancement of tumor growth in rats. Lancet, 847-849, Oct. 16, 1971.

9. Lunde, M. N., and Gelderman, A. H. (1971): Resistance of AKR mice to lymphoid leukemia associated with a chronic protozoon infection, Besnoitia Jellisoni. J. Natl. Cancer Inst., 47:485-488.

10. Mackaness, G. B. (1964): The immunological basis of acquired cellular resistance. J. Exp. Med., 120:105-114.

11. Remington, J. S., and Ruskin, J. (1969): A common mechanism of immunity for intracellular infections. J. Clin. Res., 17:156.

12. Nathan, C. F., Karnovsky, M. L., and David, J. R. (1971): Alterations of macrophage functions by mediators from lymphocytes. J. Exp. Med., 133:1356-1361.

13. Simon, Harvey B., and Sheagren, John H. (1972): Enhancement of macrophage bactericidal capacity by antigenically stimulated immune lymphocytes. Cell. Immunol., 4:163-174.

14. Hibbs, John B. (1974): Heterocytolysis by macrophages activated by bacillus Calmette-Guerin: Lysosome exocytosis into tumor cells. Science, 184:468-471.
15. Simmons, S. R., and Karnovsky, M. L. (1973): Iodinating ability of various leukocytes and their bactericidal activity. J. Exp. Med., 138:44-63.
16. Strauss, R. R., Friedman, H., Mills, L., and Zayon, G. (1975): Suppression of murine virus leukaemogenesis by thioglycollate, a bacteriological culture medium that affects macrophage peroxidase. Nature, 255:343-344.
17. Van Furth, R., Hirsch, J. G., and Fedorko, M. E. (1970): Morphology and peroxidase cytochemistry of mouse promoncytes, monocytes and macrophages. J. Exp. Med., 132:794-805.
18. Katelay, J. R., Kamo, I., Kaplan, G., and Friedman, H. (1974): Suppressive effect of leukemia virus infected lymphoid cells on in vitro immunization of normal splenocytes. J. Natl. Cancer Inst., 53:1371-1379.
19. Strauss, R. R., Paul, B. B., Jacobs, A. A., and Sbarra, A. J. (1972): The in vitro bactericidal and associated metabolic activities of mouse spleen cells. Infect. Immun., 5:114-119.
20. Strauss, R. R., Paul, B. B., Jacobs, A. A., Simmons, C., and Sbarra, A. J. (1970): The metabolic and phagocytic activities of leukocytes from children with acute leukemia. Cancer Res., 30:480-488.
21. Paul, B. B., Strauss, R. R., Jacobs, A. A., and Sbarra, A. J. (1970): Function of H_2O_2, myeloperoxidase, and hexose monophosphate shunt enzymes in phagocytizing cells from different species. Infect. Immun., 1:338-344.
22. Jerne, N. K., and Nordin, A. A. (1963): Plaque formation in agar by single antibody producing cells. Science, 140:405-407.
23. Marbrook, J. (1967): Primary immune response in cultures of spleen cells. Lancet, 2:1279-1281.
24. Ceglowski, Walter S., and Friedman, H. (1968): Immunosuppression by leukemia viruses, I. Effect of Friend disease virus on cellular and humoral hemolysin responses of mice to a primary immunization with sheep erythrocytes. J. Immunol., 101:594-604.
25. Beck, F., Lloyd, J., and Griffith, A. (1967): Lysosomal enzyme inhibition by trypan blue: A theory of teratogenesis. Science, 157:1180-1182.
26. Beck, W. S. (1958): Occurrence and control of the phosphogluconate oxidation pathway in normal and leukemic leukocytes. J. Biol. Chem., 232:271-283.
27. Strauss, R. R., Paul, B. B., and Sbarra, A. J. (1968): Effect of phenylbutazone on phagocytosis and intracellular killing by guinea pig polymorphonuclear leucocytes. J. Bacteriol., 96:1982-1990.
28. Belding, M. E., Klebanoff, S. J., and Ray, C. G. (1970): Peroxidase mediated virucidal system. Science, 167:195-196.

29. Klebanoff, S. J. (1972): Relationship of metabolism to function. In: Polymorphonuclear Leukocyte Molecular Basis of Electron Transport, Miami Winter Symp., 4: 275-300.

30. Clark, R. A., Klebanoff, S. J., Einstein, A. B., and Fefer, A. (1975): Peroxidase-H_2O_2-halide system: Cytotoxic effect on mammalian tumor cells. Blood, 45:161-170.

31. Edelson, P. J., and Cohn, Z. A. (1975): Peroxidase-mediated mammalian cell cytoxicity. J. Exp. Med., 138:318-323.

32. Fishman, Marvin (1969): Induction of antibodies in vitro. Ann. Rev. Microbiol., 23:199-222.

33. Mendelson, J., and Dick, V. (1971): Production of interferon by murine peritoneal leukocytes: Enhancement by mineral oil. J. Infect. Dis., 123:351-355.

Control of Neoplasia by Modulation of the Immune System, edited by M. A. Chirigos. Raven Press, New York 1977.

SPLENIC PROTEOLYTIC ENZYMES AND RESISTANCE TO VIRAL INFECTIONS

Phyllis S. Roberts and William Regelson

Department of Medicine, Division of Medical Oncology, Virginia Commonwealth University, Medical College of Virginia, Richmond, Virginia 23298

INTRODUCTION

It is well established that viruses are involved in the etiology of many animal cancers. Herpes viruses have been strongly implicated in the development of cancers in man and other animals (1, 2), and the diseases induced by the murine leukemia virus systems resemble human leukemia. In fact, Friend leukemia virus (FLV) disease of mice has been used as a model for studying virus-induced leukemogenesis (3-5). FLV induces a neoplastic condition in mice that is characterized by enlargement of the spleen, starting soon after infection. Several studies have shown that mice infected with FLV have suppressed immune responses (6-13), as do humans with leukemia (14-19).

The factors conferring resistance to FLV disease are not completely understood and are very complex, with several genes playing a role in this phenomenon (3, 20, 21). The $Fv-1^n$ or $Fv-1^b$ locus determines whether the mouse will be susceptible to the N-tropic or B-tropic "helper" virus, whereas the $Fv-2^s$ or $Fv-2^r$ locus determines whether the mouse will be susceptible to the spleen focus-forming virus (SFFV). These genes appear to act at a very early stage in the infectious process, perhaps when the virus penetrates the target cell or with early events associated with virus replication. In addition, H-2 (histocompatibility-2) gene also seems to influence susceptibility to FLV infection, probably influencing relatively late events during the development of the disease. Another group of genes, that of the hereditary anemias, significantly influences response to Friend virus, possibly by affecting the quality or quantity of target cells available to the virus. Finally, other unknown genes may be involved, because from a genetic basis it is not understood why strain A and BALB/c mice differ in their degree of susceptibility to FLV disease (3).

No gene product, either a protein or an enzyme, has been shown to be involved in conferring resistance to FLV infection, although a number of splenic enzymes have been found to be decreased, increased, or unchanged as this disease progresses (22-27). We found that when NYLAR mice were infected with N-tropic FLV disease, their splenic proteolytic enzyme activity (measured at pH 8 with ester substrates) decreased as the disease progressed but their splenic tributyrinase activity remained unchanged (unpublished data).

Proteases functioning under neutral or slightly alkaline conditions have been found in the human spleen and in mast cells in the spleen. Using histochemical methods, Li, Lung, and Crosby (28) showed that the neutrophils and the mast cells in human spleens contain a chymotrypsin-like protease and the mast cells a trypsin-like enzyme. A trypsin-like enzyme was also found by Ende and Auditore (29) in a human mastocytotic spleen and in a canine mastocytoma. LoSpalluto, Fehr, and Ziff (30) postulated that although proteases that are active at acid pH may be concerned with the catabolism of proteins, a protease they partially purified from a lysosome-containing granule fraction of human spleen and optimally active between pH 7 and 8, may play a key role in the immune response. This enzyme, differing from the cathepsins in several ways, degraded human immunoglobulin G as well as other proteins.

TAME and BAME (p-toluenesulfonyl- and benzoyl-L-arginine methyl ester) are substrates for proteolytic enzymes that function at slightly alkaline pH. Chymotrypsin hydrolyzes BAME but not TAME, but other proteolytic enzymes (trypsin, thrombin, plasmin, etc.) hydrolyze both TAME and BAME. Several years ago we observed that splenic homogenates from healthy adult DBA/2 and NYLAR mice, known to be very susceptible to N-tropic FLV disease, had very low levels of an enzyme(s) that hydrolyzes TAME and BAME optimally at pH 8.0, whereas splenic homogenates from healthy adult BALB/c and C57BL/6 mice, resistant to N-tropic FLV disease, had much higher levels of this enzyme(s). To investigate this further, we selected mice from four groups (3),

Group 1: $Fv-1^n$, $Fv-2^r$ (C57L, C58),
Group 2: $Fv-1^b$, $Fv-2^r$ (C57BL/6, C57BL/10),
Group 3: $Fv-1^b$, $Fv-2^s$ (BALB/c, A), and
Group 4: $Fv-1^n$, $Fv-2^s$ (DBA/2, Ha/ICR, C3H/He, C3H/Bi),

in order to determine whether the levels of TAME and/or BAME activities in splenic homogenates were related to resistance to FLV disease or to the presence of the Fv-1 or Fv-2 gene. Both C3H/He and C3H/Bi were also tested, because the former is slightly susceptible but the latter very susceptible to Gross leukemia virus yet both are $Fv-1^n$, $Fv-2^s$, and $H-2^k$ (3). In addition, splenic homogenates from several strains of mice were centrifuged and the TAME and BAME activities of the supernatant and residue fractions were determined, and these data are also reported here.

It has been shown that Pyran copolymer (a synthetic polyanionic immunopotentiator) injected i.v. into BALB/c mice makes them more susceptible to FLV disease but i.p. injections make them more resistant (31). If the levels of TAME and/or BAME activities in splenic homogenates were decreased by i.v. injections of Pyran and increased by i.p. injections, this would be additional evidence that proteolytic enzymes may play a role in resistance to FLV disease. BALB/c mice, therefore, were injected either i.v. or i.p. with Pyran and the levels of TAME and BAME activities in the splenic homogenates were determined and these data are also reported here.

After this work was completed the resistance of various strains of mice to Herpes simplex virus type 1 (HSV-1) was reported (32). Because we had determined the levels of splenic enzymes that hydrolyze TAME and BAME in several of the same strains, the relationship between these enzymatic activities and resistance to HSV-1 disease is also discussed here.

MATERIALS AND METHODS

TAME, BAME, and Tris(2-amino-2-hydroxymethyl-1,3-propanediol) were purchased from Sigma Chemical Co. Pyran copolymer (XA124-177) was kindly given to us by Dr. D. Breslow, Hercules, Inc., Wilmington, Delaware. The purest grade available of all the other chemicals was obtained commercially.

Some strains of mice were purchased from Jackson Laboratories, Microbiologics Laboratories, or Blue Spruce Farms, and all the other were kindly given to us by Mammalian Genetics and Animal Production Section, National Cancer Institute, Bethesda, Maryland. The mice were kept in our animal rooms for at least 1 week, maintained on Purina Lab Chow and water ad libitum and then killed by cervical dislocation. The spleens were immediately removed, weighed, and kept at -17°C until homogenized with cold 0.15 M NaCl (Potter-Elvehjem homogenizer with a Teflon pestle), adding 1.5 ml of saline per 70 mg of spleen wet weight when individual spleens were used or per 140 mg of spleen when two or three spleens were homogenized together. In the latter case an aliquot of the homogenate was removed and diluted with one part of cold saline for testing and the remainder was centrifuged (3,000 rpm, 10 min, 4°C) and the residue washed three times with saline. The washings were added to the supernatant fraction and the residue was resuspended in saline.

Protein was determined in duplicate by the Lowry method using a LabTrol standard (Dade Division, American Hospital Supply Corp., Miami, Florida). Rates of hydrolysis of TAME and BAME were determined in duplicate, immediately after homogenization or after the centrifugation and washings, at 37°C in 0.25 M Tris-HCl buffer, pH 8.0, with 0.02 M TAME or BAME present at the start of the rate measurements by a modification of the Hestrin method (33,34). Tris buffer (0.04 ml, 1.25 M Tris) was mixed with 0.12 ml of homogenate, supernatant, or residue and after 4 min at 37°C TAME or BAME (0.04 ml, 0.1 M) was added. Alkaline hydroxylamine reagent (0.4 ml, 1 part 4 M $NH_2OH \cdot HCl$ and 1 part 6 N NaOH) was either added immediately (for the zero time readings) or was added after 60 min of reaction and the tubes were then placed at room temperature for 20 min. The HCl·TCA reagent (0.2 ml of 43.5% HCl and 15% trichloracetic acid) was then added and after an additional 20 min the tubes were centrifuged (3,000 rpm, 20 min). A 0.5-ml aliquot of the supernatant was removed and added to 3 ml of $FeCl_3$

reagent (0.14 M $FeCl_3$ after adjustment with HCl to pH 1.2). The optical
densities were read at 525 nm against blanks that contained all the same
solutions as did the tests but to which the HCl·TCA reagent was added before
the alkaline hydroxylamine reagent. Controls for spontantaneous hydrolysis
of TAME and BAME (substituting saline for homogenate, supernatant, or
residue) were done in duplicate at the same time as the tests, and the change
in optical density found after 60 min was subtracted from the test values.

Pyran copolymer was dissolved with heating in 0.15 M NaCl, cooled, and
brought to pH 7.2 with NaOH, and 0.2 ml was injected i.v. or i.p. (25 mg of
Pyran/kg) into 6-week-old male BALB/c mice daily for 5 consecutive days.
Control mice were injected at the same times with 0.2 ml of 0.15 M NaCl,
i.v. or i.p. All mice, 5 per group, were killed by cervical dislocation on
the sixth day (31). The spleens were removed, weighed, and kept at -17°C
until individually homogenized and tested as described above.

RESULTS

Table 1 shows that homogenates of individual spleens from various strains
of 7- to 9-week old mice differ greatly in the ability to hydrolyze TAME at
pH 8.0, the rates varying from 57.1 nm of TAME hydrolyzed/min/mg of
protein (C57L/J) to 3.5 (DBA/2L), but the ability to hydrolyze BAME does
not vary as greatly, ranging from 28.1 (C57L/S) to 4.3 (DBA/2L). In addition, sex does not appear to affect the enzymatic levels significantly (Table 1,
C57BL/6 and Ha/ICR).

The highest levels of TAME and BAME activities are found in homogenates
from group 1 spleens (Table 1), slightly lower levels in homogenates from
group 2, and significantly lower levels in homogenates from groups 3 and 4,
with two exceptions. BALB/c spleens have much higher activities than do
A/J or A/HeS spleens, and spleens from C3H/MAI mice (a C3H/Bi strain)
have much higher levels of TAME activity than do C3H/He spleens.

The data in Table 1 do not show any correlation between the ability of
splenic homogenates to hydrolyze TAME and/or BAME and the Fv-1 or Fv-2
gene. Neither does there appear to be a correlation between the levels of
these activities and the H-2 haplotype, because C57L is H-2^b and C58 is
H-2^k yet splenic homogenates from these strains have about the same
enzymatic activities. In addition, if resistance to N-tropic FLV disease
depends on the level of an enzyme(s) in the spleen that hydrolyzes TAME
and/or BAME, we would have expected the resistant A and A/He spleens to
have much higher and the susceptible C3H/MAI spleens to have much lower
levels of these activities than were found.

Nevertheless, splenic homogenates from five strains of mice that are
resistant to N-tropic FLV disease have high levels of TAME and BAME
activities (C57L, C58, C57BL/10, C57BL/6, and BALB/c), and splenic
homogenates from three strains that are susceptible to this infection have
significantly lower levels (C3H/He, Ha/ICR, and DBA/2). In addition, we
found previously that spleens from susceptible NYLAR mice also have low
levels of TAME and BAME activity, and we also found low levels in spleens
from susceptible AKR mice (see Table 3).

TABLE 1. The hydrolysis of TAME and BAME by homogenates of
individual spleens from various strains of mice

Group	Strain[a]	Age	Sex	No. of tests	nmoles Ester hydrolyzed/ min/mg protein ± a.d. TAME	BAME
1	C57L/J	7 w, 1 d	M	9	57.1 ± 7.8	21.9 ± 5.4
	C57L/S	9 w	M	8	52.3 ± 4.8	28.1 ± 1.1
	C58/J	9 w, 1 d	M	6	51.5 ± 6.9	27.4 ± 3.6
2	C57BL/10J	9 w, 4 d	M	10	44.7 ± 5.8	23.4 ± 5.9
	C57BL/6J	8 w, 4 d	M	10	43.4 ± 6.3	20.5 ± 6.5
	C57BL/6L	9 w	F	10	41.4 ± 3.6	22.9 ± 3.3
3	BALB/cJ	8 w, 4 d	M	11	36.6 ± 8.4	19.3 ± 2.7
	BALB/cL	9 w	M	11	32.6 ± 3.9	23.0 ± 2.5
	A/J	9 w, 1 d	M	6	20.6 ± 6.2	—
	A/HeS	9 w	M	11	13.1 ± 2.4	9.1 ± 1.9
4	C3H/MAI	9 w, 1 d	M	10	40.6 ± 7.7	21.1 ± 6.3
	C3H/HeJ	8 w, 3 d	M	8	21.4 ± 3.2	15.2 ± 3.9
	C3H/HeT	7 w, 2 d	M	10	21.1 ± 3.2	14.8 ± 3.5
	Ha/ICR	6 w, 6 d	M	9	16.1 ± 3.4	15.3 ± 5.3
		9 w	F	10	19.4 ± 2.8	18.1 ± 4.0
	DBA/2L	9 w, 1 d	F	10	3.5 ± 1.1	4.3 ± 1.1

[a] J, Jackson Laboratories; S, Simonson Laboratories; L, Laboratory
Supply Co., Inc.; MAI, Microbiologics Laboratories; T, Texas Inbred Mice;
Ha/ICR from Blue Spruce Farms.

In further studies, the distribution of enzymatic activities was studied
using spleens from three strains of mice resistant to N-tropic FLV disease
(C57L, C57BL/6, and BALB/c) and two susceptible strains (Ha/ICR and
DBA/2) as well as spleens from C3H/He and A/He mice. In addition, spleens
from susceptible AKR mice were also tested for reasons discussed below.
Spleens (two or three) from one strain were homogenized together in saline,
centrifuged, washed, and tested as described (Materials and Methods).
From three to five separate experiments were performed on spleens from
each strain, and the averaged values are shown in Tables 2 and 3 (the sex
and age of the mice are shown in Table 1).

Table 2 shows the average weights of the mice and of their spleens, the
percent protein in the spleens as well as the percent recovery of protein and
enzymatic activities after the centrifugation and washing procedure.

TABLE 2. The averaged weights of the mice and the spleens and the percent protein and enzymatic activities recovered in the supernatant and residue fractions

Strain	Averaged values ± a.d.				Percent recovered in supernatant plus residue		
	Mouse weight (g)	Spleen weight (mg)	Percent protein in spleen	Total protein in H^a (mg)	Protein	TAME	BAME
C57L/S	25.8 ± 0.3	93.8 ± 7.8	11.4	28.0 ± 1.3	82	91	76
C57BL/6L	19.4 ± 0.6	95.2 ± 10.0	11.7	27.3 ± 3.8	79	77	87
BALB/cL	21.7 ± 0.6	123.3 ± 3.2	13.2	32.5 ± 2.1	78	80	66
A/HeS	20.3 ± 0.5	99.8 ± 9.3	13.0	30.6 ± 1.1	86	112	69
C3H/HeT	22.8 ± 0.6	101.8 ± 12.2	12.7	31.4 ± 6.1	81	62	79
Ha/ICR	29.8 ± 1.3	120.9 ± 7.2	12.2	29.5 ± 4.8	94	108	72
DBA/2L	20.4 ± 1.1	124.5 ± 5.9	12.7	31.7 ± 3.3	76	97	109

[a] H = Homogenate.

TABLE 3. Hydrolysis of TAME and BAME by splenic homogenates from various strains of mice and by the residue and supernatant fractions of the homogenates

| | nmoles ester hydrolyzed/min/mg wet weight spleen | | | | | |
| Strain | nm TAME/min/mg spleen | | | nm BAME/min/mg spleen | | |
	Homogenate	Supernatant	Residue	Homogenate	Supernatant	Residue
C57L/S	6.38	3.83	1.98	3.31	1.17	1.33
C57BL/6L	5.00	2.83	1.04	2.38	1.23	0.85
BALB/cL	3.97	2.01	1.15	3.09	0.99	1.06
A/HeS	1.75	0.68	1.27	1.47	0.39	0.63
C3H/HeT	2.74	1.22	0.49	1.88	0.94	0.54
Ha/ICR	2.60	1.40	1.42	2.12	0.17	1.35
DBA/2L	0.28	0.19	0.08	0.64	0.45	0.25
AKR[a]	2.05	0.72	0.98	0.47	0.20	0.55

[a] Charles River Breeding Laboratories, 9-week-old females.

Frequently a gelatinous material, found after the residue was washed, was discarded. This probably accounts for the low protein recovery, averaging about 82%, and it may also partially account for the varying recoveries of TAME and BAME activities, averaging about 85% but with a considerable spread in several cases. Instability of the enzymes during centrifugation and washings may also have contributed to the low recoveries found in some cases. These fluctuations in recovery of activities, however, cannot be responsible for the wide differences in activities shown in Table 3.

It can be seen in Table 3 that the levels of TAME activity vary with the strain tested and follow the same order in the homogenate as in the supernatant fraction. The three resistant strains (C57L, C57BL/6, and BALB/c), as was also seen in Table 1, have significantly more activity than do any of the other strains. The resistant A/He and the susceptible AKR spleens have much lower levels of TAME activity, particularly in the supernatant fraction, and still lower levels are found only with DBA/2 spleens. Therefore, with the exception of spleens from A/He mice, the levels of TAME activity in the splenic homogenates and in the supernatant fraction are high when resistant mice are tested and low when susceptible mice are tested. In contrast, the levels of TAME activity found in the residue fraction do not show this pattern, because Ha/ICR and AKR residue fractions have higher or almost as high levels of TAME activity as do C57BL/6 and BALB/c residue fractions.

The highest levels of BAME activity (Table 3) are also found in the homogenate and supernatant fraction from C57L, C57BL/6, and BALB/c spleens, but almost as much activity is found in the homogenate from Ha/ICR spleens and in the supernatant fraction from C3H/He spleens. Very low BAME activity is found in the supernatant fraction from the other strains tested (A/He, Ha/ICR, DBA/2, and AKR). The BAME activity of the residue fraction from Ha/ICR spleens is as high as found in the C57L and higher than in the C57BL/6 or BALB/c residue fraction. These data, therefore, show that resistance to N-tropic FLV disease does not correlate with the level of BAME activity in the supernatant or residue fraction.

Because i.p. injections of Pyran copolymer into BALB/c mice make them more resistant to NB-tropic FLV disease but, in contrast, i.v. injections make them more susceptible (31), we injected Pyran or saline (controls) into healthy BALB/c mice (for experimental details see Materials and Methods) and determined the levels of TAME and BAME activities in the individual splenic homogenates. The data, the average of 5 spleens per group, are shown in Table 4, where it can be seen that spleens from mice injected with saline, i.v. or i.p., or with Pyran i.p. weigh about 100 mg but the spleens of mice injected with Pyran i.v. are more than twice as large, averaging 260 mg.

Comparing the control mice, it can also be seen in Table 4 that spleens from mice injected with saline i.p. have about 30% more total TAME activity than spleens from mice injected with saline i.v. but about the same BAME activity. The specific TAME activity (nm of TAME/min/mg weight of spleen or mg of splenic protein), however, is about the same after i.v. or i.p. injections, but the specific BAME activity is significantly increased with saline i.v. injections. Possibly i.v. injections produce greater stress in

TABLE 4. The effects of i.p. or i.v. injections of Pyran copolymer on the weight, protein content, and enzymatic activities of spleens from BALB/c mice

Averaged values	Saline injections		Pyran injections	
	i.p.	i.v.	i.p.	i.v.
Spleen weight, mg	109.0	93.2	110.0	260.0
Protein percent	14.4	12.3	12.7	11.9
Total activity: nm Ester/min/spleen				
TAME	594	455	737	421
BAME	333	379	453	270
Specific activity: nm ester/min/mg spleen				
TAME	5.46	4.88	6.71	1.62
BAME	3.06	4.07	4.13	0.95
Specific activity: nm ester/min/mg protein				
TAME, ± a.d.	37.7 ± 3.5	40.3 ± 5.6	54.0 ± 5.1	13.9 ± 2.3
BAME, ± a.d.	21.4 ± 1.5	33.7 ± 4.7	32.9 ± 4.2	8.1 ± 0.6

the mice than do i.p. injections, causing increased synthesis or release of an enzyme that hydrolyzes BAME.

A different picture is seen when the data obtained after Pyran i.p. or i.v. injections are compared (Table 4). Despite the fact that spleens from mice injected with Pyran i.v. are much larger and contain correspondingly more protein, they contain less total TAME and BAME activities than do spleens from mice injected with Pyran i.p. The specific TAME and BAME activities, therefore, are much lower in spleens from mice injected with Pyran i.v. than with Pyran i.p.

When comparing spleens from mice injected i.p. with saline or Pyran, it can be seen (Table 4) that after Pyran the spleens contain more total TAME and BAME activities and have higher specific activities than do spleens after saline. In contrast, comparing spleens from mice injected i.v. with saline or Pyran shows that although the total TAME activity is about the same in both groups, the total BAME activity is significantly lower after Pyran i.v. However, due to the much larger size and greater total protein content of these spleens, the specific activities of both TAME and BAME are much lower than after saline i.v. injections.

These data show that spleens of mice injected with Pyran i.p. have a higher concentration of an enzyme(s) that hydrolyzes TAME and BAME than do mice injected with saline i.p. In addition, spleens of mice injected with

Pyran i.v. have a much lower concentration of this enzyme(s) than do spleens of mice injected with saline i.v. Because it has been shown that i.p. injections of Pyran increase the resistance of mice to NB-tropic FLV infection but i.v. injections of Pyran make them more susceptible (31), it seems very likely that the level of an enzyme(s) that hydrolyzes TAME and BAME optimally at slightly alkaline pH plays a role in conferring resistance to FLV infection.

After this work was completed we learned that 11 strains of 3- to 4-month-old male mice had been tested for their resistance to HSV-type 1 (32, and personal communication with Dr. Lopez). We had already determined the levels of TAME and BAME activity in splenic homogenates and in the supernatant and residue fractions in five of the strains they had studied. It can be seen (Table 3) that there is an excellent correlation between the level of BAME activity in the supernatant fraction and the resistance of mice to HSV-1 infection. The very resistant C57BL/6 mice have the highest level of BAME activity (1.23 nm of BAME/min/mg of spleen), the moderately resistant BALB/c and C3H/He have lower levels (0.99 and 0.94, respectively) and the moderately susceptible DBA/2 and A/He have still lower levels (0.45 and 0.39, respectively). Because of this correlation, we then tested the very susceptible AKR strain, and as can be seen (Table 3), they have the lowest level of BAME activity in the supernatant fraction (0.20 nm/min/mg of spleen). These data, therefore, strongly suggest that the level of an enzyme(s) that hydrolyzes BAME and is present in the supernatant fraction of splenic homogenates plays a role in the resistance of mice to HSV-1 infection.

DISCUSSION

The data presented here indicate strongly that proteolytic enzymes, active at neutral to slightly alkaline pH and present in the spleen, may play a role in the resistance of mice to viral infections.

The levels of BAME activity in the supernatant fraction of splenic homogenates from the six strains of mice of varying resistance to HSV-1 infection that were tested decreased as the resistance decreased, with the lowest levels found in susceptible spleens and the highest levels in resistant spleens. Although additional strains of mice should be tested, these data strongly suggest that a proteolytic enzyme that hydrolyzes BAME plays a role in conferring resistance to this disease.

The data relating the level of TAME activity in splenic homogenates and in the supernatant fraction with resistance to N-tropic FLV disease is not as clean-cut because exceptions were found. Homogenates from susceptible C3H/MAI (a C3H/Bi strain) had much more TAME activity than did homogenates from the other susceptible strains tested (C3H/He, DBA/2, Ha/ICR, AKR, and NYLAR), and homogenates from A and A/He spleens as well as the supernatant fraction from A/He spleens had much lower levels of TAME activity than did the other resistant strains tested (C58, C57L, C57BL/10, C57BL/6, and BALB/c). Possibly the C3H/MAI mice are not susceptible and the A and A/He mice are not resistant to N-tropic FLV disease, because it has been pointed out (3) that reports by various investigators regarding the resistance of the C3H and A strains (as well as of the BALB/c and AKR strains) to FLV disease have been conflicting. These different findings have usually been ascribed to the use of divergent strains of virus or to the use of different substrains of the mice. It would be important to study again the levels of TAME activity in the supernatant fraction of splenic homogenates from several C3H and A strains at the same time that the susceptibility to N-tropic FLV infection is determined.

In some preliminary experiments we found several enzymes that hydrolyze TAME and/or BAME in the supernatant fraction of splenic homogenates from C57BL/6 mice. The supernatant was placed on a Sephadex G-100 column and eluted with buffered saline (0.05 M Tris-HCl, pH 7.2, in 0.15 M NaCl). After the void volume, four peaks of enzymatic activity were found, two hydrolyzing only TAME, one only BAME, and one both TAME and BAME. It may be, therefore, that only one or two of these enzymes is involved with resistance to FLV disease. Possibly this fraction from C3H/MAI mice, if truly susceptible to this infection, lacks or has low levels of the enzyme(s) important for resistance but has high levels of the other enzymes. By the same reasoning, if the A strain is resistant, its splenic supernatant fraction may have adequate levels of the enzyme(s) concerned with resistance but may lack or have low levels of enzymes that are not important for resistance to this disease. These possible explanations for the exceptions found in the levels of TAME activity using C3H and A spleens need to be investigated in order to establish or refute the hypothesis that adequate levels of a proteolytic enzyme(s) are important for resistance to FLV disease.

We have also found that when homogenates from DBA/2 spleens were mixed with homogenates from C57BL/6 spleens, the rates of hydrolyzing either TAME or BAME were much lower than when the C57BL/6 homogenates were tested alone. These results indicate that an inhibitor(s) of TAME and BAME activities is present in DBA/2 splenic homogenates. Further evidence for the presence of an inhibitor(s) was found when splenic homogenates from BDF_1 (C57BL/6 X DBA/2) mice were tested. When the protein content (due entirely to the concentration of splenic homogenate) during enzymatic testing was 6 mg/ml or more, far lower rates of hydrolysis were found than when the protein content was 3 or 4 mg/ml. Decreased activity with increased protein concentration was not found when testing C57BL/6 or BALB/c homogenates, indicating the absence of significant concentrations of inhibitor(s) in these spleens. It is possible, therefore, that an inhibitor(s) of a proteolytic enzyme, present in higher concentration in the spleens of susceptible than of resistant mice, plays a role in blocking resistance to FLV infection, but this remains to be investigated.

Other data presented here also support the hypothesis that a proteolytic enzyme(s) plays a role in resistance to FLV disease. Because injections of Pyran copolymer i.p. increase the resistance of BALB/c mice to N-B-tropic FLV but i.v. injections decrease their resistance (31), healthy BALB/c mice were injected with Pyran, i.p. or i.v. As shown here, i.p. injections increased the concentration in splenic homogenates of an enzyme(s) that hydrolyzes TAME and BAME but i.v. injections decreased the concentration. The highest levels of TAME activity were found in homogenates from mice injected with Pyran i.p. and the lowest levels in homogenates from mice injected with Pyran i.v.

Although the specific activity of the enzyme(s) hydrolyzing TAME did not change significantly when control mice were injected with saline either i.p. or i.v., the specific activity of the enzyme(s) hydrolyzing BAME increased with i.v. injections so that the BAME activity in homogenates from mice injected i.v. with saline was about the same as that found when mice were injected with Pyran i.p. The stress of i.v. saline injections may be responsible for the increased BAME activity, yet despite the stress of i.v. Pyran injections, the BAME and TAME activities fell to very low levels. Because only BAME activity is increased by injections of saline i.v. but both TAME and BAME activities are decreased greatly by injections of Pyran i.v., and both TAME and BAME activities are increased by injections of Pyran i.p. but not by saline i.p., it may be that more than one enzyme is involved in resistance to FLV disease. One of these hydrolyzes BAME primarily or only and its concentration is increased due to a nonspecific stressful situation whereas the other one hydrolyzes TAME and possibly BAME also.

By what mechanism(s) Pyran copolymer produces its effects on the splenic enzyme levels is not known. Larger amounts of Pyran probably accumulate in the spleen when it is injected i.v. than i.p. and if Pyran inhibits the hydrolysis of TAME and BAME by splenic enzymes the decreased levels found after Pyran i.v. might be explained. We, therefore, varied the concentration of Pyran added to in vitro assays of splenic homogenates from untreated BALB/c mice and found that Pyran did not inhibit either the TAME or the BAME activity, so another explanation must be sought.

SUMMARY

Individual frozen spleens from various strains of mice reported to be resistant or susceptible to N-tropic FLV disease were homogenized with cold 0.15 M NaCl and the protein content as well as the ability to hydrolyze TAME and BAME (in 0.25 M Tris-HCl buffer, pH 8.0, at 37°C) were determined. Homogenates, prepared from two or three spleens of each strain, were centrifuged (3,000 rpm, 10 min, 4°C) and the homogenate, supernatant, and washed residue fractions were also tested under the same conditions.

No correlation was found between the level of TAME or BAME activity of the residue fraction and resistance to FLV disease, but the TAME activity of the homogenate and of the supernatant fraction correlated with resistance to this disease, with some exceptions. High levels of TAME activity were found when testing spleens from resistant C58, C57L, C57BL/10, C57BL/6, and BALB/c mice and much lower levels when testing spleens from susceptible DBA/2, Ha/ICR, C3H/He, AKR, and NYLAR mice. However, low levels were found in spleens from resistant A and A/He mice and high levels in spleens from susceptible C3H/MAI mice (a C3H/Bi strain). Several possible explanations for these discrepancies were suggested and remain to be investigated.

Several enzymes that hydrolyze TAME and/or BAME were found in the supernatant fraction of splenic homogenates from C57BL/6 mice. In addition, splenic homogenates from DBA/2 mice contain an inhibitor(s) of the

TAME and BAME activity in C57BL/6 spleens. It was suggested, therefore, that an inhibitor may also be involved in blocking resistance to FLV infection.

Injections of Pyran copolymer i.p. into BALB/c mice increased the levels of enzyme(s) in the spleen that hydrolyze TAME and BAME, whereas i.v. Pyran injections decreased these levels greatly. Because it has been shown by others that injections of Pyran i.p. into BALB/c mice make them more resistant to NB-tropic FLV disease but i.v. Pyran injections make them more susceptible to this disease, it was concluded that proteolytic enzymes, active at slightly alkaline pH, play a role in resistance to FLV disease.

The susceptibility of various strains of mice to HSV-1 infection has been reported by others. We had tested six of these strains and found that resistance to HSV-1 correlates with the level of BAME activity in the supernatant fraction of splenic homogenates, the highest levels found when testing the resistant C57BL/6 mice, slightly lower levels with the moderately resistant BALB/c and C3H/He mice, still lower levels with the moderately susceptible DBA/2 and A/He mice, and the lowest level with the susceptible AKR mice. It was concluded that a proteolytic enzyme in the spleen that hydrolyzes BAME at a slightly alkaline pH is involved with resistance to HSV-1 infection.

ACKNOWLEDGMENTS

This investigation was supported in part by the Colonial Heights Kiwanis Club Cancer Research Fund and by a National Institutes of Health grant, General Research Support Grant, to the Medical College of Virginia, Health Sciences Division, Virginia Commonwealth University. We gratefully acknowledge generous gifts of mice of many strains by Mammalian Genetics and Animal Production Section, National Cancer Institute, Bethesda, Maryland. This work would not have been possible without the excellent technical assistance of Mr. Kenneth I. Perlstein, Dr. Douglas E. Heritage, Ms. Georgia B. Schuller, and Mr. Richard G. May, all of whom we thank.

REFERENCES

1. Deinhardt, F. W., Falk, L. A., and Wolfe, L. G. (1974): Adv. Cancer Res., 19:167.
2. Rapp, F. (1974): Adv. Cancer Res., 19:265.
3. Lilly, F., and Pincus, T. (1973): Adv. Cancer Res., 17:231.
4. Rich, M. A., and Siegler, R. (1967): Ann. Rev. Microbiol., 21:529.
5. Moloney, J. B. (1964): Ann. Rev. Med., 15:383.
6. Salaman, M. H., and Wedderburn, N. (1966): Immunology, 10:445.
7. Millian, S. J., and Schaeffer, M. (1968): Cancer, 21:989.
8. Wedderburn, N., and Salaman, M. H. (1968): Immunology, 15:439.
9. Ceglowski, W. S., and Friedman, H. (1969): Nature, 224:1318.
10. Hirano, S., Ceglowski, W. S., Allen, J. L., and Friedman, H. (1969): J. Natl. Cancer Inst., 43:1337.

11. Chakrabarty, A. K., Friedman, H., and Ceglowski, W. S. (1970): Cancer Res., 30:617.
12. Flickinger, J. T., and Gentile, J. M. (1971): Can. J. Microbiol., 17:481.
13. Dracott, B. N., Wedderburn, N., and Salaman, M. H. (1972): J. Gen. Virol., 14:77.
14. Larson, D. L., and Tomlinson, L. J. (1953): J. Clin. Invest., 32:317.
15. Ultmann, J. E., Fish, W., Osserman, E., and Gellhorn, A. (1959): Ann. Intern. Med., 51:501.
16. Aisenberg, A. C. (1964): N. Engl. J. Med., 270:617.
17. Brody, J. I., and Beizer, L. H. (1966): Ann. Intern. Med., 64:1237.
18. Miller, D. G. (1962): Ann. Intern. Med., 57:703.
19. Heath, R. B., Hamilton, F. G., and Malpas, J. S. (1964): Br. J. Haematol., 10:365.
20. Lilly, F. (1972): J. Natl. Cancer Inst., 49:927.
21. Steeves, R. A. (1975): J. Natl. Cancer Inst., 54:289.
22. Silber, R., Cox, R. P., Haddad, J. R., and Friend, C. (1964): Cancer Res., 24:1892.
23. Bertino, J. R., Gabrio, B. W., and Huennekens, F. M. (1960): Biochem. Biophys. Res. Commun., 3:461.
24. Silber, R., Gabrio, B. W., and Huennekens, F. M. (1963): J. Clin. Invest., 42:1913.
25. Bertino, J. R., Silber, R., Freeman, M., Alenty, A., Albrecht, M., Gabrio, B. W., and Huennekens, F. M. (1963): J. Clin. Invest., 42:1899.
26. Turner, D. M., and Dawson, P. J. (1970): Br. J. Cancer, 24:371.
27. Price, F. W., and Mirand, E. A. (1971): J. Surg. Oncol., 3:17.
28. Li, C. Y., Lung, T. Y., and Crosby, W. H. (1972): J. Histochem. Cytochem., 20:1049.
29. Ende, N., and Auditore, J. V. (1962): Am. J. Clin. Pathol., 38:501.
30. LoSpalluto, J. J., Fehr, K., and Ziff, M. (1970): J. Immunol., 105:886.
31. Schuller, G. B., Morahan, P. S., and Snodgrass, M. (1975): Cancer Res., 35:1915.
32. Lopez, C., and O'Reilly, R. (1975): Fed. Proc., 34:869.
33. Roberts, P. S. (1958): J. Biol. Chem., 232:285.
34. Roberts, P. S. (1960): J. Biol. Chem., 235:2262.

Control of Neoplasia by Modulation of the Immune System, edited by M. A. Chirigos. Raven Press, New York 1977.

CORRELATION OF ABNORMAL PROFILES OF NUCLEOLYTIC
ACTIVITY TO CANCER

W. Jefferson Pendergrast, Jr., Walter P. Drake, Morton Schmukler, and
Michael R. Mardiney, Jr.

Section of Immunology and Cell Biology and Section of Enzymology and
Drug Metabolism, National Institutes of Health, National Cancer
Institute, Baltimore Cancer Research Center,
Baltimore, Maryland 21211

INTRODUCTION

Our laboratory has become increasingly interested in the correlation of abnormal profiles of nucleolytic activity to cancer. This was initially stimulated by our earlier in vitro work characterizing the effectiveness of synthetic polyribonucleotides in amplifying immune responsiveness. In these studies, the double-stranded complex of polyadenylic and polyuridylic acid (poly A:U) was shown to be a powerful modulator of lymphocyte responsiveness within the blastogenesis system (1-4). Having demonstrated that poly A:U amplified cell-associated immunity in vitro, we sought to evaluate its effectiveness in vivo as an immune adjuvant in a host with the genetic propensity to develop cancer. We chose the AKR mouse for study because this strain suffers from vertical transmission of oncogenic virus culminating in clinical leukemia at approximately 6 months of age and death by 10 months of age. With poly A:U, we sought to enhance the known ongoing immune response to both oncogenic virus and tumor and thereby increase longevity (5, 6).

Beginning at 7 weeks of age, AKR mice were divided into groups of 25 and were treated with weekly doses of poly A:U or weekly injections of saline. Table 1 represents the survival rates and median survival times of two groups. Weekly s.c. injection of 1,500 μg of poly A:U significantly increased the long-term survival of these mice. At 38 weeks, when more than 50% of the control animals had died, not a single mouse receiving 1,500 μg of poly A:U had succumbed to the leukemia. Moreover, at week 62, when all control animals had been dead for 3 months, 32% of the 1,600 μg poly A:U group

TABLE 1. Survival of AKR mice treated with poly A:U [a]

| | Age | Percent survivors | | | | | | | | MST |
Group	(weeks)	7	26	38	42	46	55	62	66	(weeks) [b]
Poly A:U (1,500 µg)		100	100	100	84	60	52	32	8	55
Saline		100	100	44	36	4	0	0	0	37

[a] Seven-week-old AKR/J mice were randomized into groups of 25 and treated with the indicated dose of poly A:U or weekly injections of saline.

[b] Median survival time.

were still alive. This synthetic polyribonucleotide proved to be therapeutically effective and demonstrated no obvious toxicity (7).

Our initial bias in the AKR system was that poly A:U was acting as an immune adjuvant. An alternative argument was that poly A:U might have altered nucleic acid metabolism in the AKR mouse. As an approach to test this hypothesis, we evaluated the effect of this synthetic polyribonucleotide on modulating ribonuclease activity in the AKR thymus — the target organ of initial neoplastic transformation. We found that high doses of poly A:U did not alter nuclease activity in the thymus of AKR mice. However, the ribonuclease levels were significantly elevated when compared to a strain of mice with a low incidence of spontaneous tumors — the C57BL/6. The identification of elevated nucleolytic activity in the AKR strain stimulated us to look at other strains of mice with a genetic propensity to develop cancer.

RIBONUCLEASE ACTIVITY IN THE THYMUS AND WHITE BLOOD CELLS OF GENETICALLY CANCER-PRONE MICE

We chose to look at the ribonuclease activity in the thymus and peripheral white blood cells of the AKR and five other strains of genetically cancer-prone mice (8) at 8 weeks of age before anticipated onset of neoplasia (Table 2).

The AKR, SJL, RF, C58, PL, and C3H/He are characterized by a high incidence of spontaneous tumors and were considered "high-incidence" strains for the purpose of this study. Three strains of mice, C57BL/6, Balb/c, and DBA/2, were used as controls because they represented classic examples of strains which have low incidences of spontaneous neoplasia. The NZB strain served as an additional control because although such mice were infected with a similar C-type RNA virus associated with leukemia in the AKR strain,

TABLE 2. Incidence of neoplasm-induced death in various mouse strains

Strain	Sex	Cause of death	Incidence with cancer (%)	Age at onset of Disease (months)	Mean life-span (months)
High incidence					
AKR	F	Leukemia, lymphocytic	91	8	9
SJL	F	Reticulum cell	91	13	13
RF	F	Reticulum cell	62	—	$14\frac{1}{2}$
C58	F	Leukemia, lymphocytic	90	10	$11\frac{1}{2}$
PL	F	Leukemia, lymphocytic	50	—	$14\frac{1}{2}$
		All tumors	71		
C3H/He	F	Mammary carcinoma	60–100	8.8	11
Low incidence					
C57BL/6	F	Few nonspecific tumors	14[a]	Late	22
Balb/c	F	Few nonspecific tumors	29[a]	Late	19
DBA/2	F	Mammary carcinoma	30[a]	14	$23\frac{1}{2}$
NZB	F	Glomerulonephritis Autoimmune	—	4	10–12

[a] Although microscopic foci of neoplastic transformation were present in the indicated percentage of aged animals at autopsy, in general, the tumors did not cause death.

TABLE 3. Thymus and WBC-associated RNase activity

	Thymus RNase		WBC RNase	
Strain	Mean (U/mg)	P Value[a]	Mean (U/ml)	P Value[a]
Low incidence tumor				
C57BL/6	2.8	—	2.4	—
Balb/c	3.5	—	2.5	—
DBA/2	2.3	—	3.0	—
NZB	3.1	—	2.6	—
High incidence tumor				
AKR	15.8	<0.001	5.0	<0.001
SJL	6.7	<0.001	2.9	NS
RF	17.9	<0.001	4.8	<0.001
C58	9.8	<0.001	2.5	NS
PL	5.1	<0.001	5.9	<0.001
C3H/He	3.2	NS	5.2	<0.001

[a] p value was determined by Student's t-test in which the activity for the high-incidence tumor strains was compared to the total combined data of the control strains, C57BL/6, Balb/c, DBA/2, and NZB. NS indicates not significantly different from controls. More detailed data can be found in ref. 8.

NZB mice effectively restrict neoplastic development and die instead of an immune complex nephritis resulting in part from the production of antibodies to this virus.

Statistical analysis of five such experiments is represented in Table 3. The AKR, SJL, RF, C58, and PL strains of mice were found to have statistically significant elevations in thymus-associated ribonuclease activity directed against poly U compared to low-incidence strains.   The four strains, AKR, RF, PL, and C3H/He, had elevated white blood cell-associated ribonuclease activity also directed against poly U. The C3H/He strain, in which 60% may develop a mammary carcinoma, had increased white blood cell-associated ribonuclease activity, although thymus-associated activity was equivalent to "low-incidence" strains. Again, activity of the NZB and low-incidence control mice were significantly lower than high-incidence strains.

This study demonstrated that ribonuclease activity can be a biochemical marker which distinguishes those strains of mice which are prone to develop spontaneous cancer from those strains in which gross cancer is infrequent and rarely the cause of death (8).

TABLE 4. Plasma-associated RNase activity against poly U[a]

Strain	Tumor	Type	Mean activity (μ/mg)	p Value
C57BL/6	—	—	708	—
C57BL/6	C1498	Myeloid leukemia	1,900	(<0.001)
C57BL/6	BW10232	Adenocarcinoma	1,283	(<0.001)
C3H/He	—	—	688	—
C3H/He	6C3HED	Lymphosarcoma	1,816	(<0.001)
C3H/He	C3HBA	Adenocarcinoma	1,200	(<0.001)
Balb/C	—	—	725	—
Balb/C	S180	Sarcoma	1,716	(<0.001)
Balb/C	H-P	Melanoma	1,925	(<0.001)

[a] The nuclease activity against poly U and poly C in the thymus and spleen homogenates and poly C in the plasma can be found in ref. 9. Spleens, thymi, and plasma were harvested around the median survival time and the significance of the difference observed in tumor-bearing animals was determined by Student's t-test.

RIBONUCLEASE ACTIVITY IN THE THYMUS, PLASMA, AND SPLEEN OF TUMOR-BEARING MICE

We also sought to determine if abnormal nuclease activity could be demonstrated in tumor-bearing mice. Six transplantable tumors were evaluated in three different strains of mice (9). The ribonuclease activities against poly U and poly C were measured in the spleen, thymus, and plasma from the tumor-bearing mice and compared to their nontumor-bearing counterparts (Table 4). Elevated activity against polyuridylic acid was observed in the plasma of all tumor-bearing mice. Although not at all inclusive, ribonuclease levels in both the spleen and thymus were generally altered as well (9).

At this point, our studies demonstrating the association between abnormal nucleolytic activity in cancer prone and tumor-bearing mice stimulated us to pursue investigation of serum nuclease levels in cancer patients.

RIBONUCLEASE ACTIVITY IN THE SERUM OF CANCER PATIENTS

The study of serum ribonuclease changes in man and its association with various human disease states, including cancer, is not new (10). Our murine studies however, suggested that we should reexplore this area. We concluded that most elevations of human serum ribonuclease activity occurred in diseases in which the common feature was a compromise in renal function. In addition, we felt, as suggested by Fink, that studies in which yeast RNA was used as a substrate might not give as much information as those in which synthetic substrates were utilized (11). Fink et al. stated that the degradation of native RNA by serum nucleases could represent the sum of various enzymes with one or more specificities. One could then visualize that the elevated activity of one nuclease system could be obscured by the decreased activity of another. Therefore, the overall serum ribonuclease activity directed against yeast RNA could appear within a normal range, even though marked alteration of a specific enzyme level had occurred. The use of a battery of pure synthetic substrates should more readily reflect any changes in specific enzyme activity, thereby providing greater specificity and sensitivity for measuring alterations of nuclease activity.

Outpatients at the Baltimore Cancer Research Center were evaluated for abnormal serum ribonuclease activity (12). In our study, only cancer patients whose BUN and serum creatinines were within normal ranges were studied. The malignancies among the 100 patients studied were acute nonlymphocytic leukemia (ANLL), Hodgkins disease (HD), nonHodgkins lymphoma (NHL), and brain tumors (BT). Control serum samples were obtained from 30 healthy donors of both sexes and of an age range similar to that of the patients. Each sample was evaluated for nucleolytic activity against six synthetic poly-nucleotides: polyadenylic acid (poly A), polyuridylic acid (poly U), polycytidylic acid (poly C), polyguanylic acid (poly G), polyadenylic·polyuridylic acid (poly A:U) and polyguanylic·polycytidylic acid (poly G:C).

The mean nuclease activity for patients in the four disease categories is represented in Table 5. The predominant serum activity was that directed against poly C, poly U, and poly A:U. The mean ribonuclease activity was significantly elevated in all four disease categories when poly C or poly U were used as substrates. When poly A:U was used as the substrate, the mean ribonuclease levels were elevated in ANLL, HD, and NHL, but not with BT.

However, evaluation of data by this type of averaging tends to obscure the more important question of what patients were identified as abnormal by this assay. Table 6 answers this question. This table represents the percent of patients that had abnormal nuclease activity against one or more substrates for each disease category. Abnormally elevated activity against one substrate did not necessarily indicate elevated activity against all. For example, 8 of 15 patients with ANLL exhibited elevated activity against poly U, 9 with poly C, and 7 with poly A:U. However, when the data for all three substrates are considered together, 10 or 67% of the ANLL patients exhibited abnormal nuclease activity against at least one substrate. Similarly, 73% of HD, 67% of NHL, and 46% of BT patients had abnormal ribonuclease activity against at least one substrate.

TABLE 5. Comparison of mean RNase activity for cancer patients

Group	Number	Assay against poly U		Assay against poly C		Assay against poly A:U	
		Mean activity (μ/ml)	$p^{\underline{a}}$	Mean activity (μ/ml)	$p^{\underline{a}}$	Mean activity (μ/ml)	$p^{\underline{a}}$
Normal	30	53.3	—	933	—	6.4	—
ANLL	15	72.9	<0.001	1,564	<0.001	10.0	<0.001
HD	22	67.6	<0.01	1,458	<0.001	9.3	<0.001
NHL	27	68.9	<0.01	1,487	<0.001	7.8	<0.01
BT	26	68.5	<0.01	1,257	<0.005	5.9	not significant

$^{\underline{a}}$ p value determined by Student's t-test.

TABLE 6. Number of patients with elevated nuclease activity as measured against either poly U, poly C, or poly A:U

Malignancy	Total No.	No. with abnormal SRNase			Total no. abnormal	Percent elevated[a]
		Poly U	Poly C	Poly A:U		
ANLL	15	8	9	7	10	67
HD	22	8	13	8	16	73
NHL	27	5	18	6	18	67
BT	26	8	10	2	12	46

[a] Percent patients with elevated activity directed against any of the three substrates tested.

The mean nuclease activity for patients with ANLL, HD, and NHL was statistically elevated over that observed for healthy normal controls. There was no absolute correlation between elevated nuclease activity and patient relapse or remission status.

In conclusion, these studies are strong evidence that the level and profile of nucleolytic activity is an important biochemical marker for either the propensity to develop cancer or the presence of cancer. We are actively pursuing this relationship.

SUMMARY

There appears to be a definite association between abnormal nucleolytic activity and cancer. The potential link between elevated nuclease levels and the preneoplastic state was suggested when six strains of mice genetically predisposed to develop cancer were studied. In all six strains, there was elevated ribonuclease activity before the onset of clinically detectable disease (8). We examined RNase activity in six transplantable murine tumors, and found that ribonuclease levels were significantly elevated in all tumor bearing mice (9). The animal studies stimulated us to study serum ribonuclease levels in cancer patients. We found that the mean serum ribonuclease levels for patients with ANLL, HD, NHL, and BT were significantly elevated over that observed for healthy controls (12).

REFERENCES

1. Chess, L., Levy, C. C., Schmukler, M., and Mardiney, M. R., Jr. (1972): Amplification of immunologically induced lymphocyte proliferation by double stranded synthetic polynucleotides. In: Proceedings of the Seventh Leukocyte Culture Conference, edited by F. Daguillard, pp. 105-118. Academic Press, London, New York.

2. Chess, L., Levy, C. C., Schmukler, M., Smith, K., and Mardiney, M. R., Jr. (1974): The effect of synthetic polynucleotides on immunologically induced tritiated thymidine incorporation. Transplantation, 14:748-755.

3. Graziano, K. D., Levy, C. C., Schmukler, M., and Mardiney, M. R., Jr. (1974): Parameters for effective use of synthetic double stranded polynucleotides in the amplification of immunologically induced lymphocyte tritiated thymidine incorporation. Cell. Immunol., 11:47-56.

4. Mardiney, M. R., Jr., Chess, L., Levy, C. C., Schmukler, M., and Smith, K. (1974): Use of double stranded synthetic polynucleotides in amplifying immunologically induced lymphocyte proliferation. In: Recent Results in Cancer Research, edited by G. Mathe and R. Weiner, Vol. 47, pp. 330-337. Springer-Verlag, Paris.

5. Oldstone, M. B., Aoki, T., and Dixon, F. J. (1972): The antibody response of mice to murine leukemia virus in spontaneous infection: Absence of classical immunological tolerance. Proc. Natl. Acad. Sci. (U.S.A.), 69:134-138.

6. Markham, R. V., Jr., Sutherland, J. C., Cimino, E. F., Drake, W. P., and Mardiney, M. R., Jr. (1972): Immune complexes localized in the renal glomeruli of AKR mice: The presence of MuLV gs-1 and C-type RNA tumor virus gs-3 determinants. Eur. J. Clin. Biol. Res., 17:11-15.

7. Drake, W. P., Cimino, E. F., Mardiney, M. R., Jr., and Sutherland, J. C. (1974): Prophylactic therapy of spontaneous leukemia in AKR mice by polyadenylic-polyuridylic acid. J. Natl. Cancer Inst., 52:941-944.

8. Drake, W. P., Pokorney, D. R., Chipman, S., Levy, C. C., and Mardiney, M. R., Jr. (1975): Elevated ribonuclease activity in the thymus and white blood cells of genetically cancer prone mice. J. Exp. Med., 141:918-923.

9. Drake, W. P., Kopyta, L. P., Levy, C. C., and Mardiney, M. R., Jr. (1975): Alterations in ribonuclease activity in the plasma, spleen and thymus of tumor-bearing mice. Cancer Res., 35:322-324.

10. Hisada, T. (1969): Changes in ribonuclease activity in serum and urine during the course of surgical treatment for digestive organ cancer and other diseases. Iryo, 23:613-625.

11. Fink, K., Adams, W. S., and Skoog, W. A. (1971): Serum ribonuclease in multiple myeloma. Am. J. Med., 50:450-457.

12. Drake, W. P., Schmukler, M., Pendergrast, W. J., Jr., Davis, A. S., Lichtenfeld, J. L., and Mardiney, M. R., Jr. (1975): Abnormal profile of human nucleolytic activity as a test for cancer. J. Natl. Cancer Inst., 55:1055-1059.

*Control of Neoplasia by Modulation
of the Immune System,* edited by
M. A. Chirigos. Raven Press, New
York   1977.

IMMUNOTHERAPEUTIC EFFICACY OF NEURAMINIDASE-TREATED ALLOGENEIC MYELOBLASTS IN PATIENTS WITH ACUTE MYELOCYTIC LEUKEMIA

*,[†] J. George Bekesi, *,[†]James F. Holland, **Raphael Fleminger,
[‡] Jerome Yates, and **Edward S. Henderson

*Department of Neoplastic Diseases, Mount Sinai School of Medicine and
Hospital of the City University of New York, New York, New York
10029, and
**Roswell Park Memorial Institute, New York State Department of Health,
Buffalo, New York 14203

INTRODUCTION

Neuraminidase of <u>Vibrio cholerae</u> origin has been used successfully in increasing the immunogenicity of a variety of spontaneous and experimental tumors (1-8). The immunoprotection evoked by the stimulation from the neuraminidase-treated tumor cells was found to be specific for the particular tumor and can be transferred by either sera or splenic lymphocytes into unimmunized syngeneic mice (4, 7, 8-15).

Cytoreductive chemotherapy, known to be effective in the treatment of children with acute lymphocytic leukemia, has been demonstrated to be effective in murine leukemia virus (MuLV)-induced spontaneous leukemia in AKR mice to a certain degree, but cure does not occur (12-14, 16-18). When such chemotherapy was followed by neuraminidase-treated leukemic cells of

[†] Formerly at Roswell Park Memorial Institute, New York State Department of Health, Buffalo, New York 14203.

[‡] Present address: Department of Medicine, University of Vermont, Burlington, Vermont 05401.

splenic or thymic origin as an immunogenic stimulant, a significant percentage (>35%) of leukemic AKR mice were apparently cured of the disease, only to relapse at a remote time from a presumptive new leukemogenic event (12-14, 19).

It has also been demonstrated that neuraminidase treated E_2G leukemic cells which, like the AKR leukemia, are Gross virus-induced, but are completely different at the H_2 genetic locus from AKR mice, were as effective as the syngeneic AKR leukemic cells in prolonging the survival of leukemic AKR mice (13,14,19). These data indicated the existence of a cross-reacting common viral membrane antigen, and suggested that if similar etiology existed for human acute leukemia it would not be essential to use autologous leukemia cells for immunization. Indeed, the data provided the basis for using neuraminidase-treated allogeneic myeloblasts in human immunotherapeutic investigation.

This chapter demonstrates the therapeutic advantage of combining neuraminidase-treated allogeneic myeloblasts with a highly effective remission inducing and sustaining chemotherapeutic protocol in the treatment of acute myelocytic leukemia compared to the use of chemotherapy alone.

MATERIALS AND METHODS

Chemotherapy

The chemoimmunotherapy program has been predicated on the maximal chemotherapeutic reduction of leukemic body burden. This was achieved by induction therapy with a regimen of cytosine arabinoside continuously administered intravenously for 7 days at 100 mg/m²/day and daunorubicin at a dose of 45 mg/m² by direct injection on days 1, 2, and 3 as described by Yates et al. (20). All patients were 60 years of age or less. These drugs led to remission in approximately 70% of the patients. All received cyclical maintenance chemotherapy every 4 weeks. This consisted of 5-day courses of injections of Ara-C 100 mg/m² every 12 hr in addition to 6-thioguanine, cyclophosphamide, CCNU, or daunorubicin sequentially with each course in a 4-month cycle.

Immunotherapy with Neuraminidase-Treated Allogeneic Myeloblasts

Collection

Patients became eligible for collection of myeloblasts if they satisfied the following criteria: no previous chemotherapy, total WBC higher than 25,000 per μl, greater than 70% myeloblasts in the peripheral blood, absence of clinical sepsis, no active major bleeding, no antibiotics being administered, and voluntary consent. All bloods were shown before use to contain no detectable hepatitis-associated antigen. Leukopheresis on an AMINCO cell separator commenced immediately upon satisfying the criteria to avoid any undue delay in the treatment of leukemic patients. Of the 14 patients leuko-phoresed, none showed important side effects from the procedure which was performed in 1 to 4 hr.

The myeloblasts were collected in transfer bags containing acid citrate-dextrose solution. After cessation of the leukophoresis, the myeloblasts were separated from contaminating red blood cells by sedimentation at 37°C for 1 to 2 hr in the presence of one volume of special freezing media containing 10 units of heparin per milliliter of buffy coat. Because of their cryosensitivity, granulocytes were removed by passage through glass beads or nylon wool if they constituted greater than 3% of the cell population. After sedimentation, the myeloblasts were mixed with special freezing media containing 15 to 20% autologous or AB plasma and 10% dimethylsufoxide to yield a final cell concentration of 4 to 6 X 10^7 cells/ml. Myeloblasts were frozen in transfer bags by programmed freezing (Union Carbide Biological Freezer) at a tem-perature drop of 0.5 to 1°C/min until -38°C was reached, and then rapidly to -85°C. The frozen cells were immediately stored in the vapor phase of liquid nitrogen.

Treatment of Myeloblasts with Neuraminidase

Myeloblasts were rapidly thawed prior to immunization in a 37° C water bath and washed three times with mixed salt and glucose media at 4° C. The best purification and recovery of myeloblasts was achieved on an albumin-sucrose gradient. Myeloblasts retrieved from liquid nitrogen storage were layered over a 22% human albumin gradient supported by 45% sucrose (1:3) to separate the viable from nonviable blast cells. Yields ranged between 30 to 95% with a 90 to 98% viability of the supernatant myeloblasts. After pur-ification, the blast cells were washed at 4°C three times with salt-glucose medium. They were then incubated with vibrio cholerae neuraminidase. The incubation mixture contained 25 units of enzyme per 5 X 10^7 cells/ml in sodium acetate buffer at pH 5.6 for 50 min at 37°C. The neuraminidase used for this study has been purified 2,500 to 3,000-fold and was free of other enzymes and bacterial endotoxins. After incubation the neuraminidase was removed from the surface of the leukemic cells by sodium EDTA to chelate calcium ions, essential for the attachment of neuraminidase to the receptor sites. The cells were then washed three times with the mixed salt and glucose media. After the last centrifugation the cells were suspended in mixed salt and glucose media and used as immunogen within 30 min.

Immunization with Neuraminidase-Treated Myeloblasts

Immunization with neuraminidase-treated allogeneic myeloblasts was performed by intradermal injections in approximately 48 sites. In order to obtain maximum exposure to the immunogen, sites were widely spread in the supraclavicular, infraclavicular, arm, forearm, parasternal, lateral, thoracic, suprainguinal, and femoral regions draining into several node bearing areas (Fig. 1).

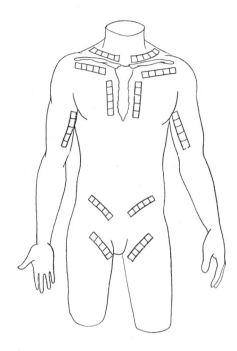

FIG. 1. Immunization diagram for neuraminidase-treated allogeneic myeloblasts.

A dose-dependent cellular titration was initially performed with each immunization with 0.5, 1.5, 2.5 X 10^8, and 0 cells. The total immunization load was about 10^{10} cells from a single donor. In addition, as a control injection, heat-denatured neuraminidase (500 units/site), X-irradiated myeloblasts, and the supernatant of the incubation fluid were also injected in some patients. Delayed hypersensitivity response to neuraminidase-treated myeloblasts was measured at 48 hr, and the induration in millimeters was recorded.

Immunological Assessment of Patients

<u>Skin testing with recall antigens.</u> The immunocompetence of patients in the chemo- and chemoimmunotherapy arms of the protocol was measured by the delayed cutaneous hypersensitivity response to five recall antigens: PPD (Parke Davis and Co.); dermatophytin 0 and candida (Hollister-Stier Laboratories); streptokinase-streptodornase (Lederle Laboratories); and mumps (Eli Lilly Co.). All recall antigens were applied in the volar forearm by intradermal inoculation in a volume of 0.1 ml through a 27-gauge needle. Delayed hypersensitivity response to antigens was read at 48 hr in the same manner as for neuraminidase-treated myeloblasts. Skin tests were considered clinically positive if the diameter of the induration was 5 mm or greater. Skin tests were applied 48 hr before the first immunotherapy with the neuraminidase-treated allogeneic myeloblasts.

Lymphocyte Blastogenesis

T- and B-lymphocyte function of peripheral blood lymphocytes was determined by monitoring the in vitro lymphocyte blastogenesis induced by selected T- and B-cell mitogens: phytohemagglutinin (PHA) for T-cells, and pokeweed mitogen (PWM). Peripheral venous blood was drawn in preservative-free heparin, and the lymphocytes were purified by the Ficoll-Hypaque sedimentation technique. After washing three times with RPMI 1640 medium, 100,000 viable peripheral lymphocytes were cultured in each of five replicate wells of Falcon microplates using RPMI 1640 medium supplemented with 20% heat-inactivated human AB sera.

The cells were cultured with $0.15\,\mu g$ per well of high-purity PHA (Burroughs Wellcome Co.) or with $30\,\mu g$ per well of PWM (Grand Island Biological Co.). Control cultures which were incubated without mitogens were also prepared in five replicate wells. The cultures were incubated at $37^\circ C$ in a humidified atmosphere containing 5% CO_2 in air. Lymphocyte blastogenesis was determined by measuring the level of DNA biosynthesis upon addition of $1\,\mu Ci$ of ^3H-TdR to each well (New England Nuclear Co.) 18 hr prior to termination of the culture. After 66 or 90 hr, the cells were harvested with a Mash II automatic harvester and the amount of ^3H-TdR incorporation was determined in a Packard liquid scintillation spectrometer.

The E-binding rosette technique (21) was used for the quantification of the T-lymphocyte population before and during immunotherapy.

Quantification of Total and Neuraminidase-Susceptible Sialic Acid

For estimation of total cellular sialic acid, normal human lymphocytes, acute lymphocytic, and acute myelocytic leukemic cells were purified on human serum albumin, and then washed three times with 50 volumes of physiological saline containing 0.005 M EDTA. Normal and leukemic cells were homogenized in 9 volumes of 95% ethanol for 2 min in a Virtis homogenizer. After centrifugation at 2,000 X g for 20 min, the residue was resuspended in 30 ml of acetone at room temperature for 60 min and then recentrifuged as above. This procedure was repeated twice. The acetone-defatted and air-dried sample was suspended in 5 to 10 ml of 0.1 N H_2SO_4 and hydrolyzed for 1 hr at $80^\circ C$. The procedure was repeated twice. After centrifugation, the supernatants were pooled, neutralized, and the clear supernatant was quantitatively transferred to a Dowex 2 X 8 (acetate) resin column. After column purification, total and neuraminidase-susceptible sialic acid was determined as previously described, using the thiobarbituric acid method (23).

Biostatistics

Analysis of the remission duration and survival of patients in the chemotherapy and chemoimmunotherapy groups was made by the generalized Kruskal Wallis test proposed by Breslow (22).

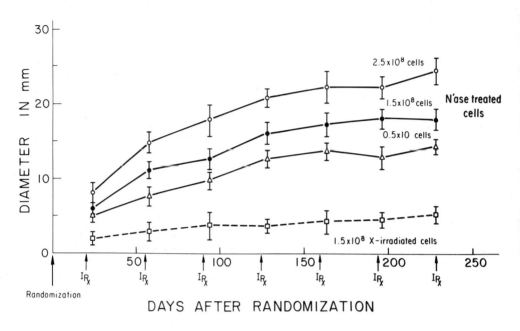

FIG. 2. Delayed hypersensitivity response from intradermal immunization with neuraminidase-treated allogeneic myeloblasts. Induration was measured 48 hr after immunization and recorded as $\pm$ SD of mean induration.

RESULTS

Normal and tumor cells used in this study have the following protein-bound N-acetylneuraminic acid content: acute myelocytic leukemia 0.36 μmoles, acute lymphocytic leukemic 0.23 μmoles, and normal human lymphocytes 0.33 μmoles per 10^9 cells.

Analysis of the major subcellular fractions of human myeloblasts showed the following distribution of protein-bound sialic acid: plasma membrane 76%, microsome (smooth and rough endoplasmic reticulum) 11%, mitochondria 5%, and nuclear fraction 8%. These data clearly indicate that the major portion of protein-bound sialic acid is localized on the surface membrane of leukemic myeloblasts.

Effect of Neuraminidase-Treated Allogeneic Myeloblasts on the Remission
Duration of Previously Treated AML Patients: A Phase I
Immunotherapy Study

A small group of patients with acute myelocytic leukemia who had relapsed at least once from previous antileukemic therapy were successfully reinduced by a regimen of cytosine arabinoside continuously administered intravenously for 7 days at 100 mg/m^2 and daunorubicin at a dose of 45 mg/m^2 by direct injection on days 1, 2, and 3. After attaining complete remission, 6 patients received cyclical sustaining chemotherapy plus sham immunization using only physiological saline. The remaining 7 patients were immunized with neuraminidase-treated myeloblasts at 48 sites monthly.

Figure 2 shows that the response to neuraminidase-treated myeloblasts at 48 hr as measured by the indurations was directly proportional to the number of myeloblasts injected per site. Furthermore, an increase in response occurred with continued immunization. Immunotherapy with treated myeloblasts produced no local lesions other than delayed-type hypersensitivity reactions, and none of the patients developed chills, fever, ulcerations, or adenopathy. No reaction was apparent at the site of injection of physiological saline, heat-denatured neuraminidase, or from the supernatant of the cell incubation media. Although the number of patients entered in this immunotherapeutic study was not large, the data presented in Fig. 3 clearly show the therapeutic advantage of immunotherapy using neuraminidase-treated myeloblasts even in previously treated AML patients. Remission durations were twice as long as that of patients in the control group.

Immunological status of patients in both groups was measured by skin testing with a battery of five recall antigens. Patients in the chemotherapy regimen showed no quantitative or qualitative change to recall antigens after randomization. There was, however, a considerable improvement in the response of patients receiving immunotherapy as measured by their increase in positive response to three recall antigens, mumps, candida, and varidase, and in one subject to PPD (Fig. 4).

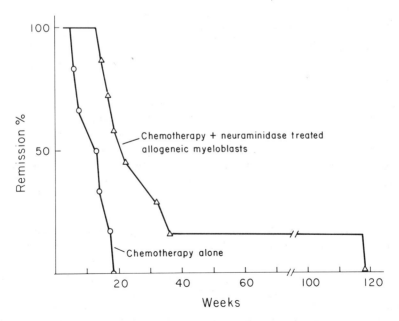

FIG. 3. Remission duration of previously treated AML patients immunized with neuraminidase-treated allogeneic myeloblasts.

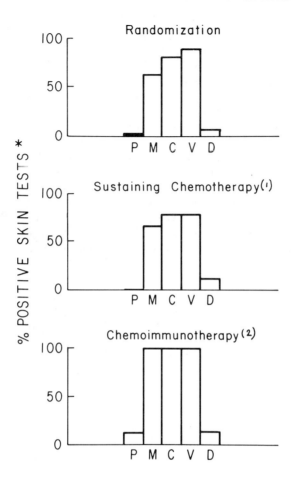

FIG. 4. Positive delayed hypersensitivity response to recall antigens in previously treated AML patients immunized with neuraminidase-treated allogeneic myeloblasts. PPD, P; mumps, M; candida, C; varidase, V; and dermatophytin, D. *Skin test diameter at 48 hr > 5 mm. (1) Skin test was done after the second course of sustaining chemotherapy. (2) Skin test was done after the second course of sustaining chemoimmunotherapy.

Immunotherapy with Neuraminidase-Treated Allogeneic Myeloblasts in Patients with Previously Untreated Acute Myelocytic Leukemia

Based on the improved remission duration attained with active immunotherapy in previously treated AML patients, a controlled clinical study was initiated.

Seventeen patients previously untreated with AML were induced into complete remission by cytosine arabinoside and daunorubicin. Beginning on day 8 after the first sustaining course of chemotherapy, and on day 15 of each

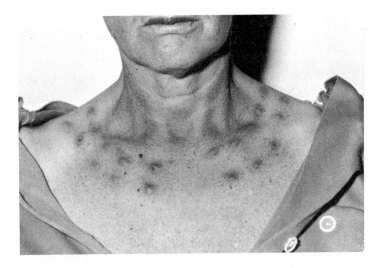

FIG. 5. Hypersensitivity reaction to neuraminidase-treated myeloblasts at 48 hr.

cycle thereafter, patients were randomly allocated to receive either chemotherapy alone, or chemotherapy plus neuraminidase-treated myeloblasts. A volume of 0.2 ml containing 2 to 2.5 X 10^8 neuraminidase-treated myeloblasts was given intradermally in at least 48 loci as indicated on the immunization diagram (Fig. 1). Strong delayed cutaneous hypersensitivity reaction to neuraminidase-treated myeloblasts was observed at each immunization site measuring 8 to 30 mm in diameter. The biopsies of the cutaneous reactions show extensive immunoblastic infiltration (Fig. 5). No hypersensitivity reaction was noted at the site of heat-denatured neuraminidase, or supernatant of the incubation media. The data in Fig. 6 compare patients receiving chemotherapy alone to those treated with immunotherapy in addition. The duration of remission among patients treated with chemoimmunotherapy is significantly longer (p = 0.0008). Six of 9 patients in the immunotherapy group are still in remission at 78 to 132 weeks as compared to 1 of 8 patients in the control group. Similarly, immunotherapy had a direct impact on the survival of AML patients (Fig. 7). Seven of 8 patients who were maintained on chemotherapy alone died within 24 months after clinical diagnosis of their disease compared with the death of 3 of 9 chemoimmunotherapy patients.

Immunological Status of AML Patients in the Chemoimmunotherapy Protocol

The immunocompetence of patients in this study was measured by the cutaneous hypersensitivity response to recall antigens. The initial skin test and sensitization was accomplished at the time of randomization of patients into the protocol. The results presented in Table 1 represent three different periods when skin tests were done. Of the patients tested at randomization, 15 of 17 gave positive delayed hypersensitivity response to at least two recall

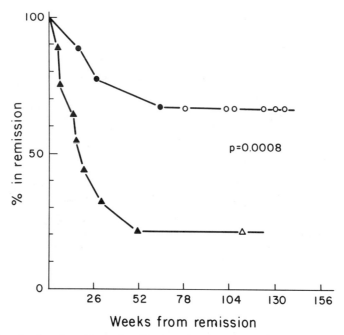

FIG. 6. Remission duration of patients with acute myelocytic leukemia immunized with neuraminidase-treated allogeneic myeloblasts. Patients treated with sustaining chemotherapy alone —▲—▲—; patients who received sustaining chemotherapy plus neuraminidase-treated myeloblasts —●—●—; open symbols indicate patients still in remission.

antigens. Patients in the chemotherapy regimen showed no qualitative nor quantitative change in their response to recall antigens after randomization, whereas both qualitative and quantitative increase in response to recall antigens was noted among chemoimmunotherapy patients.

Table 2 summarizes the percentage and absolute number of T-lymphocytes as determined at 4°C and 37°C by the E-binding rosette technique. Patients in the chemotherapy regimen at the time of randomization, as well as 3 months later, have significantly lower percentage and absolute number of T-lymphocytes at both temperatures compared to normal subjects. Patients who received chemoimmunotherapy show an increased level of T-lymphocytes after 3 months of chemoimmunotherapy, both in percentage and in absolute number.

Table 3 summarizes the lymphoblastogenesis of normal and remission lymphocytes by PHA and pokeweed mitogens (PWM). Maximum stimulation occurred at 0.15 mg/well for PHA and 30 µg/well for PWM for normal as well as remission lymphocytes. Both mitogens showed depressed stimulation of lymphocytes obtained at the time of randomization compared to normal subjects, and no improvement in patients who had received three courses of chemotherapy alone. Lymphocytes showed progressively higher stimulation of both mitogens after the third and sixth courses of chemoimmunotherapy (p = 0.0001 for both mitogens).

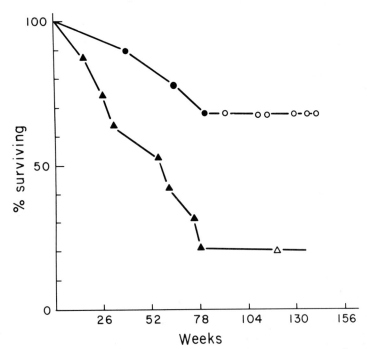

FIG. 7. Improved survival duration of patients with acute myelocytic leukemia immunized with neuraminidase-treated allogeneic myeloblasts. Patients treated with sustaining chemotherapy alone —▲—▲—; patients treated with sustaining chemotherapy plus neuraminidase-treated myeloblasts —●—●—; open symbols indicate patients still in remission.

TABLE 1. Positive delayed hypersensitivity response to recall antigens in AML patients immunized with neuraminidase-treated allogeneic myeloblasts

Antigens	Positive skin tests/total number of skin tests [a]					
	Sustaining therapy			Immunotherapy		
	At induction	At 3rd course	At 6th course	At induction	At 3rd course	At 6th course
PPD	0/8	0/6	0/3	0/9	1/9	1/8
Mumps	5/8	5/6	2/3	6/9	8/9	8/8
Candida	5/8	4/6	2/3	6/9	8/9	8/8
Varidase	6/8	4/6	3/3	6/9	9/9	8/8
Dermatophytin	1/8	1/6	0/3	1/9	1/9	2/8
No. of patients tested still in remission	8	6	3	9	9	8

[a] Skin test diameter at 48 hr > 5 mm.

TABLE 2. T-Lymphocyte subpopulation in AML patients immunized with neuraminidase-treated allogeneic myeloblasts

Status	At induction		After three courses			
	Percent T-cells[a]	Absolute T-lymphocytes	Percent T-cells[a]	p[b]	Absolute T-lymphocytes	p[b]
At 37°C						
Normal subjects, N = 35	32.5 ± 1.4[c]	868 ± 71	—	—	—	—
Chemotherapy	19.3 ± 1.2	187 ± 22	21.2 ± 1.8	0.75	213 ± 26	0.45
Chemoimmunotherapy	20.8 ± 1.3	198 ± 27	29.3 ± 2.0	0.004	401 ± 38	0.002
At 4°C						
Normal subjects, N = 35	74.4 ± 1.2[c]	1,986 ± 251	—	—	—	—
Chemotherapy	41.9 ± 2.2	402 ± 35	55.6 ± 2.7	0.02	456 ± 26	0.06
Chemoimmunotherapy	40.3 ± 1.9	338 ± 54	67.5 ± 3.9	0.001	798 ± 39	0.001

[a] Determined by the E-binding rosette technique.

[b] Probability that occurred by chance.

[c] Mean ± SE.

TABLE 3. PHA- and PWM-induced lymphoblastogenesis of peripheral lymphocytes from AML patients immunized with neuraminidase-treated allogeneic myeloblasts

Status	Normal subjects		Chemotherapy			Chemoimmunotherapy		
	cpm	SI	cpm	SI	p[b]	cpm	SI	p[b]
PHA[a]								
At induction	83,856 ± 7,237[c]	141	26,086 ± 3,332	44	—	31,715 ± 4,264	53	—
After 3rd course	83,856 ± 7,237	141	30,289 ± 3,877	51	0.7	49,244 ± 9,322	83	0.008
After 6th course	83,856 ± 7,237	141	35,073 ± 5,988	56	0.6	65,185 ± 8,265	110	0.001
PWM[d]								
At induction	79,200 ± 6,369[c]	91	20,016 ± 3,468	23	—	22,189 ± 2,976	25	—
After 3rd course	79,200 ± 6,369	91	21,687 ± 2,342	27	0.9	40,523 ± 6,529	47	0.003
After 6th course	79,200 ± 6,369	91	29,139 ± 3,866	34	0.7	54,950 ± 9,622	67	0.001

[a] Maximum stimulation 0.15 μg/well.

[b] Significance between at induction vs. during chemo- or chemoimmunotherapy of AML patients.

[c] Mean ± SE.

[d] Maximum stimulation 30 μg/well.

DISCUSSION

Varying degrees of success have been demonstrated by immunization of experimental animals with X-irradiated syngeneic tumor cells with or without BCG (13, 24-31). Similarly, improved remission duration and survival of leukemic patients have been reported after immunization with X-irradiated ALL or AML blast cells with or without BCG (32-41). Based on data obtained from immunoprophylaxis and chemoimmunotherapeutic experiments in mice with transplantable and spontaneous tumors (1-15, 19), we have tested the proposition that neuraminidase-treated myeloblasts could be an effective immunogen in the treatment of patients with acute myelocytic leukemia.

Initially, after successful chemotherapeutic remission induction, we attempted to immunize patients with neuraminidase-treated autologous myeloblasts. This practice turned out to be impractical because it became apparent that the number of patients who could enter this clinical trial were limited due to: (a) low peripheral blood cell counts; (b) those with high leukocyte counts who would not consent to participate in the clinical investigation; and (3) those too ill to be subjected to leukopheresis.

Our experimental data (13, 14, 19) as well as observations by others (42-54) indicate the presence of a common leukemia-associated and viral membrane antigen on leukemic cells and on remission lymphocytes. The assumption for a cross-reacting antigen in leukemia is supported by the findings that solid tumors of the same histological type have common tumor-specific antigens (52). Furthermore, we have demonstrated that neuraminidase-treated allogeneic E_2G leukemia cells carrying membrane antigens from the Gross leukemia virus (MuLV) were as efficacious in maintaining leukemic AKR mice in remission as were syngeneic AKR leukemic cells (13, 14, 19). Based on these observations, we initiated the use of neuraminidase-treated allogeneic myeloblasts as immunogen in patients with acute myelocytic leukemia.

Thirteen previously treated and 17 untreated patients with acute myelocytic leukemia were entered into this study. The patients were first induced into complete remission by intensive chemotherapy. Of the 13 previously treated patients, 6 received sustaining chemotherapy, and the remaining 7 patients were immunized with neuraminidase-treated allogeneic myeloblasts. The 17 previously untreated patients were allocated at random to receive no immunotherapy or immunotherapy with neuraminidase-treated myeloblasts.

Improved remission duration, as a direct result of immunotherapy with neuraminidase-treated myeloblasts, was demonstrated for the previously treated AML patients in the phase I clinical study. This observation was particularly significant because these patients were subjected, in addition to the cyclic courses of sustaining chemotherapy, to at least two intensive induction courses. Thus, their immunological responsiveness was more compromised than that of the previously untreated AML patients.

In the controlled clinical study, highly significant beneficial therapeutic effects of immunotherapy with neuraminidase-treated myeloblasts was demonstrated in previously untreated AML patients. Of the control patients receiving sustaining chemotherapy alone, the median remission duration was about 5.5 months. Six of 9 patients receiving chemoimmunotherapy are still in remission at 16 to 36 months. Similarly, chemoimmunotherapy has a direct impact on the survival of leukemic patients. Seven of 8 patients on chemotherapy alone have died, as compared to the death of only 3 of 9 patients in the immunotherapy protocol. These observations establish the effectiveness of immunotherapy with neuraminidase-treated allogeneic myeloblasts for the treatment of patients with acute myelocytic leukemia.

Immunocompetence of leukemic patients in the chemoimmunotherapy study was monitored by delayed-type hypersensitivity responses to five recall antigens. Of the patients tested before randomization, 25 of 30 gave positive response to at least two recall antigens; thus they were considered to be immunologically competent. Patients receiving sustaining chemotherapy showed no quantitative or qualitative change in their reactivity to recall antigens. There was, however, a considerable improvement in the response of patients in the immunotherapy regimen to mumps, candida, and varidase.

Direct impact of immunotherapy with neuraminidase-treated myeloblasts on the percentage and absolute T-lymphocytes was noted after the third course of chemoimmunotherapy. Compared to the values obtained at the time of randomization, the difference is statistically significant ($p = 0.004$ at $37^\circ C$ and $p = 0.001$ at $4^\circ C$).

Similarly, increased lymphocyte response to PHA and PW mitogens was noted among patients receiving immunotherapy. After the third course of immunization, both mitogens showed significantly higher stimulation for patients who received immunotherapy during remission as compared to their own response at the time of induction or to the patients who received chemotherapy alone.

It can be concluded from the in vivo and in vitro tests that AML patients immunized with neuraminidase-treated myeloblasts have a higher level of immunocompetence than control patients receiving chemotherapy alone. These findings correlate well with the improved remission duration and survival as a result of the immunotherapy.

SUMMARY

A successful chemoimmunotherapy trial was conducted in patients with acute myelocytic leukemia using neuraminidase-treated allogeneic myeloblasts as immunogen. Thirteen previously treated and 17 untreated patients with AML were allocated in two groups following successful remission induction using cytosine arabinoside and daunorubicin. All received cyclical maintenance chemotherapy. Patients designated to receive immunotherapy were injected intradermally in approximately 48 sites close to different lymph node drainage areas every 28 days with 5 to 10 X 10^9 neuraminidase-treated myeloblasts. Induration diameters at 48 hr after immunization usually exceeded 15 mm. Biopsies of cutaneous reactions have shown immunoblastic infiltration. Of the 13 patients who received previous antileukemic therapy, 7 immunized patients had more than twice the remission duration of the 6 controls. For 8 of 17 previously untreated AML patients the median remission duration on chemotherapy alone was 22 weeks, whereas those receiving chemoimmunotherapy have not yet reached the median at 78 weeks. Difference between the two groups is highly significant, p = 0.0008. Immunized patients showed significantly improved immunocompetence as compared to the controls treated with chemotherapy alone. The in vitro findings are in good agreement with and might be causally related to the extended remission duration and survival.

ACKNOWLEDGMENTS

This work was supported in part by grant and contracts Ca-1-5936-02, CA-5834, NCI Special Cancer Virus Program No. 1-CB-43879, and NCI Immunotherapy Program No. 1-CP-43225.

We express our appreciation to the Behring Institute-Behringwerke Ag. Marburg, West Germany, for supplying the highly purified neuraminidase for part of this study.

We thank Barbara Phelps and Robert Schechter for excellent technical assistance and Ronnie Schneider for preparation of this manuscript.

REFERENCES

1. Sanford, B. H. (1967): An alteration in tumor histocompatibility induced by neuraminidase. Transplantation, 5:1273-1279.
2. Sanford, B. H., and Codington, J. F. (1971): Further studies on the effect of neuraminidase on tumor cell transplantability. Tissue Antigens, 1:153-161.
3. Currie, G. A., and Bagshawe, K. D. (1968): The role of sialic acid in antigenic expression: Further studies of the Landschutz ascites tumor. Br. J. Cancer, 22:843-853.
4. Bekesi, J. G., St-Arneault, G., and Holland, J. F. (1971): Increase of leukemia L1210 immunogenicity by Vibrio cholerae neuraminidase treatment. Cancer Res., 31:2130-2132.
5. Bagshawe, K. D., and Currie, G. A. (1968): Immunogenicity of L1210 murine leukemia cells after treatment with neuraminidase. Nature, 218:1254-1255.
6. Simmons, R. L., Rios, A., and Ray, P. K. (1971): Effect of neuraminidase on the growth of a 2-methyl-cholanthrene-induced fibrosarcoma in normal and immunosuppressed syngeneic mice. J. Natl. Cancer Inst., 47:1087-1094.
7. Bekesi, J. G., St-Arneault, G., Walter, L., and Holland, J. F. (1972): Immunogenicity of leukemia L1210 cells after neuraminidase treatment. J. Natl. Cancer Inst., 49:107-118.
8. Sethi, K. K., and Brandis, H. (1973): Neuraminidase induced loss in the transplantability of murine leukemia L1210 induction of immunoprotection and the transfer of induced immunity to normal DBA/2 mice by serum and peritoneal cells. Br. J. Cancer, 27:106-113.
9. Sethi, K. K., and Teschner, M. (1974): Neuraminidase induced immunospecific destruction of transplantable experimental tumors. Postepy Hig. Med. Doswialdczaine, 28:103-120.

10. Rios, A., and Simmons, R. L. (1973): Immunospecific regression of various syngeneic mouse tumors in response to neuraminidase treated tumor cells. J. Natl. Cancer Inst., 51:637-644.

11. Rios, A., and Simmons, R. L. (1974): Active specific immunotherapy of minimal residual tumor: Excision plus neuraminidase treated tumor cells. Intern. J. Cancer, 13:71-81.

12. Bekesi, J. G., and Holland, J. F. (1974): Combined chemotherapy and immunotherapy of transplantable and spontaneous murine leukemia in DBA/2 and AKR mice in investigations and stimulation of immunity in cancer patients. Recent Results Cancer Res., 47:357-369.

13. Bekesi, J. G., Roboz, J. P., and Holland, J. F. (1975): Immuno-therapy with neuraminidase treated murine leukemia cells after cyto-reductive therapy in leukemic mice. In: Modulation of Host Immune Resistance in the Prevention or Treatment of Induced Neoplasias, edited by M. A. Chirigos. Natl. Cancer Inst. Monogr.

14. Bekesi, J. G., Roboz, J. P., Walter, L., and Holland, J. F. (1974): Stimulation of specific immunity against cancer by neuraminidase treated tumor cells. Symposium on Neuraminidase. Behringwerke-Mitt., 55:309-321.

15. Simmons, R. L., and Rios, A. (1972): Immunospecific regression of methyl-cholanthrene fibrosarcoma using neuraminidase. III. Syner-gistic effect of BCG and neuraminidase treated tumor cells. Ann. Surg., 176:188-194.

16. Skipper, H. E., Schabel, F. M., Jr., and Trader, M. W. (1972): Basic and therapeutic trial results obtained in the spontaneous AKR leukemia (lymphoma) model end of 1971. Cancer Chemother. Rep., 56:273,314.

17. Skipper, H. E., Schabel, F. M., Jr., Trader, M. W., and Lester, M. W., Jr. (1969): Response to therapy of spontaneous first passage and long passage lines of AKR leukemia. Cancer Chemother. Rep., 53:345-366.

18. Ungaro, P. C., Drake, W. P., and Mardiney, M. R., Jr. (1973): Repetitive administration of BCG in prevention and treatment of spontan-eous leukemia in AKR mice. J. Natl. Cancer Inst., 50:125-128.

19. Bekesi, J. G., Roboz, J. P., Zimmerman, E., and Holland, J. F. (1976): Treatment of spontaneous leukemia in AKR mice with chemo-therapy, immunotherapy and interferon. Cancer Res., 36:631-639.

20. Yates, J. W., Wallace, H. J., Ellison, R. R., and Holland, J. F. (1973): Cytosine arabinoside (NSC #63878) and daunorubicin (NSC #83142) therapy in acute nonlymphocytic leukemia. Cancer Chemother. Rep., 57:81-84.

21. Wykren, J., and Fudenberg, H. J. (1973): Thymus-derived rosette forming cells in various human disease states: Cancer, lymphoma bacterial and viral infections and other diseases. J. Clin. Invest., 52:106-113.

22. Breslow, N. A. (1970): Generalized Kruskal-Wallis test for comparing K samples subject to unequal patterns of censorship. Biometricka, 57:579-594.

23. Aiuti, F., Cerottini, J. C., Coombs, R. R. A., et al. (1974): Special technical reports. Identification, enumeration and isolation of B and T lymphocytes from human peripheral blood. Scand. J. Immunol., 3:521-532.

24. Haddow, A., and Alexander, P. (1964): An immunological method of increasing the sensitivity of primary sarcomas to local irradiation with x-rays. Lancet, 1:452-457.

25. Alexander, P., Bensted, J., Delarme, E. J., Hall, J. G., and Hodgett, J. (1969): The cellular immune response to primary sarcomata in rats. II. Abnormal responses of nodes draining the tumor. Proc. Roy. Soc., 174:237-251.

26. Alexander, P., and Hall, J. G. (1970): The role of immunoblasts in host resistance and immunotherapy of primary sarcomata. Adv. Cancer Res., 13:1.

27. Alexander, P., Connell, D. I., and Mikulska, Z. B. (1966): Treatment of a murine leukemia with spleen cells or sera from allogeneic mice immunized against the tumor. Cancer Res., 26:1508.

28. Laterjet, R. (1964): Action inhibitrice d'extraits leucemiques isologues irradies sue la leucemogenese spontanee de la souris AKR. Ann. Inst. Pasteur, 107:1.

29. Revesz, L. (1960): Detection of antigenic differences in isologous host-tumor systems by pretreatment with heavily irradiated tumor cells. Cancer Res., 20:443.

30. Mathe, G., Pouillart, P., and Lapeyrague, F. (1969): Active immunotherapy of L1210 leukemia applied after the graft of the tumor cells. Br. J. Cancer, 23:814-824.

31. Mathe, G., Weiner, R., Pouillart, P., Schwarzenberg, L., Jasmin, C., Schneider, M., Hayat, M., Amiel, J. L., DeVassal, F., and Rosenfield, C. (1973): BCG in cancer immunotherapy: Experimental and clinical trials of its use in treatment of leukemia minimal and/or residual disease. Natl. Cancer Inst. Monogr., 39:165-175.

32. Mathe, G., Amiel, J. L., Schwarzenberg, L., Schneider, M., Schlumberger, J. R., Hayat, M., and DeVassal, F. (1969): Active immunotherapy for acute lymphoblastic leukemia. Lancet, 1:697-699.

33. Mathe, G., Amiel, J. L., Schwarzenberg, L., Schneider, M., Cahan, A., Hayat, M., DeVassal, F., and Schlumberger, J. R. (1970): Methods and strategy for the treatment of acute lymphoblastic leukemia. Recent Results Cancer Res., 30:109-137.

34. Hamilton-Fairley, G., Crowther, D., Guyer, J. G., Hardisty, R. M., Kay, H. E. M., Knapton, P. J., McElwain, T. J., and Parr, I. B. (1970): Active immunotherapy in the treatment of leukemia and other malignant diseases. Recent Results Cancer Res., 30:138-141.

35. Leventhal, B. G., LePourhiet, A., Hlaterman, R. H., Henderson, E. S., and Herberben, R. B. (1973): Immunotherapy in previously treated acute lymphatic leukemia. Natl. Cancer Inst. Monogr., 39:177-187.

36. Sokol, J. E., Aungst, C. W., and Grace, J. T., Jr. (1973): Immunotherapy of chronic myelocytic leukemia. Natl. Cancer Inst. Monogr., 39:195-198.

37. Powles, R. L. (1973): Immunotherapy of acute myelogenous leukemia in man. Natl. Cancer Inst. Monogr., 39:243-247.
38. Powles, R. L. (1973): Immunotherapy for acute myelogenous leukemia. Br. J. Cancer, 28(Suppl. I):262-265.
39. Powles, R. L., Growther, D., Bateman, C. J. T., Beard, M. E. J., McElwain, T. J., Russell, J., Lister, T. A., Whitehouse, J. M. A., Wrigley, P. F. M., Pike, M., Alexander, P., and Hamilton-Fairley, G. (1973): Immunotherapy for acute myelogenous leukemia. Br. J. Cancer, 28:365-376.
40. Gutterman, J. U., Hersh, E. M., Rodriguez, V., McCredie, K. B., Mavligit, G., Reed, R., Burgess, M. A., Smith, T., Gehan, E., and Bodey, G. P., Sr. (1974): Chemoimmunotherapy of adult acute leukemia, prolongation of remission in myeloblastic leukemia with BCG. Lancet, 2:1405-1409.
41. Vogler, W. R., and Chan, Y. K. (1974): Prolonging remission in myeloblastic leukemia by Tice strain Bacillus Calmette Guerin. Lancet, 2:128-131.
42. Viza, D. C., Bernard-Degani, R., Bernard, C., and Harris, R. (1969): Leukemia antigens. Lancet, 2:493-494.
43. Powles, R. L., Balchin, L. A., Hamilton-Fairley, G., and Alexander, P. (1971): Recognition of leukemia cells as foreign before and after autoimmunization. Br. Med. J., 1:1820-1825.
44. Gutterman, J. U., Hersh, E. M., McCredie, K. B., Bodey, G. P., Rodriguez, V., and Freireich, E. J. (1972): Lymphocyte blastogenesis to human leukemia cells and their relationship to serum factors. Immunocompetence and prognosis. Cancer Res., 32:2524-2529.
45. Fridman, W. H., Kourisky, F. M. (1969): Stimulation of lymphocytes by autologous leukemic cells in acute leukemia. Nature, 224:277-279.
46. Oren, M. E., and Herberman, R. B. (1971): Delayed cutaneous hypersensitivity reactions to membrane extracts of human tumor cells. Clin. Exp. Immunol., 9:45-56.
47. Leventhal, B. G., Halterman, R. H., Rosenberg, E. B., and Herberman, R. B. (1972): Immune reactivity of leukemia patients autologous blast cells. Cancer Res., 32:820-825.
48. Herberman, R. B., and Rosenberg, E. B. (1976): Cellular cytotoxicity reactions to human leukemia associated antigens. Proc. Fifth Int. Symp. Comp. Leukemia Res. (in press).
49. Rosenberg, E. B., Herberman, R. B., Levine, P. H., Halterman, R. H., McCoy, J. L., and Wunderlich, J. R. (1972): Lymphocyte cytotoxicity reactions to leukemia-associated antigens in identical twins. Int. J. Cancer, 9:648-658.
50. Ortiz de Landazuri, M., and Herberman, R. B. (1972): Specificity of cellular immune reactivity to virus-induced tumors. Nature, 238:18.
51. Wahren, B. (1966): A quantitative investigation of the G (gross) antigen in preleukemic and leukemic cells. Exp. Cell Res., 42:230-242.
52. Herberman, R. B., Rosenberg, E. B., Halterman, R. H., McCoy, J. L., and Leventhal, B. G. (1972): Cellular immune reaction to human leukemia. Natl. Cancer Inst. Monogr., 35:259-266.

53. Harris, R. (1973): Leukemia antigens and immunity in man. Nature, 241:95-100.
54. Bach, M. L., Bach, F. H., and Joo, P. (1969): Leukemia associated antigens in the mixed lymphocyte culture test. Science, 166:1520-1522.
55. Hellstrom, I., Hellstrom, K. E., Sjogren, H. D., and Warner, G. A. (1971): Demonstration of cell-mediated immunity to human neoplasms of various histological types. Int. J. Cancer, 7:1-16.

Subject Index